Contemporary Rheumatology

Series Editor

Yasser El Miedany, Gravesend, UK

Everyday rheumatologists are faced with new challenges pertaining to the management of both common as well as uncommon rheumatic disorders. The series, Contemporary Rheumatology, will explore new frontiers in rheumatology. It will cover both basic and clinical sciences and provide a state-of- the art approach to the diagnosis and management of different inflammatory as well as non-inflammatory conditions. This series will highlight emerging fields, treatments, and research in rheumatology from precision medicine to the use of cannabinoids in treatment of rheumatic diseases. By gathering key information on state-of-the-art care for practitioners of rheumatology, this series aims to support clinicians in developing new treatment plans for patients diagnosed with rheumatic diseases typically treated with more traditional approaches. In addition to demystifying newer technology and research in rheumatology, this series will also explore connections between rheumatic diseases and other disorders and medical specialties, such as osteoporosis in renal failure, the genetic factors to rheumatic diseases, and the bridge between rheumatic disease and sexual health. Patients with rheumatic conditions may be at increased risk for other chronic diseases, and it is crucial to those patients to have informed clinicians across specialties. These volumes will enable physicians outside the realm of rheumatology to better treat patients in their care who also suffer from rheumatic diseases. Research in rheumatology moves quickly, and there is continued focus on advancements in research and treatment. This series provides space in the rheumatology book program at Springer to track progress made in the field with series editor Dr. Yasser El Miedany, a leader in rheumatology, and continually provide state-of-the-art titles in the area.

Yasser El Miedany • Rahma A. Elziaty
Editors

Capillaroscopy

Case-Based Nailfold Imaging for the Modern Rheumatologist

Springer

Editors
Yasser El Miedany
Canterbury Christ Church University
Canterbury, UK

Rheumatology and Rehabilitation
Ain Shams University
Cairo, Egypt

King's College
London, UK

Rahma A. Elziaty
Internal Medicine Department
Rheumatology Division
Faculty of Medicine
Ain Shams University
Cairo, Egypt

ISSN 2662-7531 ISSN 2662-754X (electronic)
Contemporary Rheumatology
ISBN 978-3-032-22965-6 ISBN 978-3-032-22966-3 (eBook)
https://doi.org/10.1007/978-3-032-22966-3

This Springer imprint is published by the registered company Springer Nature Switzerland AG
The registered company address is: Gewerbestrasse 11, 6330 Cham, Switzerland

To my father, Dr. Ahmed Elziaty; my mother, Dr. Samira Hassanin; my sister, Dr. Samira Elziaty; and my brother, Eng. Mohamed Elziaty—your encouragement shaped my path, your love fueled my work, and your belief turned effort into achievement. This book is yours as much as it is mine.

Dr. Rahma A. Elziaty

Foreword

Capillaroscopy has become an indispensable tool in the field of connective tissue diseases. For those of us dedicated to understanding and managing systemic sclerosis and related disorders, it represents far more than a diagnostic technique, it is an extension of our clinical practice. The ability to visualize the microcirculation offers a unique window into disease processes that were once invisible to the clinician's eye.

Within the EUSTAR community and beyond, capillaroscopy continues to play a central role in the diagnosis and early detection of systemic sclerosis and other connective tissue diseases. Early detection is, now more than ever, a crucial step in patient care, allowing us to intervene before irreversible damage occurs. Moreover, as ongoing research explores its potential in monitoring disease progression and therapeutic response, capillaroscopy stands at the intersection of clinical observation and scientific innovation.

Learning and mastering this technique is therefore essential for anyone interested, whether closely or remotely, in connective tissue diseases. It remains a vital skill that bridges bedside clinical evaluation and pathophysiological understanding.

This book, *100 Cases in Capillaroscopy*, provides a unique and practical approach to learning. Through real clinical scenarios, readers are guided step by step in interpreting findings, integrating them into the broader context of patient care. The combination of detailed case descriptions, clear images, and interpretive guidance makes it an invaluable resource, both for trainees and for experienced clinicians who wish to refine their expertise.

By linking theory with practice, this collection brings capillaroscopy to life in a way that is educational, contextualized, and deeply relevant to daily clinical work. It embodies the spirit of the EUSTAR community: collaboration, rigor, and the shared goal of improving the lives of patients with systemic sclerosis and other connective tissue diseases.

I warmly thank all those who contributed to this work and those who continue to advance the field through research, teaching, and clinical excellence. This book is both a testament to our collective effort and a tool for the next generation of clinicians and researchers.

I hope it aligned with your expectations.

Marie-Elise Truchetet, MD, PhD
EUSTAR President, Rheumatology Department
Centre de référence des maladies auto-immunes
systémiques rares RESO, Immunology Lab
ImmunoConcept (UMR CNRS 5164),
Bordeaux University Hospital
Bordeaux, France

Preface

From the earliest days of medical observation, the microcirculation has presented a hidden, yet profoundly revealing, world. For decades, the flicker of blood flow within the nailfold capillaries has offered a unique window into the systemic health of our patients, a visual and dynamic assessment that stands apart from every other diagnostic tool. As the clinical applications of nailfold capillaroscopy (NFC) have expanded, so too has the need for a comprehensive, authoritative, and practical resource that captures the current state of this evolving field. It is with this vision that we embarked on the journey to create this book.

This volume is born from a simple but powerful premise: that a picture is worth a thousand words, and in medicine, a well-interpreted image can guide a thousand decisions. Our goal was to create more than just a textbook; we set out to build a definitive clinical atlas that bridges the crucial gap between microscopic findings and real-world clinical experience. This book is a testament to the idea that the intricate patterns of the nailfold are not isolated curiosities, but critical biomarkers for diagnosis, prognosis, and therapeutic monitoring.

To achieve this, we have assembled an extraordinary team of leading international experts, each a pioneer in their respective fields of microcirculation research and clinical practice. Their collective wisdom and vast experience have shaped a work that is both academically rigorous and clinically accessible. The collaborative spirit of these authors has allowed us to move beyond the traditional focus on systemic sclerosis and Raynaud's phenomenon, offering a holistic view of NFC's utility across a wide range of conditions, including inflammatory arthritis, dermatomyositis, lupus, and even non-rheumatic diseases. Dedicated chapters on pediatric applications, advanced techniques, and self-assessment further solidify this book's position as a comprehensive guide for both the novice and the seasoned practitioner.

Our hope is that this book will serve as an indispensable companion for rheumatologists, internists, dermatologists, fellows, and students. May it illuminate the subtle signs of disease that lie just beneath the surface, empowering you to better understand your patients' conditions and, in turn, provide more precise and compassionate care. This is a journey into the heart of microvascular medicine, and we are honored to have you join us.

London, UK
1 August 2025

Yasser El Miedany

Contents

Contributors

Cansu Aglar-Backeberg Rhineland-Palatinate Rheumatology Center, Bad Kreuznach, Germany

Luisa Arcarese Clinical Immunology and Rheumatology Unit, Fondazione Policlinico Campus Bio-Medico di Roma, Rome, Italy

Veronica Batani Vita-Salute San Raffaele University, Milan, Italy
Unit of Immunology, Rheumatology, Allergy and Rare Diseases (UnIRAR), Inflammation, Fibrosis and Ageing Initiative (INFLAGE), IRCCS Ospedale San Raffaele, Milan, Italy
Leeds Institute of Rheumatology and Muscoloskeletal Medicine, University of Leeds. Leeds, Regno Unito, UK
Department of Medical and Surgical Sciences for Children and Adults, University of Modena and Reggio Emilia, Modena, Italy

Pietro Bearzi Clinical Immunology and Rheumatology Unit, Campus Bio-Medico University of Rome, Rome, Italy
Center of Experimental Rheumatology, Department of Rheumatology, University Hospital Zurich, University of Zurich, Zürich, Switzerland

Francesco Bonomi Department of Internal Medicine, University Hospital Careggi, Florence, Italy

Marco Matucci Cerinic Vita-Salute San Raffaele University, Milan, Italy
Unit of Immunology, Rheumatology, Allergy and Rare Diseases (UnIRAR), Inflammation, Fibrosis and Ageing Initiative (INFLAGE), IRCCS Ospedale San Raffaele, Milan, Italy

Antonio Ciancio Rheumatology Unit, Department of Precision Medicine, University of Campania "Luigi Vanvitelli", Naples, Italy

Maria De Santis Rheumatology and Clinical Immunology, IRCCS Humanitas Research Hospital, Rozzano, Milan, Italy
Department of Biomedical Sciences, Humanitas University, Pieve Emanuele, Milan, Italy

Francesco Del Galdo Leeds Institute of Rheumatic and Musculoskeletal Medicine, University of Leeds, Leeds, UK
NIHR Leeds Biomedical Research Centre, Leeds Teaching Hospitals Trust, Leeds, UK

Marco Di Battista Leeds Institute of Rheumatic and Musculoskeletal Medicine, University of Leeds, Leeds, UK
Rheumatology Unit, University of Pisa, Pisa, Italy

Yasser El Miedany Canterbury Christ Church University, Canterbury, UK
Rheumatology and Rehabilitation, Ain Shams University, Cairo, Egypt
King's College, London, UK

Rahma A. Elziaty Internal Medicine Department, Rheumatology Division, Faculty of Medicine, Ain Shams University, Cairo, Egypt

Yazmin Espinosa Rheumatology and Immunology Department, Hospital Roberto Del Río, Santiago, Chile

Ivan Foeldvari Hamburg Centre for Pediatric and Adolescent Rheumatology, Hamburg, Germany

Giulio Forte Rheumatology Unit, Department of Precision Medicine, University of Campania "Luigi Vanvitelli", Naples, Italy

Noémie Gensous CHU de Bordeaux, Internal Medicine and Clinical Immunology Department, Bordeaux, France

Roberto Giacomelli Clinical Immunology and Rheumatology Unit, Fondazione Policlinico Campus Bio-Medico di Roma, Rome, Italy
Clinical Immunology and Rheumatology Unit, Campus Bio-Medico University of Rome, Rome, Italy

Walter Hermann Department of Rheumatology and Clinical Immunology, Kerckhoff-Klinik GmbH, Bad Nauheim, Germany

Giulia Lanaia Clinical Immunology and Rheumatology Unit, Campus Bio-Medico University of Rome, Rome, Italy

Vasiliki Liakouli Rheumatology Unit, Department of Precision Medicine, University of Campania "Luigi Vanvitelli", Naples, Italy

Marco Minerba Clinical Immunology and Rheumatology Unit, Campus Bio-Medico University of Rome, Rome, Italy
Leeds Institute of Rheumatic and Musculoskeletal Medicine, University of Leeds, Leeds, UK

Nathalie Morel CHU de Bordeaux, Rheumatology Department, Bordeaux, France

Francesca Motta Rheumatology and Clinical Immunology, IRCCS Humanitas Research Hospital, Rozzano, Milan, Italy
Department of Biomedical Sciences, Humanitas University, Pieve Emanuele, Milan, Italy

Nicola Ortalli Leeds Institute of Rheumatic and Musculoskeletal Medicine, University of Leeds, Leeds, UK

Zeynep Özcan Hamburg Centre for Pediatric and Adolescent Rheumatology, Hamburg, Germany

Silvia Bellando Randone Department of Experimental and Clinical Medicine, University of Florence, Florence, Italy
Division of Rheumatology and Scleroderma Unit, University Hospital Careggi, Florence, Italy

Chiara Salvolini Clinical Immunology and Rheumatology Unit, Campus Bio-Medico University of Rome, Rome, Italy

Sophie Skopinski CHU de Bordeaux, Internal Medicine and Clinical Immunology Department, Bordeaux, France

Antonio Tonutti Rheumatology and Clinical Immunology, IRCCS Humanitas Research Hospital, Rozzano, Milan, Italy
Department of Biomedical Sciences, Humanitas University, Pieve Emanuele, Milan, Italy

Konstantinos Triantafyllias Rhineland-Palatinate Rheumatology Center, Bad Kreuznach, Germany

Marie-Elise Truchetet CHU de Bordeaux, Rheumatology Department, Bordeaux, France

Antonia Valenzuela Clinical Immunology and Rheumatology Department, Pontificia Universidad Catolica de Chile, Santiago, Chile

Cases Chapter

Nadia ben Abdelhafidh Faculty of Medicine of Tunis, Tunis El Manar University, Tunis, Tunisia
Internal Medicine and Clinical Immunology Department, Principal Military Hospital of Tunis, Tunis, Tunisia

Houssem Abida Faculty of Medicine of Tunis, Tunis El Manar University, Tunis, Tunisia
Internal Medicine and Clinical Immunology Department, Principal Military Hospital of Tunis, Tunis, Tunisia

Mohammed Hassan Abu-Zaid Rheumatology and Rehabilitation Department, Faculty of Medicine, Tanta University, Tanta, Egypt

Svetlana Agachi Rheumatology and Nephrology Discipline, Nicolae Testemiţanu University, Chişinău, Republic of Moldova

Faida Ajili Faculty of Medicine of Tunis, Tunis El Manar University, Tunis, Tunisia
Internal Medicine and Clinical Immunology Department, Principal Military Hospital of Tunis, Tunis, Tunisia
Research Unit for Autoimmune Diseases UR17DNO2, Principal Military Hospital of Tunis, Tunis, Tunisia

Elvira Díez Álvarez Department of Rheumatology, Complejo Asistencial Universitario de León, León, Spain

Doaa M. Ashour Department of Ophthalmology, Faculty of Medicine, Ain Shams University, Cairo, Egypt

Sofia Azevedo Rheumatology Department, Unidade Local de Saúde da Região de Aveiro, Aveiro, Portugal
CIRA, Centro de Investigação em Reumatologia de Aveiro, Aveiro, Portugal

Marius Cadar Rheumatology, Department of Medical and Cardiovascular Sciences, Sapienza University, Rome, Italy

Maria João Cadório Rheumathology Department, Coimbra's Local Health Unit, Coimbra, Portugal

Claudia Cobilinschi Department of Rheumatology, "Sf. Maria" Clinical Hospital, Carol Davila University of Medicine and Pharmacy, Bucharest, Romania

Sara Alves Costa Rheumathology Department, Coimbra's Local Health Unit, Coimbra, Portugal

Caroline Evers Department of Rheumatology, University Hospital Zurich, Zurich, Switzerland

Hanan Ewais Internal Medicine Department, Rheumatology Division, Faculty of Medicine, Ain Shams University, Cairo, Egypt

Ignacio González Fernández Department of Rheumatology, Complejo Asistencial Universitario de León, León, Spain

Hela Ghedira Faculty of Medicine of Tunis, Tunis El Manar University, Tunis, Tunisia
Clinical Hematology Department, Principal Military Hospital of Tunis, Tunis, Tunisia

Laura-Maria Groşeanu Department of Rheumatology, "Sf. Maria" Clinical Hospital, Carol Davila University of Medicine and Pharmacy, Bucharest, Romania

Nour El Houda Gueddiche Faculty of Medicine of Tunis, Tunis El Manar University, Tunis, Tunisia
Internal Medicine and Clinical Immunology Department, Principal Military Hospital of Tunis, Tunis, Tunisia
Research Unit for Autoimmune Diseases UR17DNO2, Principal Military Hospital of Tunis, Tunis, Tunisia

Miriam Retuerto Guerrero Department of Rheumatology, Complejo Asistencial Universitario de León, León, Spain

Rasha M. Hammoda Internal Medicine Department, Rheumatology Division, Faculty of Medicine, Ain Shams University, Cairo, Egypt

Waleed Hassan Rheumatology and Rehabilitation Department, Faculty of Medicine, Benha University, Benha, Egypt

Sherif Ismail Rheumatology and Rehabilitation, Internal Medicine Department, Medical Research and Clinical Studies Institute, National Research Center, Cairo, Egypt

Jacopo Landro Rheumatology, Department of Medical and Cardiovascular Sciences, Sapienza University, Rome, Italy

Minrui Liang Department of Rheumatology, Huashan Hospital, Fudan University, Shanghai, China

Maria Lungu Rheumatology and Nephrology Discipline, Nicolae Testemițanu University, Chișinău, Republic of Moldova
Timofei Moşneaga Republican Clinical Hospital, Chișinău, Republic of Moldova

Nada Mahmoud Internal Medicine Department, Rheumatology Division, Faculty of Medicine, Ain Shams University, Cairo, Egypt

Carolina Mazeda Rheumatology Department, Unidade Local de Saúde da Região de Aveiro, Aveiro, Portugal
CIRA, Centro de Investigação em Reumatologia de Aveiro, Aveiro, Portugal
EpiDoC Unit – NOVA Medical School, NOVA University, Lisbon, Portugal

Carina Mihai Department of Rheumatology, University Hospital Zurich, Zurich, Switzerland

Amine Ben Moussa Faculty of Medicine of Tunis, Tunis El Manar University, Tunis, Tunisia
Clinical Hematology Department, Principal Military Hospital of Tunis, Tunis, Tunisia

Fathi Msadak Faculty of Medicine of Tunis, Tunis El Manar University, Tunis, Tunisia
Clinical Hematology Department, Principal Military Hospital of Tunis, Tunis, Tunisia

Ahmed Nassar Department of Dermatology, Venereology and Andrology, Faculty of Medicine, Ain Shams University, Cairo, Egypt

Valeria Riccieri Rheumatology, Department of Medical and Cardiovascular Sciences, Sapienza University, Rome, Italy

Maria João Salvador Rheumathology Department, Coimbra's Local Health Unit, Coimbra, Portugal

Tânia Santiago Rheumathology Department, Coimbra's Local Health Unit, Coimbra, Portugal

Cristiana Sieiro Santos Center for Musculoskeletal Research, School of Biological Sciences, Faculty of Biology, Medicine and Health, University of Manchester, Manchester, UK

Merna M. Sidky Internal Medicine Department, Rheumatology Division, Faculty of Medicine, Ain Shams University, Cairo, Egypt

João Teixeira Dermatology Department, Coimbra's Local Health Unit, Coimbra, Portugal

Carolina Teles Department of Internal Medicine, Hospitais da Universidade de Coimbra, Local Health Unit of Coimbra, Coimbra, Portugal
Faculty of Medicine, University of Coimbra, Coimbra, Portugal

Simona Truglia Rheumatology, Department of Medical and Cardiovascular Sciences, Sapienza University, Rome, Italy

Carlos Valera-Ribera Department of Rheumatology, Hospital Universitario Dr. Peset, Valencia, Spain

Mary Wadie Department of Internal Medicine, Faculty of Medicine, Cairo University, Kasr Alainy, Egypt

Chapter 1
Introduction: The Microcirculation as a Window to Systemic Disease

Yasser El Miedany

The human microcirculation, an intricate network of arterioles, capillaries, and venules, forms the fundamental interface for nutrient and oxygen exchange, waste removal, and immune cell trafficking within tissues. Far from being a mere passive conduit, this extensive vascular bed, spanning approximately 10 billion capillaries in the human body, is a dynamic and highly responsive system critical for maintaining cellular homeostasis and overall organ function. Its delicate structure and physiological responsiveness make it exceptionally vulnerable to insult and, conversely, an invaluable mirror reflecting systemic pathological processes [1, 2].

In the realm of systemic autoimmune diseases, microvascular involvement is not merely a secondary consequence but frequently a *cardinal pathological feature*, often preceding overt clinical symptoms or organ damage. These chronic inflammatory conditions, characterized by a dysregulated immune response targeting the body's own tissues, exert profound effects on the endothelium, leading to widespread microvascular dysfunction and structural abnormalities [3]. Diseases such as Systemic Sclerosis (SSc), Systemic Lupus Erythematosus (SLE), Dermatomyositis (DM), and Sjögren's Syndrome (SS) consistently demonstrate a spectrum of microvascular changes, ranging from functional disturbances like vasospasm to severe structural damage, including capillary loss, disorganization, and obliterative vasculopathy. This microvascular pathology contributes significantly to disease manifestations, including tissue ischemia, inflammation, and ultimately, irreversible organ damage [4].

A quintessential example of compromised microcirculation in rheumatic disease is *Raynaud's phenomenon (RP)*. RP, a paroxysmal digital vasospasm, is a common

Y. El Miedany (✉)
Canterbury Christ Church University, Canterbury, UK

Rheumatology and Rehabilitation, Ain Shams University, Cairo, Egypt

King's College, London, UK

Y. El Miedany, R. A. Elziaty (eds.), *Capillaroscopy*, Contemporary Rheumatology,
https://doi.org/10.1007/978-3-032-22966-3_1

and often debilitating symptom experienced by up to 10% of the general population. While frequently benign (primary RP), it is a highly predictive early manifestation of underlying systemic autoimmune disease (secondary RP), particularly SSc [5]. The ability to distinguish between primary and secondary RP is of paramount clinical importance, as the latter signals a higher risk of disease progression and severe organ complications. This distinction hinges critically on the assessment of microvascular integrity, positioning microvascular evaluation as a cornerstone in the early diagnostic work-up of connective tissue diseases [4].

The Rationale for Noninvasive Microvascular Assessment

The profound and often early involvement of the microcirculation in systemic autoimmune diseases underscores the imperative for effective and accessible assessment tools. Direct visualization of microvessels offers unparalleled advantages, serving as a powerful diagnostic, prognostic, and monitoring instrument. Firstly, it facilitates *early detection* of microvascular damage, often years before the onset of overt clinical symptoms of a systemic condition. This early insight allows for timely intervention, potentially altering disease trajectory and preventing irreversible organ damage [6]. Secondly, the nature and extent of microvascular abnormalities can serve as crucial *prognostic indicators*, predicting the risk of future organ complications or disease progression in patients already diagnosed with conditions like SSc [7]. Thirdly, repeated microvascular assessment can aid in *monitoring disease activity* and evaluating the efficacy of therapeutic interventions, providing objective evidence of microvascular health changes. Finally, observing microvascular pathology in vivo offers a unique opportunity to *understand the pathophysiology* of these complex diseases in their earliest stages, informing research into disease mechanisms and novel therapeutic targets [8].

Among the various methods available for assessing microcirculation, *nailfold capillaroscopy (NFC)* stands out as the premier cost-effective and reproducible technique. By allowing direct visualization of capillaries at the nailfold cuticle, NFC provides an immediate and invaluable "window" into the systemic microvasculature. Its simplicity, coupled with its ability to reveal characteristic pathological patterns, has solidified its role as a fundamental tool in rheumatological practice and research [9].

This introductory chapter will delve into the intricate world of nailfold capillaroscopy. We will first explore its historical evolution, tracing its origins from early observations to the sophisticated digital imaging techniques used today. Subsequently, a detailed discussion on the methodology and technical aspects of NFC will be provided, emphasizing the importance of standardized procedures. The chapter will then differentiate between normal physiological variations and distinct pathological patterns, with particular emphasis on the highly characteristic "scleroderma pattern." A significant portion will be dedicated to elaborating on the specific clinical utility and findings of NFC across various rheumatic diseases, highlighting its diagnostic and prognostic value. Finally, we will address the current limitations and challenges faced in NFC implementation, concluding with a forward-looking perspective on emerging technologies and future research directions that promise to further enhance its role in the comprehensive management of systemic autoimmune diseases.

Understanding Nailfold Capillaroscopy: From Bench to Bedside

Definition and Basic Principles

Nailfold capillaroscopy (NFC) is a noninvasive, safe, and easily repeatable investigative technique that allows for the direct visualization and examination of the microcirculation in the periungual (nailfold) area. It provides a unique "window" into the peripheral microvasculature, enabling clinicians and researchers to assess the morphology, density, and functional characteristics of the terminal capillary loops. This direct observation offers invaluable insights into systemic microvascular changes that often reflect underlying pathological processes, particularly in the context of systemic autoimmune diseases [9].

The rationale for selecting the nailfold as the primary site for microvascular assessment lies in its distinct anatomical and physiological advantages. The capillaries in the nailfold are uniquely arranged *parallel to the skin surface*, unlike those in other parts of the body, which run perpendicularly. This parallel orientation, combined with the relative transparency of the epidermis and nail cuticle, allows for excellent optical access to the terminal capillary loops. Furthermore, the nail fold is an accessible and relatively stable anatomical region, making it ideal for repeated examinations and photographic documentation without undue patient discomfort. The integrity of these tiny blood vessels is highly sensitive to both local and systemic vascular disturbances, making them a crucial indicator of microcirculatory health. The mechanism of visualization relies on the principles of *light transmission and magnification*. A light source illuminates the nailfold, and the capillaries, filled with red blood cells, become visible through a magnified optical system. This magnification reveals the intricate details of capillary morphology, enabling the detection of abnormalities such as dilation, tortuosity, loss of capillaries, and the presence of microhemorrhages [10].

Historical Perspective and Evolution

The concept of observing capillaries in vivo dates back centuries, making capillaroscopy one of the oldest methods of microvascular assessment. Early observations can be traced to the *seventeenth century*, when pioneering scientists like Marcello

Malpighi, using rudimentary microscopes, described the intricate capillary networks in various tissues, including the nailfold. However, it was only in the early twentieth century that interest in nailfold capillaries gained momentum as a diagnostic tool in clinical medicine.

The true clinical utility of NFC began to emerge with the development of more advanced optical instruments. Early capillaroscopes were often simple light microscopes adapted for nailfold examination. A pivotal moment came in the mid-twentieth century with the work of *Dr. E. Carwile LeRoy and Dr. Giles G. Maricq* at the Medical University of South Carolina. Their extensive research, particularly in the 1970s and 1980s, systematically characterized the distinct capillaroscopic patterns in systemic sclerosis (SSc) and other connective tissue diseases. Maricq's seminal work on identifying the "scleroderma pattern" (initially referred to as "scleroderma-type" abnormalities) laid the foundation for using NFC in the differential diagnosis of Raynaud's phenomenon and in the early identification of SSc.

Following this, *Professor Maurizio Cutolo* and his group in Genoa, Italy, along with numerous international collaborators, played a crucial role in standardizing capillaroscopy techniques and interpretation. Their contributions have been instrumental in developing widely accepted scoring systems, defining normal ranges, and establishing the inter- and intra-observer reliability of the method. The transition from basic magnifying lenses to modern *wide-field capillaroscopes* (typically providing 200x magnification) and subsequently to *videocapillaroscopy* marked a significant leap. Videocapillaroscopy, by integrating digital cameras and software, allowed for real-time image capture, high-resolution documentation, quantitative analysis, and the dynamic observation of blood flow, thereby greatly enhancing the diagnostic precision and research capabilities of NFC [11].

What Makes NFC in Rheumatic Diseases Different?

In the evolving landscape of rheumatology, where the pursuit of early diagnosis and personalized medicine is paramount, nailfold capillaroscopy (NFC) stands out not merely as a diagnostic tool but as a transformative lens into the systemic pathology of rheumatic diseases. The innovative utility of NFC lies in its capacity to provide a dynamic, real-time assessment of the microcirculation, a unique attribute that fundamentally distinguishes it from other standard investigative methods [9]. NFC's importance is grounded in its ability to serve as a tangible link between systemic inflammation and its tangible, morphological consequences, making it an indispensable asset in modern rheumatology.

The core importance of NFC in rheumatic diseases stems from its unique ability to capture a critical stage of disease development that is often invisible to other tests: subclinical microvascular damage. In conditions like systemic sclerosis (SSc), NFC can detect the characteristic "scleroderma pattern" (e.g., giant capillaries, avascular areas) years before the full clinical criteria for the disease are met, particularly in patients presenting with isolated Raynaud's phenomenon [12]. This provides a crucial window for early therapeutic intervention, which is essential for improving long-term outcomes. Furthermore, NFC patterns in conditions like dermatomyositis (DM) and mixed connective tissue disease (MCTD) provide prognostic information, with specific findings correlating with the risk of severe organ involvement, such as interstitial lung disease (ILD) [13, 14]. NFC is thus not just a diagnostic tool but a powerful biomarker for risk stratification and disease trajectory prediction.

What makes NFC different from other investigative tools is its noninvasive, high-resolution visualization of the "live" microcirculation. Unlike a tissue biopsy, which is invasive, provides a static snapshot of a single site, and is not suitable for repeated monitoring, NFC offers a dynamic, pain-free, and repeatable assessment of the microvascular bed. It captures not just the structure but also the flow and integrity of small vessels, providing direct evidence of endothelial dysfunction and microangiopathy [15]. This distinguishes it from:

Blood Tests (e.g., ESR, CRP, autoantibodies): While essential, these tests are non-specific indicators of systemic inflammation or markers of autoimmunity. They tell clinicians that inflammation is present, but not where or how it is impacting the physical structures of the body. NFC provides a direct, morphological correlate of this systemic inflammation.

Imaging Modalities (e.g., MRI, CT, Ultrasound): These tools are invaluable for assessing macrovascular structures or specific organs, but they are expensive, often non-portable, and generally not designed for the routine, high-magnification visualization of the microcirculation that NFC provides at the bedside [16]. NFC offers a cost-effective, accessible method for a systemic microvascular check, which can then guide the decision for more expensive, targeted organ imaging.

In essence, NFC functions as a microvascular barometer for the entire body, with the nailfold acting as an accessible and representative site. Its ability to serve as a critical bridge between a patient's symptoms (like Raynaud's) and the underlying systemic pathology makes it an indispensable tool for diagnosis, prognosis, and therapeutic monitoring in rheumatic diseases. By leveraging this unique visual biomarker, clinicians can achieve a more comprehensive, holistic, and timely understanding of a patient's disease state, a foundational step toward the goal of true precision medicine.

Educational Value and Practical Impact

Capillaroscopy is often underestimated in training curricula. This was the first clue to produce this book in an attempt to bridge such a gap between textbook knowledge and real-world application by adopting a case-based approach. Trainees are frequently challenged by questions such as: When should I perform capillaroscopy? What am I looking for? How do I interpret these findings in light of uncertain clinical presentations? The cases presented in this book serve to answer those questions, providing hands-on exposure to practical scenarios.

The real-life case scenarios presented here are not only diagnostic stories—they are educational modules designed to strengthen clinical confidence and interpretive skill. For trainees and early-career clinicians, capillaroscopy often appears to be a "black box" of unfamiliar images and uncertain meaning. By walking through real cases with visual documentation, structured interpretation, and clinical correlation, we hope to demystify the process and encourage wider use of capillaroscopy in practice.

Importantly, the visual nature of capillaroscopy makes it an excellent teaching tool. Comparing normal and abnormal findings, understanding variations across diseases, and observing serial changes in the same patient are all powerful learning experiences. Therefore, we encourage institutions to integrate capillaroscopy images into bedside teaching, case conferences, and multidisciplinary rounds.

Capillaroscopy should not be limited to experts in systemic sclerosis. Its learning curve is reasonable with adequate exposure, and its diagnostic yield can be significant, even in general rheumatology clinics. The use of standardized terminology, scoring systems, and pattern classification (e.g., EULAR definitions, staging) has made it easier to teach and implement [17].

We also encourage clinicians to save and compare serial images, not only for documentation but also for teaching. The visual progression of capillary damage—or healing—is compelling for both patients and colleagues and can be a powerful motivator for clinical action or adherence to therapy.

A Tool of Empathy and Communication

An often-overlooked value of capillaroscopy is its role in patient education and engagement. Unlike many diagnostic tools, capillaroscopy offers immediate visual feedback. Showing a patient their own capillaries—and explaining what the changes mean—can be a powerful moment of education and emotional connection. It helps patients understand their disease on a tangible level and reinforces the importance of treatment adherence and lifestyle modification [7].

In this way, capillaroscopy is not just a scientific tool—it represents a communication channel between the clinician and the patient, enabling shared understanding and trust. In a field like rheumatology, where many diseases are invisible and symptoms subjective, this kind of visual communication can be especially meaningful.

Limitations and Challenges in Nailfold Capillaroscopy

Despite its remarkable utility as a noninvasive tool for assessing microvascular health in rheumatic diseases, nailfold capillaroscopy (NFC) is not without its limitations and faces several ongoing challenges that impact its widespread adoption, standardization, and ultimate diagnostic precision. Recognizing these constraints is crucial for accurate interpretation of findings and for guiding future advancements in the field.

Operator Dependency and Training

A significant challenge in NFC is its inherent *operator dependency*. The quality of the examination and the accuracy of its interpretation are highly contingent upon the skill and experience of the operator. Proper technique, including precise focusing, consistent lighting, and systematic scanning of the nailfold, requires dedicated training. Furthermore, the ability to correctly identify and classify subtle capillaroscopic abnormalities, differentiate physiological variations from pathological changes, and apply scoring systems accurately demands extensive experience and continuous learning. The lack of widely accessible, standardized, and robust training programs globally contributes to variability in skill levels and, consequently, in the reliability of NFC findings across different clinics or research centers [18].

Standardization Across Centers

Closely related to operator dependency is the broader issue of *standardization across different centers*. Variability can arise from multiple factors: differences in equipment (e.g., dermatoscope vs. wide-field vs. videocapillaroscope, varying magnifications and light sources), diverse examination protocols (e.g., number of fingers examined, specific fields of view, image acquisition settings), and inconsistencies in interpretation criteria. While international efforts, notably by EULAR (European League Against Rheumatism) [17] and other consensus groups [19], have made significant strides in proposing standardized guidelines, their universal adoption and rigorous adherence remain an ongoing challenge. This lack of complete standardization can hinder the comparison of findings between studies and limit the generalizability of research outcomes.

Quantitative Scoring Systems

Another area of challenge lies in the *lack of a universally adopted and validated quantitative scoring system for all purposes*. While several semiquantitative and quantitative scoring systems exist (e.g., the Scleroderma Capillary Abnormality Score and microangiopathy severity scores), many are complex, time-consuming, or primarily developed for specific research questions rather than routine clinical use. There is no single, widely accepted, simple yet comprehensive scoring system that can reliably quantify all aspects of microvascular damage (e.g., density, morphology, tortuosity, blood flow) across the spectrum of rheumatic diseases, making it difficult to objectively compare findings or track subtle changes over time. More recently, the fast track pathway was developed to discriminate between scleroderma and non-scleroderma patterns using a simple rule of thumb [20].

Influence of External Factors

NFC results can be significantly influenced by various *external factors* that alter microvascular appearance or blood flow, leading to potential misinterpretation:

- *Temperature:* Cold environments can induce vasospasm, leading to reduced capillary visibility and apparent density, mimicking pathological changes. Conversely, excessive warmth might lead to increased flow and dilation.
- *Medications:* Vasoactive drugs (e.g., calcium channel blockers, phosphodiesterase-5 inhibitors, decongestants) can directly affect capillary caliber and blood flow.
- *Trauma:* Even minor mechanical trauma to the nailfold (e.g., occupational microtrauma, cuticle manipulation during manicures, or habitual nail biting) can cause microhemorrhages, capillary disorganization, or even capillary dropout, leading to nonspecific abnormalities that can be mistaken for disease-related changes.
- *Nail Polish:* Opaque nail polish can obscure visualization, necessitating its removal prior to examination [17, 19].

Technical Difficulties

Certain anatomical and physiological factors can pose *technical difficulties* during NFC:

- *Thick Cuticles:* Overgrown or thickened cuticles can obscure the underlying capillary loops, making adequate visualization challenging.
- *Periungual Skin Pigmentation:* In individuals with darker skin tones, increased melanin content in the epidermis can reduce the transparency of the nailfold, impeding clear visualization of the capillaries and potentially requiring higher illumination or more specialized equipment.
- *Nail Damage/Abnormalities:* Nail abnormalities (e.g., onycholysis, dystrophy) or local infections can also interfere with the clear visualization of the nailfold.
- *Edema:* Significant periungual edema can distort the view and make capillary assessment difficult [17, 19].

Diagnostic Accuracy Limitations

It is crucial to recognize that NFC is *not a standalone diagnostic tool*. While it provides invaluable information about the microcirculation, its findings must always be interpreted in conjunction with a comprehensive clinical assessment, patient history, physical examination findings, and relevant laboratory data (e.g., autoantibody profiles, inflammatory markers). A "scleroderma pattern," for instance, is highly suggestive of SSc but does not, in isolation, constitute a definitive diagnosis. Its presence should prompt further investigations rather than replacing them [17, 19].

Limited Dynamic Assessment

While videocapillaroscopy offers the advantage of dynamic blood flow visualization, most routine NFC examinations provide a *static snapshot* of the microcirculation at a given moment. This limits the ability to fully capture the dynamic processes of vasospasm, reperfusion injury, or subtle changes in blood flow over short timeframes. While longitudinal studies with repeated assessments provide valuable insights into disease progression, the technique does not typically provide continuous, real-time physiological monitoring of microvascular function [17, 19].

In conclusion, while NFC offers a powerful and unique glimpse into the microvasculature, its practical application is tempered by operator-dependent variability, challenges in universal standardization, the influence of transient external factors, and certain technical difficulties. Acknowledging these limitations is essential for responsible clinical application and for guiding future research efforts toward refining the technique, enhancing its objectivity, and maximizing its diagnostic and prognostic potential.

Future Directions and Emerging Technologies

The landscape of nailfold capillaroscopy (NFC) is continuously evolving, driven by advancements in imaging technology, computational power, and a growing understanding of microvascular pathology. Future directions aim to overcome current limitations, enhance objectivity, improve accessibility, and integrate NFC more deeply into the realm of personalized medicine and comprehensive disease management.

Picture Analysis

The most transformative wave of innovation in NFC is undoubtedly the integration of *Artificial Intelligence (AI) and Machine Learning (ML)*. The inherently visual and pattern-based nature of capillaroscopic assessment makes it an ideal candidate for AI-driven analysis.

- *Automated image analysis, pattern recognition, and scoring:* AI algorithms, particularly deep convolutional neural networks (CNNs), are being developed to automatically detect and quantify capillary features (e.g., counting capillary loops, measuring diameters, identifying hemorrhages, and recognizing giant capillaries or avascular areas). For example, the CAPI-Detect algorithm [21], leveraging machine learning trained on expert-annotated images, has shown high accuracy in classifying scleroderma patterns (early, active, and late) and distinguishing them from normal or nonspecific patterns.
- *Improved reproducibility and reduced operator dependency*: By automating the analytical process, AI can significantly reduce the inter- and intra-observer variability inherent in manual interpretation, leading to more standardized and reproducible results across different centers and operators. This addresses a major limitation of current NFC practice.
- *Identification of subtle patterns not evident to the human eye:* AI models can discern complex relationships and subtle visual cues within capillaroscopic images that may not be perceptible to the human eye. This could potentially lead to the identification of novel biomarkers or risk factors for disease progression, uncovering insights previously overlooked.

Advanced Imaging Modalities

Beyond conventional wide-field and videocapillaroscopy, advanced imaging modalities are emerging to provide a more comprehensive view of the microvasculature.

- *Optical Coherence Tomography (OCT) for 3D reconstruction and deeper tissue assessment:* OCT is a noninvasive optical imaging technique that provides high-resolution, cross-sectional images of biological tissues. Its application in NFC allows for *3D reconstruction* of the capillary network, offering a volumetric understanding of capillary architecture that is not possible with 2D methods. Beyond simple reconstruction, advanced OCT techniques (e.g., OCT angiography) can visualize blood flow *within* the capillaries and deeper vessels, assessing microvascular density and function. This offers the potential to quantify microvascular alterations with greater precision and explore pathological changes in underlying dermal layers [22].

- *Integration with other imaging techniques:* Future research may explore the integration of NFC with other microvascular imaging techniques, such as laser Doppler flowmetry (to quantify blood flow) or thermography (to assess temperature changes), to provide a more holistic assessment of microcirculatory function and structure.

Integration with Multi-Omics Data

A compelling future direction lies in the *integration of capillaroscopic findings with multi-omics data* (genomics, proteomics, and metabolomics). This "systems biology" approach aims to connect the observable microvascular phenotype with underlying molecular mechanisms.

- *Combining capillaroscopic findings with genetic, proteomic, and metabolomic data for personalized medicine and refined prognostication:* By correlating specific capillaroscopic patterns (e.g., severe capillary loss) with genetic predispositions, circulating protein biomarkers, or metabolic profiles, researchers can develop more precise diagnostic and prognostic models. This multidimensional data integration holds the promise of ushering in *personalized medicine* in rheumatology, allowing for tailored risk stratification, prediction of treatment response, and optimization of therapeutic strategies based on an individual's unique biological signature [23].

Tele-Capillaroscopy and Remote Monitoring

Technological advancements are paving the way for more accessible and continuous monitoring through *tele-capillaroscopy and remote patient management.*

- *Feasibility and utility of remote capillaroscopy for accessible care in underserved areas:* With the development of user-friendly, portable capillaroscopes and secure telehealth platforms, NFC could be performed remotely, either by patients themselves (with guidance) or by local healthcare providers, and images transmitted to specialists for interpretation. This would significantly improve access to specialized microvascular assessment for patients in rural or underserved areas, reducing geographical barriers to care [24].
- *Potential for continuous or more frequent monitoring:* Remote NFC could enable more frequent monitoring of microvascular changes, allowing for earlier detection of disease flares or progression and providing more dynamic insights into disease activity outside of routine clinic visits.

Role in Therapeutic Monitoring

Finally, a critical future application of NFC is its development into a reliable *biomarker for therapeutic monitoring*.

- *Developing validated methods for using capillaroscopy to assess treatment response and guide therapy adjustments:* While NFC is well-established for diagnosis and prognosis, its role in monitoring treatment efficacy is still evolving. Future research focuses on identifying specific capillaroscopic parameters (e.g., changes in capillary density, reduction in giant capillaries, normalization of blood flow) that reliably reflect response to immunomodulatory or vasoactive therapies. Such validated measures could guide clinicians in adjusting treatment regimens, tapering glucocorticoids, or escalating therapy in nonresponders [25].
- *Predicting flare-ups or disease progression:* By establishing longitudinal changes in capillaroscopic patterns as indicators of impending disease flares or accelerating progression, NFC could serve as an early warning system, prompting timely interventions to prevent irreversible organ damage.

Briefly, the future of nailfold capillaroscopy is bright, with emerging technologies like AI, advanced imaging, and multi-omics integration poised to revolutionize its capabilities. These innovations promise to enhance its objectivity, accessibility, and utility, firmly embedding NFC as an indispensable tool in the precise diagnosis, prognostic stratification, and personalized management of patients with systemic rheumatic diseases.

References

1. Somani A, Steiner ME, Hebbel RP. The dynamic regulation of microcirculatory conduit function: features relevant to transfusion medicine. Transfus Apher Sci. 2010;43(1):61–8. https://doi.org/10.1016/j.transci.2010.05.010.
2. Gutterman DD, Chabowski DS, Kadlec AO, Durand MJ, Freed JK, Ait-Aissa K, Beyer AM. The human microcirculation: regulation of flow and beyond. Circ Res. 2016;118(1):157–72. https://doi.org/10.1161/CIRCRESAHA.115.305364.
3. Xiang Y, Zhang M, Jiang D, Su Q, Shi J. The role of inflammation in autoimmune disease: a therapeutic target. Front Immunol. 2023;14:1267091. https://doi.org/10.3389/fimmu.2023.1267091.
4. Hysa E, Pizzorni C, Sammorì S, Gotelli E, Cere A, Schenone C, Ferrari G, Campitiello R, Gerli V, Paolino S, Sulli A, Smith V, Cutolo M. Microvascular damage in autoimmune connective tissue diseases: a capillaroscopic analysis from 20 years of experience in a EULAR training and research referral centre for imaging. RMD Open. 2023;9(3):e003071. https://doi.org/10.1136/rmdopen-2023-003071.
5. Haque A, Hughes M. Raynaud's phenomenon. Clin Med (Lond). 2020;20(6):580–7. https://doi.org/10.7861/clinmed.2020-0754.
6. Linnemann B, Erbe M. Raynaud's phenomenon - assessment and differential diagnoses. Vasa. 2015;44(3):166–77. https://doi.org/10.1024/0301-1526/a000426.

7. Kubo S, Smith V, Cutolo M, Tanaka Y. The role of nailfold videocapillaroscopy in patients with systemic sclerosis. Immunol Med. 2018;41(3):113–9. https://doi.org/10.1080/25785826.2018.1531189.
8. Masi S, Rizzoni D, Taddei S, Widmer RJ, Montezano AC, Lüscher TF, Schiffrin EL, Touyz RM, Paneni F, Lerman A, Lanza GA, Virdis A. Assessment and pathophysiology of microvascular disease: recent progress and clinical implications. Eur Heart J. 2021;42(26):2590–604. https://doi.org/10.1093/eurheartj/ehaa857.
9. Komai M, Takeno D, Fujii C, Nakano J, Ohsaki Y, Shirakawa H. Nailfold capillaroscopy: a comprehensive review on its usefulness in both clinical diagnosis and improving unhealthy dietary lifestyles. Nutrients. 2024;16(12):1914. https://doi.org/10.3390/nu16121914.
10. Anyfanti P, Angeloudi E, Dara A, Arvanitaki A, Bekiari E, Kitas GD, Dimitroulas T. Nailfold videocapillaroscopy for the evaluation of peripheral microangiopathy in rheumatoid arthritis. Life (Basel). 2022;12(8):1167. https://doi.org/10.3390/life12081167.
11. Araújo FC, Rocha ML. Nailfold capillaroscopy: from the early ages to the early diagnosis of systemic sclerosis. ARP Rheumatol. 2022;1(3):188–9.
12. Smith V, Ickinger C, Hysa E, Snow M, Frech T, Sulli A, Cutolo M. Nailfold capillaroscopy. Best Pract Res Clin Rheumatol. 2023;37(1):101849. https://doi.org/10.1016/j.berh.2023.101849.
13. Sebastiani M, Triantafyllias K, Manfredi A, González-Gay MA, Palmou-Fontana N, Cassone G, Drott U, Delbrück C, Rojas-Serrano J, Bertolazzi C, Nuño L, Giannini M, Iannone F, Vicente EF, Castañeda S, Selva-O'Callaghan A, Trallero Araguas E, Emmi G, Iuliano A, Bauhammer J, Miehle N, Parisi S, Cavagna L, Codullo V, Montecucco C, Lopez-Longo FJ, Martínez-Barrio J, Nieto-González JC, Vichi S, Confalonieri M, Tomietto P, Bergner R, Sulli A, Bonella F, Furini F, Scirè CA, Bortoluzzi A, Specker C, Barsotti S, Neri R, Mosca M, Caproni M, Weinmann-Menke J, Schwarting A, Smith V, Cutolo M, American and European Network of Antisynthetase Syndrome Collaborative Group. Nailfold capillaroscopy characteristics of antisynthetase syndrome and possible clinical associations: results of a multicenter international study. J Rheumatol. 2019;46(3):279–84. https://doi.org/10.3899/jrheum.180355.
14. Shenavandeh S, Rashidi F. Nailfold capillaroscopy changes with disease activity in patients with inflammatory myositis including overlap myositis, pure dermatomyositis, and pure polymyositis. Reumatologia. 2022;60(1):42–52. https://doi.org/10.5114/reum.2022.114109.
15. Chojnowski MM, Felis-Giemza A, Olesińska M. Capillaroscopy - a role in modern rheumatology. Reumatologia. 2016;54(2):67–72. https://doi.org/10.5114/reum.2016.60215.
16. Cutolo M, Smith V. State of the art on nailfold capillaroscopy: a reliable diagnostic tool and putative biomarker in rheumatology? Rheumatology. 2013;52(11):1933–40. https://doi.org/10.1093/rheumatology/ket153.
17. Smith V, Herrick AL, Ingegnoli F, Damjanov N, De Angelis R, Denton CP, Distler O, Espejo K, Foeldvari I, Frech T, Garro B, Gutierrez M, Gyger G, Hachulla E, Hesselstrand R, Iagnocco A, Kayser C, Melsens K, Müller-Ladner U, Paolino S, Pizzorni C, Radic M, Riccieri V, Snow M, Stevens W, Sulli A, van Laar JM, Vonk MC, Vanhaecke A, Cutolo M, EULAR Study Group on Microcirculation in Rheumatic Diseases and the Scleroderma Clinical Trials Consortium Group on Capillaroscopy. Standardisation of nailfold capillaroscopy for the assessment of patients with Raynaud's phenomenon and systemic sclerosis. Autoimmun Rev. 2020;19(3):102458. https://doi.org/10.1016/j.autrev.2020.102458.
18. Gracia Tello B, Ramos Ibañez E, Fanlo Mateo P, Sáez Cómet L, Martínez Robles E, Ríos Blanco JJ, Marí Alfonso B, Espinosa Garriga G, Todolí Parra J, Ortego Centeno N, Callejas Rubio JL, Freire Dapena M, Marín Ballvé A, Selva-O'Callaghan A, Guillén Del Castillo A, Simeón Aznar CP, Fonollosa PV. The challenge of comprehensive nailfold videocapillaroscopy practice: a further contribution. Clin Exp Rheumatol. 2022;40(10):1926–32. https://doi.org/10.55563/clinexprheumatol/6usce8.
19. El Miedany Y, Ismail S, Wadie Fawzy M, Müller-Ladner U, Giacomelli R, Liakouli V, Hermann W, Fathy N, El Gaafary M, Fouad NA, Saber S, Abu-Zaid MH. Towards a consensus on the clinical applications and interpretations of the nailfold capillaroscopy standards in

clinical practice: an initiative by the Egyptian Society of Microcirculation. Arch Rheumatol. 2022;38(3):451–60. https://doi.org/10.46497/ArchRheumatol.2023.9875.
20. Smith V, Vanhaecke A, Herrick AL, Distler O, Guerra MG, Denton CP, Deschepper E, Foeldvari I, Gutierrez M, Hachulla E, Ingegnoli F, Kubo S, Müller-Ladner U, Riccieri V, Sulli A, van Laar JM, Vonk MC, Walker UA, Cutolo M, EULAR Study Group on Microcirculation in Rheumatic Diseases. Fast track algorithm: how to differentiate a "scleroderma pattern" from a "non-scleroderma pattern". Autoimmun Rev. 2019;18(11):102394. https://doi.org/10.1016/j.autrev.2019.102394.
21. Lledó-Ibáñez GM, Sáez Comet L, Freire Dapena M, Mesa Navas M, Martín Cascón M, Guillén Del Castillo A, Simeon CP, Martinez Robles E, Todolí Parra J, Varela DC, Maldonado G, Marín A, Pérez Abad L, Aramburu J, Vela L, Ramos Ibáñez E, Del Carmelo Gracia Tello B. CAPI-detect: machine learning in capillaroscopy reveals new variables influencing diagnosis. Rheumatology (Oxford). 2025;64(6):3667–75. https://doi.org/10.1093/rheumatology/keaf073.
22. Fujimoto JG, Pitris C, Boppart SA, Brezinski ME. Optical coherence tomography: an emerging technology for biomedical imaging and optical biopsy. Neoplasia. 2000;2(1-2):9–25. https://doi.org/10.1038/sj.neo.7900071.
23. Molla G, Bitew M. Revolutionizing personalized medicine: synergy with multi-omics data generation, main hurdles, and future perspectives. Biomedicine. 2024;12(12):2750. https://doi.org/10.3390/biomedicines12122750.
24. Ingegnoli F, Gualtierotti R, Lubatti C, Zahalkova L, Meani L, Boracchi P, Zeni S, Fantini F. Feasibility of different capillaroscopic measures for identifying nailfold microvascular alterations. Semin Arthritis Rheum. 2009;38(4):289–95. https://doi.org/10.1016/j.semarthrit.2007.10.008.
25. Cutolo M, Sulli A, Pizzorni C, Smith V. Capillaroscopy as an outcome measure for clinical trials on the peripheral vasculopathy in SSc-is it useful? Int J Rheumatol. 2010;2010:784947. https://doi.org/10.1155/2010/784947.

Chapter 2
Basics of Nailfold Caillaroscopy

Walter Hermann and Rahma A. Elziaty

Introduction to Microcirculation and the Nailfold

Capillaroscopy has emerged as a fundamental noninvasive imaging method used to examine the microvasculature, particularly in the periungual area. This technique allows clinicians to directly visualize capillary morphology, providing valuable insights into systemic vascular and autoimmune conditions. Its growing clinical application, especially in rheumatology, stems from its ability to support early diagnosis, disease classification, and monitoring of progression in connective tissue diseases such as systemic sclerosis [1].

The nailfold region is particularly suited for capillaroscopic examination due to the horizontal alignment of capillary loops relative to the skin surface. This unique anatomical feature allows for direct visualization of the capillary architecture, size, density, and morphology. Normal capillary patterns are relatively uniform, consisting of hairpin-shaped loops arranged in parallel rows. Deviations from this pattern—such as capillary enlargement, hemorrhages, avascular zones, and bushy or ramified neoangiogenic loops—can indicate pathological changes associated with rheumatological illnesses like systemic sclerosis, dermatomyositis, and mixed connective tissue disease [2].

The method is easy to perform, cost-effective, and well-tolerated by patients. However, interpretation requires proper training and an understanding of both normal anatomical variants and pathological findings. Artifacts related to improper

W. Hermann (✉)
Department of Rheumatology and Clinical Immunology, Kerckhoff-Klinik GmbH, Bad Nauheim, Germany
e-mail: w.hermann@kerckhoff-klinik.de

R. A. Elziaty
Internal Medicine Department, Rheumatology Division, Faculty of Medicine, Ain Shams University, Cairo, Egypt

Y. El Miedany, R. A. Elziaty (eds.), *Capillaroscopy*, Contemporary Rheumatology,
https://doi.org/10.1007/978-3-032-22966-3_2

technique, environmental temperature, or pressure application may mimic disease and should be carefully differentiated. To address these concerns, the development of standardized terminology and scoring systems by international groups such as European League Against Rheumatism (EULAR) and the Scleroderma Clinical Trials Consortium has greatly improved the reliability and reproducibility of capillaroscopic assessments [2, 3].

Technological advancements have significantly improved capillaroscopic capabilities. Modern digital videocapillaroscopy systems offer high-resolution imaging, image storage, and quantitative analysis, enhancing both clinical practice and research applications [2]. These developments have led to better standardization, allowing for more consistent interpretation and reporting of findings across institutions. In addition, international working groups have published guidelines on terminology, scoring systems, and capillary morphology interpretation to improve diagnostic accuracy and reduce interobserver variability [3].

The aim of this chapter is to provide a foundational understanding of capillaroscopy for clinicians and trainees. It will cover essential concepts, including basic equipment and techniques, the normal capillary architecture, pathological findings, the interpretation of commonly encountered patterns, and the role of capillaroscopy in clinical decision-making. The chapter will also address potential artifacts, limitations, the role of capillaroscopy in follow-up and monitoring, and the growing importance of standardized reporting systems in clinical and research settings.

As the field continues to evolve with the integration of artificial intelligence, digital quantification tools, and novel disease associations, capillaroscopy remains a valuable component of the modern diagnostic arsenal in autoimmune and vascular medicine. A thorough grasp of its fundamentals empowers clinicians to make more timely and informed decisions for patients presenting with early or atypical symptoms of systemic disease.

Overview of the Microcirculation

The microcirculation is the functional unit of the circulatory system composed of arterioles, capillaries, and venules, with vessel diameters typically under 100 μm. It plays a critical role in oxygen and nutrient delivery, waste removal, immune surveillance, and thermoregulation [4, 5]. This intricate vascular network ensures the proper exchange between blood and tissues and adapts dynamically to metabolic needs.

At the core of the microcirculation are capillaries, the smallest and most numerous vessels, which can be morphologically categorized into three major types, each adapted to specific tissue functions [4]:

Continuous Capillaries

These are the most common type, characterized by uninterrupted endothelial lining and tight junctions. They are found in muscle, skin, lungs, and the central nervous system. In the brain, its specialized structure contributes to the blood-brain barrier.

Fenestrated Capillaries
These possess pores (fenestrations) in the endothelial cells that increase permeability to small molecules and are typically located in organs involved in filtration or absorption, such as the kidneys, endocrine glands, and intestines.

Discontinuous (Sinusoidal) Capillaries
These have large openings in the endothelium and a discontinuous basement membrane, allowing the passage of cells and large molecules. They are found in the liver, bone marrow, and spleen, facilitating the exchange of blood cells and proteins.

Regulation of microcirculatory blood flow is mediated by myogenic tone, autonomic nervous system activity, and metabolic signals, in addition to endothelial factors such as nitric oxide and prostacyclins [5]. The endothelium acts not only as a barrier but also as a dynamic interface, responding to shear stress, inflammation, and hypoxia.

Microcirculatory dysfunction is increasingly recognized in the pathophysiology of diseases such as diabetes, hypertension, systemic sclerosis, and septic shock. Nailfold capillaroscopy offers a noninvasive window into the microcirculation, particularly useful in rheumatic diseases where structural microvascular changes (e.g., capillary dropout, hemorrhages, giant capillaries) can aid in early diagnosis and monitoring [6].

Unique Anatomy of the Nailfold Capillaries

The nailfold region provides an exceptional anatomical location for direct observation of the microvascular system. This area, situated at the base of the fingernails and toenails, is unique in that the capillaries run parallel to the skin surface, allowing for the full loop of the capillary—arterial limb, apex, and venous limb to be viewed in its entirety using simple magnification techniques. This anatomical alignment contrasts with most other skin areas, where capillaries are oriented perpendicularly and only partially visible on the surface [3].

The nailfold's epidermis is thin and relatively transparent, particularly in the eponychial region, enabling light-based imaging tools to clearly visualize the capillary network. These structural features make the nailfold one of the few areas of the human body where microcirculation can be assessed noninvasively, in real-time, and repeatedly without discomfort or harm to the patient. The capillaries themselves typically appear as homogenous, U- or hairpin-shaped loops, symmetrically arranged in parallel rows, with a normal density ranging between 7 and 14 loops per millimeter in adults [3, 7].

One of the key advantages of studying the nailfold capillaries is the relative absence of mechanical or environmental stress in this region. Unlike capillaries in the plantar or palmar skin, which are frequently exposed to pressure, shear forces, or trauma, the nailfold microvessels are well protected. This makes the nailfold an ideal location for capturing stable and reproducible microvascular images, minimizing the potential for artifacts.

In healthy individuals, the morphology of the capillaries remains remarkably consistent. However, this vascular network is highly sensitive to pathologic changes, particularly those seen in connective tissue diseases. Early structural alterations such as capillary dilation, elongation, microhemorrhages, and dropouts can be seen in autoimmune conditions like systemic sclerosis, mixed connective tissue disease, and dermatomyositis. These changes are often detectable on capillaroscopy before other clinical or serologic signs emerge, highlighting the diagnostic value of this anatomical site [7].

Furthermore, the nailfold serves not only as a diagnostic window but also as a dynamic indicator of disease activity and progression. Serial evaluation of capillary morphology in patients with systemic diseases can reveal changes over time, such as the transition from an "early" to an "active" or "late" scleroderma pattern. As such, the nailfold capillary bed is a sensitive and valuable biomarker of microvascular health in systemic autoimmune disorders [6].

Historical Perspective of Nailfold Capillaroscopy

The origins of capillaroscopy can be traced back to the seventeenth century, when Johan Christophorous Kolhaus first described the visualization of capillaries in the human nailfold using rudimentary magnifying devices. However, its clinical relevance remained limited until the ninteenth century, when Maurice Raynaud's observations on color changes in the fingers laid the foundation for the study of peripheral vascular disorders. Despite these early developments, the technique did not achieve widespread medical application until the twentieth century [8].

The turning point in nailfold capillaroscopy came with the pioneering work of Maricq and Le Roy in the 1970s. They developed the "wide-field" nailfold capillaroscopy technique, which enabled the systematic study of capillary morphology in connective tissue diseases. Their seminal publications provided the first detailed descriptions of specific microvascular changes—such as enlarged loops, hemorrhages, and capillary loss—seen in systemic sclerosis and related disorders [9]. They also introduced the concept of capillaroscopic patterns, which allowed clinicians to differentiate between normal, nonspecific, and scleroderma-like capillary changes.

This early work established the diagnostic value of capillaroscopy, particularly in patients presenting with Raynaud's phenomenon. Maricq's classification of capillaroscopic findings laid the groundwork for later standardization efforts and helped propel nailfold capillaroscopy into mainstream rheumatologic practice.

Over the past three decades, significant technological advancements—particularly the development of nailfold videocapillaroscopy (NVC)—have transformed the field. Unlike traditional light microscopy, NVC allows for higher magnification, real-time video capture, and digital storage of capillary images. These improvements have enhanced diagnostic accuracy and enabled longitudinal monitoring of disease progression [3, 6, 7].

With the growth of evidence supporting the predictive value of capillaroscopic abnormalities in systemic sclerosis and other autoimmune diseases, organizations such as the European League Against Rheumatism (EULAR) and the Scleroderma Clinical Trials Consortium (SCTC) have incorporated capillaroscopy into international diagnostic and classification guidelines. For instance, the 2013 ACR/EULAR classification criteria for systemic sclerosis explicitly include nailfold capillary abnormalities as one of the key entry points for diagnosis [10].

Beyond rheumatology, nailfold capillaroscopy has also attracted interest in other medical specialties. It has been applied in dermatology, diabetology, and even critical care, where microvascular assessment provides insights into tissue perfusion and systemic inflammatory responses [11, 12].

Today, nailfold capillaroscopy is no longer seen as an auxiliary tool but as an essential component of the rheumatologic work-up. Its historical journey—from an observational curiosity to a standardized diagnostic technique—reflects both the evolution of microvascular science and the increasing emphasis on early, noninvasive diagnostics in autoimmune medicine.

Carrying Out the Examination/Technical Requirements

Indication

The main benefit of this examination technique is that it provides an excellent differential diagnostic tool that can be used for various clinical questions [23].

Raynaud's Syndrome

The most common indication for performing a capillary microscopy is the question of whether the Raynaud's symptoms are primary (pRP) or secondary (sRP) [23, 24] (Fig. 2.1).

Known Collagenosis

A further reason to carry out the examination may be, for example, if collagenosis, such as systemic sclerosis, is already present and statements need to be made about the activity and further prognosis of the disease. Here too, capillary microscopy can provide useful information [15].

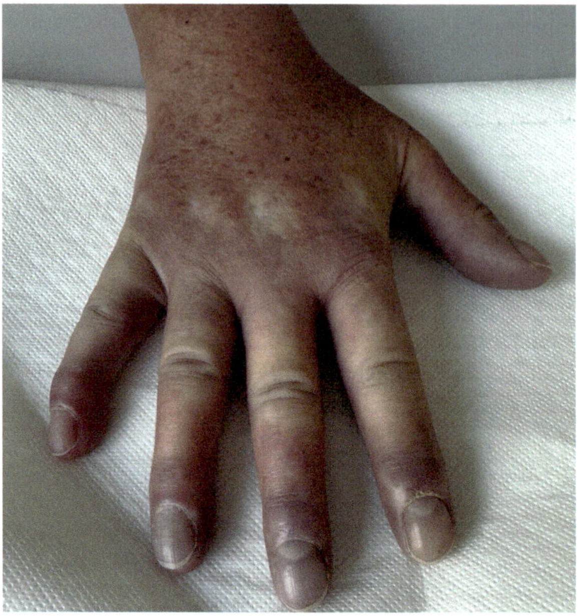

Fig. 2.1 Severe Raynaud's phenomenon in a patient with an initial diagnosis of systemic sclerosis. The investigation of Raynaud's phenomenon is one of the most common reasons for performing capillaroscopy in clinical practice. (Own illustration)

Clinically Conspicuous Findings

In some cases, clinical findings that may indicate collagenosis are also present independently of Raynaud's symptoms. These include, for example, "puffy fingers" or digital ulcerations. Here, too, capillary microscopy can provide indications that confirm the differential diagnosis of collagenosis, for example.

Other Internal Disorders

Collagenoses are known to lead to multiple internal problems. For example, interstitial lung disease can occur as the main symptom. In these cases, too, the presence of typical capillary microscopic patterns can help in the differential diagnosis and indicate a possible rheumatic process as the underlying disease.

Performing the Examination

The second and fifth fingers on both hands are examined. The thumbs are omitted from the examination. The fourth to fifth fingers of the nondominant hand are often the best for assessment. The cuticle can restrict the visibility of the capillaries and thus interfere with the examination. Its thickness decreases toward the little finger [15, 25].

The last vascularized area at the nail fold is examined. Here, the capillaries run parallel to the skin surface and can be assessed along their entire length.

Before performing capillary microscopy, cold stress, which leads to reduced blood flow in the vessels, should be avoided. For this reason, patients should have the opportunity to acclimatize for approximately 15–20 minutes in a room with a temperature of 20–23°, especially in cold outside temperatures [15].

Especially in patients with Raynaud's symptoms, exposure to cold can lead to a significant reduction in blood flow in the vessels. This naturally makes it more difficult to assess the examination [25, 26].

Manipulation of the cuticle can, for example, lead to bleeding and thus simulate the presence of microhemorrhages. For this reason, these should be avoided if possible before the examination. If there are any abnormalities, the examination can be postponed for approximately 4 weeks.

The application of nail varnish can also lead to an impairment of the ability to assess the capillaries in isolated cases (Fig. 2.2). However, the negative effect is usually less severe than feared. As a rule, there is sufficient distance between the applied nail polish and the nail fold to be assessed [26] (Fig. 2.3).

We often observe, either due to inherent factors or, for example, in people who do a lot of physical work, thickened cuticles that significantly hinder the assessability of the underlying capillaries. In cases of progressive collagen diseases with skin sclerosis, these findings can also markedly impair the quality of the examination results. Unfortunately, no effective method is known to meaningfully improve skin thickness for the examination. Therefore, skin thickness repeatedly remains a reason why capillaroscopy cannot be performed or evaluated [15].

In some cases, increased pigmentation of the skin can also lead to limited assessability during the examination.

In order to make the outer skin layers transparent and thus the capillaries visible in the first place, it is always necessary to apply an (immersion) oil. If possible, a substance with high viscosity (such as cedar oil) should be used. These substances have the advantage that they flow off more slowly, and therefore the examination can be carried out over a longer period of time without any problems. Immersion

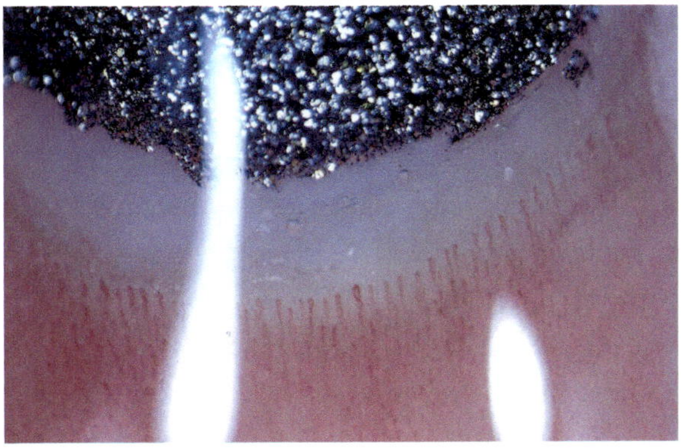

Fig. 2.2 Typical examination conditions when nail polish has been applied. It can be seen that, in most cases, there is a noticeable distance between the nail polish and the capillaries. Therefore, an assessment is usually easily possible (USB microscope). (Own image)

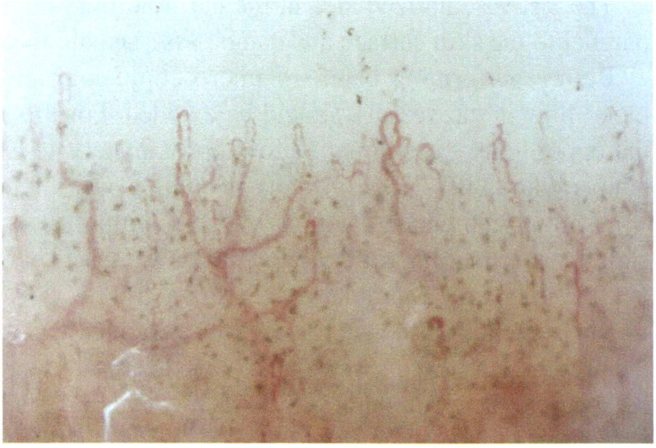

Fig. 2.3 Artifacts caused by contamination with mud (video capillaroscopy). (Own image)

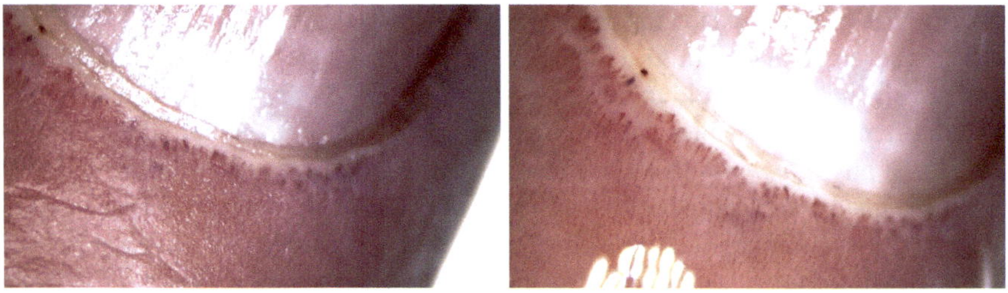

Figs. 2.4 and 2.5 Significant improvement in skin transparency after applying an oil, in this case, walnut oil. Patient with newly diagnosed systemic sclerosis. Focal areas of decreased density and caliber irregularities are visible. On the left side of the image, microhemorrhages combined with a thrombosed vessel can be seen (stereomicroscope). (Own images)

oils commonly used in microscopy can cause skin irritation in individual cases. If too little or too much oil is used, this can lead to artifacts. This often results in increased light reflection, for example, which impairs the visibility of potential pathological agents [27] (Figs. 2.4 and 2.5).

We often find exogenous microtraumas that can lead to isolated hemorrhages. This can occur more frequently after gardening or mechanical activities, for example. As a rule, these microtraumas are single-temporal and sporadic. They can therefore usually be distinguished from multiple microhemorrhages, e.g., in collagenoses.

In some cases, despite all efforts, it is not possible to achieve sufficient assessability of the capillaries. This may be the case, for example, if the skin thickness is increased due to mechanical activity or skin sclerosis [23].

Even if Raynaud's symptoms occur more on the toes than on the fingers in some patients, it does not provide any additional information if the examination is carried out on the toes. Although there may be evidence of microangiopathy here, too, this can also be detected in a similar form on the hands due to the systemic nature of the disease. The skin on the toes is generally much thicker than on the hands, making it more difficult to assess [16].

Findings

An assessment of the capillary microscopy findings should consist of two components. In the first part, a descriptive, in some cases also quantitative, assessment of the aspects present is required. This includes statements on the morphology of the capillaries, their density, extracapillary changes, and, if necessary, the blood flow [17–21].

Based on these findings, a qualitative, evaluative judgment should then be made, which classifies the described aspects medically.

One way of documenting this is to take four images of each finger at 200× magnification, covering an area of 1 mm. An alternative is, for example, to take an overview image at 50× magnification and a further exemplary image at 200× magnification for each finger [15, 27, 28].

The optimum (but also time-consuming) method is to record the findings for each individual finger. The findings can also be summarized, especially if inconspicuous aspects are present [26, 29].

Technology

There are now a large number of different types of microscopes, all of which are suitable for performing capillary microscopy, but some of which differ significantly in terms of price or image quality.

The most important prerequisite for using a device for this examination is that it must have sufficient magnification capability. Only then can the relevant findings actually be correctly recognized.

A magnification of 50× is sufficient for an overview of the examination region; for an exact diagnosis, a magnification of 100–200× should be possible. With the help of magnification on a smaller scale, you can quickly gain an initial impression of the vascularization. Conspicuous areas can be quickly identified. These should then be assessed in more detail using a larger scale. Many pathological features (such as changes in morphology, hemorrhages, or a reduction in the density of the vessels) can already be recognized during the overview [13–15].

The availability of suitable software that allows measurements and scaling of the vessels to be carried out as quickly and easily as possible is also essential for an accurate assessment. For example, it should be possible to record the number of capillaries per millimeter or the lumen of the vessels without any problems.

The images taken during the examination should be easy to save and retrieve. This is made considerably easier if the images are already assigned to the patient when they are taken. Otherwise, the images have to be assigned to the patients individually at a later date, which ultimately significantly increases working time. The presence of foot controls, for example, for making recordings, also makes things easier [26].

Purchasing a Microscope

The type of microscope to be purchased and the amount of money to be invested in this purchase ultimately depend on the objectives associated with the purchase. For centers with high numbers of examinations or for scientific publications, a (usually more expensive) high-quality microscope should be considered; if only small numbers of patients are expected, cheaper, lower-quality devices will suffice.

Video Capillary Microscopes

Video capillary microscopy has been the gold standard for capillary microscopy in recent years. Many scientific publications have been carried out with this type of device. This type of microscope generally offers very good image quality and, with the help of the associated software, excellent options for image analysis and patient-related storage of images.

Possible disadvantages of video capillary microscopy are that zooming in from low to high magnification ranges is usually not possible, and the lens must be changed (time-consuming) to change the magnification factor. Another possible source of error (which can usually be quickly rectified with practice) with all devices that are placed directly on the finger, such as video capillary microscopy, is that excessive contact pressure can reduce the blood flow in the capillaries. This can lead to the density of the vessels or their flow velocity being assessed as too low (Fig. 2.6).

Stereomicroscopes

In many cases, these are at least equivalent in quality to video capillary microscopy. They usually have a good zoom function. This means that if inconspicuous findings can be seen in the overview area, a further magnification level can often be dispensed with, thus saving time. There is no direct contact with the finger.

USB Microscopes

Video capillary microscopes and stereomicroscopes are usually quite expensive. At the other end of the price scale, you will find USB microscopes or similar low-cost devices. These are usually not originally intended for clinical examination of patients. They are mostly used for the assessment of technical devices. They are therefore not classified as medical devices. However, acceptable measurement software is often supplied with the device. Compared to the more expensive devices,

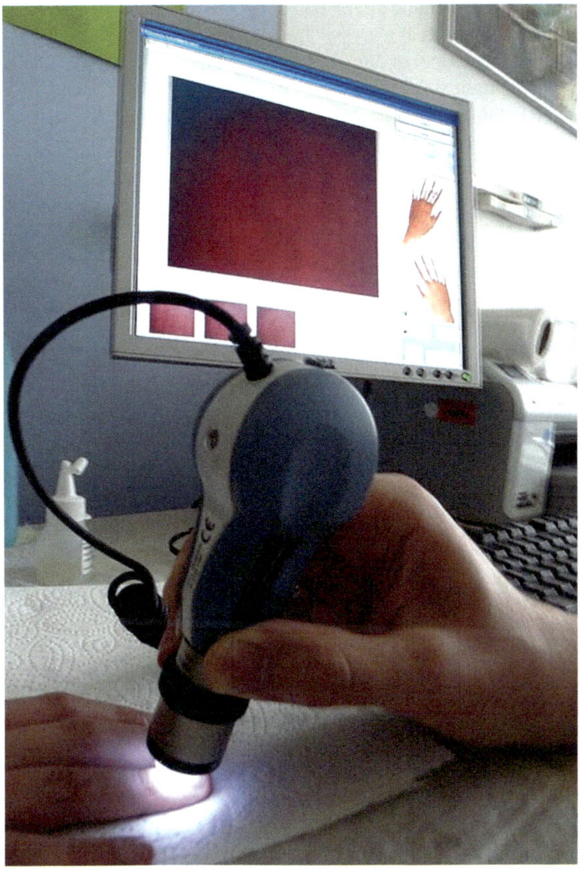

Fig. 2.6 Conducting an examination with a video capillary microscope. The device is connected directly to the computer via a USB port. It is placed on the patient's finger

there are often compromises to be made in terms of handling, image quality, and patient-related storage options. However, several studies have shown that important pathologies can often be reliably recognized even on inexpensive USB microscopes. It can be particularly useful to have such a device available for clinical routine [26].

Other Microscope Types

A whole range of other devices can now be used for capillary microscopy. In terms of price, these are usually between the microscope types already described (Fig. 2.7). In the absence of these microscopes, you will find very good image quality combined with practical storage options (Fig. 2.8).

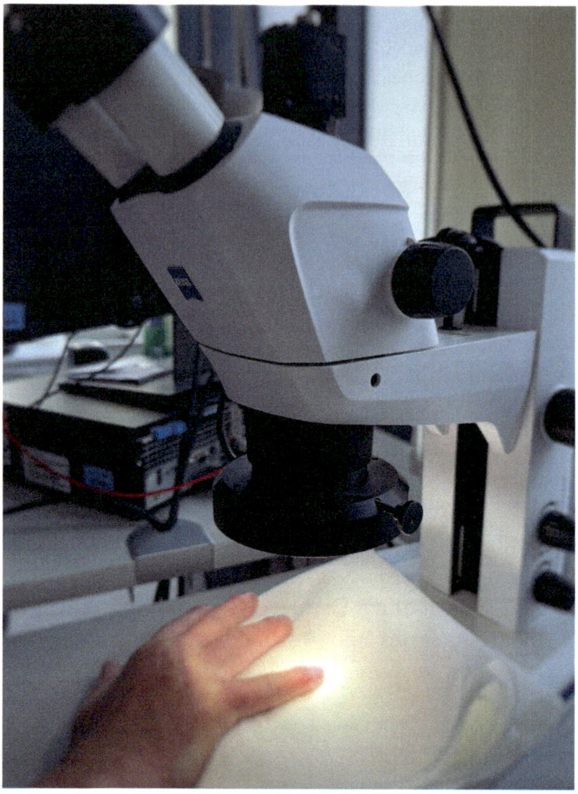

Fig. 2.7 Performing an examination with a stereomicroscope. In this case, the light source is fixed to the microscope. There is no direct contact with the patient's hand. (Own image)

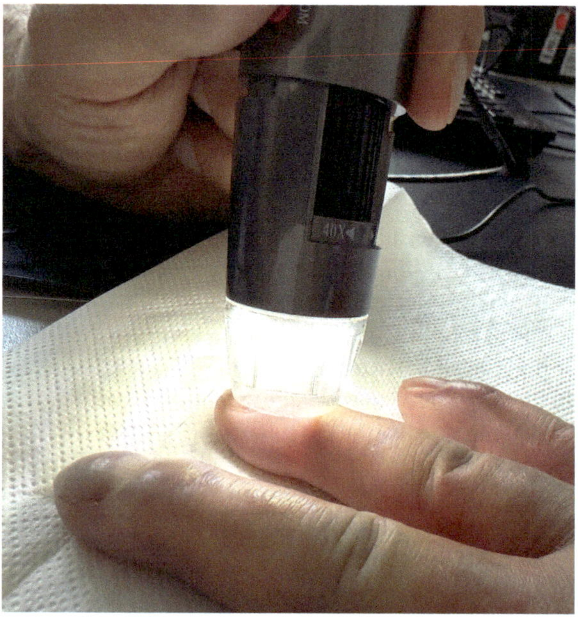

Fig. 2.8 Performing an examination with a USB microscope. The knob used to adjust the magnification is visible. There is direct contact with the patient's hand. (Own image)

Dermatoscopes

In dermatology, internal dermatoscopy is a reflected-light microscopy intended to enable a differential diagnosis between epidermal and dermal pigmentation (e.g., to rule out melanoma). It can also be used to assess the superficial vascular architecture.

As a rule, a tenfold magnification is available. This allows certain pathological changes in the nail fold to be recognized. However, due to the low magnification range, there are gaps that make reliable assessment difficult. For example, neoangiogenesis, caliber fluctuations, mild edema, or even the number of capillaries cannot always be correctly recorded.

Nevertheless, a recent study shows that dermoscopy of the nail fold can contribute well to clarifying the question of the differential diagnosis between pRP and sRP.

Capillaroscopic Findings

Morphology

The physiological lumen of a capillary varies between 8–10 μm in the afferent limb and 10–14 μm in the reference limb [27, 29].

The apex of a capillary is typically convex. Concave deformities can be considered nonspecific [22].

Multiple crossings of capillaries, as well as vessel bends without crossing, are regarded as normal findings [22].

The typical length of capillaries is around 350 μm. Occasionally, longer vessels can be observed ("elongation"). Generally, elongations are not considered pathological. However, they are important in differential diagnosis because they can initially resemble neoangiogenesis. To distinguish between them, a microscope with adequate magnification capabilities is necessary (for example, a dermatoscope cannot definitively answer this question) [15, 22].

In connection with elongation, there may be torquing or indentations of the capillaries ("shutter-like" appearance) (Fig. 2.9).

Hairpin Shape

The hairpin shape describes a specific form of capillaries where the afferent and efferent limbs run parallel to each other and are closely spaced. They cross at most once, and the apex is narrow. In approximately 70% of healthy individuals, these hairpin shapes are observed, making them the most common and simplest normal variant [26].

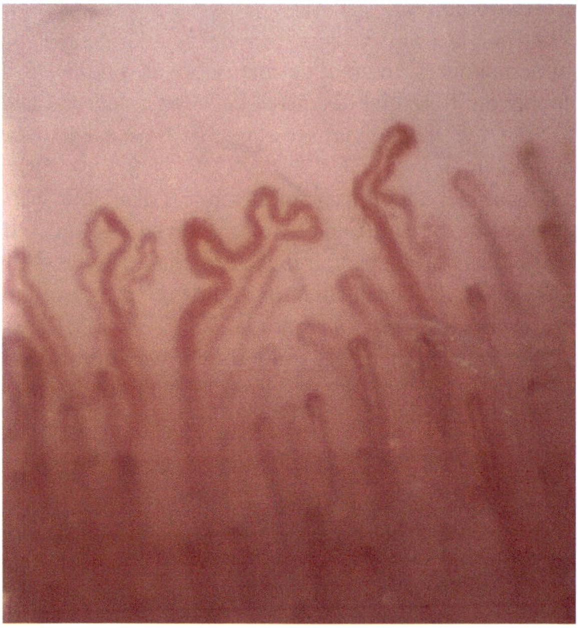

Fig. 2.9 In the center of the image, elongated capillaries with resulting nonspecific changes in the form of indentations are visible. Additionally, there are caliber irregularities as an incidental finding. The patient has undifferentiated collagenosis. (USB microscope). (Own image)

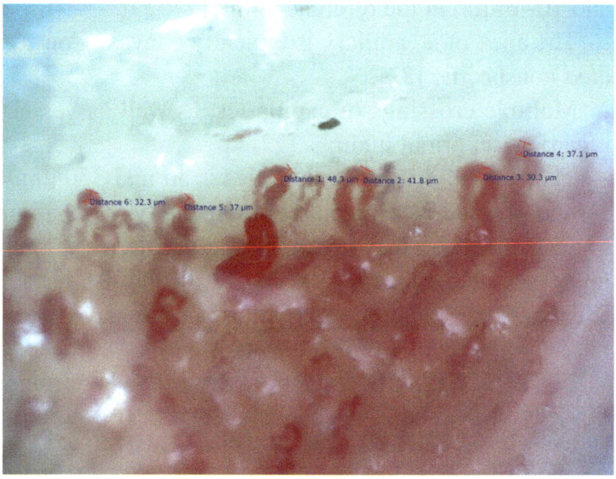

Fig. 2.10 Multiple saccular ectasias in a patient with systemic sclerosis. Since the diameter at the apex of all capillaries is less than 50 μm, they cannot be classified as "giant capillaries" (video capillaroscopy). (Own image)

Caliber Changes

The diameter of the capillaries at the apex should normally be less than 20 μm. If the diameter is larger, the change is considered nonspecific (Fig. 2.10). A diameter exceeding 50 μm is clearly pathological and is referred to as "giant capillaries," which are often seen in connection with systemic sclerosis [26] (Fig. 2.11).

Variations in caliber, meaning fluctuations in the thickness of a limb by more than 50%, are classified as nonspecific changes. However, such changes can also be observed in connection with collagen diseases.

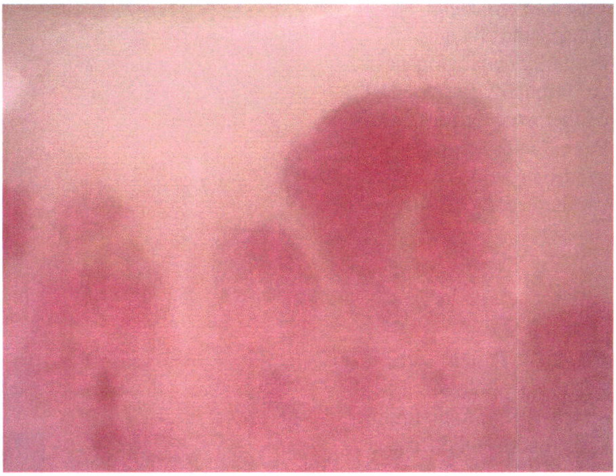

Fig. 2.11 Giant capillary as well as pronounced papilledema in combination with a focal density reduction. Patient with systemic sclerosis. Due to the limited field of view, a definitive pattern cannot be identified (video capillaroscopy). (Own image)

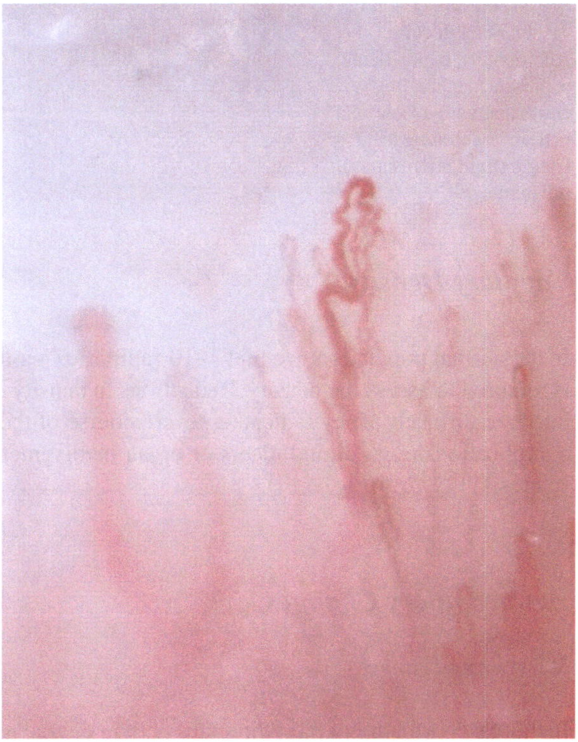

Fig. 2.12 Neoangiogenesis. Several small-caliber new blood vessels can be seen branching off from the main capillary. In this case, an unspecific finding with otherwise unremarkable capillaroscopy (USB microscope). (Own image)

Neoangiogenesis

(Usually smaller-lumen) branches emerging from a capillary indicate neoangiogenesis. The affected vessels are classically referred to as "bushy capillaries." (Fig. 2.12) They are classified as nonspecific changes and are also frequently found in collagen diseases (Fig. 2.13).

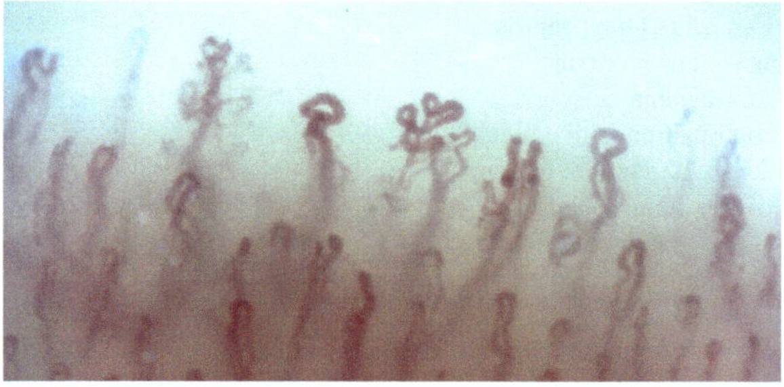

Fig. 2.13 Multiple nonspecific changes, primarily neoangiogenesis. Additionally, increased caliber irregularities. Patient with Sjögren's syndrome (video capillaroscopy). (Own image)

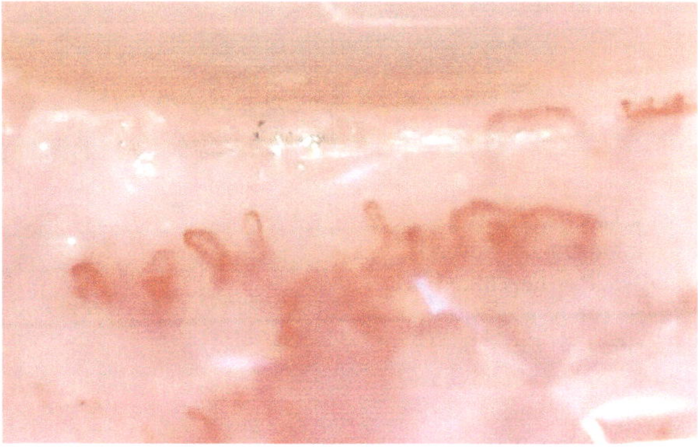

Fig. 2.14 Patient with advanced systemic sclerosis. The main finding is a pronounced diffuse reduction in capillary density combined with nonspecific changes in the vascular architecture. Additionally, papilledema is present. The finding is consistent with a "late SSc pattern," according to Cutolo (light microscopy). (Own image)

Capillary Density

In the normal population, we find 7–10 capillaries per millimeter. A calibrated scale is required to assess the density. Reductions in density can occur either focally (isolated) or diffusely. They indicate a severe course of the disease with corresponding complications (e.g., digital ulcers or organ involvement in the context of systemic sclerosis) [22, 26] (Fig. 2.14).

Extracapillary Changes

Microhemorrhages

In this case, extravascular erythrocytes or their degradation products can be detected. Causes may include trauma or capillary vascular changes. From ectatic or giant capillaries, onion-skin-like, recurrent hemorrhages often occur. While in the case of minor trauma, the hemorrhages are often isolated and single-time events, in systemic diseases, we frequently find recurrent and multiple microhemorrhages (Fig. 2.15).

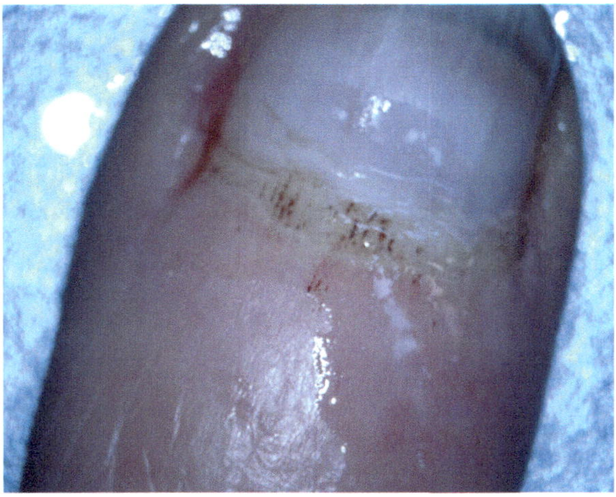

Fig. 2.15 Multiple hemorrhages visible to the naked eye in a patient with systemic lupus erythematosus (brightfield microscopy). (Own image)

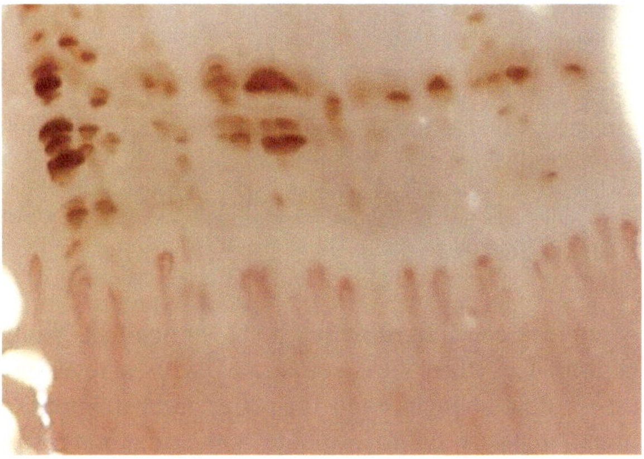

Fig. 2.16 Patient with systemic lupus erythematosus. The main finding is multiple recurrent microhemorrhages. Additionally, multiple capillary ectasias are visible (brightfield microscopy). (Own image)

Nontraumatic microhemorrhages are classified as nonspecific changes and are very commonly found in connection with collagen diseases. Their presence or absence also defines the different systemic sclerosis (SSc) patterns according to Cutolo [22, 25, 26] (Fig. 2.16).

Edema

Edema is an extracapillary dermal fluid increase caused by increased permeability of the capillaries (e.g., due to microangiopathy). Microscopically, the papilla often appears lighter; sometimes the image looks milky, and focusing on the capillaries is often insufficient due to the increased fluid deposits.This is a classic finding in advanced collagen diseases such as systemic sclerosis. Differentially, focusing can also be impaired by increased skin thickness independent of disease and can mimic the appearance of edema [25, 26].

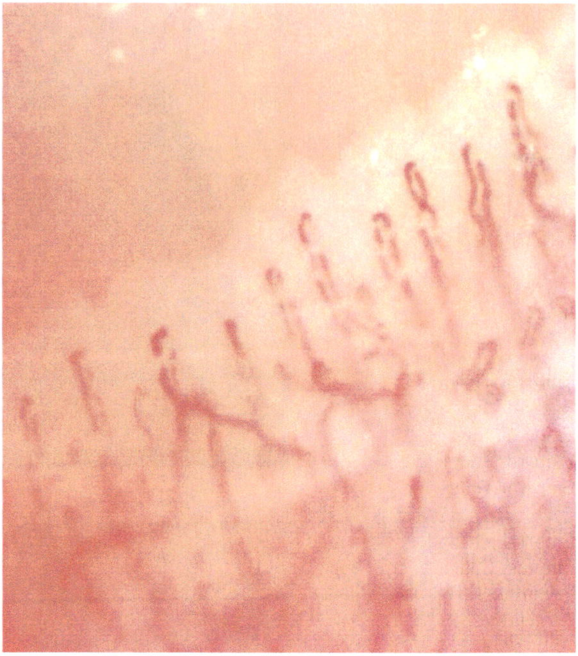

Fig. 2.17 Reduced flow in all depicted capillaries ("Sludge"). The interruption of laminar flow is clearly visible. Patient with primary Raynaud's syndrome. (Video capillaroscopy). (Own image)

Flow Changes

A reduced capillary flow is usually noticed as "sludge." This is a visible aggregation of erythrocytes, sometimes with a reversible interruption of flow. To assess flow changes (and for differential diagnosis, e.g., from caliber fluctuations), it is useful to evaluate a moving image or several sequential photos (Fig. 2.17).

Sludge can occur in both primary and secondary Raynaud's syndromes and therefore does not help clarify the differential diagnosis between these two conditions [25, 26].

Stasis/Thrombosis

Thrombosis refers to an irreversible thrombus formation with no detectable flow in the capillary. Depending on the age of the thrombus, it appears as a livid (bluish) to brownish discoloration [26].

Other Assessable Sections

Subpapillary Venous Plexus

The subpapillary venous plexus can also be observed occasionally in healthy individuals (about 30% of people) (Fig. 2.18). It is especially prominent or frequently seen in cases of reduced skin thickness (e.g., after prolonged corticosteroid use) [26] (Figs. 2.19 and 2.20).

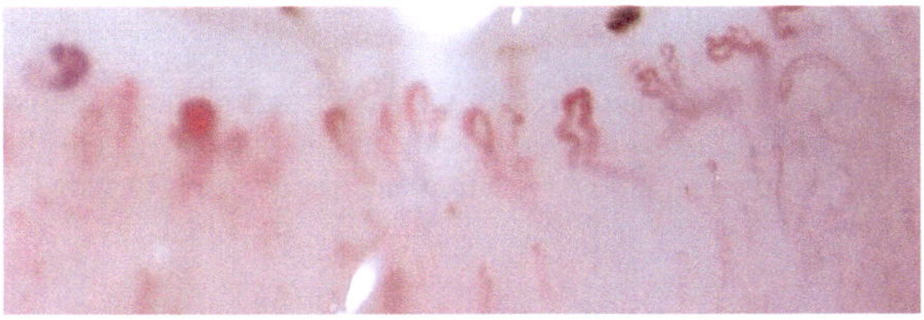

Fig. 2.18 Various abnormalities in a patient with undifferentiated connective tissue disease. The main findings include caliber irregularities, microhemorrhages, and a focal decrease in density on the right side (visible under a USB microscope). (Own image)

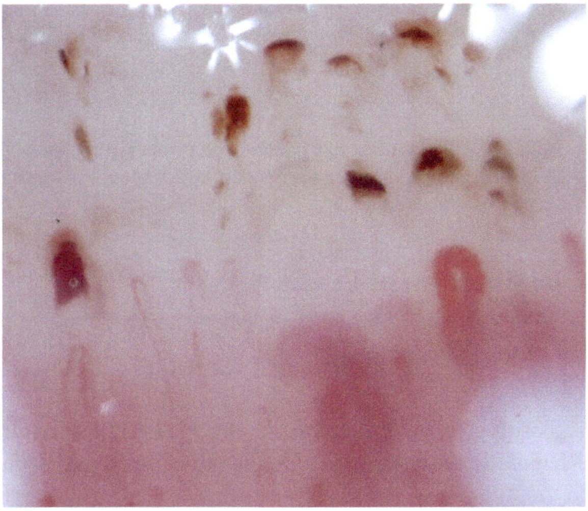

Fig. 2.19 Findings in a patient with systemic sclerosis known for 2 years. Notable are mainly caliber dilations, multiple microhemorrhages, a focal decrease in density, and papilledema. The findings are consistent with an "active SSc pattern," according to Cutolo (USB microscope). (Own image)

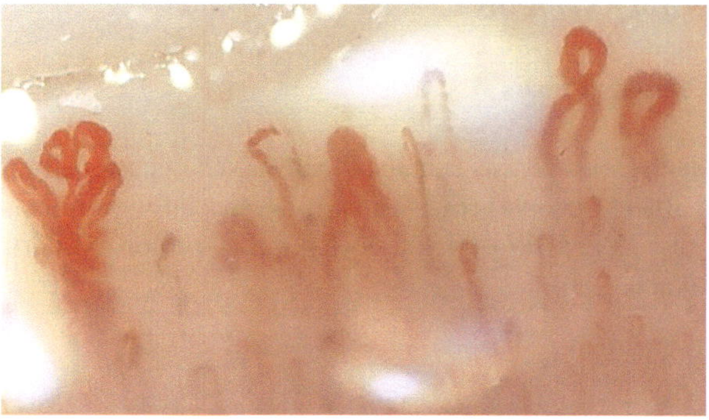

Fig. 2.20 Female patient with dermatomyositis. On the left side of the image, pronounced neoangiogenesis ("bushy capillary") is visible, along with irregularities in vessel caliber, reduced density, and, as an additional finding, a flow reduction in several vessels ("sludge") (dermatoscope). (Own illustration)

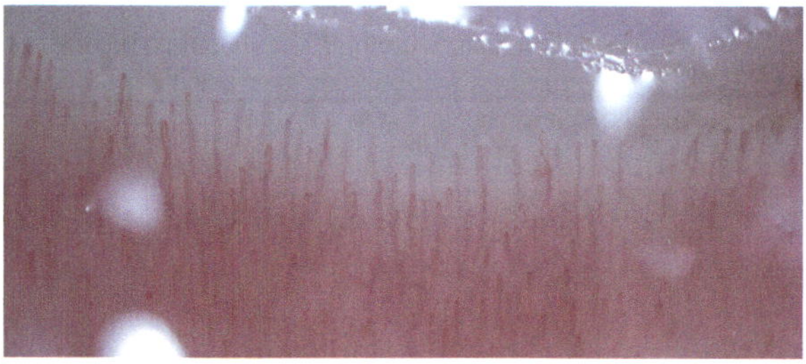

Fig. 2.21 Normal finding in a patient with primary Raynaud's phenomenon. Hairpin-shaped capillaries predominate. Neither a reduction in density nor extravascular changes are observed (USB microscope). (Own illustration)

Classification of Findings

Normal Findings

According to the guidelines of the EULAR Study Group on Microcirculation in Rheumatic Diseases, the following are considered normal [22]:

Capillary density of >7/mm
Capillary diameter at the apex of <20 μm
Apex convex in shape
Curved or crossing capillaries (Figs. 2.21 and 2.22).

In older individuals, a slight increase in crossing capillaries is occasionally described. In children, a physiological reduction in capillary density is also sometimes observed. However, very often in both age groups, no significant difference is found compared to other adults. Surprisingly, neither sex nor nicotine abuse appears to influence the capillary microscopy findings.

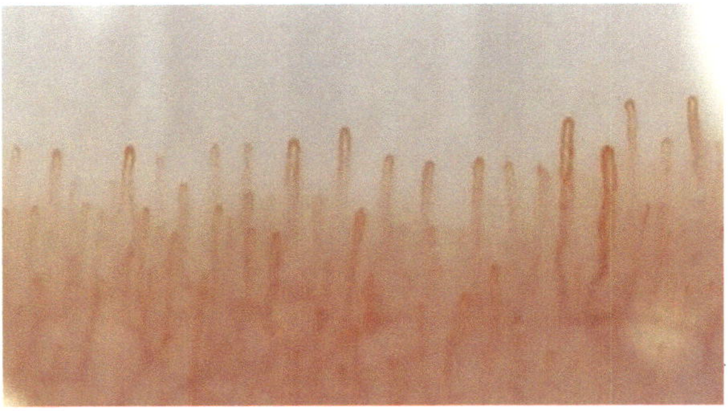

Fig. 2.22 Normal finding with predominantly hairpin-shaped capillaries. Patient with primary Raynaud's syndrome (dermatoscope). (Own illustration)

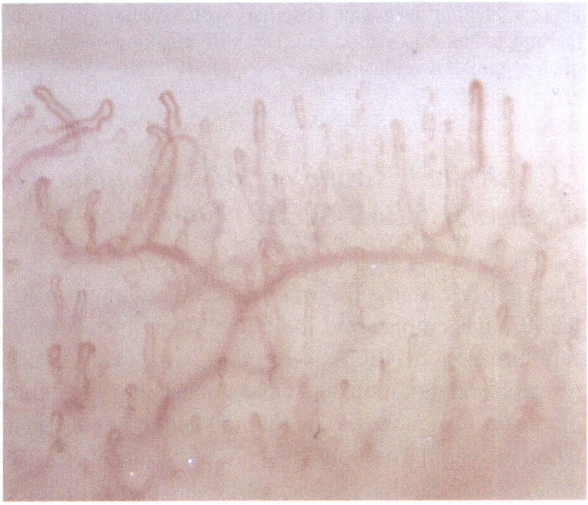

Fig. 2.23 Patient with primary Raynaud's phenomenon. Mild nonspecific caliber irregularities and a reduction in capillary flow ("sludge") with visible interruptions of continuous blood flow (e.g., in the upper right third) are visible. Additionally, the subpapillary venous plexus is clearly seen here (USB microscope). (Own illustration)

Nonspecific Findings

The following are classified as nonspecific [22]:

Reduction in capillary density (< 7/mm)
Capillary diameter at the apex of 20–50 μm
Microhemorrhages
Morphological abnormalities such as neoangiogenesis
Concave indentations at the apex
Using the frequency of nonspecific changes, various SSc (systemic sclerosis) patterns according to Cutolo can be defined (see the corresponding chapter) (Figs. 2.23 and 2.24).

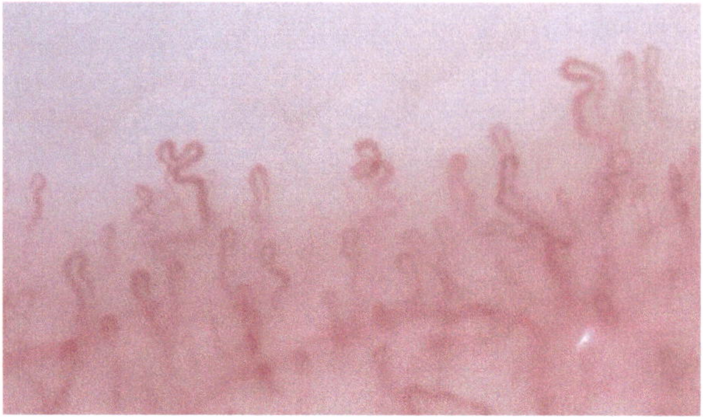

Fig. 2.24 Nonspecific changes in a patient with primary Raynaud's phenomenon. Notably, in the upper left half of the image, a capillary with a concavely shaped apex is visible. In the right half of the image, elongations of a capillary with resulting indentations of the vessel can be seen (USB microscope). (Own illustration)

EULAR Study Group on Microcirculation in Rheumatic Diseases (EULAR-SGMC) Consensus

The EULAR Study Group on Microcirculation in Rheumatic Diseases (EULAR-SGMC) has emphasized the critical need for standardized terminology in nailfold capillaroscopy (NFC) to improve diagnostic accuracy, facilitate international research collaboration, and ensure consistency in clinical reporting [3]. The absence of uniform language has historically led to confusion and variability in the interpretation of capillaroscopic images, particularly in diseases like systemic sclerosis (SSc), where capillary abnormalities are part of diagnostic and classification criteria.

In response to this need, the EULAR-SGMC working group developed a consensus-based glossary of terms to describe key microvascular abnormalities, including:

Capillary dilatation: defined as an apical diameter between 20 and 50 μm.

Giant capillaries: characterized by a homogeneously enlarged loop with an apical diameter > 50 μm.

Microhemorrhages: visible as punctate or flame-shaped dark spots adjacent to or around the capillary loops.

Avascular areas: defined as intercapillary distances exceeding 500 μm, indicating capillary dropout.

Neoangiogenesis: the presence of ramified, bushy, or bizarre capillary formations reflecting capillary regeneration.

The adoption of these definitions allows for semi-quantitative scoring systems to be implemented in both clinical and research settings. These systems often assess parameters such as capillary density, morphology, and the presence of pathological features [3].

In summary, the EULAR-SGMC consensus represents a milestone in standardizing nailfold capillaroscopy, establishing a common language for clinicians and researchers alike, and supporting its integration into routine rheumatologic practice.

Semi-Quantitative Scoring Systems

To enhance the objectivity and reproducibility of capillaroscopic evaluations, several semi-quantitative scoring systems have been developed and validated. These systems are designed to numerically assess the most relevant microvascular changes observed under nailfold capillaroscopy (NFC) in conditions such as systemic sclerosis (SSc) and Raynaud's phenomenon.

Rather than relying solely on qualitative impressions, semi-quantitative scoring assigns grades—typically on a scale from 0 to 3—to specific features such as:

Giant capillaries: large, homogeneously dilated loops with an apical diameter > 50 μm
Microhemorrhages: localized areas of capillary bleeding or extravasation
Capillary loss (avascular areas): intercapillary distances >500 μm
Neoangiogenesis: irregular, ramified, or bushy capillary formations

Each parameter is scored per digit (typically eight fingers excluding thumbs), and a mean or cumulative score is calculated. For example, the Maricq scoring system and the Cutolo semi-quantitative method are among the most widely used and allow direct comparisons between patients and over time [3].

These tools are particularly valuable in clinical research for stratifying disease severity, correlating capillaroscopic findings with organ involvement or autoantibody profiles, and evaluating treatment responses longitudinally. In clinical practice, they support early diagnosis, disease classification, and monitoring of vascular progression in systemic autoimmune conditions.

Case 1: Normal Nailfold Capillaroscopy

A 23-year-old female medical student presents for a routine clinical skills training session involving capillaroscopy. She has no history of Raynaud's phenomenon, autoimmune disease, or microvascular symptoms. She is a nonsmoker, takes no medications, and has an unremarkable family and medical history. Clinical examination is normal, with warm hands, good peripheral perfusion, and no signs of digital skin changes (Fig. 2.25).

Capillaroscopic Findings

Morphology: All capillaries demonstrated normal hairpin/U-shaped morphology. No abnormal shapes were identified. Homogeneous and orderly arrangement of capillary loops in the distal row.

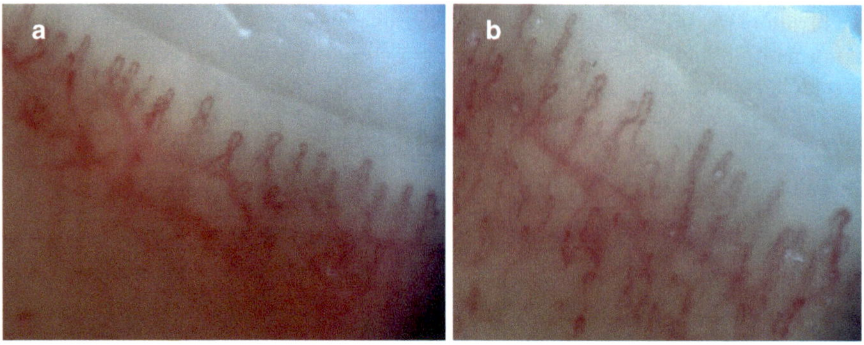

Fig. 2.25 Normal capillaroscopy showing regularly arranged hairpin-shaped capillary loops with uniform morphology. Some tortuous and crossed capillaries with convex apices are present, along with a visible subpapillary arteriovenous plexus and normal capillary density. No evidence of dilatation, hemorrhages, or avascular areas—findings consistent with a healthy microvascular structure

Capillary Density: Consistent across all examined digits, ranging between 9 and 11 capillary loops per millimeter.

Dimensions: No evidence of capillary enlargement or giant capillaries and no avascularity.

Microhemorrhages: Absent.

Subpapillary Venous Plexus: Visible in some fields, presenting as a fine vascular background without any irregularities.

Interpretation

The examination is consistent with a completely normal nailfold capillaroscopic pattern. No structural abnormalities, density variations, or microangiopathic signs are noted.

Learning Points

This case demonstrates the ideal capillaroscopic appearance of a healthy individual. It is essential for trainees and clinicians to be familiar with this "normal baseline" to accurately recognize deviations in patients with suspected connective tissue disease. Normal patterns are characterized by regularly spaced hairpin-shaped capillaries, consistent density, and the absence of any morphological alterations or hemorrhagic signs.

Case 2: Normal Nailfold with Common Physiological Variations

A 54-year-old male manual worker attends the clinic for general rheumatologic screening. He has no history of Raynaud's phenomenon, systemic autoimmune disorders, or microvascular complaints. However, he reports occasional mechanical trauma to his hands due to daily tasks and admits to mild habitual cuticle picking. He is not on any medications and has no significant medical or family history.

On examination, his hands show mild skin thickening related to occupational use but no ulcers, telangiectasia, or signs of systemic sclerosis. Peripheral pulses are intact, and capillary refill is normal (Fig. 2.26).

Capillaroscopic Findings

Capillary Morphology: General preservation of the distal row with minor irregularity in spacing. Slight tortuosity observed.

Capillary Density: Normal range in most fingers (8–10 capillaries/mm), but slightly reduced (6–7/mm) in the fifth finger bilaterally (b). "Focal decrease in density may occur due to microtrauma or poor imaging angle, not necessarily due to avascularity."

Microhemorrhages: Two tiny, dot-like hemorrhages observed near the cuticle of the index and ring fingers—likely related to minor trauma (a and b, respectively). No evidence of active bleeding or widespread hemorrhagic pattern.

Subpapillary Venous Plexus: Mildly prominent in appearance, especially in fingers exposed to greater manual strain. This feature is sometimes more visible in healthy individuals with thin skin or higher venous tone.

Interpretation

Findings are consistent with normal physiological variations. No signs of capillary enlargement, giant capillaries, avascular areas, neo-angiogenesis, or structural abnormalities suggesting secondary Raynaud's or systemic connective tissue disease.

Learning Point

Not all deviations from the "ideal" capillaroscopic pattern represent disease. Age, mechanical trauma, and individual anatomical variability can lead to minor findings

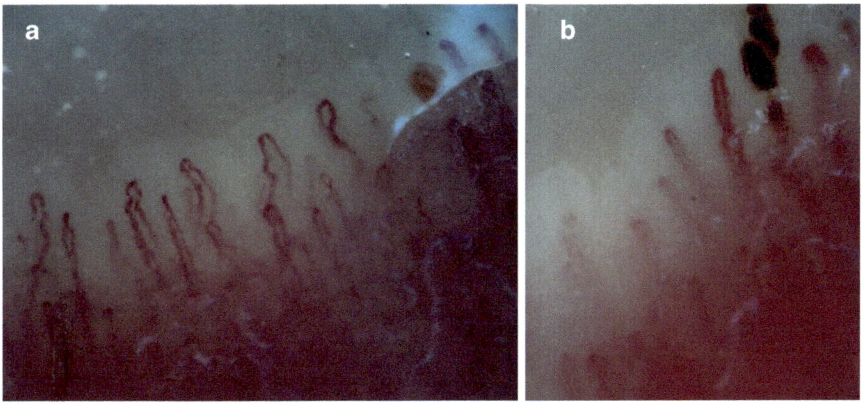

Fig. 2.26 Nailfold video capillaroscopy reveals a generally preserved distal row with mild spacing irregularities and slight tortuosity. Capillary density is mostly within normal range, with a slight focal reduction, likely due to microtrauma or imaging angle. Two small dot-like hemorrhages near the cuticles were noted (**a** and **b**, respectively)

such as tortuosity, scattered microhemorrhages, or slight density variations. These should not be overinterpreted as pathological. Proper interpretation always requires clinical context—capillaroscopy is an adjunct to, not a substitute for, clinical evaluation.

Case 3: Nonspecific Abnormalities (Capillary Dilatations)

A 30-year-old female presents with a history of Raynaud's phenomenon affecting the fingers, mainly during cold exposure. The episodes are brief, non-painful, and non-disabling. She denies joint pain, skin thickening, or any constitutional symptoms. There is no history of autoimmune disease or family history of rheumatologic disorders (Fig. 2.27).

Capillaroscopic Findings

Capillary Morphology: The architecture is preserved, and the general morphology remains uniform.

Capillary Density: The capillary density is within normal limits (typically >7 capillaries/mm).

Dimensions: few isolated capillary loops with mild dilatation, with apical diameters ranging between 20 and 30 µm.

There are no *microhemorrhages*, giant capillaries, capillary dropout, or avascular zones.

Interpretation and Discussion

These findings reflect nonspecific capillary dilatations, which may be seen in healthy individuals, especially under minor physiological or mechanical influences (e.g., exposure to cold, manual work, or minor trauma). Importantly, the absence of other features such as hemorrhages, avascular areas, or neoangiogenesis supports a non-pathological pattern.

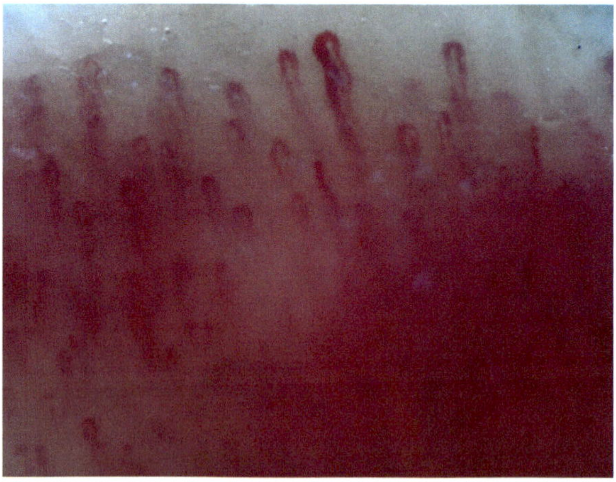

Fig. 2.27 Nailfold video capillaroscopy reveals preserved architecture with uniform morphology and normal density (≥7 capillaries/mm). Mild dilatation (20–30 µm) is noted in a few capillaries, without giant capillaries, hemorrhages, or avascular areas. These nonspecific changes do not suggest a scleroderma pattern, but clinical correlation and follow-up are recommended

Mild dilatation alone does not meet the criteria for the "scleroderma pattern." According to the 2013 EULAR Study Group on Microcirculation guidelines, dilatation should be giant (i.e., >50 µm) and typically accompanied by other features to raise concern for systemic sclerosis (SSc).

Learning Points

Understanding capillary morphology (e.g., apical diameter thresholds) is essential in distinguishing benign changes from early disease.

Clinical correlation is critical. In the absence of systemic features or serological markers, such findings are usually not concerning.

Follow-up may be warranted only if symptoms evolve or new clinical signs emerge.

Case 4: Early, Isolated Giant Capillary

A 29-year-old female presents with a 4-month history of Raynaud's phenomenon, primarily triggered by cold exposure. No history of digital ulcers, arthralgia, skin thickening, or other systemic symptoms. Clinical examination is unremarkable. Autoimmune screening is negative (Fig. 2.28).

Capillaroscopic Findings

Nailfold videocapillaroscopy reveals a predominantly normal pattern across most fingers. However, in the fourth finger of the left hand and the third finger of the right hand, there is one unequivocal giant capillary in each (measuring approximately 98 µm and 105 µm in diameter, respectively). There are no definite avascular areas, no prominent microhemorrhages, and the overall architecture remains orderly.

Interpretation

While the findings do not yet fulfill the criteria for a "scleroderma pattern," the isolated presence of giant capillaries—especially when clearly exceeding 50 µm—raises clinical suspicion. In the absence of other features, this case represents a possible preclinical phase of systemic sclerosis or another connective tissue disease.

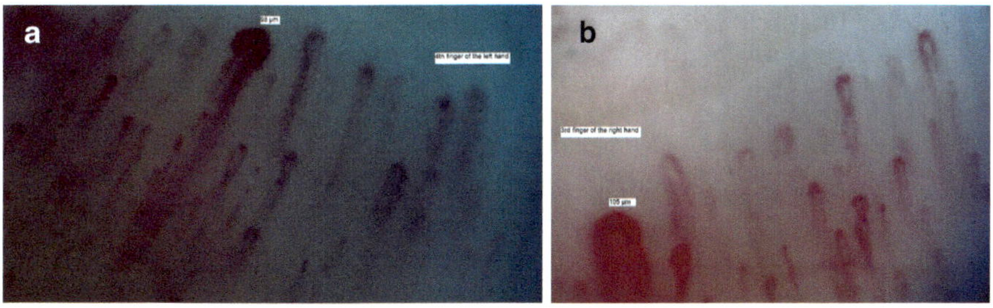

Fig. 2.28 Nailfold video capillaroscopy shows a mostly normal pattern, except for one giant capillary in the left fourth and right third fingers, measuring around 98 µm and 105 µm (**a** and **b**, respectively). No avascular areas or significant microhemorrhages are observed, with preserved overall architecture

Key Learning Points

A giant capillary is defined as a capillary loop with a diameter > 50 μm, usually with homogeneously enlarged apical portions and well-demarcated architecture.

Identifying isolated giant capillaries—especially when the rest of the capillary field is normal—can be crucial for early detection and follow-up.

This case exemplifies the value of capillaroscopy in early or preclinical autoimmune disease surveillance, even when systemic features are absent.

Regular follow-up and repeat capillaroscopy are warranted to monitor for progression toward a full scleroderma pattern.

It is suggested to repeat capillaroscopy in 6–12 months and to monitor for clinical signs of.

References

1. Lambova SN. Nailfold capillaroscopy - practical implications for rheumatology practice. Curr Rheumatol Rev. 2020;16(2):79–83.
2. Chojnowski MM, Felis-Giemza A, Olesińska M. Capillaroscopy – a role in modern rheumatology. Reumatologia. 2016;54(2):67–72.
3. Smith V, Herrick AL, Ingegnoli F, Damjanov N, De Angelis R, Denton CP, Distler O, Espejo K, Foeldvari I, Frech T, Garro B, Gutierrez M, Gyger G, Hachulla E, Hesselstrand R, Iagnocco A, Kayser C, Melsens K, Müller-Ladner U, Paolino S, Pizzorni C, Radic M, Riccieri V, Snow M, Stevens W, Sulli A, van Laar JM, Vonk MC, Vanhaecke A, Cutolo M. the EULAR Study Group on Microcirculation in Rheumatic Diseases and the Scleroderma Clinical Trials Consortium Group on Capillaroscopy. Autoimmun Rev. 2020;19(3):102458. https://doi.org/10.1016/j.autrev.2020.102458.
4. Aird WC. Phenotypic heterogeneity of the endothelium: I. Structure, function, and mechanisms. Circ Res. 2007;100(2):158–73. https://doi.org/10.1161/01.RES.0000255691.76142.4a.
5. Pries AR, Secomb TW, Gaehtgens P. Design principles of vascular beds. Circ Res. 1995;77(5):1017–23. https://doi.org/10.1161/01.res.77.5.1017.
6. Cutolo M, Sulli A, Pizzorni C, Accardo S. Nailfold videocapillaroscopy assessment of microvascular damage in systemic sclerosis. J Rheumatol. 2000;27(1):155–60.
7. Cutolo M, Sulli A, Smith V. How to perform and interpret capillaroscopy. Best Pract Res Clin Rheumatol. 2013;27(2):237–48. https://doi.org/10.1016/j.berh.2013.03.001.
8. Grover C, Jakhar D, Mishra A, Singal A. Nail-fold capillaroscopy for the dermatologists. Indian J Dermatol Venereol Leprol. 2022;88(3):300–12.
9. Maricq HR, LeRoy EC. Patterns of finger capillary abnormalities in connective tissue disease by "wide-field" microscopy. Arthritis Rheum. 1973;16(5):619–28. https://doi.org/10.1002/art.1780160506.
10. van den Hoogen F, Khanna D, Fransen J, Johnson SR, Baron M, Tyndall A, Matucci-Cerinic M, Naden RP, Medsger TA Jr, Carreira PE, Riemekasten G, Clements PJ, Denton CP, Distler O, Allanore Y, Furst DE, Gabrielli A, Mayes MD, van Laar JM, Seibold JR, Czirjak L, Steen VD, Inanc M, Kowal-Bielecka O, Müller-Ladner U, Valentini G, Veale DJ, Vonk MC, Walker UA, Chung L, Collier DH, Csuka ME, Fessler BJ, Guiducci S, Herrick A, Hsu VM, Jimenez S, Kahaleh B, Merkel PA, Sierakowski S, Silver RM, Simms RW, Varga J, Pope JE. 2013 classification criteria for systemic sclerosis: an American college of rheumatology/European league against rheumatism collaborative initiative. Ann Rheum Dis Arthritis Rheum. 2013;65(11):2737–47. https://doi.org/10.1002/art.38098. Epub 2013 Oct 3.

11. Bellando Randone S, et al. The microcirculation and rheumatic diseases. In: Cutolo, editor. Atlas of capillaroscopy in rheumatic diseases. Milano: Elsevier; 2010.
12. Carpenter P, Franco A. Atlas der Kapillaroskopie. Wiesbaden: Deutsche Abbott GmbH; 1983.
13. Cutolo M, Sulli A, Pizzorni C, Accardo S. Nailfold videocapillaroscopy assessment of microvascular damage in systemic sclerosis patients. Ann Rheum Dis. 2000;67(6):885–7.
14. Geyer M, Vasile M, Hermann W. Nagelfalzkapillarmikroskopie. Z Rheumatol. 2014;73:149–62.
15. Hasseli-Fräbel R, Hermann W, Sander O, Triantafyllias K. Kapillarmikroskopie- Grundlagen und klinische Anwendung. Z Rheumatol. 2022;81:313–22.
16. Hermann W. Kapillarmikroskopie. Z Rheumatol. 2016;75(6):586–90.
17. Imbert B, Carpentier P. Techniques for evaluating the microcirculation. In: Cutolo, editor. Atlas of Capillaroscopy in Rheumatic Diseases. Milano: Elsevier; 2010.
18. Sander O, Iking-Konert C, Ostendorf B. Taschenatlas Kapillarmikroskopie 2. Auflage. Rheumazentrum Rheinp-Ruhr (AAA); 2012.
19. Mariq HR, Le Roy EC. Patterns of finger capillary abnormalities in connective tissue disorders by "wide-field" microscopy. Arthritis Rheum. 1973;16:619–28.
20. Cutolo M, et al. Nailfold videocapillaroscopy assessment of microvascular damage in systemic sclerosis. J Rheumatol. 2000;27:155–60.
21. Smith V, Herrick AL, Ingegnoli F, et al. Standardisation of nailfold capillaroscopy for the assessment of patients with Raynaud's phenomenon and systemic sclerosis. Autoimmun Rev. 2020;19(3):102458.
22. Herrick AL, Murray A. The role of capillaroscopy and thermography in the assessment and management of Raynaud's phenomenon. Autoimmun Rev. 2018;17:465–72.
23. Cutolo M, Smith V, Sulli A. Atlas of Capillaroscopy in Rheumatic Diseases. Milano: Elsevier; 2010.
24. Sander O, et al. Kapillarmikroskopie – Durchführung und Nomenklatur. Z Rheumatol. 2010;69:253–62.
25. Sander O, Iking-Konert C, Ostendorf B. Taschenatlas Kapillarmikroskopie 2. Auflage. Rheumazentrum Rhein-Ruhr; 2012.
26. Lambova S, et al. Capillaroscopic pattern at the toes of sytsemic sclerosis patients: does it "tell" more than those oft he fingers? J Clin Rheumatol. 2011;17:311–4.
27. Sander O, Sunderkötter C, Kötter I, Wagner I, Becker M, Herrgott I, Schwarting A, Ostendorf B, Iking-Konert C, Genth ER. Capillaroscopy. Procedure and nomenclature. Z Rheumatol. 2010;69(3):252–62.
28. Klein-Weigel PF, Sunderkötter C, Sander O. Nailfold capillarsocopy microsopy- an interdisciplinary appraisal. Vasa. 2016;45:353–64.
29. Berks M, Dinsdale G, Marjanovic E, Murray A, Taylor C, Herrick AL. Comparison between low cost USB nailfold capillaroscopy and videocapillaroscopy: a pilot study. Rheumatology. 2021;60:3862–7.

Chapter 3
Raynaud's Phenomenon

Marco Di Battista, Nicola Ortalli, and Francesco Del Galdo

Introduction

In 1862, the French physician Maurice Raynaud described a group of patients presenting with what he termed "local asphyxia" and symmetrical gangrene of the extremities [1]. Since then, knowledge about the condition—now known as Raynaud's phenomenon (RP)—has expanded significantly across various domains, including pathogenesis, classification, and therapeutic approaches. Nevertheless, RP remains incompletely understood from a pathogenetic standpoint, representing an under-diagnosed condition frequently mistaken for other clinical entities. RP is sometimes still a challenge for the physician, especially in cases refractory to conventional treatments [2–4]. In this chapter, we aim to provide a thorough overview of RP, emphasizing key aspects of its diagnosis and management, as well as areas where further elucidation is needed. Through a comprehensive and structured analysis, this chapter aims to provide clinicians and researchers with an updated and nuanced understanding of RP.

M. Di Battista
Leeds Institute of Rheumatic and Musculoskeletal Medicine, University of Leeds, Leeds, UK

Rheumatology Unit, University of Pisa, Pisa, Italy

N. Ortalli
Leeds Institute of Rheumatic and Musculoskeletal Medicine, University of Leeds, Leeds, UK

F. Del Galdo (✉)
Leeds Institute of Rheumatic and Musculoskeletal Medicine, University of Leeds, Leeds, UK

NIHR Leeds Biomedical Research Centre, Leeds Teaching Hospitals Trust, Leeds, UK
e-mail: F.DelGaldo@leeds.ac.uk

Y. El Miedany, R. A. Elziaty (eds.), *Capillaroscopy*, Contemporary Rheumatology,
https://doi.org/10.1007/978-3-032-22966-3_3

Clinical Presentation

RP is a completely reversible, transient, vasospastic disorder that can affect virtually all extremities of the body with variable extent and intensity. Typically, the fingers and/or toes are affected, but not necessarily all symmetrically and not in their entirety; there may be cases limited to only some fingers and only the fingertips. Cases of involvement of the nose, ears, nipples, and even the tongue are reported [5, 6]. Despite ethnogeographic variability, this condition is more common in females, with a reported prevalence ranging from 5% to 11%, compared to 3% to 7% in males. The annual incidence rate was estimated in a U.S. study conducted over a 7-year period to be 2.2% in women and 1.5% in men [7, 8].

The clinical presentation of RP is typically characterized by episodic color changes, often described as a "triphasic" sequence: pallor, cyanosis, and rubor (Fig. 3.1). These phases correspond respectively to vasospasm-induced ischemia (white), deoxygenation of static blood following venous outflow obstruction (blue), and reactive hyperaemia upon reperfusion (red) [9]. However, not all patients exhibit the full triphasic pattern; a biphasic response—usually pallor followed by cyanosis—is common and often considered sufficient by most experts for diagnosis [10]. Uniphasic digital changes were also reported [11]. Those color changes are usually well demarcated and clearly localized to the affected digits. As a result of transient tissue ischemia secondary to vasoconstriction of the digital arteries and arterioles, these vascular episodes are often accompanied by sensory symptoms such as numbness, tingling, pain, a cold sensation, and transient functional impairment. RP is usually triggered by exposure to cold or, better yet, by a sudden change from warm to cold; other frequent triggers are emotional stress and some substances described below [2]. It is useful to underline here that the diagnosis of RP is a medical act that is based on the findings of the clinical elements just reported. Diagnostic, instrumental, and laboratory investigations are instead useful for the classification of RP.

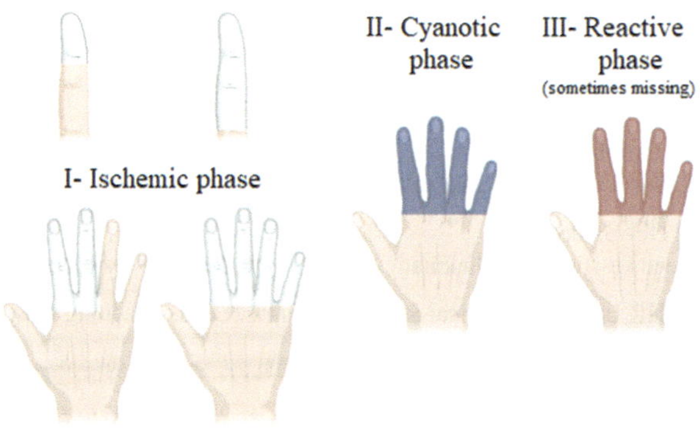

Fig. 3.1 Raynaud's typical different phases

Differential Diagnosis

RP is often confused with other vascular disorders of the extremities, such as acrocyanosis, erythromelalgia, and chilblains (see Table 3.1 for a summary of differential diagnoses). It is important to emphasize that in RP there has to be a phase of pallor, an expression of the transient ischemic event, and that this has to begin from the fingertip, then extending variably to the base of the finger.

Acrocyanosis The condition most frequently considered in the differential diagnosis of RP is acrocyanosis, which can represent a diagnostic challenge for the physician. Acrocyanosis typically presents as a painless, persistent bluish discoloration of the distal extremities, most commonly the hands, but also the feet, nose, ears, lips, and, more rarely, the nipples. The discoloration is usually symmetric and may exhibit various shades of blue or purple, often aggravated by cold exposure. While acrocyanosis closely resembles the cyanotic phase of RP, it is not paroxysmal and lacks the initial pallor phase typical of RP. Instead, the cyanosis tends to be continuous and less sharply demarcated. The condition is frequently associated with local hyperhidrosis. While both RP and acrocyanosis are exacerbated by cold and

Table 3.1 Raynaud's phenomenon differential diagnoses

	Raynaud's phenomenon	Acrocyanosis	Erythromelalgia	Chilblains (Perniosis)
Trigger	Cold, emotional stress	Cold, emotional stress	Heat, exertion, limb dependency	Cold, damp exposure
Onset	Sudden, episodic	Chronic, quite persistent	Paroxysmal, variable duration	Delayed (12–24 h after cold), seasonal
Color changes	Triphasic: pallor → cyanosis → rubor	Persistent blue/ cyanotic discoloration	Red to maroon erythema	Red to violaceous plaques, nodules
Symmetry	Either symmetric or asymmetric	Typically symmetric	Either symmetric or asymmetric	Either symmetric or asymmetric
Pain	Variable; numbness, tingling	Absent or mild discomfort	Prominent burning pain	Burning, itching, tenderness
Relief with warming	Yes	Often	Worsens with heat; relieved by cooling	Limited; lesions persist after rewarming
Lesion morphology	Diffuse color change, no distinct lesions	Diffuse discoloration	Diffuse erythema, no distinct lesions	Discrete plaques, papules, or nodules
Underlying conditions	Primary or secondary	Usually mild vascular dysregulation	Can be secondary to myeloproliferative disorders	Primary (idiopathic) or secondary (SLE)

emotional stress, acrocyanosis differs in its chronicity, symmetry, and the absence of ischemic pallor. The pathophysiology of acrocyanosis is thought to involve impaired venous return and sluggish peripheral circulation, resulting in blood pooling and increased formation of deoxygenated hemoglobin (cyanohemoglobin). Importantly, Raynaud's attacks may occasionally be superimposed on underlying acrocyanosis, further complicating the clinical picture and emphasizing the need for careful diagnostic evaluation [12, 13].

Erythromelalgia It is a rare neurovascular disorder primarily affecting the extremities and is characterized by episodes of pain, erythema, swelling, and increased skin temperature. The color changes observed in erythromelalgia are typically red to maroon, contrasting with the biphasic or triphasic pattern seen in RP. Pain is often the most prominent and disabling symptom; it may initially present as a mild burning or itching sensation and can progress to severe, intolerable burning pain. Attacks may last from minutes to several days and are usually triggered by heat, physical activity, or limb dependency. In contrast, symptoms are often alleviated by limb elevation and cooling, with immersion in ice-cold water providing such consistent relief that it is considered almost pathognomonic. Most cases of erythromelalgia are secondary and associated with underlying hematological disorders, particularly myeloproliferative neoplasms. In these cases, the pathogenesis is thought to involve platelet activation leading to arteriolar dysfunction. A primary form of the disease also exists, often linked to gain-of-function mutations in the SCN9A gene, which encodes the Nav1.7 sodium channel involved in nociceptive signaling [14, 15].

Chilblains Also known as pernio or perniosis, they are localized inflammatory skin lesions that develop in response to exposure to cold and damp (but not freezing) environments. They can be idiopathic or secondary to a number of conditions, such as infections and immune-mediated inflammatory disorders, with systemic lupus erythematosus being the commonest. Clinically, chilblains manifest as erythematous to violaceous macules, papules, or nodules on acral sites, most commonly the fingers, toes, ears, and nose. Symptoms typically begin 12–24 hours after cold exposure and include burning, pruritus, pain, and swelling. Unlike RP, the lesions of chilblains persist even after rewarming and may last for weeks, and lack a pallor phase. Instead, they produce more localized, often edematous lesions with defined morphology. Chilblain lupus presents with more persistent, potentially scarring plaques or nodules and may involve ulceration. Both primary and secondary forms involve cold-induced vascular dysfunction, but chilblain lupus also includes immune complex-mediated microvascular injury [15, 16].

Classification

RP is usually classified into two distinct subtypes: primary Raynaud's phenomenon (PRP) and secondary Raynaud's phenomenon (SRP) . This distinction is crucial in clinical practice, as it differentiates patients with an isolated benign functional vasospastic response to cold or emotional stress from those in whom RP represents the clinical expression of an underlying pathological process, most notably systemic autoimmune connective tissue diseases (CTDs).

According to a meta-analysis of observational studies on more than 33,000 participants, the pooled prevalence of PRP was 4.85% (95% CI 2.08% to 8.71%) in the general population, whereas the pooled annual incidence of PRP was 0.25% (95% CI 0.19% to 0.32%) [17]. PRP typically presents in younger individuals, often between the ages of 15 and 30, and is more common in females. It is characterized by a lack of identifiable underlying disease, a benign non-progressive course, absence of digital ischemic injury, and normal nailfold videocapillaroscopy (NVC). Notably, a family history is often reported in PRP, thus suggesting a possible yet undefined genetic predisposition [18]. Although PRP may significantly affect quality of life, it does not progress to tissue damage or systemic disease.

In contrast, SRP is often associated with underlying diseases or exogenous factors that cause vascular injury, endothelial dysfunction, or autonomic imbalance. Among these, CTDs are the most studied and clinically relevant causes. In particular, RP is among the clinical hallmarks of systemic sclerosis (SSc), and it is one of the red flags needed for the diagnosis of very early forms of the disease (VEDOSS) [19, 20]. In fact, RP is often the sentinel manifestation of SSc, reflecting the underlying systemic vasculopathic process that characterizes SSc, and can progress to irreversible structural changes and express through different manifestations such as digital ulcers or pulmonary arterial hypertension [21]. The 2013 ACR/EULAR classification criteria for SSc integrate RP and microvascular abnormalities as essential features, underscoring the importance of early identification of SRP, even in its subtle presentations [22].

Clinical and instrumental features are essential to distinguish PRP from SRP. Warning signs that raise the suspicion of SRP include onset after the age of 40, severe and frequent attacks, and incomplete resolution of symptoms between episodes. The finding of specific autoantibody positivity as well as typical alterations on NVC are obviously elements that move in the direction of SRP [23, 24]. However, it is important to remember that there may be cases of PRP that present an isolated and non-specific positivity of anti-nuclear antibodies [25]. Furthermore, non-specific capillaroscopic alterations can be found in subjects with both PRP and non-SSc-related SRP [26–28]. Recent studies emphasize that beyond clinical and laboratory markers, the lived experience of RP differs between PRP and SRP in terms of how they feel and function [29]. In a large international survey involving over 1200 individuals with RP, patients with PRP reported more neurosensory symptoms, while SRP patients were typically older, experienced more complex color changes with cyanosis being more prominent, and reported less complete resolution of symptoms between attacks [30]. Finally, it should not be forgotten that some patients may experience an evolution from PRP to SRP over time. In this regard, a prospective study of 307 patients with RP showed an annual incidence of transition to SRP of 1% [31].

However, CTDs represent only one subset of SRP. A wide array of other conditions may disrupt the physiological regulation of digital blood flow and should therefore be considered. These include hematologic and rheumatologic disorders such as cryoglobulinemia, cold agglutinin disease, and antiphospholipid syndrome; vascular occlusive diseases like atherosclerosis, thromboangiitis obliterans, and embolic events; and mechanical or traumatic causes, including carpal tunnel syndrome and hand-arm vibration syndrome. Cold injuries, notably frostbite, can also precipitate vasospastic episodes. Endocrine and metabolic abnormalities, particularly hypothyroidism, may alter vascular reactivity even in the absence of structural vascular damage, while neoplastic or paraneoplastic processes, such as paraproteinemia, can contribute through various mechanisms, including hyperviscosity or immune-mediated injury. Neurogenic compression syndromes, such as thoracic outlet syndrome, may impair sympathetic outflow to the upper extremities, further complicating the clinical picture. Finally, a wide range of pharmacologic agents are known to trigger or exacerbate RP, often by inducing vasoconstriction or endothelial dysfunction. These include non-selective beta-blockers, ergot alkaloids, amphetamines, sympathomimetic drugs, estrogens, and chemotherapeutic agents such as bleomycin and cisplatin. To better capture the spectrum of SRP, a comprehensive overview of its various forms is presented in Table 3.2, while a more detailed description of the different etiologies is provided in the subsequent section on pathogenesis.

Pathogenesis

Although the exact pathophysiological mechanism underlying RP remains unknown, it is generally accepted that episodic vasospastic attacks result from a complex interplay of multiple factors regulating peripheral blood flow. Among the theories thought to contribute to RP, we can find local vascular hyperreactivity, autonomic dysfunction with prevalence of sympathetic activity, and increased adrenergic activity. Moreover, several molecule-driven mechanisms were deeply investigated, such as endothelin-I, serotonin, thromboxane-A_2, nitric oxide (NO), and beta-adrenergic blockade, as well as lots of different exogenous factors were proved to contribute to RP. Vasospasm represents an exaggerated vasoconstrictive response that leads to the closure of the vascular lumen. The equilibrium between the tension of the arterial wall, which promotes vessel closure, and the intravascular distending pressure plays a crucial role in preserving the patency of a blood vessel [2].

Normal Thermoregulation

Cutaneous blood flow plays a fundamental role in thermoregulation by maintaining core body temperature within a narrow physiological range [32]. The regulation of vascular tone in the extremities is a complex process modulated by both endothelium--derived mediators and neurogenic mechanisms involving central and peripheral

Table 3.2 Overview of the different etiologies of secondary RP

Etiological category	Examples
Connective tissue diseases	Systemic sclerosis Undifferentiated connective tissue disease Mixed connective tissue disease Idiopathic inflammatory myopathies Systemic lupus erythematosus Sjögren's syndrome
Other inflammatory autoimmune conditions	Rheumatoid arthritis Vasculitides Sarcoidosis
Hematological and immunological disorders	Cryoglobulinemia Cold agglutinin disease Antiphospholipid syndrome
Vascular occlusive diseases	Atherosclerosis Thromboangiitis obliterans Embolic events
Mechanical and traumatic causes	Carpal tunnel syndrome Hand-arm vibration syndrome Thoracic outlet syndrome
Cold injuries	Frostbite
Endocrine and metabolic disorders	Hypothyroidism
Neoplastic or paraneoplastic syndromes	Paraproteinemic syndromes (monoclonal gammopathies, myeloma, Waldenström macroglobulinemia)
Pharmacological Agents	Non-selective beta-blockers Triptans Ergot alkaloids Nicotine Amphetamines Sympathomimetic drugs Estrogens Chemotherapeutic agents (e.g., bleomycin, cisplatin) CGRP inhibitors

pathways. During cold exposure, vasoconstriction of cutaneous vessels limits convective heat loss, thereby preventing an excessive decline in body temperature. In human skin, blood vessels are innervated by two distinct types of autonomic nerve fibers: noradrenergic fibers, which mediate vasoconstriction, and cholinergic fibers, which promote active vasodilation [33].

Low-Resistance Arteriovenous Anastomoses

In the glabrous skin of the digits, numerous thick-walled, low-resistance arteriovenous anastomoses (AVAs) allow high-volume blood flow to bypass capillary beds by shunting directly from arterioles to venules. AVAs primarily serve to regulate heat dissipation rather than to provide nutritional support to tissues. In cold conditions, the body aims to limit heat loss by vasoconstricting the AVAs, thereby reducing warm blood flow to the skin surface. This mechanism reduces non-nutritional blood flow (i.e., through AVAs) while preserving nutritional capillary perfusion in healthy individuals. Vasoconstriction of these arterioles is mediated by increased sympathetic tone, primarily through norepinephrine acting on α-adrenergic receptors located on vascular smooth muscle. This vasospastic response markedly reduces cutaneous blood flow.

AVAs are functionally connected to cutaneous capillaries, which supply the skin with nutritional blood flow. In healthy individuals, cold exposure leads to reduced flow through AVAs without significantly impairing nutritional perfusion. In contrast, patients with RP exhibit a marked reduction in both AVA and nutritional blood flow during cold exposure, contributing to the ischemic manifestations of the condition [4, 34].

Central Neurogenic Control

In PRP, the underlying defect is typically considered to involve functional dysregulation of thermoregulatory vessels, without evidence of structural vascular abnormalities or injury. In contrast, SRP arises in the context of acquired conditions, often autoimmune, that lead to vascular damage and may result in structural deterioration or loss of cutaneous vessels. There is growing evidence suggesting that the central nervous system contributes to the modulation of these exaggerated vascular responses [35]. Although the precise mechanisms underlying the abnormal vasoconstriction response to cold in RP remain incompletely understood, studies have demonstrated a selective upregulation of α_2-adrenergic receptors on vascular smooth muscle [36]. In particular, cold exposure induces an increased expression of the α_2C-adrenergic receptor subtype, which amplifies vasoconstriction in response to centrally mediated norepinephrine release [37]. This upregulation of adrenergic receptor density helps to explain the pronounced vasoconstrictive response seen in RP, which reduces both AVA shunt flow and the nutritional blood supply to the skin. While these changes are evident in PRP, they are generally more severe in RP secondary to CTDs, where structural vascular impairment further compromises blood flow.

Autonomic Dysfunction

The autonomic nervous system has increasingly gained attention as a central player in the pathogenesis of SSc, and accumulating evidence over time has highlighted its involvement in the development and modulation of RP, both in primary and secondary forms [38].

Digital vascular dysfunction, particularly in the context of SSc-RP, has been a major focus of investigation for decades. Historically, autonomic dysregulation was considered a key driver of digital vasospasm. This hypothesis was often explored using cold challenge tests, lidocaine infusion, or hand postural changes to trigger autonomic responses [39, 40]. Findings have consistently suggested that autonomic imbalance contributes to RP pathophysiology, and in SSc-RP, this imbalance appears to correlate with microvascular damage detected through NVC [41]. However, the precise nature of autonomic dysfunction remains incompletely understood. While early theories emphasized sympathetic overactivity as the predominant mechanism in RP [42], subsequent studies have called this into question, particularly in patients with SSc-RP, where sympathetic dominance may not be the prevailing feature [39, 43]. In contrast, some investigations have observed increased parasympathetic activity in association with advanced microvascular disease, such as the presence of digital ulcers or the transition toward a late capillaroscopic pattern, as well as elevated vascular endothelial growth factor levels [44]. Neurotrophic factors, including brain-derived neurotrophic factor (BDNF), have also been implicated in this context. These molecules, essential for the maintenance and plasticity of the sympathetic nervous system, are upregulated in response to ischemic stress. BDNF in particular has been proposed as a potential mediator in the shift from a primarily vasomotor sympathetic dysfunction toward a broader process involving inflammation and tissue remodeling [45]. This suggests a dynamic and evolving role for the autonomic nervous system in RP pathogenesis, influenced by both neural and vascular factors.

Local Skin Responses to Temperature

Although cold-induced vasoconstriction is primarily mediated by centrally regulated autonomic pathways, local cooling of the skin also activates several peripheral mechanisms that contribute to vascular tone modulation. These mechanisms involve the activation of temperature-sensitive ion channels, particularly the transient receptor potential (TRP) family, and the local release of vasoactive neuropeptides from sensory nerve endings. TRPM8 is a cold-sensitive ion channel expressed in a subset of sensory neurons that innervate the skin. It responds to both cold temperatures and cold-mimetic agents such as menthol. Dysfunction of TRPM8, whether inherited or acquired, may contribute to impaired thermoregulation and could represent a pathogenic mechanism underlying RP. Similarly, activation of the TRPV1 channel leads to the release of the vasodilatory neuropeptide calcitonin gene-related peptide (CGRP) and promotes NO production, both of which play essential roles in local vasodilation [46, 47].

Neurogenic vasoactive peptides, including CGRP and substance P, are localized in perivascular sensory nerve fibers, whereas NO is synthesized by endothelial cells and contributes significantly to the regulation of vascular tone. Evidence supporting the importance of CGRP in vascular reactivity comes from clinical observations:

the severity of RP has been reported to worsen in patients treated with monoclonal antibodies targeting the CGRP ligand (e.g., fremanezumab and galcanezumab) for migraine prophylaxis. Moreover, new-onset RP has been documented in a patient receiving the CGRP receptor antagonist erenumab. These findings reinforce the hypothesis that CGRP signaling plays a protective role in cutaneous vascular homeostasis, and its disruption may precipitate or exacerbate RP [48, 49].

Hereditary Aspects

Approximately 50% of individuals with PRP report a first-degree relative with similar symptoms, particularly cold sensitivity, suggesting a strong familial component. Moreover, higher concordance rates observed in monozygotic compared to dizygotic twins further support a genetic predisposition. Despite these observations, only a limited number of studies have explored candidate genes involved in the regulation of vascular reactivity in RP. Most available investigations are constrained by small cohort sizes or insufficient clinical characterization, which hampers the identification of meaningful genetic associations. Variants in genes encoding thermosensitive ion channels (e.g., *TRPM8*) and vasoactive mediators (e.g., nitric oxide synthase [*NOS*] enzymes) have been proposed as biologically plausible contributors to RP susceptibility [50, 51].

A notable study specifically evaluated the association between RP and single-nucleotide polymorphisms in genes including *TRPA1*, *TRPM8*, *CALCA*, *CALCB*, and *NOS1*. The results revealed a significant association between RP and a polymorphic variant in the *NOS1* gene in the general population. Interestingly, despite the known pathophysiological roles of TRP channels and CGRP-mediated vasodilation in RP, no significant genetic associations were found with variants in these related genes, suggesting that RP predisposition may not predominantly hinge on these pathways, and further large-scale studies are needed to clarify the genetic architecture of the condition [52]. In this context, a large genome-wide association study (GWAS) involving over 5000 RP cases and more than 400,000 controls identified three novel genetic loci associated with RP. Among these, ADRA2A, which encodes the α_2A-adrenergic receptor, and IRX1, a transcription factor involved in vascular regulation, emerged as key candidate genes. Both showed elevated expression in vascular tissues, supporting their functional relevance. These findings provide the first robust genome-wide evidence of a genetic contribution to RP, highlighting a previously underappreciated role of α_2A-adrenergic receptor signaling as a key mechanism mediating heightened catecholamine-induced vasospasm [53].

Immune-Mediated Mechanisms in Secondary RP

When considering the possible various causes of SRP, an intricate network of thermoregulatory and vascular mechanisms emerges that can be disrupted, leading to impaired blood flow to the skin and digits. The hypothesis that autoantibodies may induce RP has been investigated in experimental models: for example, antibodies targeting K10, a cytokeratin autoantigen, were shown to induce RP-like ischemia in mice [54]. Conversely, antibodies against the cold-sensitive ion channel TRPM8 were not found in patients with SSc, suggesting that the abnormal vascular reactivity observed in these patients is not due to direct immune targeting of this channel [55].

Endothelial dysfunction is a hallmark of RP in SSc, where immune-mediated injury leads to endothelial-to-mesenchymal transition, intimal fibrosis, and progressive vascular narrowing. This results in impaired production of vasodilators such as NO and prostaglandins, along with an increased release of vasoconstrictors like endothelin-1. The imbalance contributes to prolonged ischemic episodes, increased oxidative stress, and microvascular damage [56]. Associations between NVC patterns and biomarkers such as sE-selectin, endothelin-1, high-sensitivity C-reactive protein, and lipid metabolism parameters have been documented even in children and adolescents with RP [57]. A pilot study demonstrated elevated oxidative stress in both primary and secondary RP, with increased free thiol concentrations observed after cold challenge. Free thiols may exert a protective role, potentially counteracting oxidative damage in the microvasculature [58]. Furthermore, vascular injury in SSc is accompanied by platelet activation, which promotes the release of vasoconstrictive mediators such as thromboxane and serotonin. This phenomenon is increasingly recognized as a contributor to the pathogenesis of vascular complications in SSc, including RP [59].

Exogenous Factors

In addition to autoimmune diseases, numerous other conditions can mimic or precipitate vasospastic events that resemble RP. These include vasculitides, cryoglobulinemia, cold agglutinin disease, carpal tunnel syndrome, antiphospholipid syndrome, embolic disease, paraproteinaemia, frostbite, and exposure to chemotherapeutic agents such as bleomycin and cisplatin. Various metabolic or endocrine disorders—most notably hypothyroidism—can also impair vascular reactivity without causing structural vessel damage [4, 60].

Pharmacological agents are a frequent and sometimes underrecognized cause of RP. These include non-selective beta-blockers, triptans, estrogens, and vasoconstrictors such as nicotine, ergot derivatives, amphetamines, and sympathomimetic drugs [2, 61–63]. Medications used in attention-deficit/hyperactivity disorder have also been associated with RP-like symptoms [64].

Beyond biochemical and pharmacological factors, mechanical stressors such as vibration exposure represent another important cause. Occupational exposure to hand-arm vibration (e.g., from power tools) can result in vibration-induced RP, also known as vibration white finger or hand-arm vibration syndrome. The development of RP in this context is influenced by both the intensity and duration of vibration exposure, which leads to a combination of direct vascular injury and neural dysfunction [65].

Raynaud's Quantification

The evaluation and quantification of a symptom such as RP represents a challenge that has been addressed in several different ways in the literature. The subjective experience of the patient has always been taken into great consideration; therefore, patient-reported outcomes represent the main tool used in RP evaluation studies. Alongside simpler tools such as the visual analogue scale, specific questionnaires such as the Raynaud condition score have been developed and validated [66]. More recently, the ASRAP questionnaire was developed to assess the severity and impact of RP in SSc patients [67].

At the instrumental level, RP has almost always been assessed indirectly on the basis of peripheral blood perfusion or temperature. Many studies have, in fact, used infrared thermography to evaluate changes in hand temperature both in static conditions and after cold challenge [68, 69]. Similarly, peripheral perfusion has been imaged with different techniques over the years. From laser Doppler flowmetry studies that typically measure blood flow at a single point with high temporal resolution [70] to laser Doppler perfusion imaging that instead measures blood flow over a larger area with lower temporal resolution [71], we have finally arrived at laser speckle contrast analysis (LASCA). On the basis of a greater spatial and temporal resolution and also of an excellent intra- and inter-rater reliability, LASCA has been pointed out as the method of choice for the best non-invasive dynamic assessment of peripheral blood perfusion [72]. Although indirectly, all these attempts to quantify RP have had the merit of highlighting a peculiar characteristic of RP, namely the distal-dorsal difference in thermography [73] and the proximal-distal gradient in perfusion studies [74].

Finally, advances in artificial intelligence (AI) and mobile health technologies have opened new avenues for the objective quantification of RP severity. One such development is the ARTIX (Artificial Intelligence-Based Raynaud's Quantification Index)—a novel, machine learning-driven method designed to detect and quantify RP using standard mobile phone photographs. ARTIX was developed through a multistep process involving image segmentation, color decomposition, and the application of digital filters to smartphone-acquired images of the hands. This tool was validated for its ability to detect changes in fingers in response to a cold challenge in patients with both primary and secondary RP, as well as in healthy controls. Its performance was benchmarked against thermography, obtaining excellent congruence between the two methods. Although preliminary results are promising, the true utility of ARTIX in clinical practice will depend on its performance in real-life, longitudinal studies. These future investigations will determine whether ARTIX can reliably complement patient-centered self-assessment tools as a surrogate measure of RP activity and severity, particularly in remote or resource-limited settings [75].

Treatment

Non-pharmacological Interventions

Despite the presence of numerous pharmacological options, effective management of RP begins with patient education. It is, in fact, crucial that the patient behaves in such a way as to avoid or at least reduce to a minimum the situations that can trigger or worsen the RP. The patient should take all appropriate measures to protect against cold and avoid temperature differences or prolonged vibration exposure. When risky situations cannot be avoided, extremity protection (gloves, etc.) is mandatory [76]. It is then advisable to suspend or at least strongly reduce all substances that have a negative effect on peripheral circulation. It is therefore important to completely stop smoking and taking vasoconstrictive drugs such as cocaine or methamphetamines. Dietary changes involve a cessation or at least a significant reduction in the intake of substances with vasoconstrictive action, such as caffeine, theine, and taurine [5]. If the patient is taking medications that can trigger or worsen RP (e.g., beta-blockers or triptans), therapeutic alternatives should be discussed with the GP and other specialists.

Finally, exercise therapy represents a valuable component of the non-pharmacological management of RP, not least because physical activity promotes increased blood flow to the extremities. In fact, the daily use of a stress ball is generally recommended to promote blood circulation [76]. A trial on 34 SSc patients also demonstrated that exercise therapy (e.g., with an arm bicycle) can improve the microvascular endothelial function [77]. The so-called "frisbee maneuver" has also been suggested as a simple and practical technique to help interrupt or mitigate RP attacks [78].

Pharmacological Treatment

Several pharmacological agents have been reported in the literature as potentially effective in the treatment of RP. In this chapter, we will only discuss the pharmacological classes that have the strongest evidence, as outlined in the EULAR recommendations for the treatment of SSc [79]. These include calcium channel blockers, phosphodiesterase type 5 inhibitors, and prostanoids. Additionally, although supported by relatively low-quality evidence from small clinical trials, fluoxetine and losartan have shown potential benefit and may have a role in selected patients with refractory RP who do not respond adequately to conventional therapies [80, 81]. A non-exhaustive list of other drugs not discussed includes bosentan, prazosin, nitroglycerin, pentoxifylline, botulinum toxin, and surgical procedures such as sympathectomy. Figure 3.2 shows a therapeutic algorithm for RP, keeping in mind that vasoactive therapy must be tailored to the individual patient based on any comorbidities and contraindications. Combination strategies in more severe cases are possible but must be weighted carefully.

Calcium Channel Blockers (CCB) These drugs prevent or reduce calcium channels' opening, resulting in a decrease in intracellular calcium, which then leads to inhibition of vasoconstriction. Dihydropyridine-type calcium antagonists, usually nifedipine modified release or amlodipine, are the most frequently used as first-line therapy. Common side effects are headache, dizziness, nausea, palpitations, and ankle edema. In 2017, a Cochrane systematic review was conducted on 38 randomized controlled trials for a total of 982 RP patients. CCBs proved (low-to-moderate quality of evidence) to reduce the frequency, duration, and severity of RP attacks, being more effective in primary forms [82].

Phosphodiesterase-5 Inhibitors (PDE5i) Inhibition of PDE5 blocks the degradation of cyclic guanosine monophosphate, which results in increased endogenous levels of nitric oxide, which in turn causes vasodilation. Sildenafil and tadalafil are the most investigated and used drugs. Common side effects are vasomotor reactions, myalgias, allergic reactions, chest pain, dyspepsia, and nasal stuffiness. Strong evidence for the efficacy of PDE5-i comes from a 2013 meta-analysis of six clinical trials in patients with SSc [83] and a 2023 Cochrane systematic review (low quality of evidence) on a total of 411 patients with primary and secondary RP from nine clinical trials [84].

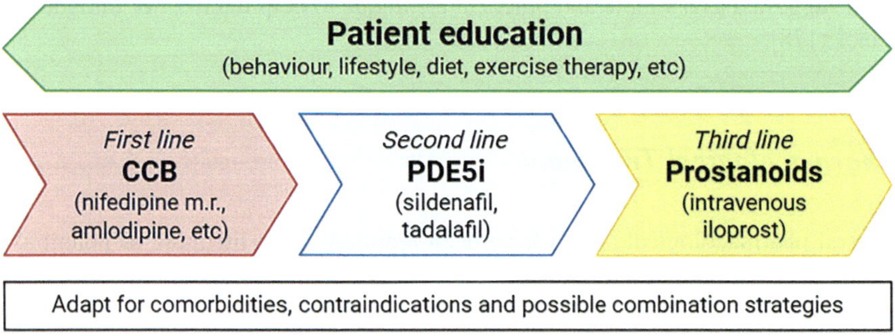

Fig. 3.2 A possible therapeutic algorithm for Raynaud's phenomenon

Prostanoids Stable synthetic analogues of prostacyclin, which stimulate adenylate cyclase, thus bringing an increase in cyclic adenosine monophosphate. Prostanoids act by inducing a powerful vasodilation and a remodeling action through the inhibition of the proliferation of vascular smooth muscle cells. In addition, they also have a mild antiplatelet action, activate fibrinolysis, block the migration of leukocytes, and reduce the release of reactive oxygen species. Intravenous iloprost is the prostanoid of choice in RP, usually as a second-line therapy following failure of oral therapy. Its efficacy in the management of RP is well confirmed by numerous trials, and a dosage between 0.5 and 2 ng/kg/min for 6–8 hours per day for 3–5 consecutive days is generally recommended [85]. However, what is the optimal dosage of intravenous iloprost is still debated. A systematic literature review and expert consensus were not able to identify the most appropriate iloprost dosage because of data heterogeneity in the different studies [86]. Moreover, real-life data collected by the tertiary referral centers are in disagreement, showing a variegated mosaic of iloprost administration [87]. Common side effects are systemic hypotension, headache, dizziness, flushing, gastrointestinal disturbance, jaw pain, and myalgia. Premedication with paracetamol and/or an antiemetic drug may help minimize adverse effects. A potential ischemic cardiac risk has been associated with prostanoids, likely due to a vascular steal effect; therefore, they are contraindicated in patients at high cardiovascular risk [88]. Selexipag, an oral selective IP prostacyclin–receptor agonist, is currently used for the treatment of pulmonary arterial hypertension but may also have a rationale in the treatment of peripheral vascular disease. Although an initial trial evaluating the efficacy of selexipag in RP did not meet its primary endpoint, several observational studies have recently reported favorable outcomes [89–91].

Clinical Cases

In this section, we present the various capillaroscopic patterns that can be observed in patients with RP due to different underlying etiologies.

1. *Primary RP*. Four different scenarios in which secondary causes were carefully excluded: a 30-year-old female (A), a 69-year-old male (B), a 33-year-old male (C), and a 50-year-old female (D). Note that the NVC pattern is essentially within normal limits or shows only mild non-specific abnormalities, such as asymmetric capillary dilations.

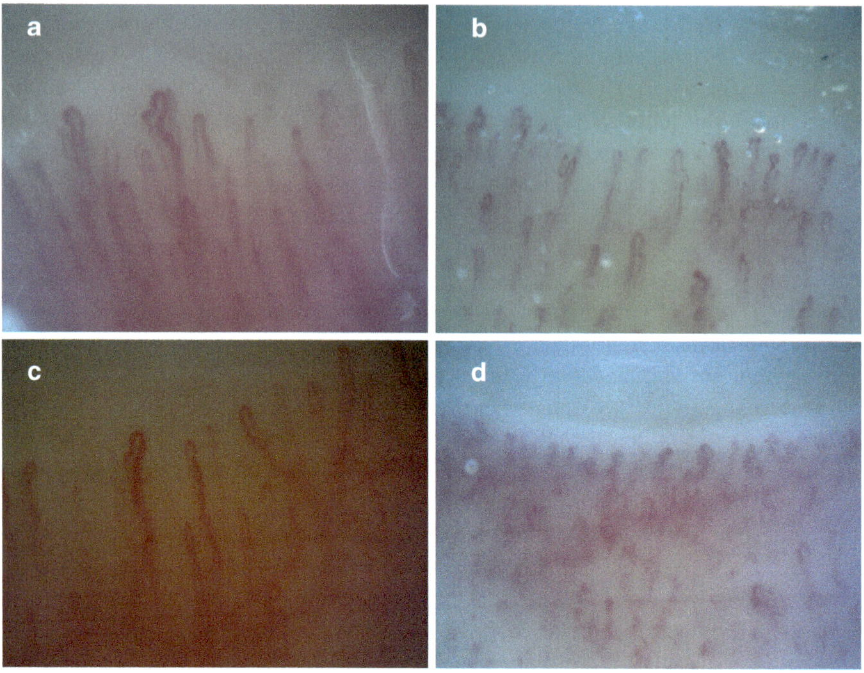

2. *Early scleroderma pattern*. Four different scenarios are shown: two VEDOSS cases (A: 45-year-old female; B: 37-year-old female) and two overt SSc cases (C: 51-year-old male; D: 67-year-old male). Note the absence of appreciable differences in the scleroderma capillaroscopic pattern between VEDOSS and overt SSc.

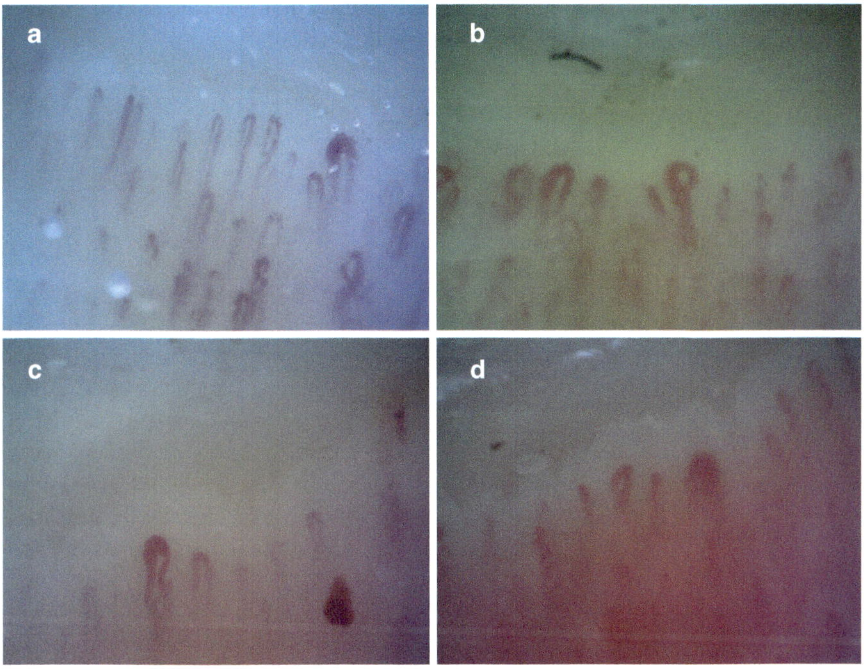

3. *Active and late scleroderma pattern*. Two patients with SSc (A: 70-year-old female—active; B: 73-year-old female—late) exhibiting severe and widespread capillaroscopic abnormalities.

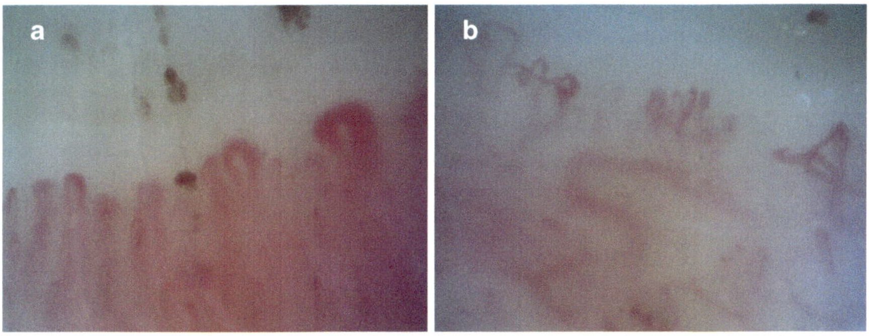

4. *Other connective tissue diseases*. In patients with dermatomyositis, NVC patterns resembling the scleroderma pattern can be observed (A: 63-year-old female), and in some cases, a characteristic bushy neoangiogenesis may be present (B: 79-year-old female). In contrast, patients with polymyositis and RP typically show absent or only mild non-specific abnormalities on NVC (C: 67-year-old male). In mixed connective tissue disease, a wide spectrum of NVC

findings can be observed, ranging from a scleroderma-like pattern (D: 59-year-old male) to normal findings (E: 60-year-old female).

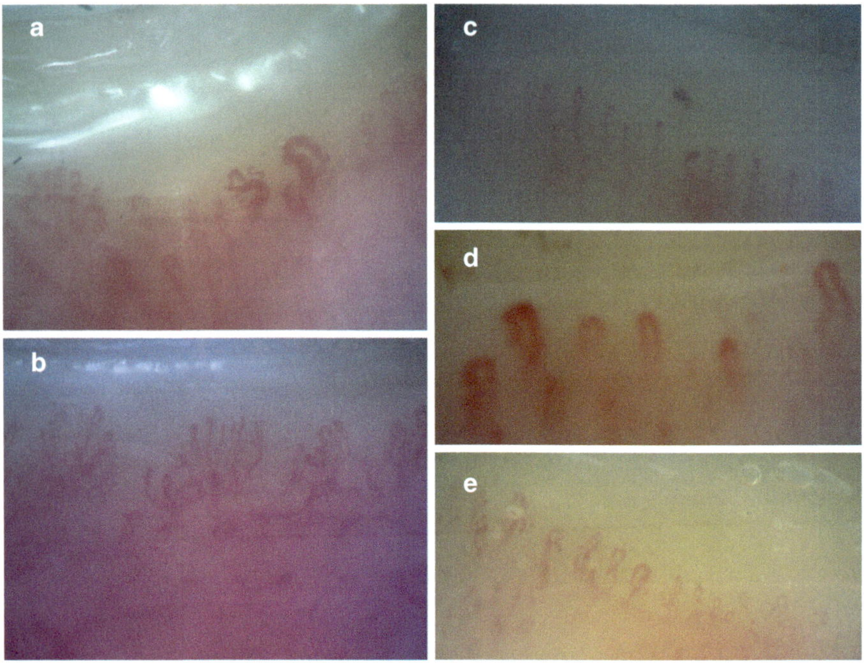

5. *Thromboangiitis obliterans*. A 46-year-old male patient with Buerger's disease, presenting with RP among his symptoms, exhibited a scleroderma-like pattern on NVC. According to the literature, microvascular abnormalities in such cases may improve following smoking cessation and treatment with prostanoids [92].

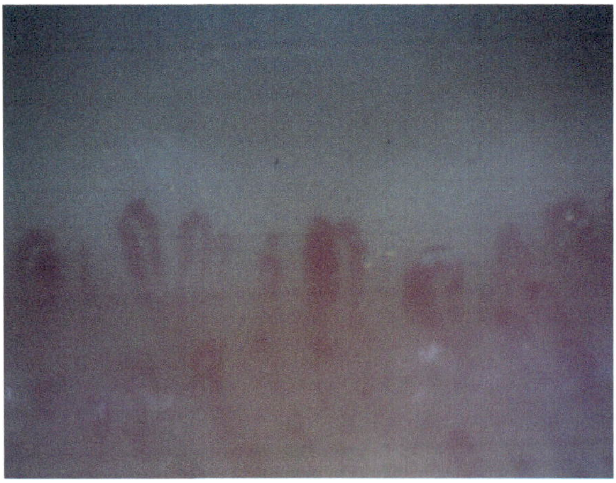

6. *Other forms of secondary RP*. Six different scenarios of secondary RP in which no or only mild non-specific NVC abnormalities are typically observed. A: A 72-year-old female with cryoglobulinemia; B: A 35-year-old male with occupational exposure to vibratory tools; C: 37-year-old female with Hashimoto's hypothyroidism; D: A 68-year-old female with Waldenström's macroglobulinemia; E: A 70-year-old female with RP following the initiation of a beta-blocker; F: 60-year-old female with RP following the initiation of a triptan.

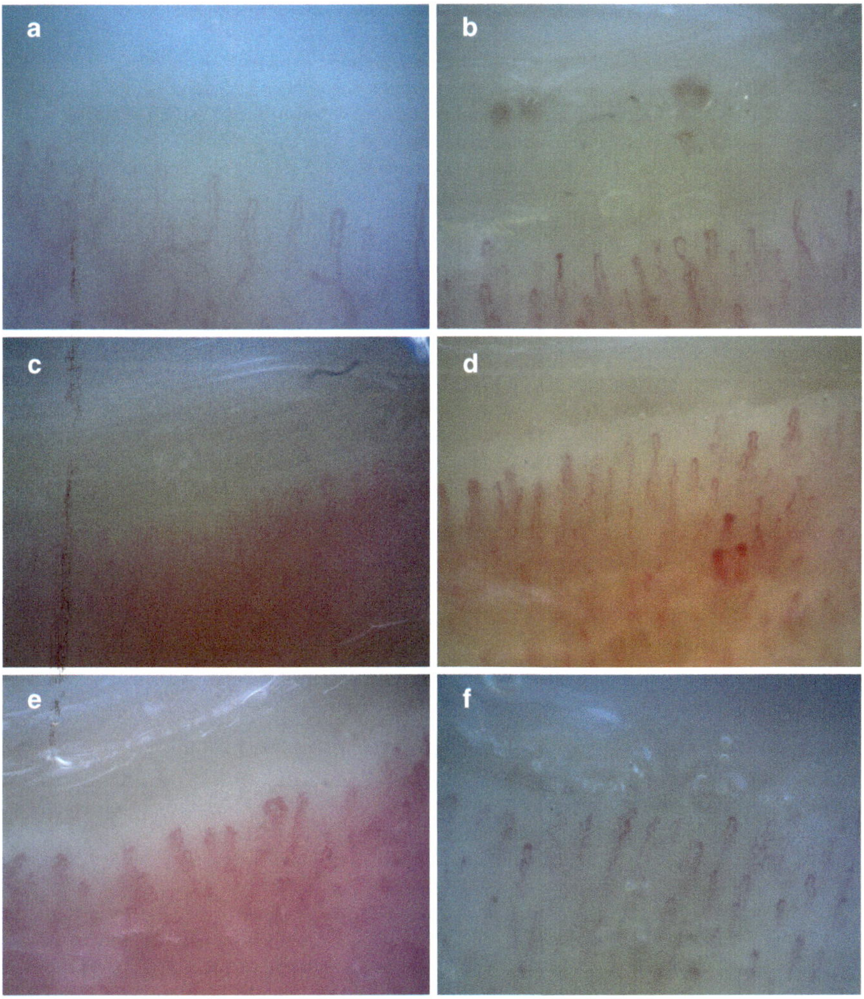

References

1. Tannahill TF. Raynaud's disease, or local asphyxia and symmetrical gangrene of the extremities. Glasgow Med J. 1888;30(6):425–9.
2. Choi E, Henkin S. Raynaud's phenomenon and related vasospastic disorders. Vasc Med. 2021;26(1):56–70.
3. Wigley FM, Flavahan NA. Raynaud's phenomenon. Campion EW, editor. N Engl J Med. 2016;375(6):556–65.
4. Herrick AL, Wigley FM. Raynaud's phenomenon. Best Pract Res Clin Rheumatol. 2020;34(1):101474.
5. Belch J, Carlizza A, Carpentier PH, Constans J, Khan F, Wautrecht JC, et al. ESVM guidelines – the diagnosis and management of Raynaud's phenomenon. Vasa. 2017;46(6):413–23.
6. Katada Y, Tanaka T. Lingual Raynaud's phenomenon. N Engl J Med. 2012;366(7):e12.
7. Maricq HR, Carpentier PH, Weinrich MC, Keil JE, Palesch Y, Biro C, et al. Geographic variation in the prevalence of Raynaud's phenomenon: a 5 region comparison. J Rheumatol. 1997;24(5):879–89.
8. Suter LG, Murabito JM, Felson DT, Fraenkel L. The incidence and natural history of Raynaud's phenomenon in the community. Arthritis Rheum. 2005;52(4):1259–63.
9. Pauling JD, Hughes M, Pope JE. Raynaud's phenomenon—an update on diagnosis, classification and management. Clin Rheumatol. 2019;38(12):3317–30.
10. Maverakis E, Patel F, Kronenberg DG, Chung L, Fiorentino D, Allanore Y, et al. International consensus criteria for the diagnosis of Raynaud's phenomenon. J Autoimmun. 2014;48–49:60–5.
11. Ingegnoli F, Gualtierotti R, Orenti A, Schioppo T, Marfia G, Campanella R, et al. Uniphasic blanching of the fingers, abnormal capillaroscopy in nonsymptomatic digits, and autoantibodies: expanding options to increase the level of suspicion of connective tissue diseases beyond the classification of Raynaud's phenomenon. J Immunol Res. 2015;2015:371960.
12. Wigley FM. The differential diagnosis of Raynaud's phenomenon. Hosp Pract. 1991;26(7):63–84.
13. Kurklinsky AK, Miller VM, Rooke TW. Acrocyanosis: the flying Dutchman. Vasc Med. 2011;16(4):288–301.
14. Mann N, King T, Murphy R. Review of primary and secondary erythromelalgia. Clin Exp Dermatol. 2019;44(5):477–82.
15. Zahn C, Puga C, Malik A, Khanna D. Painful Raynaud's mimics. Best Pract Res Clin Rheumatol. 2024;38(1):101948.
16. Dubey S, Joshi N, Stevenson O, Gordon C, Reynolds JA. Chilblains in immune-mediated inflammatory diseases: a review. Rheumatology. 2022;61(12):4631–42.
17. Garner R, Kumari R, Lanyon P, Doherty M, Zhang W. Prevalence, risk factors and associations of primary Raynaud's phenomenon: systematic review and meta-analysis of observational studies. BMJ Open. 2015;5(3):e006389.
18. Freedman RR, Mayes MD. Familial aggregation of primary Raynaud's disease. Arthritis Rheum. 1996;39(7):1189–91.
19. Denton CP, Khanna D. Systemic sclerosis. Lancet. 2017;390(10103):1685–99.
20. Bellando-Randone S, Del Galdo F, Lepri G, Minier T, Huscher D, Furst DE, et al. Progression of patients with Raynaud's phenomenon to systemic sclerosis: a five-year analysis of the European Scleroderma Trial and Research group multicentre, longitudinal registry study for Very Early Diagnosis of Systemic Sclerosis (VEDOSS). Lancet Rheumatol. 2021;3(12):e834–43.
21. Allanore Y, Distler O, Matucci-Cerinic M, Denton CP. Review: defining a unified vascular phenotype in systemic sclerosis. Arthritis Rheumatol. 2018;70(2):162–70.
22. Van Den Hoogen F, Khanna D, Fransen J, Johnson SR, Baron M, Tyndall A, et al. 2013 classification criteria for systemic sclerosis: an American college of rheumatology/European league against rheumatism collaborative initiative. Ann Rheum Dis. 2013;72(11):1747–55.

23. Pope JE. The diagnosis and treatment of Raynaud's phenomenon: a practical approach. Drugs. 2007;67(4):517–25.
24. Hughes M, Huang S, Pauling JD, Sabbagh M, Khanna D. The clinical relevance of Raynaud's phenomenon symptom characteristics in systemic sclerosis. Clin Rheumatol. 2022;41(10):3049–54.
25. Di Battista M, Morganti R, Da Rio M, De Mattia G, Della Rossa A, Mosca M. Comparison of different forms of Raynaud's phenomenon by LASCA proximal-distal gradient perfusion. Microvasc Res. 2023;148:104509.
26. Cutolo M, Sulli A, Secchi ME, Paolino S, Pizzorni C. Nailfold capillaroscopy is useful for the diagnosis and follow-up of autoimmune rheumatic diseases. A future tool for the analysis of microvascular heart involvement? Rheumatology. 2006;45(Suppl 4):v43–6.
27. Sirufo MM, Magnanimi LM, Ginaldi L, De Martinis M. The shadow zone of capillaroscopy in the classification of the Raynaud's phenomenon. Curr Med Res Opin. 2022;38(4):637–9.
28. Amaral MC, Paula FS, Caetano J, Ames PRJ, Alves JD. Re-evaluation of nailfold capillaroscopy in discriminating primary from secondary Raynaud's phenomenon and in predicting systemic sclerosis: a randomised observational prospective cohort study. Expert Rev Clin Immunol. 2024;20(6):665–72.
29. Murphy SL, Lescoat A, Alore M, Hughes M, Pauling JD, Sabbagh M, et al. How do patients define Raynaud's phenomenon? Differences between primary and secondary disease. Clin Rheumatol. 2021;40(4):1611–6.
30. Di Donato S, Huang S, Pauling JD, Del Galdo F, Sabbagh M, Khanna D, et al. Clinically relevant differences between primary Raynaud's phenomenon and secondary to connective tissue disease. Semin Arthritis Rheum. 2024;68:152521.
31. Hirschl M, Hirschl K, Lenz M, Katzenschlager R, Hutter HP, Kundi M. Transition from primary Raynaud's phenomenon to secondary Raynaud's phenomenon identified by diagnosis of an associated disease: results of ten years of prospective surveillance. Arthritis Rheum. 2006;54(6):1974–81.
32. Charkoudian N. Skin blood flow in adult human thermoregulation: how it works, when it does not, and why. Mayo Clin Proc. 2003;78(5):603–12.
33. Alba BK, Castellani JW, Charkoudian N. Cold-induced cutaneous vasoconstriction in humans: function, dysfunction and the distinctly counterproductive. Exp Physiol. 2019;104(8):1202–14.
34. Coffman JD. Total and nutritional blood flow in the finger. Clin Sci. 1972;42(3):243–50.
35. Gosk-Bierska I, Misterska-Skóra M, Wasilewska M, Bilińska M, Gosk J, Adamiec R, et al. Analysis of peripheral nerve and autonomic nervous system function and the stage of microangiopathy in patients with secondary Raynaud's phenomenon in the course of connective tissue diseases. Adv Clin Exp Med. 2018;27(11):1587–92.
36. Freedman RR, Baer RP, Mayes MD. Blockade of vasospastic attacks by α2-adrenergic but not α1-adrenergic antagonists in idiopathic Raynaud's disease. Circulation. 1995;92(6):1448–51.
37. Bailey SR, Mitra S, Flavahan S, Flavahan NA. Reactive oxygen species from smooth muscle mitochondria initiate cold-induced constriction of cutaneous arteries. Am J Physiol Heart Circ Physiol. 2005;289(1):243–50.
38. Di Battista M, Wasson CW, Alcacer-Pitarch B, Del Galdo F. Autonomic dysfunction in systemic sclerosis: a scoping review. Semin Arthritis Rheum. 2023;63:152268.
39. Freedman RR, Mayes MD, Sabharwal SC. Induction of vasospastic attacks despite digital nerve block in Raynaud's disease and phenomenon. Circulation. 1989;80(4):859–62.
40. Engelhart M, Seibold JR. The effect of local temperature versus sympathetic tone on digital perfusion in Raynaud's phenomenon. Angiology. 1990;41(9):715–23.
41. Masini F, Galiero R, Pafundi PC, Gjeloshi K, Pinotti E, Ferrara R, et al. Autonomic nervous system dysfunction correlates with microvascular damage in systemic sclerosis patients. J Scleroderma Relat Disord. 2021;6(3):256–63.
42. Engelhart M. The effect of sympathetic blockade and cooling in Raynaud's phenomenon. Clin Physiol. 1990;10:131–6.

43. Lau CS, Khan F, Brown R, Belch JJF. Digital blood flow response to body warming, cooling, and rewarming in patients with Raynaud's phenomenon. Angiology. 1995;46(1):1–10.
44. Gigante A, Margiotta D, Navarini L, Liberatori M, Barbano B, Tubani L, et al. Parasympathetic activity increases with digital microvascular damage and vascular endothelial growth factor in systemic sclerosis. Clin Exp Rheumatol. 2018;36(Suppl 113):S24–7.
45. Kasselman LJ, Sideris A, Bruno C, Perez WR, Cai N, Nicoletti JN, et al. BDNF: a missing link between sympathetic dysfunction and inflammatory disease? J Neuroimmunol. 2006;175(1–2):118–27.
46. Mccoy DD, Knowlton WM, Mckemy DD. Scraping through the ice: uncovering the role of TRPM8 in cold transduction. Am J Phys Regul Integr Comp Phys. 2011;300(6):1278–87.
47. Caterina MJ, Schumacher MA, Tominaga M, Rosen TA, Levine JD, Julius D. The capsaicin receptor: a heat-activated ion channel in the pain pathway. Nature. 1997;389(6653):816–24.
48. Breen ID, Brumfiel CM, Patel MH, Butterfield RJ, VanderPluym JH, Griffing L, et al. Evaluation of the safety of calcitonin gene-related peptide antagonists for migraine treatment among adults with Raynaud phenomenon. JAMA Netw Open. 2021;4(4):e217934.
49. Sun W, Li Y, Xia B, Chen J, Liu Y, Pang J, et al. Adverse event reporting of four anti-Calcitonin gene-related peptide monoclonal antibodies for migraine prevention: a real-world study based on the FDA adverse event reporting system. Front Pharmacol. 2024;14:1257282.
50. Cherkas LF, Williams FMK, Carter L, Howell K, Black CM, Spector TD, et al. Heritability of Raynaud's phenomenon and vascular responsiveness to cold: a study of adult female twins. Arthritis Care Res. 2007;57(3):524–8.
51. Hur YM, Chae JH, Chung KW, Kim JJ, Jeong HU, Kim JW, et al. Feeling of cold hands and feet is a highly heritable phenotype. Twin Res Hum Genet. 2012;15(2):166–9.
52. Munir S, Freidin MB, Brain S, Williams FMK. Association of raynaud's phenomenon with a polymorphism in the NOS1 gene. PLoS One. 2018;13(4):e0196279.
53. Hartmann S, Yasmeen S, Jacobs BM, Denaxas S, Pirmohamed M, Gamazon ER, et al. ADRA2A and IRX1 are putative risk genes for Raynaud's phenomenon. Nat Commun. 2023;14(1):6156.
54. Ascherman DP, Zang Y, Fernandez I, Clark ES, Khan WN, Martinez L, et al. An autoimmune basis for Raynaud's phenomenon: murine model and human disease. Arthritis Rheumatol. 2018;70(9):1489–99.
55. Shah AA, Montagne J, Oh SY, Wigley FM, Casciola-Rosen L. Pilot study to determine whether transient receptor potential melastatin type 8 (TRPM8) antibodies are detected in scleroderma. Clin Exp Rheumatol. 2015;33(91):123–6.
56. Vona R, Giovannetti A, Gambardella L, Malorni W, Pietraforte D, Straface E. Oxidative stress in the pathogenesis of systemic scleroderma: an overview. J Cell Mol Med. 2018;22(7):3308–14.
57. Gorski S, Bartnicka M, Citko A, Żelazowska-Rutkowska B, Jablonski K, Gorska A. Microangiopathy in naifold videocapillaroscopy and its relations to se- selectin, endothelin-1, and hscrp as putative endothelium dysfunction markers among adolescents with raynaud's phenomenon. J Clin Med. 2019;8(5):567.
58. Abdulle AE, van Roon AM, Smit AJ, Pasch A, van Meurs M, Bootsma H, et al. Rapid free thiol rebound is a physiological response following cold-induced vasoconstriction in healthy humans, primary Raynaud and systemic sclerosis. Physiol Rep. 2019;7(6):e14017.
59. Ntelis K, Solomou EE, Sakkas L, Liossis SN, Daoussis D. The role of platelets in autoimmunity, vasculopathy, and fibrosis: implications for systemic sclerosis. Semin Arthritis Rheum. 2017;47(3):409–17.
60. Curtiss P, Svigos K, Schwager Z, Lo Sicco K, Franks AG. Part I: Epidemiology, pathophysiology, and clinical considerations of primary and secondary Raynaud's phenomenon. J Am Acad Dermatol. 2024;90(2):223–34.
61. Fraenkel L, Zhang Y, Chaisson CE, Evans SR, Wilson PWF, Felson DT. The association of estrogen replacement therapy and the Raynaud phenomenon in postmenopausal women. Ann Intern Med. 1998;129(3):208–11.
62. Mohokum M, Hartmann P, Schlattmann P. The association of Raynaud syndrome with β-blockers: a meta-analysis. Angiology. 2012;63(7):535–40.

63. Khouri C, Blaise S, Carpentier P, Villier C, Cracowski JL, Roustit M. Drug-induced Raynaud's phenomenon: beyond β-adrenoceptor blockers. Br J Clin Pharmacol. 2016;82(1):6–16.
64. Umair HM, Sandler RD, Alunno A, Matucci-Cerinic M, Hughes M. Association between central nervous system stimulants used to treat attention deficit hyperactivity disorder (ADHD) and Raynaud's phenomenon: a scoping review. Semin Arthritis Rheum. 2021;51(6):1200–4.
65. Stoyneva Z, Lyapina M, Tzvetkov D, Vodenicharov E. Current pathophysiological views on vibration-induced Raynaud's phenomenon. Cardiovasc Res. 2003;57(3):615–24.
66. Merkel PA, Herlyn K, Martin RW, Anderson JJ, Mayes MD, Bell P, et al. Measuring disease activity and functional status in patients with scleroderma and Raynaud's phenomenon. Arthritis Rheum. 2002;46(9):2410–20.
67. Pauling JD, Yu L, Frech TM, Herrick AL, Hummers LK, Shah AA, et al. Construct validity and reliability of the Assessment of Systemic Sclerosis-Associated Raynaud's Phenomenon (ASRAP) questionnaire. Rheumatology. 2024;63(5):1281–90.
68. Pauling JD, Shipley JA, Harris ND, McHugh NJ. Use of infrared thermography as an endpoint in therapeutic trials of Raynaud's phenomenon and systemic sclerosis. Clin Exp Rheumatol. 2012;30(Suppl 71):S103–15.
69. Herrick AL, Murray A. The role of capillaroscopy and thermography in the assessment and management of Raynaud's phenomenon. Autoimmun Rev. 2018;17(5):465–72.
70. Engelhart M, Kristensen JK. Raynaud's phenomenon: blood supply to fingers during indirect cooling, evaluated by laser Doppler flowmetry. Clin Physiol. 1986;6(6):481–8.
71. Rosato E, Borghese F, Pisarri S, Salsano F. Laser Doppler perfusion imaging is useful in the study of Raynaud's phenomenon and improves the capillaroscopic diagnosis. J Rheumatol. 2009;36(10):2257–63.
72. Cutolo M, Vanhaecke A, Ruaro B, Deschepper E, Ickinger C, Melsens K, et al. Is laser speckle contrast analysis (LASCA) the new kid on the block in systemic sclerosis? A systematic literature review and pilot study to evaluate reliability of LASCA to measure peripheral blood perfusion in scleroderma patients. Autoimmun Rev. 2018;17(8):775–80.
73. Anderson ME, Moore TL, Lunt M, Herrick AL. The "distal-dorsal difference": a thermographic parameter by which to differentiate between primary and secondary Raynaud's phenomenon. Rheumatology. 2007;46(3):533–8.
74. Di Battista M, Morganti R, Tani E, Da Rio M, Della Rossa A, Mosca M. Definition and application of proximal-distal gradient finger perfusion in systemic sclerosis by laser speckle contrast analysis. Microvasc Res. 2022;140:104307.
75. Di Battista M, Colak S, Howard A, Donadoni F, Owen-Smith C, Rindone A, et al. Artificial intelligence-based Raynaud's quantification Index (ARTIX): an objective mobile-based tool for patient-centered assessment of Raynaud's phenomenon. Arthritis Res Ther. 2025;27(1):120.
76. Stöcker JK, Schouffoer AA, Spierings J, Schriemer MR, Potjewijd J, De Pundert L, et al. Evidence and consensus-based recommendations for non-pharmacological treatment of fatigue, hand function loss, Raynaud's phenomenon and digital ulcers in patients with systemic sclerosis. Rheumatology. 2022;61(4):1476–86.
77. Mitropoulos A, Gumber A, Crank H, Akil M, Klonizakis M. The effects of upper and lower limb exercise on the microvascular reactivity in limited cutaneous systemic sclerosis patients. Arthritis Res Ther. 2018;20(1):112.
78. Curtiss P, Cobos G, Lo Sicco K, Franks AG. The Frisbee maneuver: a novel method to abort acute attacks of the Raynaud phenomenon. J Am Acad Dermatol. 2018;78(3):e61.
79. Del Galdo F, Lescoat A, Conaghan PG, Bertoldo E, Čolić J, Santiago T, et al. EULAR recommendations for the treatment of systemic sclerosis: 2023 update. Ann Rheum Dis. 2024;84(1):29–40.
80. Coleiro B, Marshall SE, Denton CP, Howell K, Blann A, Welsh KI, et al. Treatment of Raynaud's phenomenon with the selective serotonin reuptake inhibitor fluoxetine. Rheumatology. 2001;40(9):1038–43.

81. Dziadzio M, Denton CP, Smith R, Howell K, Blann A, Bowers E, et al. Losartan therapy for Raynaud's phenomenon and scleroderma: clinical and biochemical findings in a fifteen-week, randomized, parallel-group, controlled trial. Arthritis Rheum. 1999;42(12):2646–55.
82. Rirash F, Tingey PC, Harding SE, Maxwell LJ, Tanjong Ghogomu E, Wells GA, et al. Calcium channel blockers for primary and secondary Raynaud's phenomenon. Cochrane Database Syst Rev. 2017;12(12):CD000467.
83. Roustit M, Blaise S, Allanore Y, Carpentier PH, Caglayan E, Cracowski JL. Phosphodiesterase-5 inhibitors for the treatment of secondary Raynaud's phenomenon: systematic review and meta-analysis of randomised trials. Ann Rheum Dis. 2013;72:1696–9.
84. Maltez N, Maxwell LJ, Rirash F, Tanjong Ghogomu E, Harding SE, Tingey PC, et al. Phosphodiesterase 5 inhibitors (PDE5i) for the treatment of Raynaud's phenomenon. Vol. 11, Cochrane Database of Systematic Reviews. John Wiley and Sons Ltd; 2023. p. CD014089.
85. Pope J, Fenlon D, Thompson A, Shea B, Furst D, Wells GA, et al. Iloprost and cisaprost for Raynaud's phenomenon in progressive systemic sclerosis. Cochrane Database Syst Rev. 1998;(2):CD000953.
86. Ingegnoli F, Schioppo T, Allanore Y, Caporali R, Colaci M, Distler O, et al. Practical suggestions on intravenous iloprost in Raynaud's phenomenon and digital ulcer secondary to systemic sclerosis: systematic literature review and expert consensus. Semin Arthritis Rheum. 2019;48(4):686–93.
87. Negrini S, Magnani O, Matucci-Cerinic M, Carignola R, Data V, Montabone E, et al. Iloprost use and medical management of systemic sclerosis-related vasculopathy in Italian tertiary referral centers: results from the PROSIT study. Clin Exp Med. 2019;19(3):357–66.
88. Bellando-Randone S, Bruni C, Lepri G, Fiori G, Bartoli F, Conforti ML, et al. The safety of iloprost in systemic sclerosis in a real-life experience. Clin Rheumatol. 2018;37(5):1249–55.
89. Denton CP, Hachulla É, Riemekasten G, Schwarting A, Frenoux JM, Frey A, et al. Efficacy and safety of selexipag in adults with Raynaud's phenomenon secondary to systemic sclerosis: a randomized, placebo-controlled, phase II study. Arthritis Rheumatol. 2017;69(12):2370–9.
90. Di Battista M, Della Rossa A, Da Rio M, De Mattia G, Morganti R, Mosca M. Preliminary clinical and laser speckle contrast analysis data on selexipag efficacy for the treatment of digital vasculopathy in systemic sclerosis. J Rheumatol. 2023;50(8):1029–31.
91. Di Battista M, Della Rossa A, Mosca M. Long-term data on efficacy and safety of selexipag for digital systemic sclerosis vasculopathy. J Rheumatol. 2024;51(9):899–903.
92. Guidelli GM, Bardelli M, Fioravanti A, Selvi E. Nailfold capillaroscopy in Buerger's disease: a useful tool? Eur J Rheumatol. 2014;49(88):81–3.

Chapter 4
Nailfold Videocapillaroscopy in Systemic Sclerosis

Luisa Arcarese, Giulia Lanaia, Marco Minerba, Chiara Salvolini, Pietro Bearzi, and Roberto Giacomelli

Introduction

SSc is a rare connective tissue disease characterized by immune activation, widespread vasculopathy, and progressive fibrosis of the skin and internal organs [1]. One of the earliest and most specific features of SSc is microvascular dysfunction, which precedes fibrotic damage and contributes to irreversible end-organ complications. The pathogenesis of microvascular damage in SSc involves endothelial injury, altered angiogenesis, and defective vascular repair mechanisms, ultimately leading to capillary rarefaction and intimal proliferation [2, 3].

L. Arcarese
Clinical Immunology and Rheumatology Unit, Fondazione Policlinico Campus Bio-Medico di Roma, Rome, Italy
e-mail: l.arcarese@policlinicocampus.it

G. Lanaia · C. Salvolini (✉)
Clinical Immunology and Rheumatology Unit, Campus Bio-Medico University of Rome, Rome, Italy
e-mail: giulia.lanaia@unicampus.it; chiara.salvolini@unicampus.it

M. Minerba
Clinical Immunology and Rheumatology Unit, Campus Bio-Medico University of Rome, Rome, Italy

Leeds Institute of Rheumatic and Musculoskeletal Medicine, University of Leeds, Leeds, UK
e-mail: marco.minerba@unicampus.it

P. Bearzi
Clinical Immunology and Rheumatology Unit, Campus Bio-Medico University of Rome, Rome, Italy

Center of Experimental Rheumatology, Department of Rheumatology, University Hospital Zurich, University of Zurich, Zürich, Switzerland
e-mail: pietro.bearzi@usz.ch

Y. El Miedany, R. A. Elziaty (eds.), *Capillaroscopy*, Contemporary Rheumatology,
https://doi.org/10.1007/978-3-032-22966-3_4

SSc vascular manifestations include Raynaud's phenomenon (RP), DUs, and PAH, while fibrotic complications typically affect the skin and lungs, manifesting as skin thickening and ILD [1]. Among diagnostic tools, NVC has emerged as a cornerstone in the early identification of microvascular damage, particularly in patients presenting with RP [3]. NVC is part of the ACR/EULAR 2013 classification criteria for SSc and also plays a pivotal role in the diagnosis of VEDOSS [4]. NVC allows the identification of characteristic capillary abnormalities, such as enlarged capillaries, microhemorrhages, capillary dropout, and neoangiogenesis, whose combination defines the "scleroderma pattern" [2]. This pattern is subdivided into early, active, and late phases, which reflect different degrees of vascular damage and are associated with disease duration, cutaneous subset, and severity of internal organ involvement [5]. Notably, NVC abnormalities in SSc are not merely diagnostic but may also have a prognostic value. Progression from early to active/late patterns has been linked to the future development of ILD, PAH, and DUs [6–8]. Specifically, capillary density has been suggested as a predictor of organ involvement in several observational studies. A reduced capillary density has been independently associated with incident ILD and PAH [9, 10].

The presence of avascular areas, megacapillaries, and microhemorrhages further refines risk stratification. In fact, avascular areas have been independently associated with mortality in SSc [11], whereas the presence of microhemorrhages and megacapillaries has been consistently associated with higher disease activity [11, 12]. Several scoring systems, including the capillaroscopic skin ulcer risk index (CSURI) and NEMO scores, have been proposed to quantify these features and predict disease complications such as DUs [13, 14].

Despite these data, a complete validation of capillaroscopic patterns as clinical biomarkers, suitable for use in both clinical trials and routine practice, is still lacking, highlighting the need for specifically designed studies to achieve definitive validation. In this clinical review, we present four different cases of SSc with longitudinal NVC follow-up, highlighting the correlation between evolving capillaroscopic patterns, internal organ involvement, and disease activity over time. These cases underline the diagnostic, prognostic, and therapeutic relevance of NVC in the real-world management of patients with SSc and strongly support the need for full scientific validation of this tool.

R. Giacomelli
Clinical Immunology and Rheumatology Unit, Fondazione Policlinico Campus Bio-Medico di Roma, Rome, Italy

Clinical Immunology and Rheumatology Unit, Campus Bio-Medico University of Rome, Rome, Italy
e-mail: roberto.giacomelli@policlinicocampus.it

Case 1: SSc Without Organ Involvement

Patient History

A 37-year-old woman was referred to our clinic in 2022 after a 2-year history of RP, with daily episodes during the cold season. The RP's attacks were also triggered by stress. The patient started to avoid cold exposure by wearing warm gloves and using hand warmers.

At the first visit, the patient reported symptoms consistent with gastroesophageal reflux disease, such as heartburn and postprandial belching. She denied a history of acral DUs, smoking, spontaneous miscarriages, joint pain or arthritis, alopecia, photosensitivity, xerostomia, xerophthalmia, or epilepsy. The examination revealed puffy fingers (PFs), consistent with early edematous changes in SSc. The modified Rodnan Skin Score (mRSS) was 5 with involvement limited to acral regions (fingers, hands, and face). Pulmonary auscultation demonstrated normal vesicular breath sounds, with no crackles or wheezes. The examination was compatible with high suspicion for SSc.

The patient showed laboratory tests previously ordered by her general practitioner. The findings included positive antinuclear antibodies (ANA) 1:320 with a homogeneous pattern without positivity for Systemic Sclerosis (SSc) specific autoantibodies, reduced complement (C) levels, and mildly elevated markers of inflammation, with a C-reactive protein (CRP) of 0.7/0.5 mg/dl and an eritrosedimentation rate (ESR) of 47/35 mm/h.

To confirm the diagnosis and assess possible organ involvement, the following tests were required: NVC, pulmonary function tests (PFT) with diffusing capacity for carbon monoxide (DLCO), high-resolution CT scan (HRCT), echocardiography, upper gastrointestinal endoscopy (esophagogastroduodenoscopy), and esophageal manometry. The patient was also required to repeat autoimmune serology, including a search for specific SSc-autoantibodies [anti-centromere (ACA), anti-Topo-I (ATA), anti-RNA pol III].

Capillaroscopic Findings

NVCs were performed by using an optical probe videocapillaroscopy equipped with a 200× contact lens and connected to image analysis software (VideoCap). The patient was inside the building for 30 min before the test, and the room temperature was 21 °C. The nailfolds of eight fingers (excluding the thumbs) were examined after a drop of immersion oil had been placed on the nailfold bed to improve the image resolution (Fig. 4.1).

The first NVC showed normal capillary density with variable length. Morphologic analysis of the capillaries revealed multiple ectasias and megacapillaries. Capillary flow was slow. Microhemorrhages were also present in two fingers. The

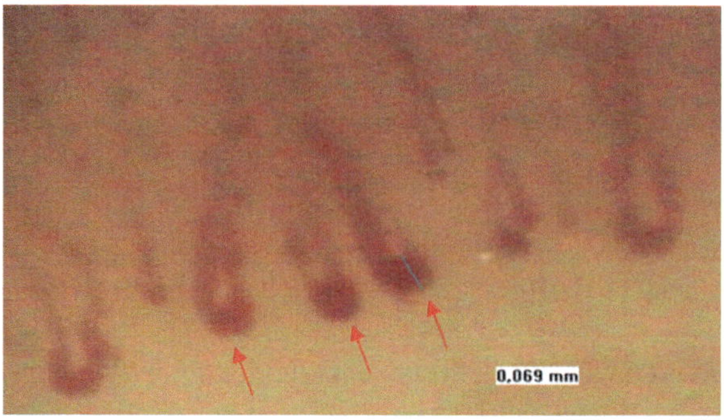

Fig. 4.1 Capillaries with preserved density, some abnormal shapes, diffused ectasias with some megacapillaries (arrows). No microhemorrhages are visible

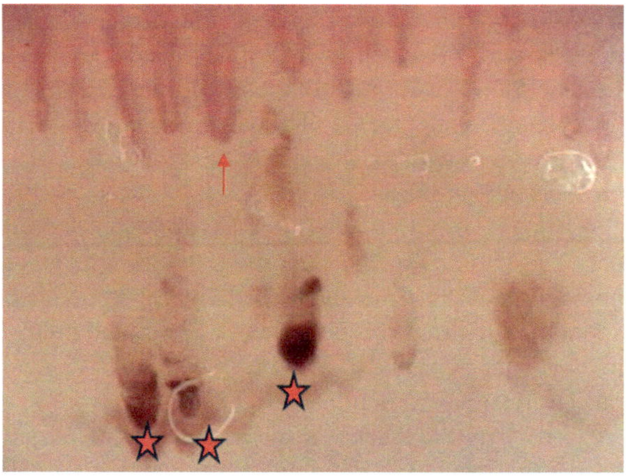

Fig. 4.2 Capillaries with preserved density, some dilations (arrow) and diffused microhemorrhages, visible as red or brown spots of hemosiderin deposits (star symbol), indicating blood leakage from disrupted capillaries

combination of few enlarged/giant capillaries, few capillary microhemorrhages, a relatively well-preserved capillary distribution, and no evident loss of capillaries was compatible with the early scleroderma pattern (Fig. 4.2).

The patient repeated the NVC 1 year later. In this case, NVC revealed a markedly altered capillary architecture, with reduced capillary density and high variability in capillary length. Morphological assessment demonstrated the presence of multiple abnormalities, including diffused ectasias, capillary morphological irregularities ("bizarre" loops), neoangiogenesis, and multiple megacapillaries involving all fingers bilaterally. The capillary flow was visible but notably sluggish and granular. The background was edematous in all examined digits, with the exception of the fifth fingers bilaterally. Additionally, multiple microhemorrhages were observed. Avascular areas were also identified. Considering the frequent giant capillaries and microhemorrhages with moderate loss of capillaries and altered capillary architecture, the capillaroscopic pattern was consistent with an active scleroderma pattern, indicative of ongoing microvascular damage and remodeling (Figs. 4.3 and 4.4).

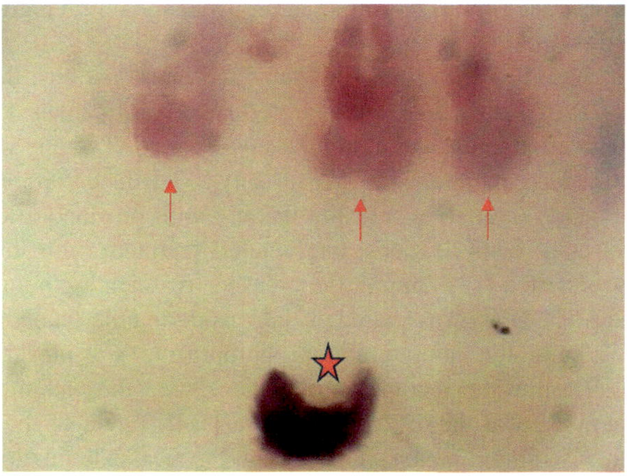

Fig. 4.3 Reduced capillary density, giant capillaries (red arrows), and detail of microhemorrhage (star symbol)

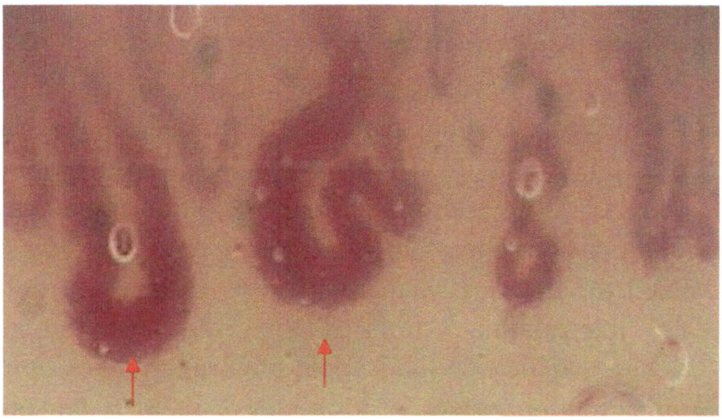

Fig. 4.4 Detail of a field in which multiple giant capillaries (red arrows) with reduced capillary density are evident

Diagnosis and Management

At the follow-up visit, a progression of skin fibrosis with bilateral involvement of the forearm was noticed: the mRSS increased from 5 to 9. The serological tests showed positivity for ATA autoantibodies, a specific SSc-related autoantibody pattern associated with diffuse skin involvement, pulmonary fibrosis, as well as poor prognosis and increased mortality [1].

PFTs revealed a forced vital capacity of 70% with a normal FEV1/FVC ratio and a mild diffusion deficit with DLCO 70% and DLCO/VA 65%, suggestive of initial pulmonary involvement later confirmed at the HRCT, showing a subtle thickening of the pulmonary interstitium involving the subpleural parenchyma bilaterally, more evident in the dependent basal regions. The gastroscopy was normal, while esophageal high-resolution manometry (HRM) revealed no post-swallow peristalsis with solids and liquids (no contractility according to the Chicago version 4) [15]. The esophagus is the most frequently involved internal organ in SSc, with a prevalence of up to 90% [16]. The absence of contractility in HRM is associated with greater severity of skin involvement and poorer lung function [17]. Echocardiography showed normal sPAP, minimal tricuspid and mitral regurgitation, and no pericardial effusion.

Based on the clinical findings and investigations, the patient fulfilled the 2013 ACR/EULAR classification criteria and was diagnosed with limited cutaneous SSc with esophageal and mild lung involvement. Therapy with nifedipine was initiated to reduce the frequency and severity of RP. Due to poor RP control, it was decided to start a course of infusion therapy with prostanoid as a second line. To prevent vascular complications, antiplatelet treatment with low-dose acetylsalicylic acid was started [18]. Immunosuppressive treatment with micofenolate mofetil at a dosage of 2 g/day was started [19]. Considering the esophageal involvement, treatment with a proton pump inhibitor (pantoprazole) was prescribed [20].

Despite the therapy, during the winter, the patient reported worsening of RP, numbness of the distal phalanx of the III finger of the right hand associated with intense fingertip pain and swelling. Physical examination showed the occurrence of a DU, so it was decided to add oral therapy with bosentan, an endothelin receptor antagonist [21]. The patient responded positively to the therapy with progressive healing of the ulcer.

NVC is a noninvasive and safe tool that allows the evaluation of the morphology of the microcirculation, and it is incorporated in the 2013 ACR/EULAR classification criteria for SSc [3, 4]. Structural microvascular abnormalities are one of the key features of SSc. Based on capillaroscopic characteristics (capillary density, capillary dimension, abnormal capillary morphology, and presence/absence of hemorrhages), the assessor can qualitatively deduce whether an image has changes specific to the "scleroderma pattern" as they occur in scleroderma spectrum diseases [3].

Characteristic capillaroscopic abnormalities or combinations of abnormalities specific to the "scleroderma pattern" include the presence of giant capillaries ("giants," i.e., capillaries with an apical diameter ≥50 μm), lowered capillary density (<7 capillaries/mm), or the combination of abnormal shapes with an extremely lowered number of capillaries [22].

Considering scleroderma patterns, the main feature distinguishing early and active is capillary density: the early pattern never presents with lowered density, while active and late patterns always present with lowered density. In addition, in the active pattern, the loss of capillaries is combined with giant capillaries.

Images can also be assessed quantitatively or semi-quantitatively, evaluating capillary characteristics (capillary density, capillary dimension, capillary morphology, and presence/absence of hemorrhages) per unit of quantity (e.g., per linear mm).

Besides the established role of NVC in the diagnosis of SSc, several studies have shown that abnormalities noted on the exam can also be of great value as a predictor of disease [7]. In an Italian-Belgian cohort study, qualitative assessment of NVC, performed at a baseline consultation, was able to predict which patients with SSc may develop novel future severe organ involvement, with the maximum OR (26.69/6.66) for the late pattern versus the normal pattern at multiple logistic regression analysis [7].

In the clinical case described, NVC revealed a progression of microvascular damage, reflected by the clinical manifestations of the disease. Specifically, the progression from early to active patterns anticipated the appearance of a DU.

DU is a frequent complication of SSc, which represents a visible manifestation of peripheral vasculopathy. Considering the early phase of the disease, with the onset of RP approximately 2 years prior, the peripheral vasculopathic manifestations serve as an important warning sign of potential disease progression. Although pulmonary involvement is currently asymptomatic, its early detection confirms the need for vigilant monitoring. Given the risk of progression to severe organ complications, a close and structured follow-up is vital to enable timely therapeutic interventions.

DUs usually occur early in the course of the disease and cause pain and functional impairment, with a negative impact on the patient's quality of life [23]. DUs can be complicated by infections, gangrene, and osteomyelitis, and in severe cases, amputation may be necessary [24]. NVC patterns have been associated with future severe peripheral vascular or lung involvement at 18–24 months, with odds ratios rising steadily through the patterns (OR 2.52 for the early, 6.37 for the active, and 16.07 for the late NVC scleroderma pattern versus the normal pattern in a multiple logistic regression analysis) [25]. In a multicenter, prospective, observational cohort study (videoCAPillaroscopy (CAP) study), the mean number of capillaries per millimeter in the middle finger of the dominant hand was a strong risk factor for new DUs at multivariable logistic regression analysis, together with DUs or critical digital ischemia at enrollment [26].

Some authors proposed a quantitative score, the "capillaroscopic skin ulcer risk index" (CSURI), in which the number of capillaries (N), megacapillary (M), and maximum diameter of megacapillary (D) are combined in the algorithm 'D × M/N2 to obtain a risk score for DUs. A multicenter validation study demonstrated high sensitivity (92.98%), specificity (81.4%), and predictive value of CSURI on the possible development of scleroderma DUs within 3 months from NVC, with an area under the curve of 0.884 (95% CI 0.835 to 0.922) [13].

This case underscores the predictive value of NVC in SSc, highlighting its role not only in identifying early microvascular damage but also in stratifying the risk of future internal organ involvement and disease progression.

When integrated into routine clinical assessment, NVC findings can guide the intensity and frequency of follow-up strategies, ultimately enabling earlier therapeutic intervention and potentially reducing the burden of irreversible organ complications.

Case 2: SSc with PAH

Patient History

Patient: A 72-year-old with repetitive daily RP and PFs in the last 5 years, associated with skin and oral telangiectasias in the last 2 years.

Laboratory investigations revealed ANA positivity (1:640) with a centromeric pattern. The other SSc-specific autoantibodies, and any kind of autoantibodies, were negative. Based on the clinical findings and investigations, the patient fulfilled the 2013 ACR/EULAR classification criteria for SSc and underwent comprehensive screening for organ involvement, including pulmonary function tests (PFTs), HRCT of the chest, esophageal barium swallow, and transthoracic echocardiography.

PFTs showed a mild reduction (70%) of diffusing capacity for DLCO, which was not fully corrected for alveolar volume (VA; DLCO/VA 78%), with preserved lung volumes (FVC 90%). Transthoracic echocardiography revealed normal left ventricular dimensions and wall thickness with preserved global systolic function and no regional wall motion abnormalities. A grade I diastolic dysfunction with an inverted E/A ratio was observed. Estimated systolic pulmonary artery pressure (sPAP) was 21 mmHg. The right chambers were normal in size and function. Chest HRCT did not show ground-glass opacities or other specific abnormalities, and the esophageal barium swallow was negative. Nifedipine 20 mg QD was started to control RP, and cardioaspirin 100 mg QD was started for primary prevention of digital ulcers.

Two years later, at the annual scleroderma assessment, the patient complained about progressively increasing dyspnea, affecting her activities of daily living (NYHA functional class II). At the same time, minimal skin fibrosis at the level of the fingers and hand dorsum was appreciable (mRSS = 4). This clinical worsening was associated with a marked increase in sPAP (33 vs 21 mmHg). A type 2 diastolic dysfunction and a slight increase in the right atrium size (20 cm^2) were also observed. Furthermore, new PFTs showed a marked DLCO decrease (45%), only moderately corrected for VA (55%), and an FVC of 80%. A blood test showed an increase in NT-proBNP to 500 pg/mL and slightly elevated urate levels (6.5 mg/dL).

Capillaroscopic Findings

NVC was performed by using an optical probe videocapillaroscopy equipped with a 200× contact lens and connected to image analysis software (VideoCap). The patient was inside the building for 30 min before the test, and the room temperature was 21°. The nailfolds of eight fingers (excluding the thumbs) were examined after a drop of immersion oil had been placed on the nailfold bed to improve the image resolution.

Baseline NVC (Fig. 4.5) showed megacapillaries (apical diameter >50 μm), reduced capillary density (5 capillary loops/mm), and the presence of microhemorrhages, as shown in Fig. 4.1. These findings were compatible with an active scleroderma pattern.

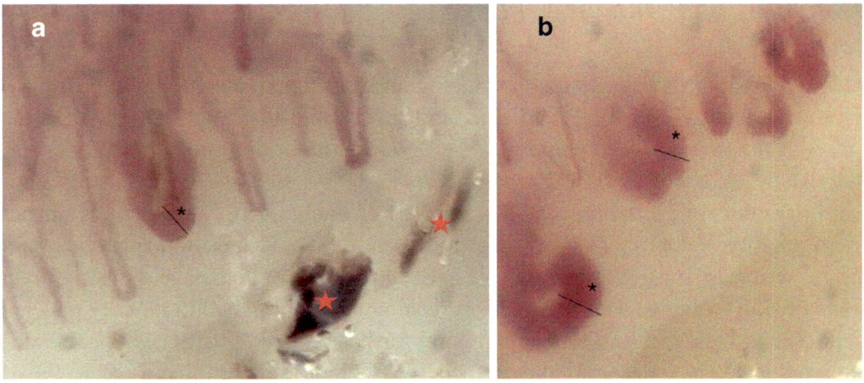

Fig. 4.5 Baseline capillaroscopy. Decreased capillary density (<7 capillary loops per mm) (**a**, **b**) with the presence of megacapillaries (*) and microhemorrhages (red stars)

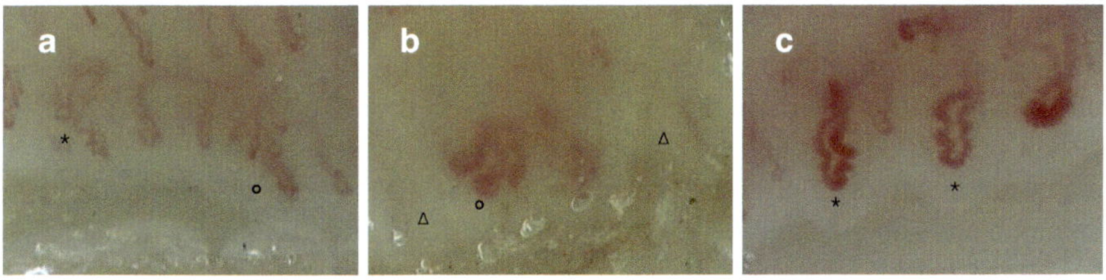

Fig. 4.6 Follow-up nailfold capillaroscopy showing decreased capillary density (**a**–**c**) with different avascular areas (Δ) (**b**). Bushy capillaries (°) (**a**, **b**) and neoangiogenesis (*) (**a**, **c**). This is compatible with a scleroderma late pattern

The follow-up NVC (Fig. 4.6) showed a further decrease in capillary density (three capillary loops), accompanied by the diffuse alteration of capillary loops and the presence of "bushy" neoangiogenesis (Fig. 4.6b, c). No megacapillaries nor microhemorrhages were present. These findings were compatible with a scleroderma late pattern.

Diagnosis and Management

Given the patient's risk factors—including anticentromere autoantibody positivity, elevated serum NT-proBNP and uric acid levels, and the time elapsed since the onset of the first non-RP symptom—the DETECT algorithm was applied to assess the risk of PAH. The DETECT score incorporates several clinical, functional, echocardiographic, and laboratory parameters, namely FVC, DLCO, Tricuspid Regurgitation Velocity (TRV), right atrium area, right axis deviation at EKG, serum urate, serum NT-proBNP, presence of anticentromere antibodies, and history/presence of skin telangiectases [27]. This screening tool is designed to identify patients with SSc at high risk for PAH who require further evaluation with right heart catheterization (RHC), the gold standard for PAH diagnosis. Following the result of DETECT screening (Step 1 = 322; Step 2 = 39 → RHC recommended), the patient underwent a right heart catheterization, showing a precapillary PAH with a mean pulmonary artery pressure (mPAP) of 30 mmHg, pulmonary artery wedge pressure (PAWP) of 15 mmHg, and pulmonary vascular resistance (PVR) of 4.5 Wood Units (WU), consistent with a precapillary pattern. Coronary angiography showed no significant epicardial coronary artery disease.

Pulmonary Hypertension (PH) (Table 4.1) includes a group of conditions characterized by elevated pulmonary arterial pressure. PH is one of the most severe vascular manifestations in SSc, especially during the late stages, and, according to the World Health Organization (WHO), it is classified into five groups: pulmonary arterial hypertension (PAH, Group 1), PH due to left heart disease (PH-LHD, Group 2), PH associated with lung diseases and/or hypoxia (PH-lung, Group 3), PH caused by pulmonary artery obstructions, including chronic thromboembolic PH (CTEPH, Group 4), and PH with unclear or multifactorial mechanisms (Group 5). SSc-PH is estimated to affect 15–18% of patients, with SSc-PAH (group 1) being the most common and showing the highest mortality. SSc-PAH is a precapillary form of PH, defined by mPAP >20 mmHg, PAWP ≤15 mmHg, and PVR ≥2 WU.

Early screening for SSc-PAH is essential, as it represents a major determinant of SSc-related mortality, alongside SSc-ILD [28]. Patients with SSc should undergo screening with yearly transthoracic echocardiography (TTE) and lung function tests [29]. These two assessments are integrated in the DETECT algorithm, which should be used to select high-risk PAH patients requiring invasive RHC [27]. The DETECT algorithm had been developed before the latest 2022 ESC/ERS Guidelines for the Diagnosis and Treatment of PH, posing RHC parameter value cutoffs for PAH at mPAP >20 mmHg and a PVR cut-off ≥2 WU. These new guidelines have decreased cutoffs (mPAP >20 mmHg vs ≥25 mmHg and PVR ≥2 WU) to include patients with mild PAH (mPAP 21–24 mmHg and PVR 2–3 WU), which indeed has been shown to have a worse prognosis compared to patients with normal mPAP (< 21 mmHg) independently of comorbid heart and lung disease [29–31]. Although the DETECT has high negative predictive value for SSc-PAH diagnosis and maintains similar performance with the updated 2022 PAH definition, its positive predictive value has been reported to be 47–53%. This suggests the need to explore methods for a better

Table 4.1 2022 WHO classification of pulmonary hypertension

WHO group	Mechanism	Clinical definition	Hemodynamic definition	Examples	In systemic sclerosis
1	Vascular remodeling of pulmonary arteries	Precapillary	mPAP >20 mmHg; PAWP ≤15 mmHg; PVR > 2 WU	Idiopathic, medications, HIV, connective tissue disorders	Very common
2	Left heart disease causing back-up of blood flow	Postcapillary	mPAP >20 mmHg; PAWP >15 mmHg	Left heart failure, aortic valve disease, mitral valve disease	Rare
		Isolated postcapillary	mPAP >20 mmHg; PAWP >15 mmHg; PVR ≤ 2 WU	Left heart failure, valvular diseases	
		Combined pre- and postcapillary	mPAP >20 mmHg; PAWP >15 mmHg; PVR > 2 WU	Left heart failure with pulmonary vascular remodeling	
3	Chronic lung disease causing hypoxemia	Precapillary	mPAP >20 mmHg; PAWP ≤15 mmHg; PVR > 2 WU	COPD, ILD, sleep apnea	Common

(continued)

Table 4.1 (continued)

WHO group	Mechanism	Clinical definition	Hemodynamic definition	Examples	In systemic sclerosis
4	Chronic thromboembolic pulmonary hypertension (CTEPH)	Precapillary	mPAP >20 mmHg; PAWP ≤15 mmHg; PVR > 2 WU	Pulmonary embolism	Rare
5	Unclear and multifactorial mechanisms	Precapillary	mPAP >20 mmHg; PAWP ≤15 mmHg; PVR > 2 WU	Sarcoidosis, chronic hemolytic anemia, thyroid disorders, sickle cell disease, splenectomy, mediastinal tumors, chronic renal failure	Rare
		Postcapillary	mPAP >20 mmHg; PAWP >15 mmHg		
		Isolated postcapillary	mPAP >20 mmHg; PAWP >15 mmHg; PVR ≤ 2 WU		
		Combined pre- and postcapillay	mPAP >20 mmHg; PAWP >15 mmHg; PVR > 2 WU		

mPAP mean Pulmonary Arterial Pressure, *PAWP* pulmonary artery wedge pressure, *PVR* Pulmonary Vascular Resistance, *WU* Wood Units

stratification of SSc-PAH risk to ameliorate early diagnosis and treatment but also reduce costs related to unnecessary RHC.

To improve the performance of the DETECT score, the incorporation of additional TTE parameters has been proposed. In this context, the 2022 ESC/ERS guidelines have included the tricuspid annular plane systolic excursion (TAPSE) to systolic pulmonary artery pressure (sPAP) ratio as part of the TTE assessment for 1-year mortality risk stratification, highlighting its role as a promising noninvasive marker for both the diagnosis of PH and mortality prediction across various cardiovascular diseases [29]. In patients with SSc-PAH, a retrospective analysis from the EUSTAR cohort demonstrated that a TAPSE/sPAP ratio of <0.55 was significantly and independently associated with the presence of PAH, up to 12 months before the diagnosis was confirmed by RHC. Furthermore, a TAPSE/sPAP ratio ≤0.32 was associated with increased all-cause mortality during a median follow-up period of 39 months [32].

The DETECT algorithm and the TAPSE/sPAP ratio demonstrate the superior performance of a multiparametric approach compared to the assessment of isolated parameters. Notably, a TTE sPAP >36 mmHg has been previously associated with reduced survival in patients with SSc. sPAP is derived from tricuspid regurgitation velocity (TRV), which represents the recommended TTE parameter for follow-up in patients with suspected or confirmed pulmonary hypertension [29]. In routine monitoring of SSc-PAH, sPAP has been extensively used for treatment follow-up and has shown comparable efficacy to other TRV-based methods for PH screening [33, 34].

Besides its relevance in the pre-disease stage, changes in the NVC pattern have been shown to occur during disease progression, with some specific findings related to SSc-PAH diagnosis [35]. Two longitudinal studies following up patients for more than 2 years showed that both specific quantitative and qualitative capillaroscopic changes are associated with SSc-PAH diagnosis (Table 4.2) [6, 10].

Sulli et al. conducted a longitudinal study involving 38 SSc patients with a median follow-up duration of 84 months, aimed at exploring the progression of NVC patterns over time. At baseline, all patients exhibited an early scleroderma NVC pattern. By the conclusion of the study period, four individuals (two showing an active NVC pattern and two with a late pattern) were diagnosed with SSc-PAH, confirmed through right heart catheterization. Analysis of the quantitative NVC changes revealed a significant association between SSc-PAH and both reduced capillary density ($p = 0.04$) and increased capillary morphological abnormalities ($p = 0.04$). However, no significant link was observed between the development of SSc-PAH and either capillary size (megacapillaries) or the presence of microhemorrhages. Regarding qualitative NVC findings, patients who transitioned from an early to either an active or late NVC pattern during follow-up were more likely to develop SSc-PAH, with statistical significance noted for both transitions ($p = 0.05$ for active pattern, $p = 0.01$ for late pattern) [10]. Accordingly, in the presented case, the patient developed during follow-up the changes mentioned above (Fig. 4.6), supporting the presence of specific NVC changes associated with SSc-PAH.

At the same time, cross-sectional studies have shown that SSc-PAH patients have significantly more severe (active/late) patterns at NVC compared to SSc patients without PAH [36, 37]. Thus supporting the role of NVC in identifying patients at risk for internal organ involvement. Similar to longitudinal studies, cross-sectional studies showed an association between SSc-PAH and decreased capillary density; this was true not only for SSc-PAH but also in rarer cases of SSc-PH, such as

Table 4.2 NFC findings significantly associated with incident SSc-PAH in longitudinal studies

Type of assessment	Characteristics	NFC changes	Conclusions
Quantitative	Density	Progressive capillary loss	Unequivocally associated with incident SSc-PAH
	Morphology	Abnormal morphology of capillary loops	Abnormal morphology at inclusion was more commonly associated with incident SSc-PAH
Qualitative	Transition to a severe NFC scleroderma pattern (active or late)	Scleroderma pattern active or late	Progression to a severe NFC pattern (active/late) was unequivocally associated with incident SSc-PAH in 2

CTEPH [36, 38]. Finally, in the semiquantitative assessment, avascular areas resulted associated with SSc-PAH and were also observed in the follow-up NVC of the case presented above (Fig. 4.6b) [36].

Recently published new treatment recommendations for SSc divide therapy into eight clinical domains, one of which is SSc-PAH. Although these domains are based on the clinical presentation of SSc, the new guidelines introduce the concept of a vascular therapeutic continuum, reflecting a shared pathophysiological mechanism underlying the vascular manifestations of SSc, namely RP, DUs, and PAH [20]. In the therapy of SSc, the vascular continuum refers to the use of the same class of drugs for different vascular manifestations, as, for example, the use of bosentan for DUs and PAH. Bosentan is a dual endothelin receptor antagonist (ERA) that prevents DU occurrence and is effective in ameliorating the clinical status of SSc-PAH patients [39].

A recent meta-analysis confirmed that bosentan is associated with a reduction in sPAP in patients with SSc. However, this effect was not sustained in studies with a follow-up period of ≥12 months. Furthermore, the interpretation of these findings remains uncertain due to substantial publication bias, suggesting that relevant data may be missing or selectively reported [34]. Consequently, whether bosentan exerts a long-term protective effect on the SSc-PAH development still remains an open question. Recent data from a retrospective multicenter study involving 727 SSc patients have provided further insight into this issue. In this study, the presence of DUs was confirmed as a risk factor for the development of PAH. Moreover, patients with DUs who received bosentan treatment exhibited a reduced incidence of PAH onset [40]. These findings support the hypothesis of a multiorgan, anti-vasculopathic effect of bosentan, which has also been demonstrated by NVC. Specifically, bosentan treatment was associated with increased capillary density and improvement of the NVC pattern [41, 42].

In the case of isolated SSc-PAH, macitentan or ambrisentan are recommended over bosentan, owing to their better pharmacodynamics and better prevention of clinical worsening [43, 44]. Moreover, current recommendations support initiating endothelin receptor antagonists (ERAs) as part of combination therapy with PDE5i, such as tadalafil, rather than as monotherapy. This approach has demonstrated superiority in improving survival outcomes in patients with PAH, including those with SSc-PAH [44, 45]. In this regard, PDE5i are drugs that can be used to treat RP and DUs, thus representing another therapeutic continuum in SSc vascular manifestations. In the case of this patient, combination therapy was started with macitentan and tadalafil. Macitentan was chosen over bosentan for the absence of DU history and better pharmacodynamics in the combination therapy with PDE5i.

In more severe cases of SSc-PAH, such as WHO functional class III/IV or with intermediate to high risk according to the ESC/ERS guidelines, the addition of riociguat, a soluble guanylate cyclase (sGC) stimulator, to ongoing therapy should be considered [46]. In parallel, intravenous prostacyclin analogues represent a valid therapeutic option for patients with the most severe forms of SSc-PAH. Beyond their established role in advanced PAH, prostacyclin analogues have also demonstrated beneficial effects on peripheral vascular manifestations of SSc, including RP and DUs, making them a valuable component of the therapeutic strategy in patients with extensive vasculopathy [20, 42]. In the current clinical case, combination therapy with macitentan and tadalafil was initiated and was well tolerated, with no adverse events observed throughout the treatment period. At the 1-year follow-up, comprehensive clinical reassessment and TTE were performed. The patient's dyspnea remained stable (NYHA functional class II), the six-minute walk test demonstrated moderate dyspnea (Borg Dyspnea Scale 3), and follow-up TTE findings were unaltered. These results support the efficacy of combination therapy in maintaining a favorable therapeutic response.

Case 3: SSc-ILD

Patient History

A 59-year-old woman presented to our hospital with a 3-year history of RP and a 1-year history of PFs, accompanied by progressing skin thickening. She also reported gastrointestinal symptoms, predominantly gastroesophageal reflux and constipation. Six months earlier, NVC performed in another center showed an "active" scleroderma pattern. Autoantibody testing showed positivity for ANA and ATA. Other laboratory tests, including complete blood count (CBC), ESR, CRP, uric acid, and NT-proBNP, were unremarkable. Based on these clinical and biological findings, a diagnosis of SSc was already established at that time. The first clinical assessment in our scleroderma unit showed skin thickness of the face, right arm, both forearms, hands, feet, and fingers, yielding a total mRSS of 11. No DUs, calcinosis, or telangiectasia were detected.

Capillaroscopic Findings

At baseline, the first NVC was performed by using an optical probe videocapillaroscopy equipped with a 200× contact lens and connected to image analysis software (VideoCap). The patient was inside the building for 30 min before the test, and the room temperature was 21 °C. The nailfolds of eight fingers (excluding the thumbs) were examined after a drop of immersion oil had been placed on the nailfold bed to improve the image resolution. The analysis revealed a mild disorganization of the capillary architecture and an initial loss of capillaries. Frequent giant capillaries (diameter >50 μm) and microhemorrhages were detected, particularly on digits II and III bilaterally. No extensive avascular areas were noted. These findings were consistent with an "active" scleroderma pattern, which has been reported to have a 97.5% specificity for the diagnosis of SSc (Fig. 4.7) [2, 47].

At 18-month follow-up, NVC showed a further reduction of capillary density, accounting for 30% in digit II of the right hand, as well as an average decrease in the number of megacapillaries (Fig. 4.8). Additionally, the presence of abnormally shaped and ramified capillaries was documented. This capillaroscopic presentation still met the criteria for an "active" scleroderma pattern, despite the changes from baseline that may suggest a possible future evolution toward a "late" scleroderma pattern.

Diagnosis and Management

In October 2023, the SSc diagnosis was confirmed. The patient fulfilled the ACR/EULAR 2013 criteria, with a total score of 21 points, resulting from skin thickening extending proximal to the metacarpophalangeal joint (nine points), PFs (two points), sclerodactyly of the fingers (four points), abnormal nailfold capillaries (two points), RP (three points), and anti-topoisomerase I positivity (three points). Skin involvement extended proximal to the right elbow, indicating a diffuse cutaneous subset of the disease [48].

The management plan included esophageal manometry to investigate the persistent reflux symptoms, likely secondary to gastrointestinal dysmotility related to scleroderma, and lung evaluation with PFT and thorax high-resolution computed tomography (HRCT) in light of the increased risk for lung involvement associated with the diffuse cutaneous subset and ATA positivity [49]. An echocardiogram was also performed to assess for potential cardiac involvement, but the absence of telangiectasias, combined with normal uric acid and NT-proBNP levels, was reassuring in this regard. Aspirin 100 mg QD, nifedipine 20 mg QD, and omeprazole 40 mg QD were introduced in the patient's therapy.

From a diagnostic perspective, the capillaroscopic findings aligned well with the clinical presentation. Increasing evidence in the literature supports the correlation between NVC abnormalities and skin involvement in SSc, as assessed by mRSS, high-frequency skin ultrasound (US), and the plicometer skin test (PST). [50]

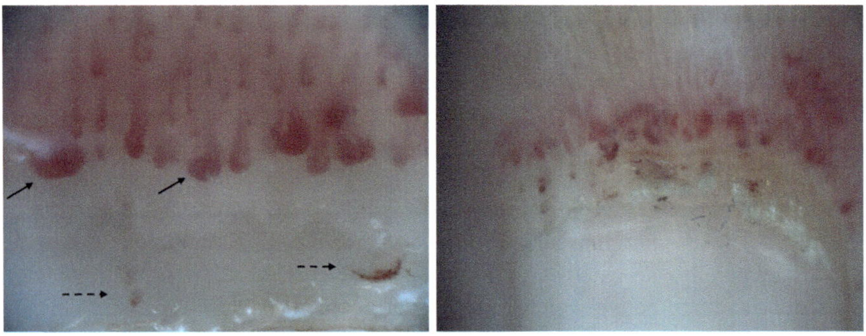

Fig. 4.7 (baseline) In 2022, NVC revealed an early and mild loss of capillaries, with frequent megacapillaries (solid arrow) and microhemorrhages (dashed arrow). The blue line refers to the apical diameter of megacapillaries. These findings are consistent with the active scleroderma pattern

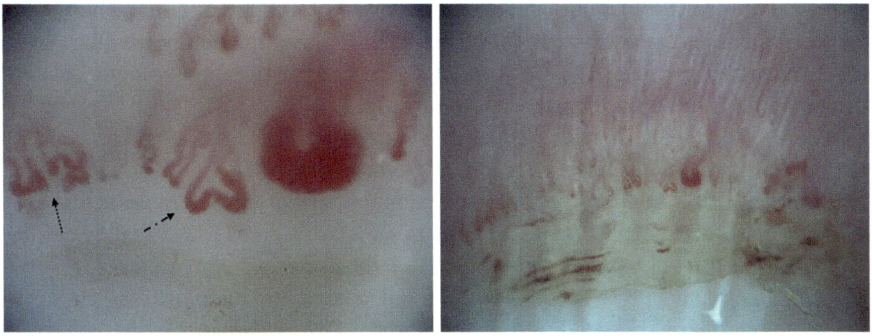

Fig. 4.8 (follow-up) NVC performed in 2023 showed a more pronounced disorganization of the capillary architecture, concomitant with a further decrease of capillary density. A reduction in megacapillaries was noted, accompanied by the emergence of abnormally shaped (dash-dot arrow) and ramified capillaries (dotted arrow). These findings are consistent with the active scleroderma pattern

Greater skin involvement has been observed in patients with active or late scleroderma patterns, which are more prevalent in the diffuse subset associated with ATA [2]. Reduced capillary density is another hallmark of ATA positivity, consistent with our case [51]. Furthermore, the median time to progression of NVC patterns has been reported to be shorter in ANA- and ATA-positive patients [5].

In our case, the baseline NVC findings could have provided prognostic insight into the subsequent disease trajectory. In fact, the presence of an active/late scleroderma pattern is a known predictive factor for both organ and skin progression, and the severity of organ involvement increases progressively from early to late NVC pattern [5, 7, 8].

At a four-month follow-up, our patient returned with worsening cutaneous and vascular symptoms: her mRSS had increased to 16, and she had developed three DUs. Gastrointestinal and pulmonary evaluations confirmed progressive internal organ involvement. Manometry revealed esophagogastric junction outflow obstruction, while PFTs showed preserved total lung capacity (TLC) and FVC, accounting for 113 and 114% of predicted, respectively; however, the DLCO was reduced (53%), and the DLCO adjusted for alveolar volume (DLCO/VA) was 58%. Thorax HRCT confirmed the diagnosis of SSc-associated interstitial lung disease (SSc-ILD), showing bilateral thickening of the interlobular and subpleural interstitium, more evident in the lower and peripheral lung regions.

The most common initial symptoms of SSc-ILD are exertional dyspnea and dry cough, although early disease may be relatively asymptomatic [52]. HRCT is the gold standard for the diagnosis of SSc-ILD, allowing for direct visualization of parenchymal lung abnormalities. The most frequent radiologic pattern is nonspecific interstitial pneumonia (NSIP), characterized by bilateral ground-glass opacities, reticulations, and traction bronchiectasis predominantly in the lower lobes [52]. HRCT is generally sufficient to distinguish between NSIP and usual interstitial pneumonia (UIP) patterns [53]. Although lung biopsy is rarely necessary, if performed, it typically reveals interstitial fibrosis with temporal homogeneity and limited inflammation, consistent with fibrotic NSIP. Less frequently, cellular NSIP or UIP may be observed [52]. However, a discrepancy between radiologic and histologic findings has been reported in several cases [54]. In SSc-ILD, PFTs typically show a restrictive pattern, with decreased FVC and/or TLC, a preserved FEV1, and a normal or increased FEV1/FVC ratio, as well as reduced DLCO. However, in the early phase of disease, lung volumes may remain normal despite radiological evidence of disease and reduced DLCO [55]. In fact, two studies found that over 60% of patients with ILD diagnosed via HRCT had normal spirometry [55, 56]. Therefore, although PFTs remain an essential part of the diagnostic assessment, they are not sufficiently sensitive to detect early ILD.

Given the patient's clinical deterioration, including worsening skin and new-onset SSc-ILD, immunosuppressive therapy with full-dose mycophenolate mofetil (MMF) at 3 g QD was initiated. MMF is a first-line treatment for SSc-ILD, supported by the Scleroderma Lung Study II (SLS II), showing the non-inferiority of MMF compared to oral cyclophosphamide in improving FVC over 24 months. In this trial, MMF had a significantly better safety and tolerability profile [19].

Following the onset of DUs, our patient was started on intravenous (IV) iloprost, administered five times per month. IV iloprost has a level A recommendation for the treatment of active DU, based on two randomized controlled trials assessing its efficacy compared to placebo [20]. Moreover, findings from a 2013 meta-analysis support the role of this drug in the prevention of new DUs (SMD 0.77 [95% CI 1.46, 0.08], $p = 0.03$) [57]. Of interest, in another study, treatment with iloprost has been associated with a significant reduction in the number of megacapillaries over time [58]. Several studies have shown that microhemorrhages and microthrombosis (NEMO score), as well as giant capillaries, are reliable indicators of disease activity in SSc, with a reported sensitivity of 95% and specificity of 85% [12, 59]. Additionally, reduced capillary density has been correlated with higher disease activity scores, such as the European Scleroderma Study Group (EScSG) index [60]. In our patient, NVC findings could have anticipated the development of DU. One study found that all patients with DU exhibited an active NVC pattern, indicating high sensitivity despite limited positive predictive value, since nearly half of patients without DU also displayed this pattern [61]. More specifically, capillary loss predicted new-onset DU (HR = 5.33) and was associated with overall disease progression (HR = 4.35), lung vascular progression (HR = 18.53), progression of skin fibrosis (HR = 4.22), and worsening of the Medsger severity score (HR = 5.26) [6]. Interestingly, patients with increasing numbers of giant capillaries over time were less likely to develop new DU (HR = 0.53). The combined assessment of giant capillaries and capillary density led to the development of the Capillaroscopic Skin Ulcer Risk Index (CSURI), which has shown high predictive value for DU onset within 3 months following NVC [13]. Similarly, the NEMO score appeared to be closely associated with DU development in SSc [14].

At follow-up in October 2023, mRSS rose to 19, and pulmonary function tests revealed a significant worsening in FVC (93% vs 114%), DLCO (43% vs 53%), and DLCO/VA (45% vs 58%). Moreover, chest HRCT showed an increased extension of parenchymal alterations, presenting as ground-glass opacities. These findings were consistent with a progression of SSc-ILD [62]. In response, antifibrotic therapy with nintedanib QD was added. The SENSCIS trial showed that nintedanib significantly reduced the annual rate of FVC decline in patients with SSc-ILD, particularly in those receiving background MMF therapy [63, 64]. A post-hoc analysis revealed that the combination of MMF and nintedanib yielded the greatest reduction in FVC decline, suggesting a complementary effect between immunosuppressive and antifibrotic mechanisms [64]. Based on these findings, this combination therapy is currently considered a preferred strategy in progressive SSc-ILD [20].

In our patient, new capillaroscopic alterations appeared in parallel with the worsening of skin fibrosis and with the progression of ILD, demonstrating that NVC findings correlate with disease activity and progression in SSc [6, 60]. Emerging evidence highlights the potential role of NVC as a predictor of SSc-ILD [65]. Two cross-sectional studies reported an inverse association between ILD and capillary density ($p = 0.008$ and $p = 0.005$), and avascular areas correlated with worse pulmonary function, reflected by lower FVC and DLCO [9, 66]. In a longitudinal study, incident SSc-ILD was linked to progressive capillary loss ($p = 0.04$) and worsening NVC pattern (0.001 from early to active, $p = 0.005$ from active to late). Additionally, esophageal involvement, as observed in our patient, also correlated with increased capillary loss and disorganization scores ($p = 0.03$) [10].

Subsequent studies confirmed these results, demonstrating a positive correlation between avascular areas and lung fibrosis, as well as the association between reduced baseline FVC and lower capillary density [66]. In another study, Pearson correlation analysis further validated the strong relationship between capillary loss and SSc-ILD ($r = 0.7255$) [67].

This case illustrates the diagnostic and prognostic utility of NVC in SSc, highlighting its potential as a promising biomarker valuable for predicting internal organ involvement and guiding treatment decisions. The integration of capillaroscopy into routine clinical practice may enhance risk stratification, enable earlier intervention, and ultimately improve patient outcomes in SSc.

Case 4: SSc Sine Scleroderma

Patient History

A 28-year-old female was first referred to the Rheumatology and Clinical Immunology Unit of a university hospital in 2011 for episodes of RP in the last 10 years. At that time, an undifferentiated connective tissue disease was diagnosed, based on the presence of RP, a strongly positive ANA (1:1280), and ACA positivity. No specific capillaroscopic abnormalities were observed. The patient was subsequently lost to follow-up after 3 years.

In 2021, at the age of 48, she was re-referred to our scleroderma clinic due to the worsening, as well as the frequency and intensity of RP. Between 2011 and 2021, she was treated with Hydroxicloroquine (HCQ) 200 mg QD and ASA 100 mg QD, which was discontinued due to gastrointestinal intolerance, and with CCBs (nifedipine 30 mg QD), which was discontinued because of adverse effects including headache, hypotension, and tachycardia.

A TTE performed in 2019 was available, showing a PASP of 25 mmHg. An upper GI endoscopy performed in 2021 showed chronic gastritis. On physical examination, no signs of cutaneous sclerosis were detected: the mRSS was 0, with no PFs or telangiectasias. An active DU was present on the second digit of the left hand. For this reason, a new NVC was performed in 2021.

Capillaroscopic Findings

Two NVC assessments were performed by using an optical probe videocapillaroscopy equipped with a 200× contact lens and connected to image analysis software (VideoCap). The patient was inside the building for 30 min before the test, and the room temperature was 21 °C. The nailfolds of eight fingers (excluding the thumbs) were examined after a drop of immersion oil had been placed on the nailfold bed to improve the image resolution. The first assessment was performed at the time of initial patient evaluation in 2011, and the second in 2021.

In 2011, the examination showed normal and homogeneous capillary distribution and density, with regular capillary flow. Capillaries maintained normal length, with diffuse and circumscribed ectasias and mild convolutions. A single pre-megacapillary (37 μm) was identified on digit IV left. No megacapillaries, neoangiogenesis, avascular areas, bizarre shapes, or ramified capillaries were observed. Rare microhemorrhages were detected. These findings were consistent with non-specific abnormalities, not classifiable within the scleroderma pattern (Fig. 4.9) [3, 22].

In 2021, at NVC, the capillary architecture demonstrated a regular and homogeneous distribution and normal density. Capillaries exhibited normal length and diffuse ectatic changes. Two megacapillaries (>50 μm) were identified on digits III right and II left. In addition, isolated microhemorrhages were observed on digits II–IV bilaterally and on digit III right. Capillary blood flow was preserved. No tortuosity, ramified capillaries, bizarre morphologies, avascular areas, or neoangiogenesis were observed. Overall, the findings were consistent with an early scleroderma pattern (Fig. 4.10) [3, 47].

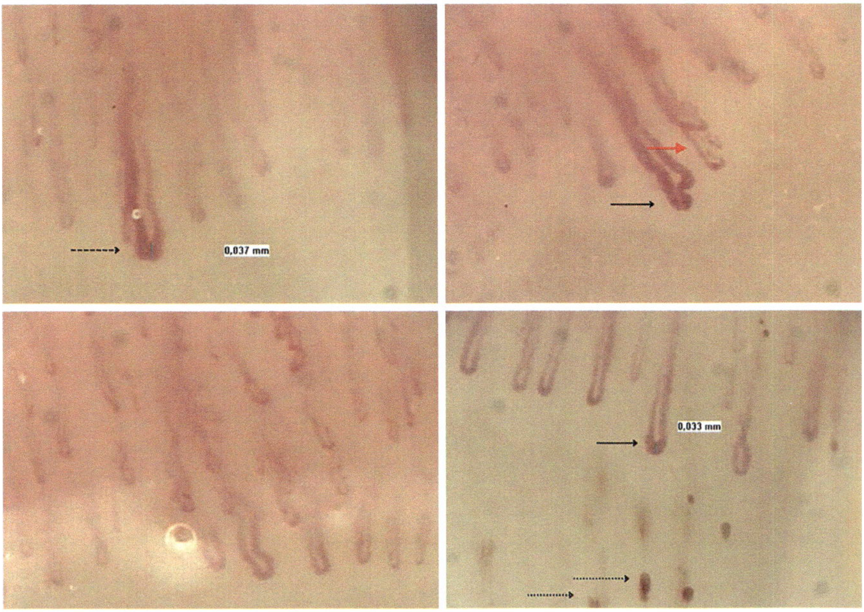

Fig. 4.9 In 2011, nailfold videocapillaroscopy revealed diffuse and circumscribed *ectasias (continuous arrow), mild convolutions (red arrow),* and rare *microhemorrhages (dotted arrow).* A single *pre-megacapillary (dashed arrow)* was identified on the fourth digit of the left hand. These findings represent nonspecific capillaroscopic abnormalities not consistent with scleroderma spectrum patterns

Diagnosis and Management

Diagnosis of SSc was confirmed, and the patient fulfilled the ACR/EULAR 2013 criteria: RP (3), ANA with ACA (3), typical NVC abnormalities (2), and active DU (2), with a total score of 10. Given the absence of cutaneous involvement and the lack of clinical features indicative of other CTD, a diagnosis of Systemic Sclerosis sine scleroderma (ssSSc) was established [68].

ssSSc was first reported by Abrams in 1954 and further described by Rodnan and Fennel in 1962 [69]. The main diagnostic criteria for ssSSc include RP or other peripheral vascular involvement, positive ANA, and involvement of one visceral organ typical of SSc without skin thickening, in the absence of another defined CTD. The etiology remains unknown, and the condition predominantly affects females [70, 71]. Clinical manifestations often include esophageal or gastric dysmotility, renal involvement, arthralgia or myalgia, and pulmonary manifestations [70, 71].

Recent data from the international EUSTAR database, published in 2023, provide further insight into the clinical characteristics and prognosis of patients with ssSSc. Among 4263 patients with SSc, 8.8% were classified as having ssSSc. In this cohort, overall survival was higher in patients with ssSSc compared to those with

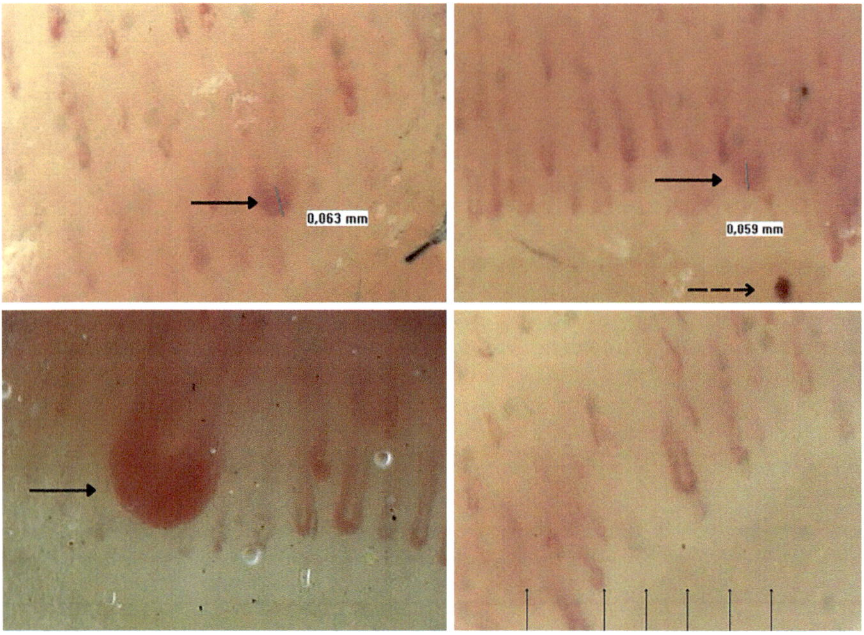

Fig. 4.10 In 2021, NVC revealed homogeneous distribution and normal density (small arrows); two *megacapillaries* (diameter > 50 μm) (thick continuous arrow) were identified on the third digit of the right hand and the second digit of the left hand. Additionally, isolated *microhemorrhages* (dashed arrow) were present. These findings are consistent with an *early scleroderma pattern*

lcSSc and dcSSc after long-term follow-up. The prevalence of ILD in ssSSc was comparable to that observed in lcSSc but significantly lower than in dcSSc. Furthermore, skin telangiectasias in ssSSc were found to be associated with diastolic dysfunction, and the presence of anti-Scl-70 antibodies represented the main independent predictor for the development of skin fibrosis in this subgroup [68].

Our patient experienced RP for several decades, but the development of microvascular abnormalities was remarkably slow, as NVC findings remained normal in 2011, and an NVC scleroderma pattern became evident many years later. This unusually indolent course of microangiopathy is consistent with data from the national registry SPRING of the Italian Society for Rheumatology, showing that a prolonged RP-to-diagnosis time frame was found to distinguish ssSSc from lcSSc as well as dcSSc, thus supporting the hypothesis that delayed capillaroscopic evolution may reflect a distinct disease trajectory, documenting a generally slower progression of microvascular damage in ssSSc [72].

The EUSTAR cohort showed that disease severity in patients with ssSSc is generally milder than in dcSSc and comparable to that observed in lcSSc. Of note, skin telangiectasias in patients with ssSSc were associated with important internal organ manifestations, such as elevated systolic pulmonary arterial pressure, diastolic dysfunction, as well as gastrointestinal symptoms, independently of age or disease duration. These findings underscore the importance of systematically evaluating even non-fibrotic skin manifestations in this subset of patients, indirectly confirming the central role of vasculopathy in the pathogenesis of these complications [68]. In this context, despite the very slow evolution to a specific scleroderma pattern and the typically indolent course of the disease, NVC may be of pivotal importance in these patients, allowing the clinician to establish the diagnosis [73, 74].

Between 2021 and 2022, the patient underwent a comprehensive multidisciplinary evaluation involving the lungs, heart, and gastrointestinal tract. PFT showed preserved lung volumes, with an FVC of 117% and an FEV_1 of 116% of predicted values, with a normal FEV_1/FVC ratio. The DLCO was 83% of predicted, and the KCO was 81%. HRTC showed no signs of lung fibrosis. TTE showed a preserved LVEF of 63%, with mild regurgitation of the pulmonary, tricuspid, and mitral valves. PASP was estimated at 28 mmHg. A 24-h Holter ECG revealed a stable sinus rhythm with an average heart rate of 91 bpm. No supraventricular or ventricular ectopic activity, significant sinus pauses, or repolarization abnormalities were detected. At HRM, 60% of the swallows were ineffective with no evidence of esophagogastric obstruction, resulting in the diagnosis of Ineffective Esophageal Motility (IEM) according to the Chicago Classification v4.0 [15].

Considering the active DUs and esophageal dysmotility, a targeted vasoactive treatment regimen was initiated, consisting of nifedipine 20 mg QD, ASA 75 mg QD, bosentan 125 mg BID, and IV prostanoid to address severe digital vasculopathy following the Wigley et al. procedure for the treatment with prostacyclin during severe RP and DUs [75]. In addition to vasoactive therapy, PPI (esomeprazole 40 mg QD) was also added for the treatment of gastroesophageal reflux [18, 20].

At long-term FU, the patient maintained sustained clinical stability. No signs of cutaneous fibrosis were observed, with a consistently unchanged mRSS. There was no development of new telangiectasias or DUs, and the patient did not report symptoms of resting dyspnea.

The patient continued long-term treatment with ASA, CCB, IV prostanoid, and ERA. Throughout the follow-up period, no clinical evidence of disease progression or emergence of new systemic or vascular complications was noted.

References

1. Volkmann ER, Andréasson K, Smith V. Systemic sclerosis. Lancet (Lond Engl). 2023;401:304–18. https://doi.org/10.1016/S0140-6736(22)01692-0.
2. Cutolo M, Pizzorni C, Tuccio M, et al. Nailfold videocapillaroscopic patterns and serum autoantibodies in systemic sclerosis. Rheumatol Oxf Engl. 2004;43:719–26. https://doi.org/10.1093/rheumatology/keh156.
3. Smith V, Herrick AL, Ingegnoli F, et al. Standardisation of nailfold capillaroscopy for the assessment of patients with Raynaud's phenomenon and systemic sclerosis. Autoimmun Rev. 2020;19:102458. https://doi.org/10.1016/j.autrev.2020.102458.
4. van den Hoogen F, Khanna D, Fransen J, et al. 2013 classification criteria for systemic sclerosis: an American college of rheumatology/European league against rheumatism col-

laborative initiative. Ann Rheum Dis. 2013;72:1747–55. https://doi.org/10.1136/annrheumdis-2013-204424.
5. Sulli A, Paolino S, Pizzorni C, et al. Progression of nailfold capillaroscopic patterns and correlation with organ involvement in systemic sclerosis: a 12 year study. Rheumatology (Oxford). 2020;59:1051–8. https://doi.org/10.1093/rheumatology/kez374.
6. Avouac J, Lepri G, Smith V, et al. Sequential nailfold videocapillaroscopy examinations have responsiveness to detect organ progression in systemic sclerosis. Semin Arthritis Rheum. 2017;47:86–94. https://doi.org/10.1016/j.semarthrit.2017.02.006.
7. Smith V, Riccieri V, Pizzorni C, et al. Nailfold capillaroscopy for prediction of novel future severe organ involvement in systemic sclerosis. J Rheumatol. 2013;40:2023–8. https://doi.org/10.3899/jrheum.130528.
8. Vanhaecke A, Cutolo M, Distler O, et al. Nailfold capillaroscopy in SSc: innocent bystander or promising biomarker for novel severe organ involvement/progression? Rheumatology (Oxford). 2022;61:4384–96. https://doi.org/10.1093/rheumatology/keac079.
9. Guillén-Del-Castillo A, Simeón-Aznar CP, Callejas-Moraga EL, et al. Quantitative videocapillaroscopy correlates with functional respiratory parameters: a clue for vasculopathy as a pathogenic mechanism for lung injury in systemic sclerosis. Arthritis Res Ther. 2018;20:281. https://doi.org/10.1186/s13075-018-1775-9.
10. Sulli A, Pizzorni C, Smith V, et al. Timing of transition between capillaroscopic patterns in systemic sclerosis. Arthritis Rheum. 2012;64:821–5. https://doi.org/10.1002/art.33463.
11. Sambataro D, Sambataro G, Zaccara E, et al. Nailfold videocapillaroscopy micro-haemorrhage and giant capillary counting as an accurate approach for a steady state definition of disease activity in systemic sclerosis. Arthritis Res Ther. 2014;16:462. https://doi.org/10.1186/s13075-014-0462-8.
12. Kayser C, Sekiyama JY, Próspero LC, et al. Nailfold capillaroscopy abnormalities as predictors of mortality in patients with systemic sclerosis. Clin Exp Rheumatol. 2013;31:103–8.
13. Sebastiani M, Manfredi A, Vukatana G, et al. Predictive role of capillaroscopic skin ulcer risk index in systemic sclerosis: a multicentre validation study. Ann Rheum Dis. 2012;71:67–70. https://doi.org/10.1136/annrheumdis-2011-200022.
14. Del Papa N, Pignataro F, Maglione W, et al. High NEMO score values in nailfold videocapillaroscopy are associated with the subsequent development of ischaemic digital ulcers in patients with systemic sclerosis. Arthritis Res Ther. 2020;22:237. https://doi.org/10.1186/s13075-020-02342-5.
15. Yadlapati R, Kahrilas PJ, Fox MR, et al. Esophageal motility disorders on high-resolution manometry: Chicago classification version 4.0©. Neurogastroenterol Motil. 2021;33:e14058. https://doi.org/10.1111/nmo.14058.
16. Miller JB, Gandhi N, Clarke J, et al. Gastrointestinal involvement in systemic sclerosis: an update. J Clin Rheumatol Pract Rep Rheum Musculoskelet Dis. 2018;24:328–37. https://doi.org/10.1097/RHU.0000000000000626.
17. Kuribayashi S, Motegi S-I, Hara K, et al. Relationship between esophageal motility abnormalities and skin or lung involvements in patients with systemic sclerosis. J Gastroenterol. 2019;54:950–62. https://doi.org/10.1007/s00535-019-01578-6.
18. Garaiman A, Steigmiller K, Gebhard C, et al. Use of platelet inhibitors for digital ulcers related to systemic sclerosis: EUSTAR study on derivation and validation of the DU-VASC model. Rheumatology (Oxford). 2023;62:SI91–100. https://doi.org/10.1093/rheumatology/keac405.
19. Tashkin DP, Roth MD, Clements PJ, et al. Mycophenolate Mofetil versus Oral Cyclophosphamide in Scleroderma-related Interstitial Lung Disease: Scleroderma Lung Study II (SLS-II), a double-blind, parallel group, randomised controlled trial. Lancet Respir Med. 2016;4:708–19. https://doi.org/10.1016/S2213-2600(16)30152-7.
20. Del Galdo F, Lescoat A, Conaghan PG, et al. EULAR recommendations for the treatment of systemic sclerosis: 2023 update. Ann Rheum Dis. 2025;84:29–40. https://doi.org/10.1136/ard-2024-226430.

21. Ross L, Maltez N, Hughes M, et al. Systemic pharmacological treatment of digital ulcers in systemic sclerosis: a systematic literature review. Rheumatology (Oxford). 2023;62:3785–800. https://doi.org/10.1093/rheumatology/kead289.
22. Smith V, Vanhaecke A, Herrick AL, et al. Fast track algorithm: How to differentiate a “scleroderma pattern” from a “non-scleroderma pattern”. Autoimmun Rev. 2019;18:102394. https://doi.org/10.1016/j.autrev.2019.102394.
23. Mouthon L, Mestre-Stanislas C, Bérezné A, et al. Impact of digital ulcers on disability and health-related quality of life in systemic sclerosis. Ann Rheum Dis. 2010;69:214–7. https://doi.org/10.1136/ard.2008.094193.
24. Guillevin L, Hunsche E, Denton CP, et al. Functional impairment of systemic scleroderma patients with digital ulcerations: results from the DUO Registry. Clin Exp Rheumatol. 2013;31:71–80.
25. Smith V, Decuman S, Sulli A, et al. Do worsening scleroderma capillaroscopic patterns predict future severe organ involvement? A pilot study. Ann Rheum Dis. 2012;71:1636–9. https://doi.org/10.1136/annrheumdis-2011-200780.
26. Cutolo M, Herrick AL, Distler O, et al. Nailfold Videocapillaroscopic features and other clinical risk factors for digital ulcers in systemic sclerosis: a multicenter, prospective cohort study. Arthritis Rheumatol (Hoboken NJ). 2016;68:2527–39. https://doi.org/10.1002/art.39718.
27. Coghlan JG, Denton CP, Grünig E, et al. Evidence-based detection of pulmonary arterial hypertension in systemic sclerosis: the DETECT study. Ann Rheum Dis. 2014;73:1340–9. https://doi.org/10.1136/annrheumdis-2013-203301.
28. Elhai M, Meune C, Boubaya M, et al. Mapping and predicting mortality from systemic sclerosis. Ann Rheum Dis. 2017;76:1897–905. https://doi.org/10.1136/annrheumdis-2017-211448.
29. Humbert M, Kovacs G, Hoeper MM, et al. 2022 ESC/ERS Guidelines for the diagnosis and treatment of pulmonary hypertension. Eur Heart J. 2022;43:3618–731. https://doi.org/10.1093/eurheartj/ehac237.
30. Karia N, Howard L, Johnson M, et al. Predictors of outcomes in mild pulmonary hypertension according to 2022 ESC/ERS Guidelines: the EVIDENCE-PAH UK study. Eur Heart J. 2023;44:4678–91. https://doi.org/10.1093/eurheartj/ehad532.
31. Galiè N, Hoeper MM, Humbert M, et al. Guidelines for the diagnosis and treatment of pulmonary hypertension: the Task Force for the Diagnosis and Treatment of Pulmonary Hypertension of the European Society of Cardiology (ESC) and the European Respiratory Society (ERS), endorsed by the International Society of Heart and Lung Transplantation (ISHLT). Eur Heart J. 2009;30:2493–537. https://doi.org/10.1093/eurheartj/ehp297.
32. Colalillo A, Hoffmann-Vold A-M, Pellicano C, et al. The role of TAPSE/sPAP ratio in predicting pulmonary hypertension and mortality in the systemic sclerosis EUSTAR cohort. Autoimmun Rev. 2023;22:103290. https://doi.org/10.1016/j.autrev.2023.103290.
33. Lv G, Li A, Tao X, et al. The accuracy and influencing factors of Doppler echocardiography in estimating pulmonary artery systolic pressure: comparison with right heart catheterization: a retrospective cross-sectional study. BMC Med Imaging. 2022;22:91. https://doi.org/10.1186/s12880-022-00806-5.
34. Bearzi P, Navarini L, Currado D, et al. Bosentan effect on echocardiographic systolic pulmonary arterial pressure in systemic sclerosis-related pulmonary hypertension: a systematic review and metanalysis. Clin Exp Rheumatol. 2024;42:1615–22. https://doi.org/10.55563/clinexprheumatol/xbdtb5.
35. Smith V, Vanhaecke A, Vandecasteele E, et al. Nailfold Videocapillaroscopy in systemic sclerosis–related pulmonary arterial hypertension: a systematic literature review. J Rheumatol. 2020;47:888–95. https://doi.org/10.3899/jrheum.190296.
36. Riccieri V, Vasile M, Iannace N, et al. Systemic sclerosis patients with and without pulmonary arterial hypertension: a nailfold capillaroscopy study. Rheumatology. 2013;52:1525–8. https://doi.org/10.1093/rheumatology/ket168.

37. Corrado A, Correale M, Mansueto N, et al. Nailfold capillaroscopic changes in patients with idiopathic pulmonary arterial hypertension and systemic sclerosis-related pulmonary arterial hypertension. Microvasc Res. 2017;114:46–51. https://doi.org/10.1016/j.mvr.2017.06.005.
38. Smits AJ, Isebia K, Combee-Duffy C, et al. Low nailfold capillary density in patients with pulmonary arterial hypertension and chronic thromboembolic pulmonary hypertension: biomarker of clinical outcome? Sci Rep. 2024;14:19467. https://doi.org/10.1038/s41598-024-69017-y.
39. Matucci-Cerinic M, Denton CP, Furst DE, et al. Bosentan treatment of digital ulcers related to systemic sclerosis: results from the RAPIDS-2 randomised, double-blind, placebo-controlled trial. Ann Rheum Dis. 2011;70:32–8. https://doi.org/10.1136/ard.2010.130658.
40. Cacciapaglia F, De Angelis R, Ferri C, et al. Pulmonary arterial hypertension incidence in patients with systemic sclerosis treated with Bosentan for digital ulcers: evidence from the SPRING-SIR Registry. J Rheumatol. 2025;52:375–82. https://doi.org/10.3899/jrheum.2024-0750.
41. Trombetta AC, Pizzorni C, Ruaro B, et al. Effects of Longterm treatment with Bosentan and Iloprost on Nailfold absolute capillary number, fingertip blood perfusion, and clinical status in systemic sclerosis. J Rheumatol. 2016;43:2033–41. https://doi.org/10.3899/jrheum.160592.
42. Cutolo M, Ruaro B, Pizzorni C, et al. Longterm treatment with endothelin receptor antagonist bosentan and iloprost improves fingertip blood perfusion in systemic sclerosis. J Rheumatol. 2014;41:881–6. https://doi.org/10.3899/jrheum.131284.
43. Li J, Yang Z-Y, Wang S, et al. Efficacy and safety of switching from bosentan or ambrisentan to macitentan in pulmonary arterial hypertension: a systematic review and meta-analysis. Front Cardiovasc Med. 2022;9 https://doi.org/10.3389/fcvm.2022.977110.
44. Galiè N, Barberà JA, Frost AE, et al. Initial use of Ambrisentan plus Tadalafil in pulmonary arterial hypertension. N Engl J Med. 2015;373:834–44. https://doi.org/10.1056/NEJMoa1413687.
45. Distler O, Ofner C, Huscher D, et al. Treatment strategies and survival of patients with connective tissue disease and pulmonary arterial hypertension: a COMPERA analysis. Rheumatology (Oxford). 2024;63:1139–46. https://doi.org/10.1093/rheumatology/kead360.
46. Rubin LJ, Galiè N, Grimminger F, et al. Riociguat for the treatment of pulmonary arterial hypertension: a long-term extension study (PATENT-2). Eur Respir J. 2015;45:1303–13. https://doi.org/10.1183/09031936.00090614.
47. Wu P-C, Huang M-N, Kuo Y-M, et al. Clinical applicability of quantitative nailfold capillaroscopy in differential diagnosis of connective tissue diseases with Raynaud's phenomenon. J Formos Med Assoc Taiwan Yi Zhi. 2013;112:482–8. https://doi.org/10.1016/j.jfma.2012.02.029.
48. LeRoy EC, Medsger TA. Criteria for the classification of early systemic sclerosis. J Rheumatol. 2001;28:1573–6.
49. Boonstra M, Ninaber MK, Ajmone Marsan N, et al. Prognostic properties of anti-topoisomerase antibodies in patients identified by the ACR/EULAR 2013 systemic sclerosis criteria. Rheumatology (Oxford). 2019;58:730–2. https://doi.org/10.1093/rheumatology/kez005.
50. Ruaro B, Pizzorni C, Paolino S, et al. Correlations between nailfold microvascular damage and skin involvement in systemic sclerosis patients. Microvasc Res. 2019;125:103874. https://doi.org/10.1016/j.mvr.2019.04.004.
51. Wildt M, Andréasson K, Hamberg V, et al. Treatment with mycophenolate mofetil is associated with improved nailfold vasculature in systemic sclerosis. Rheumatology (Oxford). 2024;63:385–91. https://doi.org/10.1093/rheumatology/kead207.
52. Liakouli V, Ciancio A, Del Galdo F, et al. Systemic sclerosis interstitial lung disease: unmet needs and potential solutions. Nat Rev Rheumatol. 2024;20:21–32. https://doi.org/10.1038/s41584-023-01044-x.
53. Desai SR, Veeraraghavan S, Hansell DM, et al. CT features of lung disease in patients with systemic sclerosis: comparison with idiopathic pulmonary fibrosis and nonspecific interstitial pneumonia. Radiology. 2004;232:560–7. https://doi.org/10.1148/radiol.2322031223.
54. Damiani A, Orlandi M, Bruni C, et al. The role of lung biopsy for diagnosis and prognosis of interstitial lung disease in systemic sclerosis: a systematic literature review. Respir Res. 2024;25:138. https://doi.org/10.1186/s12931-024-02725-1.

55. Suliman YA, Dobrota R, Huscher D, et al. Brief report: pulmonary function tests: high rate of false-negative results in the early detection and screening of scleroderma-related interstitial lung disease. Arthritis Rheumatol (Hoboken NJ). 2015;67:3256–61. https://doi.org/10.1002/art.39405.
56. Molberg Ø, Hoffmann-Vold A-M. Interstitial lung disease in systemic sclerosis: progress in screening and early diagnosis. Curr Opin Rheumatol. 2016;28:613–8. https://doi.org/10.1097/BOR.0000000000000323.
57. Tingey T, Shu J, Smuczek J, et al. Meta-analysis of healing and prevention of digital ulcers in systemic sclerosis. Arthritis Care Res. 2013;65:1460–71. https://doi.org/10.1002/acr.22018.
58. Cestelli V, Manfredi A, Sebastiani M, et al. Effect of treatment with iloprost with or without bosentan on nailfold videocapillaroscopic alterations in patients with systemic sclerosis. Mod Rheumatol. 2017;27:110–4. https://doi.org/10.1080/14397595.2016.1192761.
59. Andracco R, Irace R, Zaccara E, et al. The cumulative number of micro-haemorrhages and micro-thromboses in nailfold videocapillaroscopy is a good indicator of disease activity in systemic sclerosis: a validation study of the NEMO score. Arthritis Res Ther. 2017;19:133. https://doi.org/10.1186/s13075-017-1354-5.
60. Gheorghiu AM, Oneata R, Ancuta I, et al. Capillary loss reflects disease activity and prognosis in patients with systemic sclerosis. Exp Ther Med. 2020;20:3438–43. https://doi.org/10.3892/etm.2020.8979.
61. Lambova S, Müller-Ladner U. Capillaroscopic findings in systemic sclerosis – are they associated with disease duration and presence of digital ulcers? Discov Med. 2011;12:413–8.
62. Cottin V, Martinez FJ, Jenkins RG, et al. Safety and tolerability of nintedanib in patients with progressive fibrosing interstitial lung diseases: data from the randomized controlled INBUILD trial. Respir Res. 2022;23:85. https://doi.org/10.1186/s12931-022-01974-2.
63. Distler O, Highland KB, Gahlemann M, et al. Nintedanib for Systemic Sclerosis–Associated Interstitial Lung Disease. N Engl J Med. 2019;380:2518–28. https://doi.org/10.1056/NEJMoa1903076.
64. Highland KB, Distler O, Kuwana M, et al. Efficacy and safety of nintedanib in patients with systemic sclerosis-associated interstitial lung disease treated with mycophenolate: a subgroup analysis of the SENSCIS trial. Lancet Respir Med. 2021;9:96–106. https://doi.org/10.1016/S2213-2600(20)30330-1.
65. Smith V, Vanhaecke A, Guerra MG, et al. May capillaroscopy be a candidate tool in future algorithms for SSC-ILD: are we looking for the holy grail? A systematic review. Autoimmun Rev. 2020;19:102619. https://doi.org/10.1016/j.autrev.2020.102619.
66. Caetano J, Paula FS, Amaral M, et al. Nailfold Videocapillaroscopy changes are associated with the presence and severity of systemic sclerosis-related interstitial lung disease. J Clin Rheumatol Pract Rep Rheum Musculoskelet Dis. 2019;25:e12–5. https://doi.org/10.1097/RHU.0000000000000815.
67. Vilela VS, Vanhaecke A, da Silva BRA, et al. Is there a link between Nailfold Videocapillaroscopy and pulmonary function tests in systemic sclerosis patients? A 24-month follow-up monocentric study. J Clin Rheumatol. 2022;28:26–32. https://doi.org/10.1097/RHU.0000000000001798.
68. Lescoat A, Huang S, Carreira PE, et al. Cutaneous manifestations, clinical characteristics, and prognosis of patients with systemic sclerosis sine scleroderma: data from the international EUSTAR database. JAMA Dermatol. 2023;159:837–47. https://doi.org/10.1001/jamadermatol.2023.1729.
69. Rodnan GP, Fennell RH. Progressive systemic sclerosis sine scleroderma. JAMA. 1962;180:665–70. https://doi.org/10.1001/jama.1962.03050210027006.
70. Alghamdi M, Derbes SJ. Systemic sclerosis sine scleroderma manifested with gastrointestinal bleeding, antiphospholipid syndrome and positive anti-RNA polymerase III antibody: case report and literature review. Int Med Case Rep J. 2020;13:323–6. https://doi.org/10.2147/IMCRJ.S254859.
71. Marangoni RG, Rocha LF, Del Rio APT, et al. Systemic sclerosis sine scleroderma: distinct features in a large Brazilian cohort. Rheumatology (Oxford). 2013;52:1520–4. https://doi.org/10.1093/rheumatology/ket163.

72. De Angelis R, Ferri C, Giuggioli D, SPRING-SIR (Systemic Sclerosis PRogression INvestiGation group of the Italian Society of Rheumatology). Systemic sclerosis sine scleroderma: clinical and serological features and relationship with other cutaneous subsets in a large series of patients from the national registry 'SPRING' of the Italian Society for Rheumatology. RMD Open. 2023;9(1):e002890. https://doi.org/10.1136/rmdopen-2022-002890.
73. Tolosa-Vilella C, Morera-Morales ML, Simeón-Aznar CP, Marí-Alfonso B, Colunga-Arguelles D, Callejas Rubio JL, Rubio-Rivas M, Freire-Dapena M, Guillén-Del Castillo A, Iniesta-Arandia N, Castillo-Palma MJ, Egurbide-Arberas M, Trapiellla-Martínez L, Vargas-Hitos JA, Todolí-Parra JA, Rodriguez-Carballeira M, Marin-Ballvé A, Pla-Salas X, Rios-Blanco JJ, Fonollosa-Pla V, RESCLE Investigators, Autoimmune Diseases Study Group (GEAS). Digital ulcers and cutaneous subsets of systemic sclerosis: clinical, immunological, nailfold capillaroscopy, and survival differences in the Spanish RESCLE Registry. Semin Arthritis Rheum. 2016;46(2):200–8. https://doi.org/10.1016/j.semarthrit.2016.04.007. Epub 2016 May 18. PMID: 27312381.
74. Diab S, Dostrovsky N, Hudson M, Tatibouet S, Fritzler MJ, Baron M, Khalidi N, Canadian Scleroderma Research Group. Systemic sclerosis sine scleroderma: a multicenter study of 1417 subjects. J Rheumatol. 2014;41(11):2179–85. https://doi.org/10.3899/jrheum.140236. Epub 2014 Oct 1. PMID: 25274885.
75. Wigley FM, Seibold JR, Wise RA, McCloskey DA, Dole WP. Intravenous iloprost treatment of Raynaud's phenomenon and ischemic ulcers secondary to systemic sclerosis. J Rheumatol. 1992;19(9):1407–14. PMID: 1279170.

Chapter 5
Capillaroscopy in Dermatomyositis

Francesco Bonomi and Silvia Bellando Randone

Dermatomyositis in the Spectrum of Idiopathic Inflammatory Myopathies

Introduction

Dermatomyositis (DM) is one of the major subtypes of the idiopathic inflammatory myopathies (IIM), a heterogeneous group of rare autoimmune muscle diseases that often have multiorgan involvement [1]. DM classically presents with a subacute onset of symmetrical proximal muscle weakness accompanied by hallmark cutaneous lesions, distinguishing it clinically from polymyositis (PM) and other myositis subsets [1]. In contrast to DM, the entity of PM (muscle inflammation without skin findings) has become contested and is now considered a diagnosis of exclusion. Other IIM subgroups include immune-mediated necrotizing myopathy (IMNM), anti-synthetase syndrome (ASAS), overlap myositis (OM), and inclusion body myositis (IBM), each defined by different clinical patterns and immunopathology [2]. DM is set apart by its prominent skin manifestations and a propensity for microangiopathy, features not usually seen in pure PM. Clinical expression in DM is

F. Bonomi
Department of Internal Medicine, University Hospital Careggi, Florence, Italy
e-mail: francesco.bonomi@unifi.it

S. B. Randone (✉)
Department of Experimental and Clinical Medicine, University of Florence, Florence, Italy

Division of Rheumatology and Scleroderma Unit, University Hospital Careggi, Florence, Italy

Y. El Miedany, R. A. Elziaty (eds.), *Capillaroscopy*, Contemporary Rheumatology,
https://doi.org/10.1007/978-3-032-22966-3_5

remarkably heterogeneous: some patients have the full classic phenotype of proximal weakness with Gottron's papules and heliotrope rash, while others may have minimal to no muscle involvement or atypical features [3]. This variability often correlates with distinct myositis-specific autoantibodies (MSAs). For example, anti-Mi-2 antibodies are associated with the classic DM rash, severe weakness with very high creatine kinase levels, and a favorable response to therapy. In contrast, anti-TIF1γ (also called anti-p155) marks a subset of DM with increased risk of internal malignancy (reported in around 15–25% of these patients) and may have only mild muscle involvement [4]. Another subset is anti-MDA5-positive DM, typically presenting as clinically amyopathic dermatomyositis (CADM); these patients often lack significant muscle weakness but develop aggressive interstitial lung disease (ILD) and painful skin ulcerations [5]. Indeed, anti-MDA5 DM is characterized by severe vasculopathic features (e.g., digital infarcts, palmar papules) and a high mortality from rapidly progressive lung disease [6]. Thus, "dermatomyositis" in adults actually encompasses a spectrum of overlapping syndromes defined by autoantibodies, clinical features, and outcomes. It is also useful to contrast adult DM with juvenile dermatomyositis (JDM): both share the hallmark skin and muscle symptoms, but JDM often exhibits more severe vasculopathy, leading to a higher frequency of ulcerative skin lesions and dystrophic calcinosis in children. Conversely, malignancy is a concern predominantly in adult DM [7]. This clinical heterogeneity underscores the need to understand DM's unique pathophysiology and diagnostic markers, such as nailfold capillaroscopy (NVC), which can help differentiate DM from other myositis subtypes and guide evaluation of systemic involvement.

Pathophysiology of Dermatomyositis: Endothelial Injury, Interferon Pathways, and Autoimmunity

DM is fundamentally an immune-mediated microangiopathy. A central pathogenic event is injury to endothelial cells in muscle capillaries, which leads to capillary loss, tissue ischemia, and the characteristic perifascicular muscle fiber atrophy [8]. Immunopathology studies of DM muscle biopsies have shown deposition of the complement membrane attack complex (MAC, C5b-9) along endomysial capillaries, especially in perifascicular areas, even in early disease before lymphocytic infiltrates appear [8]. This complement activation in DM can be triggered via the classical pathway (with C1q deposition on capillaries) despite an absence of bound immunoglobulin, suggesting complement may be activated by nontraditional mechanisms [8]. The result is a membrane attack complex-mediated destruction of capillaries, causing ischemic muscle damage. In support of the role of complement, active DM patients have elevated circulating levels of complement split products (C3a, C5b-9) compared to inactive disease, and treatment with intravenous immunoglobulins (IVIG), which can inhibit complement, leads to a reduction of muscle C3/MAC deposits alongside clinical improvement [8]. The endomysial capillaries are among the earliest immune targets in DM, underlining endothelial injury as a central pathogenetic feature of the disease [9].

In parallel with humoral complement-mediated damage, DM has a prominent type I interferon (IFN) immune signature [10]. Muscle biopsies and blood samples from DM patients show marked overexpression of type I IFN-inducible genes, a pattern of "interferonopathy" that is far less pronounced in other myositis subtypes [11]. Plasmacytoid dendritic cells, the principal producers of IFN-α/β, infiltrate DM muscle tissue and likely drive local IFN production. The upregulation of IFN-stimulated genes (such as MxA and ISG15) in DM muscle correlates with disease activity and muscle fiber regeneration attempts. For instance, one study found that serum IFN-β protein (a type I IFN) was elevated in DM patients and correlated with the IFN gene signature and with cutaneous disease severity. The IFN pathway thus appears to contribute to endothelial activation and perpetuation of the immune response in DM, possibly linking to the vasculopathic features. Type II IFN-γ activity has also been noted in DM, reflecting a broad activation of cytokine pathways. In addition to IFN, other immune effector mechanisms in DM include a perimysial inflammatory infiltrate rich in CD4+ T cells and B cells and the upregulation of MHC class I on muscle fibers, but these are secondary to the initial microvascular injury [12].

The presence of myositis-specific autoantibodies (MSAs) in DM patients is another key to its pathogenesis and clinical diversity. At least five MSAs are closely associated with DM, each identifying a subset with distinct immunologic features [13]. Some evidence suggests certain MSAs might contribute to disease mechanisms: for example, TIF1γ antibodies have been hypothesized to relate to oncogenic processes or immune surveillance (explaining their link with cancer) [14]. Others, like anti-MDA5, point to the involvement of specific pathways such as innate antiviral responses; MDA5 is a cytosolic RNA sensor, and patients with anti-MDA5 DM have an extreme IFN-driven phenotype (clinically amyopathic with high IFN levels and vascular injury in skin and lung) [15]. Overall, the pathophysiology of DM appears to arise from a confluence of humoral autoimmunity (complement-fixing autoantibodies attacking endothelium), cell-mediated inflammation, and innate immune activation (IFN signaling), which together cause a small-vessel vasculopathy in muscle and skin (Fig. 5.1). This microangiopathy is the thread that links the muscle weakness, skin lesions, and systemic manifestations of DM. Notably, DM's vascular involvement is systemic; recent reviews emphasize that DM patients have an increased risk of ischemic complications such as retinal vascular occlusion and even cerebrovascular events due to their disease-related vasculitis and thrombosis tendency [16]. Understanding this mechanistic backdrop provides insight into the clinical features of DM, especially those related to vascular compromise, and the role of NVC in detecting and monitoring the microvascular changes.

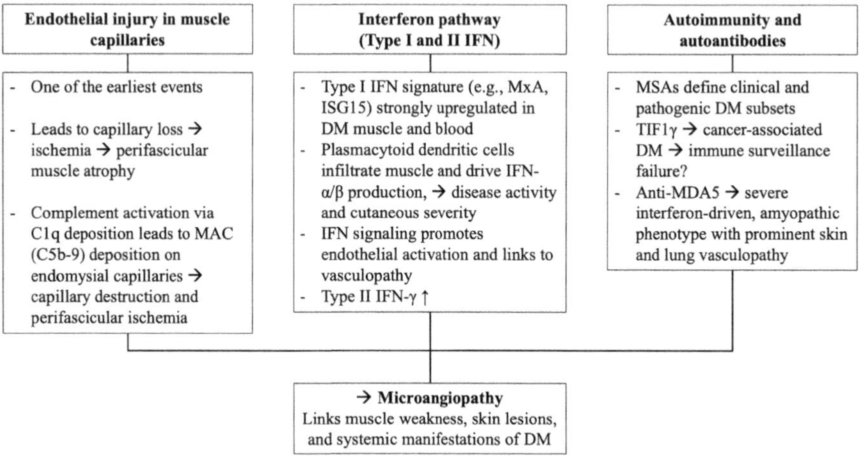

Fig. 5.1 Pathogenic triad of dermatomyositis: endothelial injury, interferonopathy, and autoimmunity. The pathophysiology of dermatomyositis (DM) arises from the interplay of three interconnected immune mechanisms. (1) Endothelial injury in muscle capillaries, mediated by complement activation and membrane attack complex (MAC) deposition, leads to capillary dropout, ischemia, and perifascicular atrophy. (2) Type I and II interferon pathways are highly upregulated in DM, driven by plasmacytoid dendritic cells and associated with disease activity, cutaneous involvement, and endothelial activation. (3) Myositis-specific autoantibodies (MSAs) define distinct DM subsets and may contribute to pathogenesis, such as anti-TIF1γ in cancer-associated DM and anti-MDA5 in severe, interferon-driven vasculopathic forms. These converging mechanisms result in a systemic microangiopathy, which underlies the muscle, skin, and organ manifestations of the disease

Vasculopathic Clinical Manifestations in Dermatomyositis

Many of the characteristic clinical manifestations of DM can be traced to its underlying vasculopathy and endothelial injury. The cutaneous findings of DM, for example, reflect both inflammation and disordered microcirculation in the skin. Gottron's papules, the raised, violaceous plaques overlying the extensor surfaces of joints, and the heliotrope rash with periorbital edema are pathognomonic skin signs [9]. These features result from interface dermatitis and complement-mediated damage in dermal capillaries, leading to edema and inflammation in sun-exposed or mechanically stressed areas of skin. Patients often have periungual erythema and dilated capillary loops at the nailfolds visible on microscopy, sometimes accompanied by splinter hemorrhages or cuticular infarcts, which are direct clinical evidence of the nailfold microangiopathy [17]. In more severe cases, especially in certain DM subsets, frank skin ulcerations can occur. Painful fingertip or periungual ulcers are most classically seen in anti-MDA5-positive DM, where they result from severe digital ischemia secondary to the small vessel vasculopathy [8]. Skin ulcers and even areas of necrosis can also be seen in long-standing juvenile DM or very active adult DM, often heralding a high degree of vascular damage. Indeed, the development of ulcerative skin lesions in DM is a red flag, as it is associated with more aggressive disease and internal involvement [9].

Raynaud's phenomenon, episodic digital ischemia causing finger blanching in the cold, is another common feature in adult DM, reflecting heightened vasospasm reactivity in the context of an abnormal microvasculature. Many DM patients experience Raynaud's, and its presence correlates with capillaroscopic abnormalities; in one cohort, those with a "scleroderma-like" capillary pattern were much more likely to have Raynaud's phenomenon noted on exam [17]. This underscores that the same microvascular dysfunction seen in nailfold capillaries extends to other vascular beds such as the digital arteries.

Beyond the skin, DM's vasculopathy can affect internal organs. ILD is one of the most significant systemic complications of DM [18]. Up to 20–40% of adult DM patients develop ILD, ranging from mild chronic interstitial changes to rapidly progressive, life-threatening pneumonitis. While the pathogenesis of myositis-associated ILD involves immune-mediated alveolitis, there is also an important vascular component: damage to pulmonary capillaries and endothelial cells (for example, via IFN-mediated mechanisms) likely contributes to the development of ILD in DM [9]. The association is especially strong in clinical subsets like anti-MDA5-positive DM, where a fulminant diffuse ILD can develop early and is the leading cause of mortality [6]. Notably, patients with DM who display a scleroderma-type nailfold capillaroscopic pattern tend to have a higher frequency of ILD, suggesting that the degree of systemic microangiopathy (as evidenced by capillary changes) parallels the risk of lung involvement [17].

Less commonly, gastrointestinal and cardiac manifestations in DM can also be linked to vasculopathy. In juvenile DM, severe vasculitis of the gastrointestinal tract can cause abdominal pain, bleeding, or even perforation (a feared complication), and this is attributed to the same process of endothelial injury and thrombosis in intestinal vessels [19]. Adult DM patients rarely exhibit such dramatic GI vasculitis, but milder gut involvement (mesenteric ischemia or hemorrhage) can occur in very active disease [19]. Cardiac involvement in DM may present as myocarditis, arrhythmias, or heart failure [20]. Some cases of DM have subclinical myocardial ischemia or fibrosis thought to result from microvascular damage to myocardial capillaries, analogous to the process in skeletal muscle. Additionally, overlap syndromes (such as patients with ASAS or mixed connective tissue disease overlap) can lead to perimyocarditis. Overall, the development of vasculopathy is associated with the most severe extramuscular manifestations of DM, including ulcerative skin lesions, ILD, gastrointestinal ischemia, and cardiac dysfunction [9]. These complications portend a worse prognosis and often require aggressive treatment. It is noteworthy that the burden of vasculopathy differs between patient groups; for instance, juvenile DM tends to have more florid vascular lesions (hence more frequent ulcers and calcinosis), whereas adult DM is more often complicated by malignancy rather than by extreme vascular phenomena [9]. Nonetheless, recognizing signs of vasculopathy in any DM patient is critical, as these signs (e.g., nailfold changes, digital ulcers, Raynaud's) should prompt a thorough search for internal involvement and aggressive management. NVC is one tool that can directly visualize this microvasculopathy, offering a window into the systemic vascular health of DM patients.

Nailfold Capillaroscopic Findings in Dermatomyositis

NVC allows noninvasive in vivo examination of the microcirculation, and in DM it reveals characteristic abnormalities reflecting the disease's microangiopathy. In fact, capillaroscopic changes are so common in DM that they have diagnostic significance; they are often termed a "scleroderma-like" pattern because of their resemblance to the capillary alterations seen in systemic sclerosis [21, 22]. The classic capillaroscopic findings in adult DM include enlarged capillaries, giant capillaries, microhemorrhages, capillary loss, and overall disorganization of the normal capillary array [21]. Capillary enlargement appears as dilated loops, sometimes dramatically expanded (>50 μm diameter) and tortuous; these "giant" capillaries are a hallmark of active microvascular damage. Frequent microhemorrhages, seen as dark spots or hemosiderin deposits around the nailfold, indicate capillary fragility and leakage [21]. With ongoing injury, capillaries are destroyed, leading to areas of avascularity (capillary dropout). Capillary density in DM is often markedly reduced compared to that of normal controls. In a prospective single-center study on 15 DM patients, about 80% had decreased nailfold capillary density at presentation [23]. The remaining capillaries can appear extremely dilated and malformed, and new "ramified" (bushy) capillaries may sprout as evidence of neovascularization in response to tissue ischemia [22]. The overall arrangement of capillaries becomes highly disorganized in DM, losing the neat parallel rows seen in healthy individuals. One analysis found a disorganized capillary architecture in ~72% of adult DM patients, versus only 4% of patients with PM [21]. The net result of these changes is the "scleroderma pattern" on capillaroscopy, defined by the presence of giant capillaries, hemorrhages, and avascular areas. Notably, this pattern is observed in a large proportion of DM patients (reported in approximately 45–82% of cases in different cohorts), whereas it is rarely observed in PM and in healthy individuals [17, 22]. PM patients typically exhibit either normal nailfold capillaries or only mild, nonspecific changes, underscoring a fundamental pathophysiologic difference: significant nailfold capillary abnormalities point strongly toward DM rather than PM [21]. Thus, NVC can help distinguish DM from other myopathies by demonstrating this microangiopathic signature.

It is important to recognize that the capillaroscopic phenotype in DM can vary with disease phase and immunological subset. Early in the disease course, capillary abnormalities tend to be most pronounced. Patients in the first months of active DM often show more giant capillaries and more severe capillary loss than those with longer-standing disease (in one study, DM patients with ≤6 months of disease had significantly lower capillary density and more frequent giant loops than those with a longer disease duration) [21]. A complete scleroderma pattern may be more evident in early, untreated disease (though one series noted this difference as a trend that did not reach statistical significance) [21]. This suggests that as disease activity decreases or the condition transitions to a chronic stage, the microvasculature may partially recover or stabilize, with the development of neovascularization (bushy capillaries) and fewer grossly giant loops. Indeed, longitudinal studies have documented that nailfold capillary density can improve and giant loops can regress over time with effective immunosuppressive therapy [16, 23]. Such findings indicate a degree of reversibility in DM-related microangiopathy, unlike systemic sclerosis, in which advanced capillary loss is typically permanent.

Additionally, distinct autoantibody-defined subsets of DM can exhibit different capillaroscopic profiles. MSAs not only correlate with clinical differences but also with the patterns seen on NFC [24]. For example, patients with anti-TIF1γ antibodies (who often have classic rash and malignancy-associated DM) tend to show a high prevalence of scleroderma-spectrum capillary changes. A recent study noted that 8 out of 10 anti-TIF1γ–positive DM patients had scleroderma-like nailfold abnormalities, including giant capillaries and hemorrhages in many cases [22]. In contrast, patients with ASAS (e.g., anti-Jo-1 antibody) or IMNM often display more nonspecific capillaroscopic changes [25]. In a multicenter cohort, a nonspecific capillary pattern (mild dilations without the full scleroderma features) was the most frequent finding in anti-Jo-1–positive patients and was statistically associated with the ASAS and ILD [25]. Those patients typically showed only mild capillary dilatation and bushy (ramified) capillaries consistent with chronic injury and repair, but not the extensive giant loops or capillary drop-out seen in classic DM [22] (Fig. 5.2). On the other hand, anti-MDA5-positive patients, who have severe vasculopathy clinically, often manifest capillaroscopic patterns of marked capillary loss with extensive microhemorrhages and disorganization [26]. These correlate with the poor-prognosis features of that subset (for instance, one report found that in MDA5-DM, the degree of capillary disarray and bleeding correlated with high serum ferritin, CRP, and KL-6 levels and with lung CT abnormalities) [27]. Another subset, anti-NXP2 antibody–positive DM (more common in juvenile cases but also seen in adults with malignancy-associated DM), has been noted to show prominent capillary dilation and dropout; in one series, all anti-NXP2 patients had enlarged capillaries and reduced density, and the majority had significant hemorrhages as well [22, 24]. Taken together, these findings illustrate that while the "active scleroderma" capillaroscopic pattern is a unifying feature of DM, its prevalence and specific components (giant loops, hemorrhages, bushy neo-vessels, etc.) can differ based on disease duration and the patient's autoantibody profile. Recognizing these patterns not only aids in diagnosis but also provides clues to the phenotype of DM one is dealing with (for instance, a DM patient with many ramified capillaries and few giant loops might have an anti-synthetase overlap, whereas one with massive capillary dropout and hemorrhages might prompt a check for anti-MDA5).

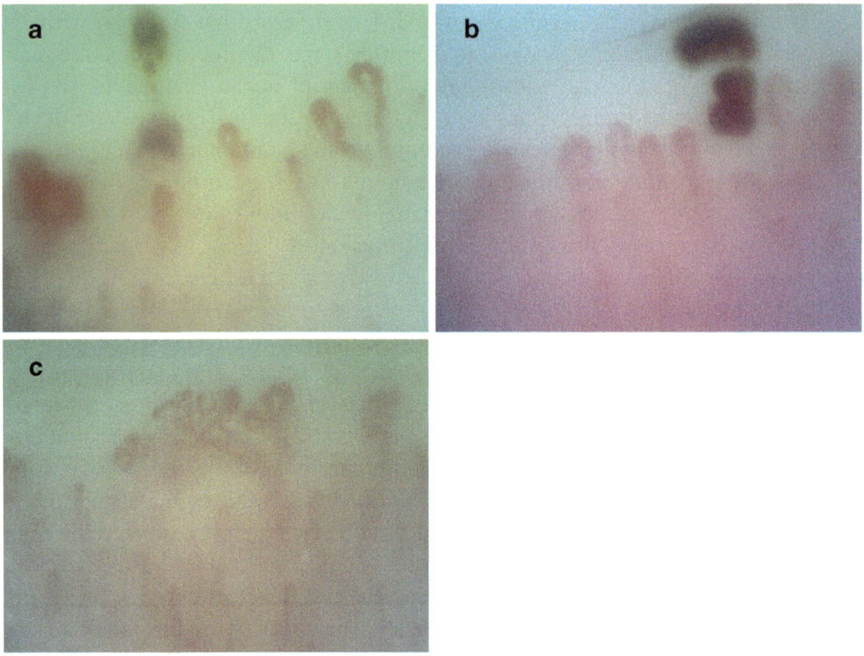

Fig. 5.2 (**a–c**) Representative nailfold videocapillaroscopy findings in dermatomyositis. (**a**) Enlarged and giant capillaries with reduced capillary density; a linear microhemorrhage resembling a "string of pearls" is visible. (**b**) Enlarged capillaries with focal microhemorrhage. (**c**) Neoangiogenesis with branching capillary loops with reduced capillary density

Clinical Utility of Nailfold Capillaroscopy in Dermatomyositis

NVC has emerged as a valuable clinical tool in the evaluation of DM, with important diagnostic, prognostic, and monitoring implications (Fig. 5.3). From a diagnostic standpoint, the presence of a scleroderma-like capillaroscopic pattern can help confirm the clinical impression of DM and distinguish it from other myositis or rheumatic differentials. In a patient presenting with, for example, only rash and vague weakness, finding multiple giant capillaries would strengthen the diagnostic impression of DM rather than PM or other causes of myopathy [21]. Likewise, in an individual with an undifferentiated connective tissue disease (UCTD) or an overlap syndrome, identifying a DM-type capillaroscopic pattern (even in the absence of skin lesions) might prompt a closer look for muscle involvement and DM-specific autoantibodies. Studies comparing IIM subtypes have indeed shown that nailfold changes can differentiate DM from PM: one prospective study comparing 29 DM patients, 23 PM, and 52 healthy controls found that no PM patients or healthy controls displayed a scleroderma pattern on NVC, whereas a majority of DM patients did [21]. Another prospective study comparing 13 CADM and 39 DM patients noted that CADM patients have a similar high prevalence of capillary abnormalities

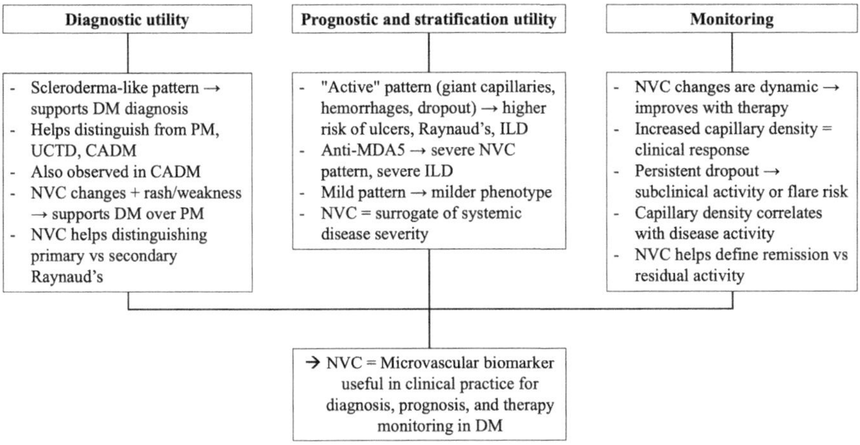

Fig. 5.3 Clinical utility of nailfold videocapillaroscopy (NVC) alterations in dermatomyositis (DM). NVC alterations serve as a valuable microvascular biomarker in DM, with applications across diagnosis, prognostic stratification, and therapeutic monitoring

as classic DM, indicating that NVC can detect microvascular changes even when muscle symptoms are minimal [17]. Moreover, nailfold capillary exams can aid in distinguishing primary Raynaud's phenomenon (where capillaries are normal) from Raynaud's secondary to DM or other systemic rheumatic diseases (where capillary dropout and giant loops would be seen). In essence, the nailfold findings serve as a tangible microvascular biomarker of DM that can increase diagnostic confidence early in the disease course.

Beyond diagnosis, capillaroscopic findings carry prognostic information in DM. Certain capillary abnormalities have been linked to more severe disease and specific complications [28]. For example, the presence of an active scleroderma-type pattern (with extensive giant capillaries, hemorrhages, and avascular areas) correlates with the co-occurrence of critical manifestations like cutaneous ulcerations, Raynaud's, and ILD [17]. In one cohort, DM patients with a scleroderma NVC pattern were significantly more likely to have ILD than those without, suggesting that NVC could help stratify the risk of ILD in DM [17]. Similarly, as mentioned, the subset of anti-MDA5 patients who have extreme nailfold changes (capillary dropout and hemorrhages) also tend to have worse prognostic indicators (high ferritin, severe ILD) [26]. These observations suggest that the extent of nailfold microangiopathy may serve as a surrogate marker for systemic disease severity in DM; patients with "milder" capillaroscopic changes may exhibit a more limited disease phenotype, whereas those with severe patterns might warrant more aggressive monitoring and therapy. There is also evidence that NVC can help predict treatment response and track disease activity over time [23, 29]. Because DM capillary abnormalities are dynamic and can improve with effective treatment, serial NVC exams can be used as an objective measure of microvascular recovery or ongoing damage. In a prospective study of adult DM patients, nearly all had abnormal nailfolds at baseline, but after a period of immunosuppressive therapy, there was a statistically significant improvement in capillary density and a reduction in giant capillary diameter and microhemorrhages [23]. Concurrently, those improvements in capillary morphology were associated with clinical disease improvement. In that study, lower capillary density and more microhemorrhages were correlated with higher disease activity scores, while patients who went into remission showed capillary density restoration [23]. Multivariate analysis confirmed that capillary density inversely tracked global disease activity, independent of traditional lab markers. This is notable because conventional biomarkers like creatine kinase (CK) or C-reactive protein (CRP) often do not reliably reflect disease fluctuations in DM. Thus, NVC provides a window into the ongoing disease process: capillary dropout signals active disease, and its persistence or worsening may predict an impending flare, whereas rising capillary counts and normalization of capillary loops could indicate a successful treatment response. Indeed, a multiethnic study reported that after treatment, DM patients showed an increase in capillary density and a decrease in avascular areas and giant capillaries, paralleling clinical improvement [25]. Such findings pave the way for using NVC in routine practice to monitor DM; for instance, a clinician might serially image the nailfolds to help decide if a patient is truly in remission or if subclinical disease activity persists in the microvasculature.

In summary, NVC in DM is far more than a research curiosity: it has practical applications in diagnosing DM, in prognostication (identifying patients at risk for severe organ involvement), and in potentially guiding therapy by monitoring microvascular changes. As a safe, noninvasive bedside tool, NVC can be repeated over time, allowing clinicians to visualize improvements or new damage to capillaries as treatment is adjusted. The strong association between NVC abnormalities and DM-specific autoantibodies further enhances its utility—for example, a scleroderma-pattern NVC in a patient initially classified as having "polymyositis" might prompt testing for a DM-specific antibody like TIF1γ or NXP2, thereby unmasking a misclassified DM overlap. Given all these advantages, NVC has become a valuable extension of the clinical examination in idiopathic inflammatory myopathies.

Having outlined the pathogenesis, clinical features, and capillaroscopic profile of DM, we now turn to illustrative clinical cases. These cases will demonstrate how NVC findings correlate with patient presentation and outcomes and how they can be applied in real-world diagnostic and management decisions for adult DM.

Case 1: Paraneoplastic-Like Anti-TIF1γ Dermatomyositis Mimicking Malignancy in a Patient with Rifampicin-Resistant Tuberculous Lymphadenitis

Clinical Presentation

A 52-year-old woman with no prior history of autoimmune disease presented to the clinic with a 6-month history of progressive cutaneous manifestations characterized by heliotrope rash and violaceous erythema of the face, as well as papular lesions over the metacarpophalangeal joints, consistent with Gottron's papules. She reported generalized fatigue and mild dysphagia for solids but denied Raynaud phenomenon, sicca symptoms, or inflammatory arthritis.

On physical examination, the heliotrope rash was clearly visible, accompanied by subtle periorbital edema. Gottron's papules were noted together with an erythematous rash over the dorsum of the hands, and on the elbows and knees. The periungual areas were erythematous, with some capillary telangiectasias. Neuromuscular assessment revealed moderate symmetrical proximal muscle weakness (MRC grade 3/5 at the hip flexors and shoulder abductors), while distal muscle strength was fully preserved. There was no muscle atrophy or fasciculations. Deep tendon reflexes were preserved and symmetric. Cardiovascular and respiratory examinations were unremarkable, with no abnormal breath sounds. No digital ulcers or joint swelling was noted. The patient appeared markedly underweight, with a height of 160 cm and a weight of 42 kg (BMI 16.4).

Diagnostic Work-Up

Initial laboratory investigations revealed a microcytic normochromic anemia (hemoglobin 9.7 g/dL), along with significantly elevated lactate dehydrogenase (LDH 719 U/L), mildly increased creatine kinase (CPK 199 U/L), and aldolase (17 U/L). Inflammatory markers were also elevated, with an erythrocyte sedimentation rate (ESR) of 54 mm/h and C-reactive protein (CRP) at 28 mg/L, suggesting ongoing systemic inflammation. Antinuclear antibodies (ANA) were positive at a titer of 1:320 with a fine speckled pattern, and myositis-specific serology confirmed marked positivity for anti-TIF1γ antibodies.

Given the prominent periungual erythema and vasculitic skin features, a NVC was performed early in the diagnostic work-up (Fig. 5.4). The exam revealed a scleroderma-like capillaroscopic pattern, characterized by reduced capillary density (<7 capillaries/mm), significant architectural disorganization, frequent giant capillaries, and bushy, ramified loops. Although no extensive avascular areas were present, the overall picture was consistent with active and severe microangiopathy. The

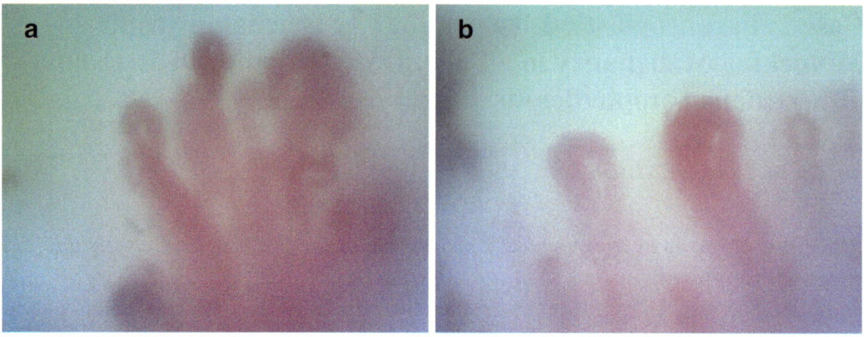

Fig. 5.4 (**a**, **b**) Nailfold videocapillaroscopy showing reduced capillary density, architectural disorganization, and giant, bushy, and ramified capillaries

identification of these capillary abnormalities further supported the diagnosis of DM and suggested prominent systemic microangiopathy.

In light of the proximal muscle weakness and elevated muscle enzymes, an MRI of the proximal lower limbs was performed. The scan revealed extensive symmetrical hyperintensity on short-tau inversion recovery (STIR) sequences involving the quadriceps, gluteal, and adductor muscle groups bilaterally. These findings were consistent with active inflammatory myositis and confirmed the muscular involvement despite the relatively mild elevation in serum CPK levels.

Given the combination of cutaneous findings, muscle inflammation, and serological positivity for anti-TIF1γ antibodies, a profile frequently associated with paraneoplastic DM, an extensive oncologic screening was promptly initiated. Contrast-enhanced thoracoabdominal imaging revealed multiple enlarged lymph nodes in the cervical, supraclavicular, and axillary regions, raising concern for underlying malignancy or an infectious granulomatous disease. The detection of lymphadenopathy in this context reinforced the need for tissue sampling and a comprehensive diagnostic evaluation to exclude an occult neoplasm.

The patient was admitted for further evaluation due to suspected lymphoma. Imaging revealed bilateral hilar and mediastinal lymphadenopathy. A lymph node biopsy ultimately confirmed tuberculous lymphadenitis with rifampicin resistance. She began second-line antitubercular therapy with a combination regimen including bedaquiline, linezolid, moxifloxacin, and isoniazid.

Therapeutic Approach

Given the active infectious process and the diagnosis of drug-resistant tuberculosis, the use of immunosuppressive therapy, such as high-dose corticosteroids, methotrexate, or mycophenolate mofetil, was initially contraindicated. However, in the context of rapidly worsening cutaneous manifestations, progressive proximal muscle weakness, and severe cachexia (with body weight declining to 36 kg), it was deemed necessary to introduce IVIG at immunomodulatory doses of 2 g/kg/month. Additionally, hydroxychloroquine (5 mg/kg/day) was introduced to manage cutaneous symptoms but was discontinued shortly thereafter due to a severe drug-induced exanthem.

Following the initiation of effective antitubercular therapy and under close supervision by infectious disease specialists, corticosteroid therapy was introduced at high doses. This resulted in progressive improvement of both cutaneous lesions and muscle strength. Once TB treatment was stabilized and lymphadenopathy regressed, methotrexate was introduced as a steroid-sparing agent, initiated at 10 mg/week subcutaneously with folic acid supplementation. A tapering schedule for corticosteroids was established, aiming to reduce long-term steroid exposure.

Progressive clinical improvement was observed over the following months. The patient reported a gradual reduction in fatigue, pruritus, and muscle weakness. Inflammatory markers normalized (CPK <200 U/L, LDH <300 U/L), and follow-up thoracic CT showed no evidence of TB reactivation or progression of lymphadenopathy. Cutaneous involvement remained mild and clinically stable, with faint erythema persisting over the dorsal knuckles and subtle residual heliotrope discoloration around the eyelids.

Discussion

This case illustrates the complex management of DM in the presence of a coexisting chronic infectious disease, such as multidrug-resistant tuberculosis. The delay in the use of conventional immunosuppressants posed significant therapeutic challenges, with reliance on IVIG and corticosteroids for disease control. The presence of anti-TIF1γ antibodies, usually associated with cancer-associated myositis, raised the initial concern for malignancy, which was ruled out after comprehensive evaluation. Instead, the coexistence of TB lymphadenitis, rare in high-income countries, underscores the importance of thorough differential diagnosis in patients presenting with lymphadenopathy and systemic inflammation.

The early detection of a scleroderma-like capillaroscopic pattern provided essential support for the diagnosis of DM and justified further histopathological investigations. Beyond its diagnostic utility, the NVC findings were reflective of an underlying systemic vasculopathy. The observed microangiopathy—marked by capillary rarefaction, ramified loops, and microhemorrhages—mirrored the vascular pathology seen both in the skin, with periungual erythema and vasculitic features, and in the muscle, as evidenced by cachexia and MRI findings consistent with active inflammatory infiltration. This case underscores the clinical relevance of NVC not only in diagnosis but also in capturing systemic microvascular disease burden—serving as a valuable adjunct in complex cases where conventional diagnostic or serological parameters may be inconclusive.

Case 2: Dermatomyositis with Anti-NXP2, Calcinosis, Severe Capillaroscopic Changes, and Chronic Course

Clinical Presentation

A 48-year-old woman presented with a one-year history of progressive muscle weakness and recurrent skin ulcerations on the lower limbs and gluteal region. The patient reported the initial appearance of firm, painful subcutaneous nodules, later confirmed as calcifications, with gradual extension. She also reported severe fatigue and diffuse myalgias but denied Raynaud's phenomenon, sicca syndrome, or dysphagia. At presentation, she was significantly limited in her daily activities due to pain and fatigue.

Her past medical history was unremarkable, and no family history of autoimmune or neuromuscular diseases was noted.

On physical examination, there was marked hypotrophy of the proximal musculature in both upper and lower limbs, particularly affecting the thighs and pelvic girdle. Manual muscle testing revealed significant proximal weakness, with strength graded as 2/5 in the deltoids, iliopsoas, and quadriceps bilaterally. Distal strength was preserved, and there were no fasciculations or distal atrophy. Deep tendon reflexes were present and symmetric, and no sensory deficits were elicited. The most striking cutaneous finding consisted of multiple firm calcified subcutaneous nodules involving the lateral and posterior aspects of the thighs, as well as the gluteal region. Several of these lesions were associated with overlying skin ulceration, with areas of crusting, erythema, and signs of chronic inflammation. There was no joint swelling or tenderness suggestive of active arthritis. Nailfolds were erythematous, but digital ulcers and telangiectasias were absent. Cardiopulmonary examination was unremarkable with a normal heart and clear lung auscultation. Abdominal and neurological examinations were otherwise within normal limits.

Diagnostic Work-Up

Laboratory tests revealed mild normocytic anemia (Hb 10.4 g/dL), elevated CK (1480 U/L), LDH (520 U/L), and aldolase (13 U/L). CRP and ESR were slightly elevated. ANA was positive at 1:160 with a speckled pattern. Myositis-specific antibody testing returned positive for anti-NXP2 antibodies.

Electromyography (EMG) of proximal muscles showed findings consistent with irritable myopathy, including small-amplitude, short-duration, polyphasic motor unit potentials, with spontaneous fibrillation potentials and positive sharp waves, most prominent in the quadriceps and deltoid muscles.

MRI of the thighs revealed diffuse hyperintensity on STIR and T2-weighted sequences predominantly involving the vastus lateralis, biceps femoris, and adductor groups bilaterally. These changes were indicative of active muscle inflammation, without evidence of fatty replacement or advanced fibrosis.

To confirm the diagnosis histologically, a biopsy of the left quadriceps muscle was performed. Histopathologic examination revealed classic features of DM, including perifascicular atrophy, perivascular and endomysial inflammatory infiltrates composed primarily of CD4+ T lymphocytes and macrophages, and scattered necrotic fibers undergoing myophagocytosis. No inclusion bodies or rimmed vacuoles were observed.

High-resolution computed tomography (HRCT) of the chest excluded ILD, showing preserved parenchymal architecture without ground-glass opacities, reticulations, or traction bronchiectasis. Echocardiography showed normal cardiac chamber dimensions and function, with no pericardial effusion or regional wall motion abnormalities.

Given the association between anti-NXP2 positivity and malignancy, an extensive neoplastic work-up was undertaken. Mammography and pelvic ultrasound revealed no abnormalities, and a contrast-enhanced thoracoabdominal CT scan showed no suspicious lesions or lymphadenopathy. The overall evaluation excluded an occult neoplasm at the time of diagnosis.

NVC revealed important microangiopathy characterized by enlarged bushy capillaries and markedly reduced capillary density, consistent with a "scleroderma pattern" (Fig. 5.5). Although not specific for DM, these findings supported extensive microvascular involvement, providing additional prognostic stratification, especially in light of the extensive calcinosis.

Radiographs of thighs and pelvis confirmed the presence of extensive, sheet-like calcifications of the soft tissues, with some phlebolith-like structures and no bone involvement. CT imaging supported the extent and depth of calcium deposits, reaching the interfascial planes of the thigh muscles.

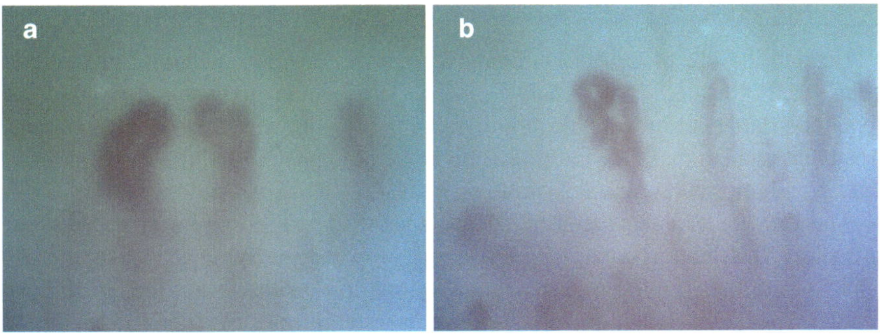

Fig. 5.5 (**a**, **b**) Nailfold videocapillaroscopy showing enlarged and bushy capillaries and reduced capillary density

Therapeutic Approach

The patient was initially treated with intravenous methylprednisolone pulses (1 g/day for 3 days), followed by oral prednisone 1 mg/kg/day. Methotrexate (20 mg/week subcutaneously) with folic acid supplementation was added 2 weeks later. After 6 months, disease activity persisted with progressive calcinosis and only minimal improvement in muscle strength; treatment was switched to mycophenolate mofetil (2 g/day), with a partial response.

Due to refractory calcinosis and persistently elevated muscle enzymes, IVIG (2 g/kg/month) was administered. This led to stabilization of muscle strength and subjective improvement in fatigue and pain, although calcinosis remained unchanged.

During the second year of follow-up, the patient experienced a flare of cutaneous ulcers and pain; treatment was escalated with rituximab (two 1-g doses 2 weeks apart). This induced partial control of the skin component and halted the progression of calcinosis.

Supportive treatments included intensive physiotherapy, pain control, and surgical consultation for possible excision of calcified masses, although no surgical intervention was ultimately performed.

Discussion

This case illustrates a severe, chronic course of DM associated with anti-NXP2 antibodies, complicated by extensive calcinosis, prominent vasculopathy, and significant functional impairment. Anti-NXP2 positivity has been linked to more severe myositis and a higher frequency of calcinosis, particularly in juvenile forms but also in adults.

The presence of severe microangiopathy on NVC, although not pathognomonic, supported the concept of an aggressive vasculopathic phenotype. This aligned with recent studies showing that endothelial dysfunction may contribute to ectopic calcification in DM, especially when chronic inflammation and tissue ischemia are present.

Despite the use of multiple immunosuppressive agents—including glucocorticoids, methotrexate, mycophenolate mofetil, IVIG, and rituximab—the calcinosis remained stable but irreversible, highlighting the importance of early diagnosis and treatment escalation. IVIG and rituximab proved effective in stabilizing the disease course and improving muscle symptoms.

This case underscores the need for a personalized, multidisciplinary approach in refractory DM, with special attention to vasculopathy markers such as capillaroscopy and antibody profiling. A structured follow-up plan was established, including regular clinical assessments every 3–4 months to monitor disease activity and treatment response. Given the initial severity of capillaroscopic abnormalities, repeat NVC is planned annually or in the event of clinical flare to assess microvascular recovery or progression. Although initial oncologic screening was negative, ongoing vigilance is warranted due to anti-NXP2 positivity; repeat malignancy screening (including imaging and age-appropriate cancer screening tests) will be considered annually or if new clinical signs suggest neoplasia.

Case 3: Classic Dermatomyositis with Anti-Mi-2 Antibodies and Reversible Scleroderma-Like Capillaroscopic Pattern

Clinical Presentation

A 45-year-old woman presented to our outpatient rheumatology clinic complaining of progressive fatigue and proximal muscle weakness that had developed insidiously over the previous 4 months. She described a gradual reduction in her ability to perform daily activities, including climbing stairs, rising from a seated position, and lifting objects above shoulder level. In addition to muscular symptoms, she reported the onset of a purplish rash over her upper eyelids and scaly red plaques over the backs of her hands and elbows. These cutaneous lesions had been present for several weeks and were exacerbated by sun exposure, though they were neither painful nor pruritic. She denied joint pain, Raynaud's phenomenon, dysphagia, or respiratory symptoms.

Her past medical history was unremarkable, and she was not on any regular medications. She was a nonsmoker and had no family history of autoimmune or neuromuscular diseases.

On physical examination, the patient appeared well, afebrile, with normal vital signs. A typical heliotrope rash with subtle periorbital edema was observed, along with erythematous-violet facial discoloration, consistent with photosensitive dermatosis. Gottron's papules were evident over the metacarpophalangeal and proximal interphalangeal joints, as well as over the elbows and knees, where flat-topped, violaceous papules were accompanied by mild desquamation. No digital ulcers, telangiectasias, or signs of vasculopathy were observed at the fingertips. There were no oral ulcers or alopecia. Manual muscle testing revealed symmetrical weakness of the deltoids and hip flexors, graded 4/5 on the Medical Research Council scale, without pain on movement or significant atrophy. Distal muscle groups were preserved. Cardiac and pulmonary auscultation revealed no abnormalities, and the remainder of the physical examination was unremarkable.

Diagnostic Work-Up

Laboratory tests showed a hemoglobin level of 11.8 g/dL, with normal white cell and platelet counts. Serum CK was markedly elevated at 3950 U/L, and LDH was 678 U/L. Aldolase was also elevated (15 U/L), while liver and renal function tests were within normal limits. ESR was 49 mm/h, and Crp was modestly increased at 13 mg/L. ANA was positive at a titer of 1:640 with a speckled pattern.

A myositis-specific autoantibody panel was obtained and revealed positivity for anti-Mi-2 antibodies. All other tested autoantibodies were negative.

The thighs' MRI demonstrated diffuse, symmetrical STIR hyperintensity affecting the quadriceps, adductors, and gluteal muscles, indicative of active inflammatory myopathy. EMG confirmed a myopathic pattern, with small-amplitude, polyphasic motor unit potentials and fibrillation potentials, especially in proximal muscle groups. A quadriceps muscle biopsy was considered but ultimately deferred due to the concordant clinical, serological, and radiological findings.

HRCT of the chest showed no ILD or pleural effusions, and pulmonary function tests, including diffusing capacity for carbon monoxide, were normal. Transthoracic echocardiography did not reveal any structural or functional cardiac abnormalities. A malignancy screening, including mammography, pelvic ultrasound, and abdominal imaging, was negative.

As part of the systemic evaluation, a NVC was performed (Fig. 5.6). Despite the absence of Raynaud phenomenon, the exam revealed clear microvascular abnormalities. The capillaroscopic pattern was consistent with an active scleroderma-like pattern, characterized by the presence of several giant capillaries. Some microhemorrhages were also noted. The overall architecture was relatively preserved, without significant neoangiogenesis or severe disorganization. Although such a pattern is more typically associated with systemic sclerosis, similar changes have been described in DM and are believed to reflect active microvascular injury, particularly in the early inflammatory phases. In this patient, the NVC findings supported the

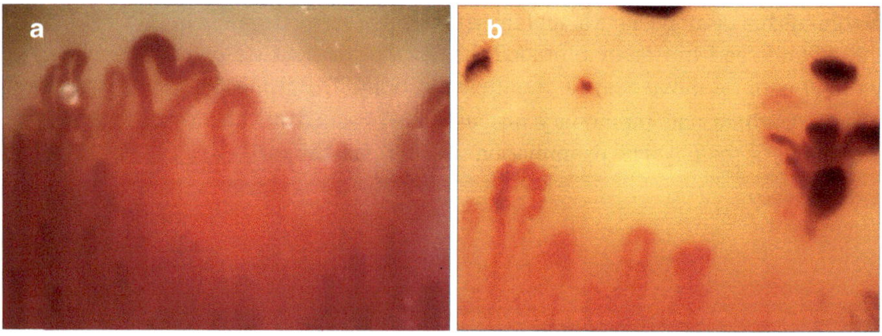

Fig. 5.6 (**a**, **b**) Nailfold videocapillaroscopy showing giant and enlarged capillaries. Microhemorrhages are also observed

presence of systemic vasculopathy and added weight to the diagnosis of inflammatory myopathy.

Therapeutic Approach

The patient began treatment with intravenous methylprednisolone (1 g/day for 3 days), followed by oral prednisone at 1 mg/kg/day. Due to the severity of muscle involvement and significant elevation of CPK, she was also started on two monthly cycles of IVIG at a dose of 2 g/kg per cycle, divided over 3 days. After stabilization of acute symptoms and mild improvement in muscle strength, methotrexate was introduced at a dose of 15 mg per week subcutaneously, with folic acid supplementation, to serve as a steroid-sparing agent.

Within 1 month of starting treatment, the patient reported a dramatic improvement in muscle strength, energy levels, and skin appearance. The heliotrope rash faded significantly, and Gottron's papules became less prominent. Her CPK dropped to 620 U/L by week 4 and normalized (<200 U/L) by week 10. Prednisone was gradually tapered by 10 mg every 2–3 weeks, and methotrexate was increased to 20 mg/week. The patient tolerated treatment well and experienced no infectious or gastrointestinal complications.

Six months after therapy initiation, the patient underwent repeat NVC. The exam revealed a clear regression of previous abnormalities: microhemorrhages had resolved completely, giant capillaries were no longer visible, and capillary density had improved to approximately 9 capillaries per millimeter. The capillary loops had regained a more regular, parallel orientation with only rare dilated loops and no signs of neoangiogenesis. This improvement paralleled the favorable clinical response, supporting the notion that capillaroscopic changes may reflect not only disease activity but also therapeutic efficacy.

At the one-year follow-up, the patient remained in complete clinical and biochemical remission. She continued methotrexate (20 mg/week) and low-dose prednisone (5 mg/day), without recurrence of skin lesions or muscle symptoms. Follow-up MRI of the thighs showed complete resolution of inflammatory edema, and pulmonary function remained normal. She resumed full-time work and regular physical activity without restrictions.

Discussion

This case exemplifies a typical presentation of classic DM associated with anti-Mi-2 antibodies, which is frequently characterized by prominent cutaneous manifestations, significant but reversible muscle involvement, and excellent responsiveness to immunosuppressive therapy. The anti-Mi-2 phenotype is often associated with a lower risk of systemic complications such as ILD or malignancy and carries a generally favorable prognosis when treated promptly. Importantly, NVC proved a valuable noninvasive tool in this case. It supported the diagnosis during the initial work-up and mirrored the resolution of disease activity over time. Although traditionally associated with systemic sclerosis, capillaroscopic patterns may provide important insights into the vascular pathophysiology of DM and help monitor therapeutic response in selected patients.

Case 4: Clinically Amyopathic Dermatomyositis with Anti-MDA5 Antibodies and Rapidly Progressive ILD

Clinical Presentation

A 38-year-old man was referred to our clinic for evaluation of persistent low-grade fever, joint pain, and progressive cutaneous lesions affecting the hands. His symptoms had begun approximately 3 weeks prior, with the insidious onset of symmetrical arthralgias involving the wrists and metacarpophalangeal joints. Soon thereafter, he developed painful papular eruptions over the palms and lateral aspects of the fingers, followed by shallow ulcerations on the distal fingertips. Despite the systemic and cutaneous symptoms, he denied muscle weakness, fatigue, dysphagia, Raynaud's phenomenon, or sicca symptoms.

His past medical history was unremarkable, with no prior diagnoses of autoimmune, pulmonary, or dermatologic conditions. He was a nonsmoker, with no relevant occupational exposures and no family history of connective tissue disease or ILD.

On physical examination, the patient appeared in good general condition but was febrile (temperature 37.8 °C) and reported localized pain in the fingers. Cutaneous inspection revealed multiple violaceous macules and papules along the palmar surfaces and lateral aspects of the digits, particularly over the hypothenar eminences and the lateral sides of the index and middle fingers, consistent with palmar papules. The periungual areas showed erythema and subtle telangiectasias. Several shallow, painful ulcerations were present on the distal aspects of the second and third digits bilaterally, with signs of incipient ischemic damage. There was no evidence of heliotrope rash, Gottron's papules, poikiloderma, or scalp involvement. Neuromuscular examination revealed full strength (MRC grade 5/5) in all proximal and distal muscle groups of both upper and lower extremities. No muscle atrophy, tenderness, or abnormal tone was observed. Deep tendon reflexes were preserved and symmetric. Cardiac examination was normal. Pulmonary auscultation revealed fine bibasilar crackles, raising concern for early interstitial involvement. No lymphadenopathy or organomegaly was noted on abdominal palpation.

Diagnostic Work-Up

Laboratory investigations demonstrated elevated markers of systemic inflammation, with an ESR of 48 mm/h and CRP at 6.2 mg/dL. Serum ferritin was markedly elevated at 720 ng/mL, raising suspicion for a hyperinflammatory state. Muscle enzymes were within normal limits, with CK at 98 U/L and aldolase in the normal range, consistent with the clinically amyopathic phenotype. Complete blood count and metabolic panel, including liver and renal function tests, were unremarkable.

Autoimmune serologies revealed a positive ANA titer of 1:640 with a fine-speckled cytoplasmic pattern. Myositis-specific antibody testing confirmed strong positivity for anti-MDA5 antibodies, supporting the diagnosis of a vasculopathic subtype of CADM.

Given the periungual erythema and digital ulcerations, a NVC was performed and revealed severe microangiopathy (Fig. 5.7). The capillaroscopic findings included a markedly reduced capillary density (less than 5 capillaries per mm) and disorganized capillary architecture with frequent ramified and bushy capillaries. Numerous giant capillaries were observed, some with bizarre morphology, and focal dropout zones were noted. These alterations were highly suggestive of a scleroderma-like pattern with active and destructive features, reinforcing the systemic vasculopathic nature of the disease.

Pulmonary function tests (PFTs) revealed a restrictive ventilatory defect, with a forced vital capacity (FVC) of 72% of predicted and a markedly reduced diffusing capacity for carbon monoxide (DLCO) at 54%. These findings, in conjunction with clinical signs and auscultatory findings, prompted urgent imaging of the chest. Chest HRCT showed extensive bilateral ground-glass opacities with associated subpleural reticulations, predominantly in the lower lobes. The radiological pattern was consistent with an early fibrosing process and supported the diagnosis of rapidly progressive ILD (RP-ILD).

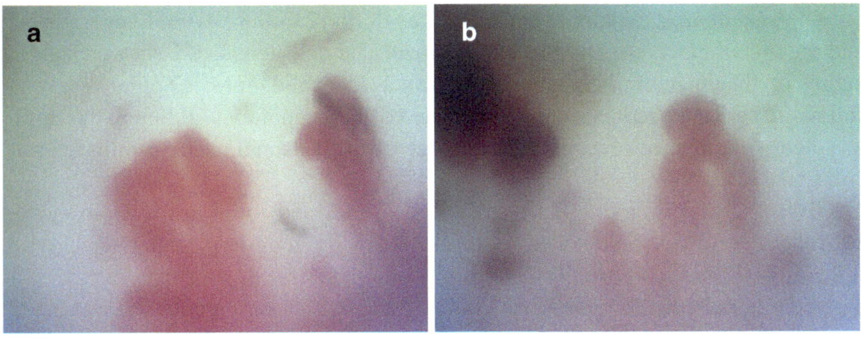

Fig. 5.7 (**a**, **b**) Nailfold videocapillaroscopy showing reduced capillary density and disorganized capillary architecture with ramified, bushy, and giant capillaries

No additional signs of organ involvement were identified, and tumor screening was not pursued further given the serological profile and absence of malignancy-associated features.

Therapeutic Approach

In light of the rapidly progressive clinical picture, high ferritin levels, and serological confirmation of anti-MDA5 positivity, we initiated an aggressive immunosuppressive regimen without delay. The patient received intravenous methylprednisolone at a dose of 1 gram daily for three consecutive days, followed by a transition to oral prednisone at 1 mg/kg/day. This was aimed at rapidly controlling both cutaneous vasculopathy and pulmonary inflammation.

Given the known poor prognosis of anti-MDA5-positive RP-ILD and supported by growing evidence favoring early multi-agent therapy, we instituted IVIG at a total dose of 2 g/kg administered over 5 days. In parallel, calcineurin inhibitor therapy was started with tacrolimus, titrated to maintain therapeutic trough levels between 5 and 10 ng/mL. The decision to use tacrolimus rather than cyclosporine was based on its superior tolerability and pulmonary efficacy profile.

In view of the extent of radiological involvement and the markedly elevated ferritin, an independent negative prognostic factor in this disease subset, we also initiated monthly intravenous cyclophosphamide at a dose of 1 g/m^2, planning a total of six infusions. The aim was to maximize early control of lung inflammation and prevent irreversible fibrosis.

Trimethoprim-sulfamethoxazole prophylaxis (800/160 mg thrice weekly) was instituted to prevent Pneumocystis jirovecii pneumonia, given the intensity of the immunosuppressive regimen. The patient was closely monitored for signs of cytopenias, hepatotoxicity, and infectious complications. A baseline ophthalmologic evaluation and laboratory screening for latent infections (including hepatitis B, C, and tuberculosis) had been completed prior to therapy.

After 2 months of therapy, the patient reported partial improvement in dyspnea but a persistent need for supplemental oxygen during exertion. Arthralgias resolved, and the digital ulcers began to re-epithelialize. The repeated HRCT showed stabilization of the interstitial findings without new consolidations. Capillaroscopy at follow-up showed a reduction in the number of giant capillaries, although the capillary density remained low, and the presence of tortuous and bushy capillaries was still noted (Fig. 5.8).

Given the improvement and tolerability, we decided to transition from cyclophosphamide to mycophenolate mofetil (MMF) for long-term maintenance at a dose of 1000 mg twice daily. Tacrolimus was continued. Oral prednisone was tapered gradually to 10 mg/day. PFTs after 4 months showed modest improvement in DLCO (now 60%), and the patient no longer required oxygen at rest, though it was still necessary for moderate exertion.

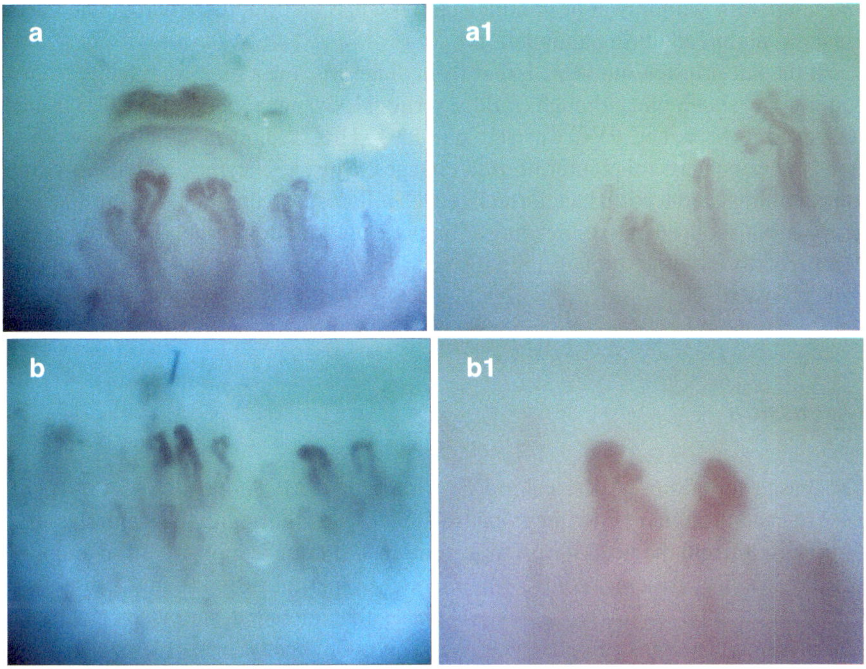

Fig. 5.8 (**a**, **b**) Nailfold videocapillaroscopy performed after 2 months of treatment showing persistently low capillary density, a reduction in the number of giant capillaries, and persistent tortuous capillaries

Six months into follow-up, however, a flare of cutaneous lesions occurred during a temporary interruption of MMF due to intercurrent infection and planned vaccination. The patient developed new periorbital erythema, palmar erythematous patches, and recurrence of painful fingertip ulcers. This relapse was accompanied by increased fatigue and mild hypoxemia on minimal exertion. HRCT performed shortly thereafter demonstrated new ground-glass opacities and increased fibrotic changes in the basal segments of the lower lobes, especially on the left side. DLCO declined to 55%. Capillaroscopy again revealed active microangiopathy with new hemorrhages and further capillary dropout.

Given this relapse, we reinforced immunosuppression with the reintroduction of MMF at full dosage, and prednisone was increased to 0.5 mg/kg/day. The potential benefit of initiating antifibrotic therapy was discussed with the patient. Following thorough counselling regarding efficacy and side effect profile, oral nintedanib was initiated at 150 mg twice daily. In the months following the initiation of nintedanib, the patient developed gastrointestinal side effects, including nausea and diarrhea, managed with dietary adjustments, probiotics, and intermittent antiemetics. Despite these adverse effects, nintedanib was maintained at a full dose. The patient experienced further infectious complications, including bronchitis requiring antibiotics and temporary withdrawal of immunosuppressants. Oxygen therapy remained necessary at night and during ambulation.

At the latest follow-up visit, 1 year from diagnosis, the patient was stable from a respiratory standpoint, though mild exertional dyspnea persisted. DLCO had improved to 68%, and FVC was stable at 83%. HRCT showed no new consolidations but persistent subpleural fibrotic changes. Muscle enzymes remained within normal limits, and ferritin had normalized. Capillaroscopy continued to show severe dropout but reduced active bleeding. The patient's functional status was improved compared to baseline, though limitations in physical exertion and residual digital pain persisted.

Discussion

This case exemplifies a classical presentation of anti-MDA5-positive CADM with RP-ILD and prominent microangiopathy. It highlights the aggressive natural course of the disease and the need for prompt, combined immunosuppressive and supportive therapy. The patient's course was marked by partial response and subsequent stabilization after an early aggressive phase that included steroids, calcineurin inhibitors, IVIG, and cyclophosphamide. The maintenance phase with MMF and tacrolimus, and more recently with nintedanib, underscores the role of long-term disease control and fibrosis modulation.

Despite the absence of significant myositis, the severe pulmonary and vascular involvement confirmed the necessity of early intervention. NVC proved useful not only as a diagnostic clue but also as a marker of disease activity and response to therapy. The patient's course was complicated by infectious episodes and drug-related intolerance, both of which required dynamic adjustments in management. Nevertheless, the multidisciplinary approach enabled stabilization of pulmonary function and gradual improvement in the cutaneous and systemic disease burden, offering a cautious but encouraging outlook in a condition typically associated with a high mortality risk.

Case 5: Antisynthetase Syndrome with Anti-Jo-1 Antibodies and Non-Sclerodermiform Capillaroscopic Findings

Clinical Presentation

A 52-year-old man was referred to our rheumatology department for evaluation of chronic myalgias, inflammatory arthritis, and progressive dyspnea on exertion. The symptoms had evolved gradually over the previous 18 months and were initially attributed to post-viral fatigue and mechanical joint pain. However, over the past year, the patient had developed episodes of low-grade fever, morning stiffness lasting more than 1 h, and symmetric joint swelling involving the wrists, metacarpophalangeal, and proximal interphalangeal joints. He also reported episodic color changes of the fingers triggered by cold exposure, with pallor followed by cyanosis and hyperemia, consistent with Raynaud's phenomenon. Muscle strength was reported to be variably impaired, particularly in the proximal lower limbs, though not associated with frank atrophy or functional limitation. There were no cutaneous ulcerations, digital pitting scars, or heliotrope rashes.

The patient had a remote smoking history and no family history of connective tissue diseases or pulmonary conditions. He had previously been treated with NSAIDs and short courses of corticosteroids with partial benefit, but symptoms recurred promptly after tapering.

At presentation, physical examination revealed mild interphalangeal synovitis with soft tissue swelling and tenderness on palpation. Auscultation of the lungs demonstrated faint end-inspiratory crackles at the bases. There were no rales, wheezes, or signs of congestive heart failure. Muscle strength was normal on formal testing (5/5), although tenderness of the thighs and shoulders was reported. No telangiectasias, sclerodactyly, or cutaneous lesions suggestive of DM or systemic sclerosis were identified. Nailfolds appeared erythematous but intact.

Diagnostic Work-Up

Initial laboratory investigations showed normocytic anemia (hemoglobin 11.2 g/dL), elevated ESR (64 mm/h), and mildly increased CRP (11.5 mg/L). Muscle enzymes were modestly elevated, with CK at 465 U/L and aldolase at 10 U/L. ANA was positive at 1:1280 with a cytoplasmic pattern. Immunoblot testing revealed strong positivity for anti-Jo-1 antibodies. Testing for other myositis-specific and myositis-associated antibodies was negative.

Pulmonary function tests demonstrated a restrictive ventilatory pattern with a forced vital capacity (FVC) of 68% and a reduced diffusing capacity for carbon monoxide (DLCO) at 58%. A high-resolution computed tomography (HRCT) scan of the chest revealed bilateral, basal-predominant ground-glass opacities with subtle reticulation and traction bronchiectasis—consistent with the nonspecific interstitial pneumonia (NSIP) pattern. There were no signs of honeycombing or pleural effusion. Cardiac evaluation, including transthoracic echocardiography, was unremarkable.

A NVC was performed to evaluate for microvascular changes and to assess possible overlap with systemic sclerosis (Fig. 5.9). The examination revealed moderately dilated capillary loops and a few ramified capillaries but no megacapillaries, microhemorrhages, or avascular areas. The capillary density was preserved, with 8–9 capillaries per millimeter, and the overall architecture remained regular. These findings were not suggestive of a scleroderma pattern and instead supported a nonspecific microangiopathy. In the differential diagnosis of inflammatory myopathies

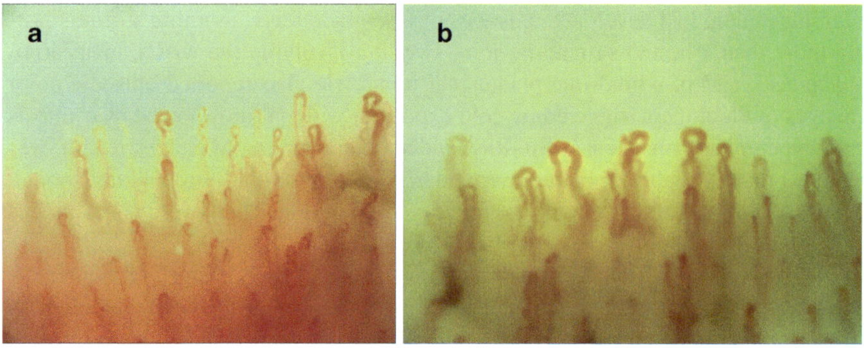

Fig. 5.9 (**a**, **b**) Nailfold videocapillaroscopy showing dilated capillary loops. Preserved capillary density, with no evidence of megacapillaries, microhemorrhages, or avascular areas

and connective tissue diseases with ILD, the absence of a sclerodermiform pattern was useful in reinforcing the diagnosis of antisynthetase syndrome rather than systemic sclerosis or overlap syndromes.

Therapeutic Approach

With a clinical picture dominated by arthritis, myalgias, ILD, Raynaud's phenomenon, and anti-Jo-1 positivity, the diagnosis of antisynthetase syndrome was established. The patient was started on oral prednisone at an initial dose of 0.75 mg/kg/day. Given the presence of chronic ILD and evidence of active inflammation, mycophenolate mofetil (MMF) was introduced as a steroid-sparing agent, starting at 500 mg twice daily and progressively titrated to 1000 mg twice daily. Prophylaxis for Pneumocystis jirovecii was initiated with trimethoprim-sulfamethoxazole, and calcium and vitamin D supplementation were prescribed.

The patient responded gradually to therapy, with resolution of low-grade fever and improvement of joint symptoms over the first month. Muscle enzymes normalized within 2 months, and dyspnea on exertion improved modestly. Follow-up HRCT at 6 months showed stability of the fibrosing changes with no progression, and PFTs revealed a slight increase in FVC to 74% and in DLCO to 62%. No digital ulcers developed, and Raynaud's symptoms remained manageable with cold protection and low-dose calcium channel blockers.

Repeat capillaroscopy at 12 months confirmed the stability of the microvascular pattern. Capillary density was preserved, and there was no evolution toward avascularity or neoangiogenesis. This remained consistent with a nonspecific pattern and contributed to distinguishing this patient's disease course from the fibrotic vasculopathy typical of systemic sclerosis.

After 18 months, the patient remained clinically stable on low-dose prednisone (5 mg/day) and full-dose MMF, with preserved pulmonary function and control of articular symptoms. No additional immunosuppressive agents were required.

Discussion

This case exemplifies the presentation of antisynthetase syndrome with anti-Jo-1 antibodies and chronic NSIP-pattern ILD, associated with systemic inflammatory features such as fever, arthritis, and Raynaud's phenomenon. Unlike systemic sclerosis or MDA5-associated DM, the patient's capillaroscopic findings were nonspecific and nonprogressive. The absence of megacapillaries, microhemorrhages, and capillary dropout supported the diagnosis of antisynthetase syndrome and proved useful in the differential diagnosis, particularly in excluding sclerodermiform overlap.

Although the prognosis in antisynthetase syndrome is highly variable, early identification and treatment remain essential in preventing irreversible pulmonary damage. In this case, the timely initiation of combined immunosuppression with prednisone and MMF led to a stable clinical and functional trajectory over the first 2 years of follow-up. The absence of cutaneous vasculopathy, a relatively mild elevation of muscle enzymes, and the radiological stability of ILD suggest a more indolent course compared to more aggressive vasculopathic phenotypes. Nonetheless, regular monitoring, particularly of lung function and capillaroscopic findings, remains crucial in anticipating disease evolution.

Final Discussion

NVC has emerged as a critical tool in the evaluation of DM, offering a unique window into the systemic microangiopathy that underpins many of its clinical manifestations. As highlighted throughout this chapter, DM is not only a myopathic disorder but also a disease of the microvasculature, with endothelial injury, complement activation, and IFN-mediated inflammation as central pathological mechanisms. The changes observed on NVC—giant capillaries, microhemorrhages, capillary loss, and architectural disorganization—mirror this vasculopathic process and provide valuable clinical insight.

Capillaroscopic findings in DM are diagnostically informative, particularly in distinguishing DM from polymyositis and other myositis subsets. The presence of a scleroderma-like pattern, though not exclusive to DM, is uncommon in other idiopathic inflammatory myopathies and may guide clinicians toward the correct diagnosis, even in cases with atypical or incomplete clinical presentations. Moreover, NVC can support the diagnosis of amyopathic or hypomyopathic forms of DM, where conventional muscle markers may be less informative.

From a prognostic standpoint, capillaroscopic abnormalities have been associated with disease severity and specific systemic complications, such as ILD, cutaneous ulceration, and calcinosis. In particular, severe microangiopathy, marked by extensive avascular areas, hemorrhages, and capillary dropout, tends to identify patients at higher risk of aggressive disease, especially in anti-MDA5- and anti-NXP2-positive subsets. In this regard, NVC can aid in risk stratification and help guide therapeutic decisions, prompting early initiation of aggressive immunosuppression in high-risk phenotypes.

Importantly, capillaroscopic changes in DM are dynamic and potentially reversible. Unlike systemic sclerosis, where the progression of capillary loss often reflects irreversible vascular damage, patients with DM may demonstrate significant improvement in capillary density and morphology with effective treatment. This responsiveness makes NVC a promising tool for monitoring disease activity and therapeutic response. Longitudinal studies and illustrative cases in this chapter confirm that changes in capillary morphology can parallel clinical improvement, offering a noninvasive and repeatable biomarker of treatment efficacy.

Finally, the integration of capillaroscopic findings with autoantibody profiling and clinical phenotype allows for a more nuanced understanding of DM heterogeneity. The observed differences in NVC patterns across DM subsets, such as anti-Mi-2, anti-TIF1γ, anti-MDA5, and anti-NXP2, support the concept that vascular injury in DM is shaped by distinct immunological pathways. This stratification has the potential to inform personalized therapeutic strategies and future research into pathogenesis and targeted interventions.

In conclusion, NVC should be considered an essential component of the diagnostic and monitoring toolkit in DM. Its ability to detect subclinical microvascular involvement, predict systemic complications, and monitor treatment response underscores its value in both routine practice and clinical research. As our understanding of the immunopathogenesis of DM deepens, NVC will likely play an increasingly prominent role in tailoring care to individual patient phenotypes.

References

1. Lundberg IE, Fujimoto M, Vencovsky J, Aggarwal R, Holmqvist M, Christopher-Stine L, et al. Idiopathic inflammatory myopathies. Nat Rev Dis Primers. 2021;7:86.
2. Lundberg IE, de Visser M, Werth VP. Classification of myositis. Nat Rev Rheumatol. 2018;14:269.
3. Mainetti C, Terziroli Beretta-Piccoli B, Selmi C. Cutaneous manifestations of dermatomyositis: a comprehensive review. Clin Rev Allergy Immunol. 2017;53:337–56.
4. Okiyama N, Fujimoto M. Cutaneous manifestations of dermatomyositis characterized by myositis-specific autoantibodies. F1000Res. 2019;8:F1000 Faculty Rev-1951.
5. Fornaro M, Girolamo F, Giannini M, Coladonato L, Capuano A, Capodiferro M, et al. Clinical, histologic and prognostic features of clinically amyopathic dermatomyositis. Clin Exp Rheumatol. 2024;42:288–94.
6. Lu X, Peng Q, Wang G. Anti-MDA5 antibody-positive dermatomyositis: pathogenesis and clinical progress. Nat Rev Rheumatol. 2024;20:48–62.

7. Oldroyd AGS, Callen JP, Chinoy H, Chung L, Fiorentino D, Gordon P, et al. International guideline for idiopathic inflammatory myopathy-associated cancer screening: an international myositis assessment and clinical studies group (IMACS) initiative. Nat Rev Rheumatol. 2023;19:805–17.
8. Kamperman RG, van der Kooi AJ, de Visser M, Aronica E, Raaphorst J. Pathophysiological mechanisms and treatment of dermatomyositis and immune mediated necrotizing myopathies: a focused review. Int J Mol Sci. 2022;23:4301.
9. McLellan K, Papadopoulou C. Update on biomarkers of vasculopathy in juvenile and adult myositis. Curr Rheumatol Rep. 2022;24:227–37.
10. Gasparotto M, Franco C, Zanatta E, Ghirardello A, Zen M, Iaccarino L, et al. The interferon in idiopathic inflammatory myopathies: different signatures and new therapeutic perspectives. A literature review. Autoimmun Rev. 2023;22:103334.
11. Kao L, Chung L, Fiorentino DF. Pathogenesis of dermatomyositis: role of cytokines and interferon. Curr Rheumatol Rep. 2011;13:225–32.
12. Bolko L, Jiang W, Tawara N, Landon-Cardinal O, Anquetil C, Benveniste O, et al. The role of interferons type I, II and III in myositis: a review. Brain Pathol. 2021;31:e12955.
13. Betteridge Z, McHugh N. Myositis-specific autoantibodies: an important tool to support diagnosis of myositis. J Intern Med. 2016;280:8–23.
14. Fiorentino D, Casciola-Rosen L. TIF1 autoantibodies in dermatomyositis shed insight into the cancer-myositis connection. Arthritis Rheum. 2012;64:346–9.
15. Fuzzi E, Gatto M, Zen M, Franco C, Zanatta E, Ghirardello A, et al. Anti-MDA5 dermatomyositis: an update from bench to bedside. Curr Opin Rheumatol. 2022;34:365–73.
16. Xu H, Qian J. Vasculopathy in dermatomyositis. Chin Med J (Engl). 2024;137:247–9.
17. Bogojevic M, Markovic Vlaisavljevic M, Medjedovic R, Strujic E, Pravilovic Lutovac D, Pavlov-Dolijanovic S. Nailfold Capillaroscopy changes in patients with idiopathic inflammatory myopathies. J Clin Med. 2024;13:5550.
18. Long K, Danoff SK. Interstitial lung disease in polymyositis and dermatomyositis. Clin Chest Med. 2019;40:561–72.
19. Matas-Garcia A, Milisenda JC, Espinosa G, Cuatrecasas M, Selva-O'Callaghan A, Grau JM, et al. Gastrointestinal Involvement in dermatomyositis. Diagnostics (Basel). 2022;12:1200.
20. Zhu H, Li R, Tan H, Ding T, Yuan Y, Wen Z, et al. Cardiac involvement in idiopathic inflammatory myopathies. J Inflamm Res. 2025;18:3879–88.
21. Manfredi A, Sebastiani M, Cassone G, Pipitone N, Giuggioli D, Colaci M, et al. Nailfold capillaroscopic changes in dermatomyositis and polymyositis. Clin Rheumatol. 2015;34:279–84.
22. Flatley EM, Collins D, Lukowiak TM, Miller JH. Nailfold microscopy in adult-onset dermatomyositis in association with myositis antibodies. Arch Dermatol Res. 2024;317:34.
23. Johnson D, van Eeden C, Moazab N, Redmond D, Phan C, Keeling S, et al. Nailfold Capillaroscopy abnormalities correlate with disease activity in adult dermatomyositis. Front Med (Lausanne). 2021;8:708432.
24. Kubo S, Todoroki Y, Nakayamada S, Nakano K, Satoh M, Nawata A, et al. Significance of nailfold videocapillaroscopy in patients with idiopathic inflammatory myopathies. Rheumatology (Oxford). 2019;58:120–30.
25. Torres-Ruiz J, Pinal-Fernandez I, Selva-O'Callaghan A, Campbell B, Muñoz-Braceras S, Mejía-Domínguez NR, et al. Nailfold capillaroscopy findings of a multicentric multiethnic cohort of patients with idiopathic inflammatory myopathies. Clin Exp Rheumatol. 2024;42:367–76.
26. Sugimoto T, Mokuda S, Kohno H, Ishitoku M, Araki K, Watanabe H, et al. Nailfold capillaries and myositis-specific antibodies in anti-melanoma differentiation-associated gene 5 antibody-positive dermatomyositis. Rheumatology (Oxford). 2022;61:2006–15.
27. Wakura R, Matsuda S, Kotani T, Shoda T, Takeuchi T. The comparison of nailfold videocapillaroscopy findings between anti-melanoma differentiation-associated gene 5 antibody and anti-aminoacyl tRNA synthetase antibody in patients with dermatomyositis complicated by interstitial lung disease. Sci Rep. 2020;10:15692.

28. Selva-O'Callaghan A, Fonollosa-Pla V, Trallero-Araguás E, Martínez-Gómez X, Simeon-Aznar CP, Labrador-Horrillo M, et al. Nailfold capillary microscopy in adults with inflammatory myopathy. Semin Arthritis Rheum. 2010;39:398–404.
29. Mugii N, Hamaguchi Y, Horii M, Fushida N, Ikeda T, Oishi K, et al. Longitudinal changes in nailfold videocapillaroscopy findings differ by myositis-specific autoantibody in idiopathic inflammatory myopathy. Rheumatology (Oxford). 2023;62:1326–34.

Chapter 6
Rheumatologic Overlap Syndromes

Konstantinos Triantafyllias and Cansu Aglar-Backeberg

Introduction

Raynaud's phenomenon (RP) is a frequent clinical feature of altered microcirculation, and it is a common manifestation in autoimmune connective tissue diseases (CTDs), with a prevalence widely ranging from 11% to 90% according to the considered CTD [1]. Nailfold capillaroscopy (NFC) stands as an indispensable, noninvasive tool in rheumatology, providing a direct window into microvascular health. While its utility in distinguishing primary from secondary Raynaud's phenomenon and in the early diagnosis and prognosis of systemic sclerosis (SSc) is well-established [2], its role in the complex realm of overlap rheumatic disorders is increasingly recognized as pivotal for comprehensive patient assessment. This chapter delves into the specific and often challenging capillaroscopic patterns observed in two key overlap syndromes: Mixed Connective Tissue Disease (MCTD) and Anti-Synthetase Syndrome (ASyS), highlighting how NFC contributes to their diagnostic refinement and prognostic stratification.

Mixed connective tissue disease (MCTD), characterized by overlapping features of SSc, Systemic Lupus Erythematosus (SLE), polymyositis/dermatomyositis (PM/DM), and rheumatoid arthritis (RA), often presents a heterogeneous clinical picture [3]. Nailfold capillaroscopy findings in MCTD are similarly diverse, reflecting the variable microvascular involvement characteristic of this syndrome. While a "scleroderma-like" pattern (featuring giant capillaries, hemorrhages, and architectural disorganization) is frequently observed in MCTD, it often presents with less severity and progression compared to definite SSc [4]. Importantly, other patterns, including nonspecific changes (e.g., bushy capillaries, dilated capillaries without significant disorganization) or even normal findings, can also be seen [5]. To date, there are few reports in the literature on the capillaroscopic picture in MCTD

K. Triantafyllias (✉) · C. Aglar-Backeberg
Rhineland-Palatinate Rheumatology Center, Bad Kreuznach, Germany

Y. El Miedany, R. A. Elziaty (eds.), *Capillaroscopy*, Contemporary Rheumatology,
https://doi.org/10.1007/978-3-032-22966-3_6

patients and its relationship to organ involvement. Compared to SSc, the typical pattern of changes within the nail shaft vessels has not yet been confirmed in MCTD. The relationship between changes in capillaroscopic imaging and organ changes in patients with MCTD has also not been clearly confirmed [6]. Earlier data revealed that patients with MCTD had a significantly higher incidence of certain microvascular lesions. Lesions such as giant capillaries, branching capillaries, or dilated capillaries were found more frequently compared to the control group. A reduction in the number of capillaries was also significantly more frequently observed. Reduced capillary density count proved to be a significant predictor for the diagnosis of MCTD in the study group [7, 8, 9]. The relationship between clinical symptoms (collected based on classification criteria) and parameters assessed by capillaroscopic imaging in MCTD patients revealed that patients with PAH are more likely to have a prominent subpapillary plexus and branched capillaries. Patients with sclerodactyly are statistically significantly more likely to have a reduced number of vessels and more likely to have avascular areas; a scleroderma-like pattern was also more frequently present. In addition, the number of capillaries was reported to be a significant predictor of sclerodactyly [10]. This section explores these distinct capillaroscopic presentations in MCTD, discussing their clinical presentation, correlations (e.g., association of specific patterns with sclerodactyly or pulmonary arterial hypertension), and how NFC assists in distinguishing MCTD from its constituent diseases, particularly in early stages or in patients with less defined clinical phenotypes. The unique combination of features, such as the frequent presence of bushy capillaries alongside scleroderma-like changes, may offer specific clues to the underlying MCTD diagnosis, contributing to a more precise diagnostic algorithm.

Anti-synthetase syndrome, a distinct subset of idiopathic inflammatory myopathies characterized by the classic triad of arthritis, myositis, and interstitial lung disease (ILD) [11, 12], It is also characterized by the presence of anti-aminoacyl-tRNA synthetase antibodies. Raynaud phenomenon (RP), fever, and mechanic's hands are other relevant but less prevalent accompanying features [13]. The most frequent anti-aminoacyl-tRNA synthetase (ARS) antibody is the anti-Jo1, whereas other ARS specificities are less commonly detected (for example, anti-PL-7, -PL-12, -EJ, -OJ, -KS, -YRS, and -Zo) [14]. and a constellation of clinical features, including myositis and interstitial lung disease (ILD).

While microvascular involvement is a hallmark of inflammatory myopathies, particularly dermatomyositis, the capillaroscopic features of the anti-synthetase syndrome have been less extensively characterized. AENEAS (the American and European NEtwork of Anti-synthetase Syndrome) is an international collaborative group that aims to study AS thoroughly and better understand its clinical and pathophysiological features [15]. A multicenter study carried out by this group on anti-synthetase syndrome patients revealed that those patients with the disease have abnormal NVC patterns, confirming that vasculopathy is a typical manifestation of this rare condition. This chapter elucidates the observed NFC patterns in anti-synthetase syndrome, which often include a combination of enlarged and giant capillaries, disorganization, and sometimes avascular areas, akin to a "scleroderma-like" pattern, even in the absence of overt SSc [16, 17]. Crucially, the presence and severity of capillaroscopic abnormalities in anti-synthetase syndrome, including a reduced capillary density or increased ramified capillaries, have been correlated with specific clinical manifestations, such as the presence and severity of ILD [18]. This underscores NFC's potential as a valuable, noninvasive biomarker for risk stratification and monitoring of disease activity in anti-synthetase syndrome patients, guiding therapeutic decisions and predicting prognosis, particularly concerning lung involvement.

In essence, nailfold capillaroscopy serves as a vital diagnostic and prognostic adjunct in these complex overlap rheumatic disorders. By systematically analyzing the microvascular patterns unique to MCTD and ASSD, clinicians can achieve greater diagnostic certainty and stratify patients based on microangiopathic risk. Further standardized, longitudinal studies leveraging advanced imaging and AI-driven analysis are crucial to fully unlock the predictive power of NFC in these heterogeneous conditions.

Mixed Connective Tissue Disease (MCTD)

Introduction MCTD

MCTD is an autoimmune rheumatic disorder defined by overlapping clinical manifestations of systemic lupus erythematosus, systemic sclerosis (SSc), polymyositis, and rheumatoid arthritis [19, 20]. Elevated levels of anti-U1 ribonucleoprotein antibodies (anti-U1-RNP) are also associated with the presence of MCTD [19].

Kahn and Appelboom [21], Sharp [22], and Kasukawa [23], as well as Alarcón-Segovia and Villarreal [24], established classification and diagnostic criteria for MCTD. The criteria of Alarcón-Segovia and Villarreal are often used in clinical practice due to their broad applicability in a clinical setting [19] (Table 6.1).

In addition to these criteria, MCTD presents with clinical manifestations typical of the overlapping connective tissue diseases. The most common clinical features include fibrosing alveolitis, pulmonary hypertension, esophageal dysmotility, pleurisy, and pericarditis [25]. Nailfold microvascular abnormalities have also been observed in patients with MCTD, suggesting potential diagnostic or prognostic relevance [10].

Table 6.1 Classification criteria for MCTD

Criteria	
Serological	Positive anti-RNP titer ≥1:1600
Clinical	Synovitis or myositis +2 of the following
	Edema of the hands
	Raynaud's phenomenon
	Acrosclerosis/Sclerodactyly

Adapted from Alarcón-Segovia and Villarreal [24] and Pepmueller [19]

NVC in MCTD

Changes in the nailfold capillaries are among the earliest findings in scleroderma-associated conditions: systemic sclerosis (SSc), dermatomyositis, and undifferentiated and mixed connective tissue disease [4].

In SSc, alterations in the microvascular network correlate with disease progression and the degree of organ impairment [26, 27]. Therefore, NVC is utilized for diagnostic evaluation, disease staging, and monitoring treatment response in patients with SSc [4]. A few studies have investigated whether patients with MCTD also exhibit relevant nailfold capillaroscopic patterns and correlations with organ involvement [10, 29, 31].

In a study by Ornowska et al. [10], NVC was performed on 43 patients with MCTD, including 36 (83.72%) women and 7 (16.28%) men, to detect characteristic capillary changes. All patients were admitted to the Connective Tissue Disease Department at the Institute of Geriatrics, Rheumatology, and Rehabilitation (NIGRiR) in Warsaw, Poland, between 2020 and 2022. The inclusion of the patients was based on the classification criteria by Alarcón-Segovia and Villarreal [24] and Kasukawa [23]. All patients had Raynaud's phenomenon, and the median disease duration was 136.72 months. Capillary changes were defined according to the Cutolo assessment criteria [10, 28]. Moreover, an effort was made to determine whether a specific type of microvascular lesion correlates with organ involvement [10].

Significant findings included SSc patterns ($n = 20$, p-value $= 0.0003$), dominated by the early pattern ($n = 10$), whereas none were observed in the control group [10].

Regarding morphological changes of the capillaries, the presence of giant capillaries ($n = 19$, $p = 0.0005$) and branched capillaries ($n = 14$, $p = 0.005$) was recognized. None were found in the control group [10] (see cases 1–3 for exemplary images of patients with MCTD).

Furthermore, a reduction of capillary density ($p < 0.0001$) was detected [10] (see cases 2 and 3 for exemplary images of patients with MCTD).

Notably, MCTD patients with sclerodactyly ($n = 10$) showed a lower capillary density (5.6 ± 1.4 vs. 7.2 ± 1.2, $p = 0.002$), more frequent avascular areas ($n = 4$, 40% vs. $n = 2$, 6%; $p = 0.006$), and a higher prevalence of the SSc pattern ($n = 8$, 80% vs. $n = 12$, 36%; $p = 0.02$). Furthermore, the presence of branching capillaries was significantly associated with pulmonary arterial hypertension ($n = 2$, 100% vs.

$n = 7$, 17%; $p = 0.005$), as well as with a prominent subpapillary plexus ($n = 2$, 100% vs. $n = 12$, 29%; $p = 0.04$) [10].

Paolino et al. [6] conducted a retrospective study analyzing morphological capillary alterations in patients with mixed connective tissue disease (MCTD) over a 3-year period and compared these changes with those observed in patients with systemic sclerosis (SSc) . The study included ten patients with MCTD (eight women, two men) and ten patients with SSc (all women), with comparable disease duration (5 years) and mean age (51 years). During the follow-up period, no significant capillary changes were observed in the MCTD cohort [6].

At baseline (T0), a systemic sclerosis (SSc) capillaroscopic pattern was observed in 70% of MCTD patients, while the remaining 30% showed no morphological capillary changes. Among those with an SSc pattern, the most frequently observed abnormalities—ranked from highest to lowest—were branching vessels, reduced capillary density, microhemorrhages, and megacapillaries. Importantly, dilated capillaries were found in all MCTD patients. Throughout the 3-year follow-up of MCTD patients, NVC revealed no relevant progression of microangiopathy. In comparison, capillary abnormalities were significantly higher in patients with SSc: microhemorrhages ($p = 0.05$), dilated capillaries ($p = 0.04$), and megacapillaries ($p < 0.02$) [6].

In a study by Chebbi et al. (2021), NVC was performed in 27 MCTD patients (26 women, one man) as a comparison to patients with systemic lupus erythematosus. Patient inclusion was based on the classification criteria proposed by Alarcón-Segovia and Villarreal [24] or Kahn and Appelboom [21].

Patients with MCTD showed a more reduced average capillary density (5.1 ± 1.7/mm) as compared to patients with RNP-positive SLE (7.3 ± 1.4/mm), $p < 0.01$. Giant capillaries (MCTD: 3.4 ± 4.9 and RNP-positive SLE: 0.3 ± 0.9, $p < 0.01$), enlarged capillaries (MCTD: 16.6 ± 10.3 and RNP-positive SLE: 8.5 ± 9.1, $p = 0.01$), and avascular areas were more frequently observed in patients with MCTD [9].

Moreover, Bernardino et al. [7] conducted a retrospective analysis of clinical data from patients who attended the NVC clinic of an autoimmune diseases unit between 2011 and 2017. Inclusion criteria comprised a confirmed diagnosis of different connective tissue diseases, including MCTD ($n = 38$, 33 women and five men), based on the Alarcón-Segovia and Villarreal classification criteria (1987).

In this study, 97.37% of MCTD patients suffered from Raynaud's phenomenon. In the NVC of these patients, the following morphological capillary patterns were observed: SSc pattern (68.42%), non-scleroderma NVC changes (28.95%), and normal capillaries (2.63%). The observed SSc pattern could be classified into early ($n = 10$), active ($n = 12$), and late ($n = 4$) patterns. Quantitative analysis of NVC demonstrated a decreased capillary density (6.47/mm) and avascular areas (21.05%) in patients with MCTD. Moreover, giant capillaries (68.42%), enlarged capillaries (84.21%), hemorrhages (63.16%), and neoangiogenesis (39.47%) were found [7].

In the aforementioned analyses, no specific MCTD pattern could be described. [6, 7, 9, 10]. However, various abnormalities have been observed in some MCTD patients, with the presence of SSc patterns being one of them [6, 7, 10].

Specifically, lower capillary density is a significant predictor for diagnosing MCTD [6, 7, 9, 10].

The presence of branching capillaries observed in NVC is associated with an increased incidence of interstitial lung disease and pulmonary arterial hypertension in patients with SSc [29, 30]. There are individual reports suggesting that similar associations may also be present in patients with MCTD, although these have not been conclusively proven [7, 10, 31, 32].

Conclusion

NVC already plays an important role in the diagnosis of SSc, as well as in disease progression monitoring and the assessment of disease severity in SSc. In patients with MCTD, NVC also reveals abnormal capillaroscopic findings, such as lower capillary density, enlarged capillaries, and branching vessels, that may serve as supportive indicators for diagnosis and risk of potential organ involvement. Thus, it seems that NVC can be of value in the care of MCTD patients. However, further prospective research is required to validate NVC as a standardized diagnostic and disease monitoring tool for MCTD.

Case 1

- A 32-year-old patient with MCTD (initial manifestation in 2001), with positive anti-RNP antibodies.
- Onset of symptoms with generalized muscle weakness and pain, fatigue/exhaustion, skin sensitivity, episodes of fever, Raynaud's phenomenon, and, in the further course, joint pain—particularly affecting the shoulders, elbows, and hands.
- Status post pericardial effusion and recurrent pleural effusion (Fig. 6.1).

Case 2

- A 30-year-old patient admitted in June 2021 due to known MCTD with positive anti-RNP antibodies and an initial manifestation of the disease in March 2020.
- Symptoms/clinical signs: Painful skin lesions on the face and both ears, as well as hands and feet; fatigue; sicca; Raynaud's phenomenon; and alopecia.
- Lung function test: Mild restrictive and obstructive ventilatory impairment (Fig. 6.2).

Case 3

- A 59-year-old patient with MCTD with positive anti-U1RNP titer.
- Symptoms/clinical signs: Raynaud's phenomenon, esophageal involvement, sicca, sclerodactyly, arthralgia/myalgia, reflux (Fig. 6.3).

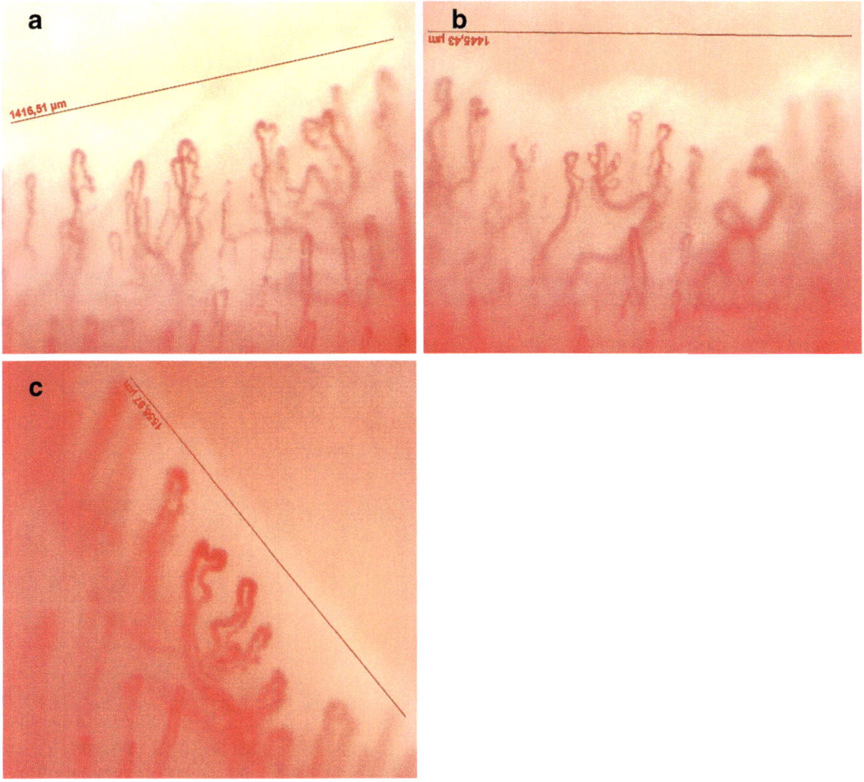

Fig. 6.1 (**a**) Presence of branched capillaries and edema. (**b**) Presence of branched capillaries and edema. (**c**) Presence of branched and mildly ectatic capillaries, as well as edema. (Source: Rhineland-Palatinate Rheumatology Center, Germany)

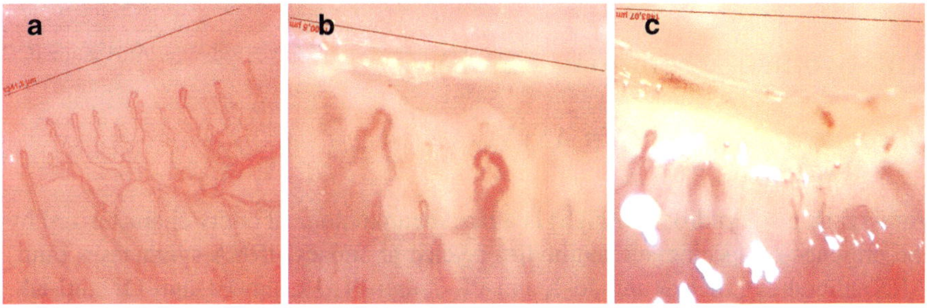

Fig. 6.2 (**a**) A Disorganization of the capillary architecture, reduced vascular density. (**b**) Reduced vascular density/avascular areas, edema, and one ectatic capillary. (**c**) Reduced vascular density/avascular areas, edema, microhemorrhages, ectatic/giant capillaries. (Source: Rhineland-Palatinate Rheumatology Center, Germany)

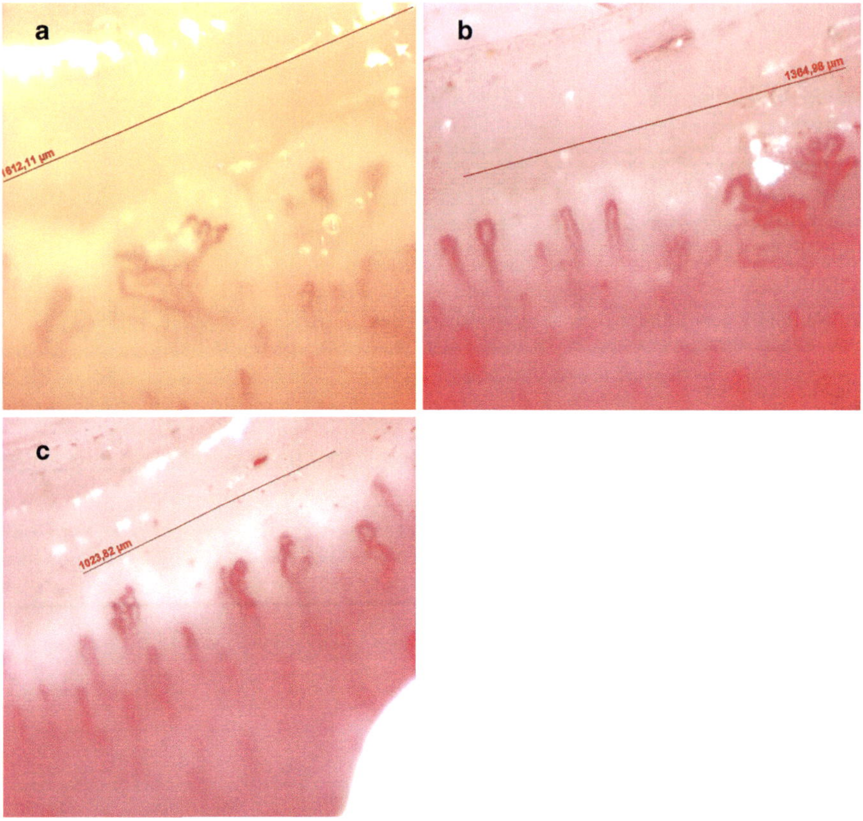

Fig. 6.3 (**a**) Presence of branched capillaries, reduced vascular density/avascular areas, and edema. (**b**) Presence of branched capillaries, reduced vascular density/avascular areas, edema, and microhemorrhages. (**c**) Presence of branched capillaries, reduced vascular density/avascular areas, and microhemorrhages. (Source: Rhineland-Palatinate Rheumatology Center, Germany)

Anti-Synthetase Syndrome (ASyS)

Introduction and NVC in ASyS

Anti-synthetase syndrome (ASyS) is a rare rheumatological entity characterized by the presence of specific autoantibodies against aminoacyl-tRNA synthetases (anti-ARS antibodies), such as anti-Jo-1, anti-PL-7, anti-PL-12, anti-EJ, anti-OJ, anti-KS, and anti-YRS, often in combination with a classic triad of arthritis, myositis, and interstitial lung disease (ILD) as well as different accompanying features like fever, Raynaud's, and mechanic's hands [33, 34]. There is limited NVC data in the literature on ASyS. Most of the information on this topic comes from the multicenter NASCAR study by Sebastiani & Triantafyllias et al. (American and European Network for Anti-synthetase Syndrome; AENEAS), which analyzed the largest cohort to date of patients with confirmed ASyS in a controlled manner.

NASCAR Study

In the international NASCAR study, the capillaroscopic features of 190 patients with ASyS (female/male ratio 3.63, mean age 49.7 ± 12.8 years, average disease duration 51.2 ± 71.4 months) were examined in comparison to control subjects. A total of 2550 nailfold capillaroscopic images of ASyS patients were analyzed. The study included patients with at least two anti-synthetase antibody-positive tests (anti-Jo1 positive in 133 patients (69.5%), anti-PL-7 positive in 19 patients (10%), anti-PL-12 in 22 patients (11.5%), anti-OJ in six patients (3%), and anti-EJ in ten patients (6%). In addition, the included patients exhibited one or more features of the classic triad: arthritis (76.5%), myositis (80.2%), and ILD (86.2%) [16].

Capillaroscopic abnormalities (giant capillaries, microhemorrhages, branching vessels, and reduction of capillary density) were observed more frequently in patients with ASyS compared to control subjects (62.1% versus 29.3%, $p < 0.001$). Giant capillaries and avascular areas were detected only in the ASyS group (59 patients, 31.1%, and 39 patients, 20.5%, respectively, $p < 0.005$), while capillary branching was more common in the ASyS group (94 patients, 49.5% vs. 5 patients, 6.7%, $p < 0.005$). (Figs. 6.4, 6.5, and 6.6).

Case 4 (ASyS)

- A 37-year-old patient with ASyS, anti-Jo-1 positive.
- Arthritis, Myositis.
- Gottron papules, heliotrope rash (Fig. 6.4).

Case 5

- A 74-year-old patient with ASyS, anti-Jo-1 positive.
- CT signs of interstitial lung disease and impaired CO diffusion.
- Rapid fatigue and dyspnea with minimal exertion (Fig. 6.5).

Case 6

- A 46-year-old patient with ASyS, antinuclear and anti-PL-12 antibodies positive, with interstitial lung disease.
- Myositis.
- Arthritis.
- Raynaud's, mechanic's hands (Fig. 6.6).

Moreover, microbleeding was found significantly more often in the ASyS group ($p = 0.008$) (Figs. 6.4 and 6.5), and differences regarding capillary density between the two groups (control group: significantly higher capillary density, $p < 0.005$) were demonstrated (Figs. 6.4 and 6.6). Interestingly, 35.3% of patients with ASyS exhibited a capillaroscopic pattern that was practically indistinguishable from the known SSc patterns [16].

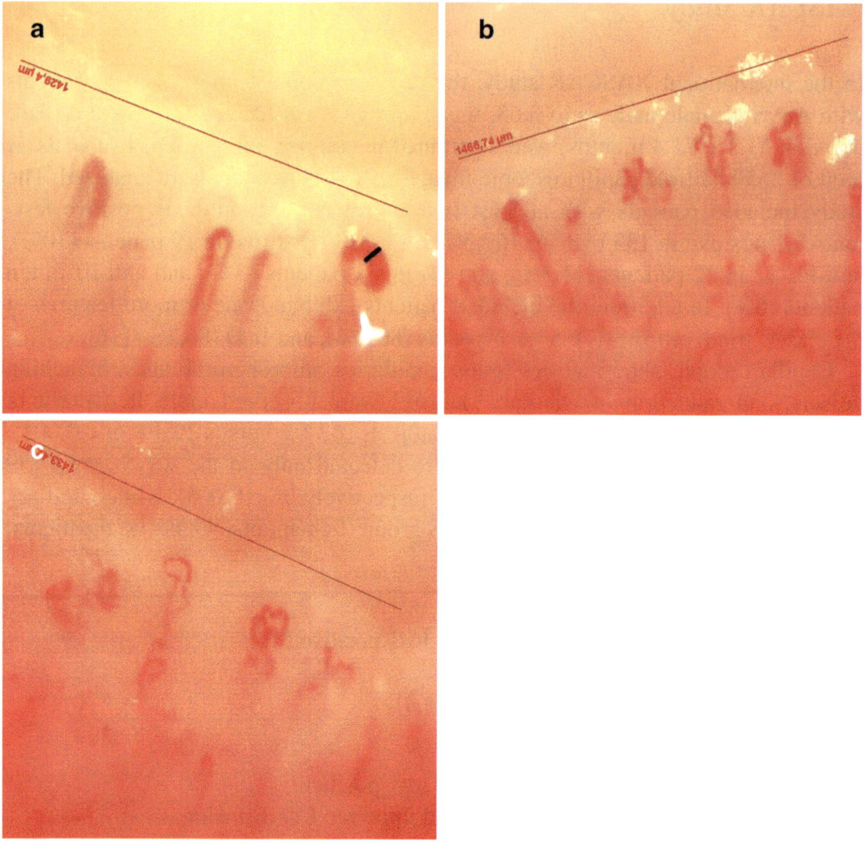

Fig. 6.4 (**a**) Presence of a giant capillary, ectasia, reduced vascular density, and avascular areas. (**b**) Presence of branched capillaries, edema, and reduced vascular density. (**c**) Presence of branched capillaries, edema, and reduced vascular density. (Source: Rhineland-Palatinate Rheumatology Center)

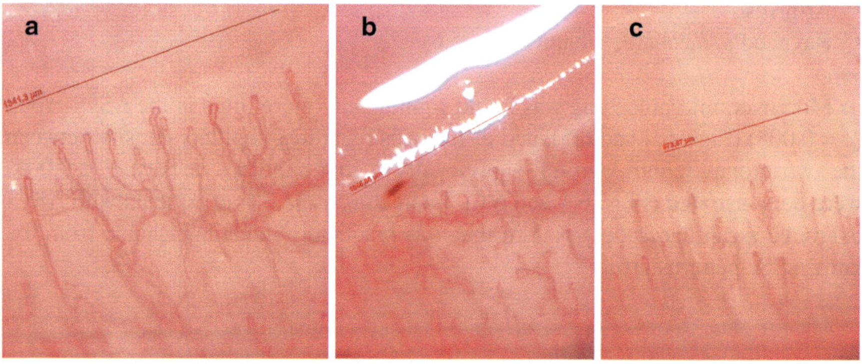

Fig. 6.5 (**a**) Presence of branched capillaries and mild edema. (**b**) Presence of microbleeding, edema, and branched capillaries. (**c**) Presence of edema, branched capillaries, and reduced vascular density. (Source: Rhineland-Palatinate Rheumatology Center, Germany)

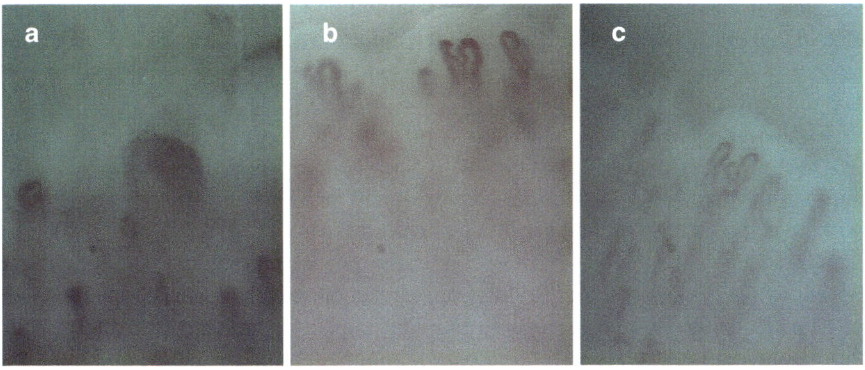

Fig. 6.6 (**a**) Giant capillary, pronounced edema, reduced vascular density. (**b**) Avascular area, branched and ectatic capillaries, pronounced edema. (**c**) Avascular area, branched capillary, edema. (Source: Rhineland-Palatinate Rheumatology Center, Germany)

Associations with Clinical Features

Capillaroscopic abnormalities were associated with the presence of interstitial lung disease (ILD) ($p = 0.02$), and branching capillaries occurred twice as frequently in patients with ILD compared to those without ILD (53.4% vs. 27.6%, $p = 0.01$). Locally reduced density (avascular areas) correlated with SSA-Ro and anti-Jo1 positivity as well as with the presence of myositis and Raynaud's phenomenon. Moreover, the SSc-like capillaroscopic pattern was associated with Jo1 antibody positivity (44% in patients with anti-Jo1 antibodies vs. 21.5% for other anti-synthetase specificities, $p = 0.002$), longer disease duration (107.1 ± 87.6 months in SSc patients vs. 84.6 ± 85.9 months without the SSc-like pattern, $p = 0.004$), and ILD occurring at a later stage of the disease [16].

This suggests that NVC could potentially serve as an early indicator for the onset of ILD in the early phase of ASyS [16]. Moreover, the various associations identified here, such as between ILD and branching capillaries or between avascular areas and myositis, may support the value of capillaroscopy as a screening tool for the occurrence of ASyS-specific clinical manifestations. Furthermore, these findings are significant in that the detection of an SSc-like pattern should broaden the rheumatological differential diagnosis to include ASyS and alert rheumatologists to the possible late onset of ILD.

Further Research

Other scarce NVC data arise mainly from a few studies and case reports that assessed other conditions such as polymyositis (PM) and dermatomyositis (DM) [36–39]. These studies reported positivity for ARS antibodies only in small subgroups, making it difficult to extract detailed and reliable data concerning the role of these antibodies. Moreover, patients in these studies were not clearly characterized as having ASyS, possibly also because there are no well-established classification criteria for this rare disease.

Furthermore, no separate ASyS subcohort analyses were performed. For instance, in one study investigating 27 patients with dermatomyositis, only four patients were anti-Jo1 positive [36]. All four patients exhibited an SSc-like pattern (two patients with an active pattern and two with a late pattern). Mugii et al. [37] were unable to demonstrate a statistically significant association between anti-ARS antibody positivity and the presence of an SSc-like capillaroscopic pattern in a very small cohort of 13 patients (29.7% of patients with SSc-like and 15.4% with normal pattern) with dermatomyositis [37]. However, the patient numbers in these studies do not allow for statistically significant conclusions.

A further small study concerning the NVC alterations in 24 patients with idiopathic inflammatory myopathies (IIM) reported a positivity of anti-Jo1 antibodies in eight patients [35]. The only abnormality reported in this small cohort of anti-Jo1–positive patients was a reduction of the capillary density in comparison to other patients. Positivity of anti-ARS was not associated with the presence of an SSc-like pattern in a study on 13 patients with DM reported by Mugii et al. [37]. In contrast, our study showed a significant association between anti-Jo1 antibodies and the SSc-like pattern [16].

Selva-O'Callaghan et al. [38] investigated 53 patients with IIM11 and reported a positivity for anti-ARS in 16 (12 positive for anti-Jo1 and four for other ARS). The comparison between patients with the 16 anti-ARS and six anti-Pm/Scl antibodies positive patients did not show statistically significant differences in regard to NVC alterations. Interestingly, in a study examining 27 patients with DM, an SSc-like pattern was recorded in all four patients who were anti-Jo1-positive [36].

In a study by Soubrier et al. [39], NVC was performed and analyzed on 43 patients (29 women and 14 men, average age 54.9 ± 17.4 years), including 12 patients with ASyS (two women and ten men, average age 62.2 ± 11.8, mean disease duration 102 ± 79 months) and the rest with DM, overlap myositis (OM) and immune-mediated necrotizing myopathy (IMNM). In addition, the NVC results of the aforementioned patients were compared to those of patients with SSc [39].

The presence of giant capillaries varied between the subgroups ($p = 0.05$). None were found in patients with ASyS (n = 1/12, 0.09%) and in IMNM patients (0%). Megacapillaries were more frequent in OM (n = 4/8, 50%) and in DM patients (n = 3/17, 17%). Furthermore, abnormal vascular structure was detected in patients with DM (11.8%) and OM (62.5%); no occurrences were observed in ASyS or IMNM patients ($p = 0.001$). Avascular zones were found in DM (11.7%) and OM (62.5%), but not in ASS and IMNM patients [39].

The results of this analysis are limited because of the small number of participants in the subgroups. As a result, it is possible that no specific NVC abnormalities were identified in the ASyS patients [39].

Conclusion

The NASCAR study described for the first time the characteristics and the frequency of SSc-like patterns in patients with ASyS, as well as their correlation with the clinical features of the disease. It demonstrated that NVC findings in ASyS can be abnormal, thereby confirming vasculopathy as a not-so-rare manifestation of this rare condition. Nailfold capillaroscopy can prove to be a valuable diagnostic tool in ASyS, as the observed changes—such as reduced capillary density and the characteristic SSc-like pattern—not only assist in diagnosing ASyS but may also serve as indicators of disease severity and progression. Further data are needed to explore the full potential of NVC in the clinical management of ASyS.

References

1. Suter LG, Murabito JM, Felson DT, et al. The incidence and natural history of Raynaud's phenomenon in the community. Arthritis Rheum. 2005;52:1259–63. https://doi.org/10.1002/art.20988.
2. van den Hoogen F, Khanna D, Fransen J, et al. 2013 classification criteria for systemic sclerosis: an American College of Rheumatology/European League against Rheumatism Collaborative Initiative. Ann Rheum Dis. 2013;72(11):1747–55.
3. Chaigne B, Scirè CA, Talarico R, Alexander T, Amoura Z, et al. Mixed connective tissue disease: state of the art on clinical practice guidelines. RMD Open. 2018;4(Suppl 1):e000783. https://doi.org/10.1136/rmdopen-2018-000783.
4. Dima A, Berza I, Popescu DN, Parvu MI. Nailfold capillaroscopy in systemic diseases: short overview for internal medicine. Rom J Intern Med. 2021;59(3):201–17. https://doi.org/10.2478/rjim-2021-0007. PMID: 33600677.
5. Cutolo M, Sulli A, Secchi ME, Olivieri M, Pizzorni C. The contribution of capillaroscopy to the differential diagnosis of connective autoimmune diseases. Best Pract Res Clin Rheumatol. 2007;21(6):1093–108. https://doi.org/10.1016/j.berh.2007.10.001.
6. Paolino S, Ferrari G, Pizzorni C, Patanè M, Smith V, Cutolo M, Sulli A. Long-term follow-up of nailfold videocapillaroscopic microvascular parameters in mixed connective tissue disease versus systemic sclerosis patients: a retrospective cohort study. Clin Exp Rheumatol. 2019;37 Suppl 119(4):102–7. Epub 2019 Oct 3. PMID: 31587695.
7. Bernardino V, Rodrigues A, Lladó A, Panarra A. Nailfold capillaroscopy and autoimmune connective tissue diseases in patients from a Portuguese nailfold capillaroscopy clinic. Rheumatol Int. 2020;40(2):295–301. https://doi.org/10.1007/s00296-019-04427-0. Epub 2019 Aug 26. PMID: 31451935.
8. Blockmans D, Vermylen J, Bobbaers H. Nailfold capillaroscopy in connective tissue disorders and in Raynaud's phenomenon. Acta Clin Belg. 1993;48(1):30–41. https://doi.org/10.1080/17843286.1993.11718282.
9. Chebbi PP, Goel R, Ramya J, Gowri M, Herrick A, Danda D. Nailfold capillaroscopy changes associated with anti-RNP antibodies in systemic lupus erythematosus. Rheumatol Int. 2022;42(8):1355–61. https://doi.org/10.1007/s00296-021-04894-4. Epub 2021 Jun 2. PMID: 34076720.
10. Ornowska S, Wudarski M, Dziewięcka E, et al. Naifold capillaroscopy in mixed connective tissue disease patients. Clin Rheumatol. 2024;43:1703–9. https://doi.org/10.1007/s10067-024-06879-7. Epub 2024 Mar 21. PMID: 38509242.

11. Chatterjee S, Prayson R, Farver C. Antisynthetase syndrome: not just an inflammatory myopathy. Cleve Clin J Med. 2013;80:655–66.
12. Dugar M, Cox S, Limaye V, Blumbergs P, Roberts-Thomson PJ. Clinical heterogeneity and prognostic features of South Australian patients with anti-synthetase autoantibodies. Intern Med J. 2011;41:674–9.
13. Lega JC, Fabien N, Reynaud Q, Durieu I, Durupt S, Dutertre M, et al. The clinical phenotype associated with myositis-specific and associated autoantibodies: a meta-analysis revisiting the so-called antisynthetase syndrome. Autoimmun Rev. 2014;13:883–91.
14. Hervier B, Devilliers H, Stanciu R, Meyer A, Uzunhan Y, Masseau A, et al. Hierarchical cluster and survival analyses of antisynthetase syndrome: phenotype and outcome are correlated with anti-tRNA synthetase antibody specificity. Autoimmun Rev. 2012;12:210–7.
15. Cavagna L, Nuño L, Scirè CA, Govoni M, Longo FJ, Franceschini F, et al. Clinical spectrum time course in anti Jo-1 positive antisynthetase syndrome: results from an international retrospective multicenter study. Medicine. 2015;94:e1144.
16. Sebastiani M, Triantafyllias K, Manfredi A, González-Gay MA, Palmou-Fontana N, Cassone G, Drott U, Delbrück C, Rojas-Serrano J, Bertolazzi C, Nuño L, Giannini M, Iannone F, Vicente EF, Castañeda S, Selva-O'Callaghan A, Trallero Araguas E, Emmi G, Iuliano A, Bauhammer J, Miehle N, Parisi S, Cavagna L, Codullo V, Montecucco C, Lopez-Longo FJ, Martínez-Barrio J, Nieto-González JC, Vichi S, Confalonieri M, Tomietto P, Bergner R, Sulli A, Bonella F, Furini F, Scirè CA, Bortoluzzi A, Specker C, Barsotti S, Neri R, Mosca M, Caproni M, Weinmann-Menke J, Schwarting A, Smith V, Cutolo M, American and European Network of Antisynthetase Syndrome Collaborative Group. Nailfold capillaroscopy characteristics of antisynthetase syndrome and possible clinical associations: results of a multicenter international study. J Rheumatol. 2019;46(3):279–84. https://doi.org/10.3899/jrheum.180355.
17. Sambataro D, Sambataro G, Libra A, Vignigni G, Pino F, Fagone E, Fruciano M, Gili E, Pignataro F, Del Papa N, Vancheri C. Nailfold videocapillaroscopy is a useful tool to recognize definite forms of systemic sclerosis and idiopathic inflammatory myositis in interstitial lung disease patients. Diagnostics (Basel). 2020;10(5):253. https://doi.org/10.3390/diagnostics10050253.
18. Pizzorni C, Ferrari G, Schenone C, et al. Nailfold capillaroscopy in undifferentiated and mixed connective diseases. Ann Rheum Dis. 2021;80:686.
19. Pepmueller PH. Undifferentiated connective tissue disease, mixed connective tissue disease, and overlap syndromes in rheumatology. Mo Med. 2016;113(2):136–40. PMID: 27311225; PMCID: PMC6139943.
20. Sharp GC, Irvin WS, Tan EM, Gould RG, Holman HR. Mixed connective tissue disease--an apparently distinct rheumatic disease syndrome associated with a specific antibody to an extractable nuclear antigen (ENA). Am J Med. 1972;52(2):148–59. https://doi.org/10.1016/0002-9343(72)90064-2. PMID: 4621694.
21. Kahn MF, Appelboom T. Syndrome de sharp. In: Kahn MF, Peltier AP, Meyer O, Piette JC, editors. Les Maladies Systemiques, vol. 3. Paris: Flammarion; 1991. p. 545–56.
22. Sharp GC. Diagnostic criteria for classification of MCTD. Amsterdam: Elsevier; 1987. p. 23–32.
23. Kasukawa R, Miyawaki S. Preliminary diagnostic criteria for classification of mixed connective tissue disease. Mixed connective tissue disease and antinuclear antibodies. Amsterdam: Elsevier; 1987. p. 41–7.
24. Alarcon-Segovia D, Villarreal M. Classification and diagnostic criteria for mixed connective tissue disease. In: Kasukawawa R, Sharp GC, editors. Mixed connective tissue disease and anti-nuclear antibodies. Amsterdam: Exerpta Medica; 1987. p. 33–40.
25. Venables PJ. Mixed connective tissue disease. Lupus. 2006;15(3):132–7. https://doi.org/10.1191/0961203306lu2283rr. PMID: 16634365.
26. Cutolo M, Sulli A, Pizzorni C, Accardo S. Nailfold videocapillaroscopy assessment of microvascular damage in systemic sclerosis. J Rheumatol. 2000;27(1):155–60. PMID: 10648032.

27. Ruaro B, Pizzorni C, Paolino S, Smith V, Ghio M, Casabella A, Alessandri E, Patané M, Sulli A, Cutolo M. Correlations between nailfold microvascular damage and skin involvement in systemic sclerosis patients. Microvasc Res. 2019;125:103874. https://doi.org/10.1016/j.mvr.2019.04.004. Epub 2019 Apr 8. PMID: 30974112.
28. Cutolo M, editor. Atlas of Capillaroscopy in rheumatic diseases. Milano: Elsevier Srl; 2010.
29. Ji LL, Wang H, Zhang XH, Zhang ZL. Correlation between nailfold capillaroscopic findings and presence of interstitial lung disease in systemic sclerosis patients. Beijing Da Xue Xue Bao. 2018;50(3):501–6. Chinese. PMID: 29930420.
30. Corrado A, Correale M, Mansueto N, Monaco I, Carriero A, Mele A, Colia R, Di Biase M, Cantatore FP. Nailfold capillaroscopic changes in patients with idiopathic pulmonary arterial hypertension and systemic sclerosis-related pulmonary arterial hypertension. Microvasc Res. 2017;114:46–51. https://doi.org/10.1016/j.mvr.2017.06.005. Epub 2017 Jun 12. PMID: 28619664.
31. Celińska-Löwenhoff M, Pastuszczak M, Pełka K, Stec-Polak M, Wojas-Pelc A, Musiał J. Associations between nailfold capillaroscopy findings and interstitial lung disease in patients with mixed connective tissue disease. Arch Med Sci. 2019;16(2):297–301. https://doi.org/10.5114/aoms.2018.81129. PMID: 32190139; PMCID: PMC7069420.
32. Todoroki Y, Kubo S, Nakano K, Miyazaki Y, Ueno M, Satoh-Kanda Y, Kanda R, Miyagawa I, Hanami K, Nakatsuka K, Saito K, Nakayamada S, Tanaka Y. Nailfold microvascular abnormalities are associated with a higher prevalence of pulmonary arterial hypertension in patients with MCTD. Rheumatology (Oxford). 2022;61(12):4875–84. https://doi.org/10.1093/rheumatology/keac165. PMID: 35285493.
33. Loganathan A, Zanframundo G, Yoshida A, Faghihi-Kashani S, Bauer Ventura I, Dourado E, et al. Agreement between local and central anti-synthetase antibodies detection: results from the Classification Criteria of Anti-Synthetase Syndrome project biobank. Clin Exp Rheumatol. 2024;42(2):277–87. https://doi.org/10.55563/clinexprheumatol/s14zq8. Epub 2024 Mar 14. PMID: 38488094.
34. Faghihi-Kashani S, Yoshida A, Bozan F, Zanframundo G, Rozza D, Loganathan A, et al. Clinical characteristics of anti-synthetase syndrome: analysis from the classification criteria for anti-synthetase syndrome project. Arthritis Rheumatol. 2025;77(4):477–89. https://doi.org/10.1002/art.43038. Epub 2024 Dec 17. PMID: 39467037; PMCID: PMC11936500.
35. Mercer LK, Moore TL, Chinoy H, Murray AK, Vail A, Cooper RG, et al. Quantitative nailfold video capillaroscopy in patients with idiopathic inflammatory myopathy. Rheumatology. 2010;49(9):1699–705.
36. Shenavandeh S, Zarei Nezhad M. Association of nailfold capillary changes with disease activity, clinical and laboratory findings in patients with dermatomyositis. Med J Islam Repub Iran. 2015;29:233.
37. Mugii N, Hasegawa M, Matsushita T, Hamaguchi Y, Horie S, Yahata T, et al. Association between nail-fold capillary findings and disease activity in dermatomyositis. Rheumatology (Oxford). 2011;50(6):1091–8.
38. Selva-O'Callaghan A, Fonollosa-Pla V, Trallero-Araguás E, Martínez-Gómez X, Simeon-Aznar CP, Labrador-Horrillo M, Vilardell-Tarrés M. Nailfold capillary microscopy in adults with inflammatory myopathy. Semin Arthritis Rheum. 2010;39(5):398–404. https://doi.org/10.1016/j.semarthrit.2008.09.003. Epub 2008 Nov 20. PMID: 19022479.
39. Soubrier C, Seguier J, Di Costanzo MP, Ebbo M, Bernit E, Jean E, Veit V, Swiader L, Salort-Campana E, Attarian S, De Paula AM, Kaplanski G, Durand JM, Harlé JR, Schleinitz N. Nailfold videocapillaroscopy alterations in dermatomyositis, antisynthetase syndrome, overlap myositis, and immune-mediated necrotizing myopathy. Clin Rheumatol. 2019;38(12):3451–8. https://doi.org/10.1007/s10067-019-04710-2. Epub 2019 Aug 22. PMID: 31440919.

Chapter 7
Systemic Lupus Erythematosus and Antiphospholipid Syndrome

Noémie Gensous, Nathalie Morel, Sophie Skopinski, and Marie-Elise Truchetet

Introduction

Raynaud's phenomenon (RP) is a common feature in autoimmune connective tissue diseases and often serves as an early clinical clue prompting further diagnostic investigations. In the context of systemic lupus erythematosus (SLE) and antiphospholipid syndrome (APS), RP raises important questions about underlying microvascular involvement and the potential for disease overlap, particularly with systemic sclerosis (SSc). Nailfold capillaroscopy (NFC) has become an increasingly valuable tool in this diagnostic process, offering a noninvasive window into the microcirculation and capillary architecture.

This article aims to explore the capillaroscopic features observed in patients with SLE and APS, highlighting the diversity and non-specificity of findings while underlining their clinical utility. Through selected illustrative case vignettes, we describe the spectrum of capillary changes seen in these diseases, including dilated capillaries, microhemorrhages, and occasional scleroderma-like patterns. We also examine the potential roles of NFC in supporting differential diagnosis, identifying overlap syndromes, and evaluating disease activity or vascular risk, even though its prognostic value in SLE remains under investigation.

N. Gensous · S. Skopinski
CHU de Bordeaux, Internal Medicine and Clinical Immunology Department, Bordeaux, France
e-mail: Noemie.gensous@chu-bordeaux.fr; sophie.skopinski@chu-bordeaux.fr

N. Morel · M.-E. Truchetet (✉)
CHU de Bordeaux, Rheumatology Department, Bordeaux, France
e-mail: nathalie.morel@chu-bordeaux.fr; Marie-elise.truchetet@chu-bordeaux.fr

Y. El Miedany, R. A. Elziaty (eds.), *Capillaroscopy*, Contemporary Rheumatology,
https://doi.org/10.1007/978-3-032-22966-3_7

Diagnosis and Management of Systemic Lupus Erythematosus (SLE)

Introduction

SLE is a chronic systemic autoimmune disease that most commonly affects young women of childbearing age with a peak incidence between 15 and 45 years and a female-to-male ratio of approximately 9:1. Worldwide occurrence of SLE exhibits a broad range, with an incidence ranging from 1.5 to 11 per 100,000 person-years and a prevalence ranging from 13 to 7713.5 per 100,000 individuals [2]. Non-Caucasian individuals, including those of African-American, African-Caribbean, American-Hispanic, and Asian ancestry, are at greater risk of SLE and of developing a more severe disease phenotype, especially regarding renal involvement.

Despite a remarkable increase in the lifespan of SLE patients during the last decades due to advances in both diagnostic approaches and therapeutic management, standardized mortality ratios are still high in this population in relation to the accumulation of organ damage and higher incidence of comorbidities such as cardiovascular events or infectious diseases [13, 27].

Diagnostic Criteria and Classification

Due to the heterogeneity of the disease, classification criteria have been revised multiple times to improve diagnostic accuracy and standardization. The most recent update, developed in 2019 by the European League Against Rheumatism (EULAR) and the American College of Rheumatology (ACR), introduced stricter guidelines to enhance both specificity and sensitivity [1]. They use positive antinuclear antibodies (ANA) (at a titer of ≥1:80) as an entry criterion and have weighted items across multiple domains, ranging from 2 (for delirium, noninfectious fever, and antiphospholipid antibodies) to 10 (for class III or IV lupus nephritis) [1].

While classification criteria are designed to standardize case categorization for research or analytical purposes, they do not serve as diagnostic criteria for SLE. Diagnosis should be established by an experienced clinician, based on a comprehensive assessment of specific combinations of clinical and immunologic features, alongside a thorough evaluation to exclude alternative explanations for the clinical presentation.

Pathogenesis

Despite extensive research, the pathophysiology of SLE remains complex and only partially understood. The etiology of the disease is unknown but is believed to develop through the interplay of susceptibility genes, epigenetic and environmental factors, immune cells, and molecules that participate in apoptosis, and innate and adaptive immune responses [26]. A key concept in the pathogenesis of SLE is the defective clearance of apoptotic cells, leading to the accumulation of apoptotic debris that elicits an abnormal immune response. It ultimately triggers the production of autoantibodies, which, upon forming immune complexes, drive chronic inflammation and tissue damage. Alongside this humoral response, excessive cytokine production, including type I interferons, further amplifies immune activation, contributing to disease progression and multiorgan involvement.

Clinical Spectrum

SLE clinical expression is remarkably heterogeneous, with a broad spectrum of symptoms encompassing almost all organs, which can vary from mild to life-threatening. The course of the disease is characterized by multisystem involvement with interchanging flares and remissions of variable duration.

The most common manifestations include malar rash, photosensitivity, polyarthralgia or arthritis, serositis, and nephropathy.

Clinical manifestations can be graded by frequency of occurrence:

- Musculoskeletal involvement (approximately 90% of patients): typically presents as nonerosive polyarthritis affecting small joints of hands, wrists, and knees, which can significantly impact quality of life.
- Mucocutaneous manifestations (occurring in 70–80% of patients), including malar rash, discoid lesions, photosensitivity, and oral ulcers, represent some of the most recognizable signs of the disease. Of note, Raynaud's phenomenon occurred frequently in this context of autoimmunity. These manifestations are specifically detailed in Table 7.1.
- Hematological manifestations (50–75% of patients), including hemolytic anemia, leukopenia, lymphopenia, and thrombocytopenia.
- Renal involvement (approximately 40–60% of patients): lupus nephritis remains one of the most severe complications, often determining long-term prognosis due to its risk of progression to chronic kidney disease and end-stage renal failure.
- Cardiopulmonary manifestations: including serositis (pleuritis in 30–50% and pericarditis in 20–30% of patients) and, less frequently, myocarditis and pulmonary hypertension.

Table 7.1 Mucocutaneous involvement is among the most common clinical manifestations in SLE patients. These include both lupus-specific and nonspecific lesions

Lupus-specific lesions	Lupus nonspecific lesions
Acute cutaneous lupus erythematosus	*Cutaneous vasculitis*
Localized or generalized	Palpable purpura
Subacute cutaneous lupus erythematosus	Urticarial vasculitis
Annular, papulosquamous	Livedo reticularis
Chronic cutaneous lupus erythematosus	Periungual telangiectasia/erythema
Classic discoid lupus erythematosus	Splinter nailfold hemorrhages
Hypertrophic discoid lupus	Ulcerations
Lupus panniculitis	Digital gangrene
Mucosal lupus erythematosus	Cutaneous infarctions
Lupus tumidus	*Raynaud's phenomenon*
Chilblain lupus	*Nonspecific bullous lesions*
	Acanthosis nigricans
	Erythema multiform
	Leg ulcers
	Lichen planus
	Alopecia
	Urticaria

- Neuropsychiatric involvement (25–40% of patients): ranging from cognitive dysfunction and mood disorders to seizures and psychosis. It represents an important diagnostic and therapeutic challenge.
- Constitutional symptoms: fever, fatigue, and weight loss.

Management of SLE

The treatment of SLE follows a personalized approach based on organ involvement and disease severity, as outlined in the 2023 EULAR guidelines [9].

General measures include smoking cessation, sun protection, regular exercise and balanced nutrition, appropriate vaccinations, weight management, and control of cardiovascular risk factors.

Hydroxychloroquine is recommended for all patients, unless rarely contraindicated. Conventional immunosuppressants are selected based on disease severity. For mild to moderate disease, options include methotrexate, azathioprine, mycophenolate mofetil, and calcineurin inhibitors. In severe forms of the disease, cyclophosphamide or mycophenolate mofetil should be considered for disease control.

Biologics represent an important advancement in SLE management. Belimumab, which targets B-lymphocyte stimulator (BLyS), can be effective across multiple disease manifestations. Anifrolumab, which blocks type I interferon receptors, has demonstrated particular efficacy for cutaneous manifestations. Rituximab, an anti-CD20 monoclonal antibody that depletes B cells, is typically reserved for severe or refractory disease states.

Targets under treatment focus on achieving either complete remission (defined as clinical SLEDAI = 0 with hydroxychloroquine and glucocorticoids ≤5 mg/day) or low disease activity (SLEDAI ≤4 with similar medication parameters), with immunosuppressive or biological agents at a stable, tolerated dose [9].

Diagnosis and Management of the Antiphospholipid Syndrome (APS)

Introduction

APS is a systemic autoimmune disorder defined by thrombotic and/or obstetrical complications occurring in individuals with persistent antiphospholipid antibodies (aPL). These antibodies are directed against phospholipid-binding plasma proteins, notably β2-glycoprotein I, and are believed to play a direct pathogenic role. APS can be primary or associated with other autoimmune diseases, most commonly SLE.

The main clinical manifestations of APS include arterial or venous thrombosis, recurrent pregnancy loss, and adverse obstetrical outcomes such as intrauterine growth restriction or severe preeclampsia. Non-thrombotic manifestations can include heart valve disease, livedo reticularis, thrombocytopenia, nephropathy, and cognitive dysfunction.

The syndrome has been recognized as a leading acquired cause of thrombophilia, especially in young patients. Its diagnosis and management remain complex due to variability in presentation and serologic patterns.

Diagnostic Criteria and Classification

The diagnosis of APS requires both clinical and laboratory criteria, as defined by the revised Sapporo (Sydney) criteria established in 2006 [16]. Clinical criteria include one or more episodes of vascular thrombosis (arterial, venous, or small-vessel) or specific obstetrical complications such as one or more unexplained deaths of a morphologically normal fetus beyond the 10th week of gestation, premature birth of a normal neonate before the 34th week due to preeclampsia or placental insufficiency, or three or more unexplained consecutive miscarriages before the 10th week. Laboratory criteria require the presence of lupus anticoagulant, anticardiolipin antibodies (IgG or IgM), or anti–β2-glycoprotein I antibodies (IgG or IgM) on two occasions at least 12 weeks apart. Transient positivity can occur due to infection or medication, which is why persistence over time is critical to establish the diagnosis.

In 2023, updated EULAR/ACR classification criteria for APS were proposed, broadening the clinical spectrum to include microvascular involvement (such as renal, pulmonary, and adrenal manifestations or livedo), hematologic features like thrombocytopenia, and cardiac valvular abnormalities (e.g., Libman–Sacks endocarditis), thus better reflecting the diverse organ involvement observed in clinical practice [3]. The traditional risk factors for venous or arterial thrombosis are taken into account, with the introduction of a weighting of the thrombotic episode according to the presence or absence of vascular risk factors [3]. Obstetrical events are better defined, with the presence of stigmata of preeclampsia and/or placental insufficiency (including the presence of intrauterine growth retardation) taking precedence over severity criteria [3].

Finally, this new classification better integrates the biological phenotype by incorporating risk stratification, particularly the concept of double and triple positivity. This high-risk profile, defined by the persistent presence of all three aPL in Antiphospholipid Syndrome (APS), is associated with more severe clinical outcomes and a poorer prognosis [3, 17]. Isolated low-titer antibodies or transient aPL positivity no longer meet the criteria for APS and carry a lower risk.

While these updated classification criteria aim to standardize research populations, they are not strictly intended to establish a diagnosis and should not replace clinical judgment in individual cases.

Pathogenesis

aPL antibodies promote a procoagulant state by multiple mechanisms. These include activation of endothelial cells, monocytes, and platelets, inhibition of endogenous anticoagulant pathways (such as the protein C pathway), and activation of complement. Experimental models have demonstrated that the passive transfer of aPL into animals can reproduce key features of APS, such as thrombosis and fetal loss [11]. Complement activation appears to play a central role in mediating these outcomes, particularly in obstetrical APS. Furthermore, β2-glycoprotein I undergoes conformational changes upon binding to anionic phospholipid membranes, exposing epitopes that are recognized by autoantibodies. These interactions are central to the pathogenic cascade. The end result is endothelial injury, thrombus formation, and impaired placental function.

Clinical Spectrum

APS can present in various forms. The most common is deep-vein thrombosis of the lower limbs, but pulmonary embolism, stroke, myocardial infarction, and renal or mesenteric thrombosis can also occur. Arterial thromboses, although less frequent, often have more devastating consequences. Obstetrical manifestations are diverse and include early or late fetal loss, preterm delivery due to placental insufficiency, and preeclampsia.

A particularly severe and rare form of the disease is catastrophic antiphospholipid syndrome (CAPS), characterized by the rapid development of thromboses, which mainly affect the microvasculature, in multiple organ systems. This life-threatening variant affects less than 1% of patients with APS and is often precipitated by suboptimal anticoagulation management, infection, trauma, or surgery [5, 21, 24].

Management of APS

Thrombotic APS

For patients with confirmed APS and a thrombotic event, long-term anticoagulation is the cornerstone of treatment. The first-line therapy is warfarin (vitamin K antagonist) with a target international normalized ratio (INR) of 2.0–3.0. In cases of arterial thrombosis, some experts recommend a higher INR target of 3.0–4.0, although supporting evidence is limited and increased bleeding risk must be considered [25].

There is an ongoing debate about the role of direct oral anticoagulants (DOACs) in APS. Studies such as the TRAPS trial [18] showed higher rates of recurrent thrombosis in high-risk APS patients treated with rivaroxaban compared to warfarin. Consequently, guidelines recommend avoiding DOACs in patients with triple positivity, arterial events, or high-risk obstetrical history.

In patients with low-risk profiles (single aPL positivity, low titer, no prior thrombosis), the role of primary thromboprophylaxis is uncertain. Low-dose aspirin (LDA) is sometimes considered in this group, particularly when additional cardiovascular risk factors are present. However, data are conflicting, and decisions must be individualized.

Management of Obstetrical APS

Pregnant women with APS require special management to optimize maternal and fetal outcomes. Those with a history of obstetrical APS but no thrombosis are generally treated with LDA combined with prophylactic low-molecular-weight heparin (LMWH). This regimen has significantly improved live birth rates [20, 22]. For women with both thrombotic and obstetrical APS, therapeutic LMWH plus LDA is used throughout pregnancy and continued postpartum.

The postpartum period carries a high risk of thrombosis and justifies extended anticoagulation (usually 6 weeks). Hydroxychloroquine, an immunomodulatory drug widely used in SLE, is under investigation for potential use in APS, particularly in refractory or high-risk obstetrical cases. Its antithrombotic and anti-inflammatory properties make it an attractive adjunct, although evidence is still emerging. Immunosuppressants and corticosteroids are not routinely used in classic APS but may be indicated in CAPS or when APS overlaps with SLE [25].

Management of Catastrophic APS

CAPS is a medical emergency requiring immediate treatment. Management typically includes full anticoagulation, high-dose corticosteroids, plasma exchange, and/or intravenous immunoglobulin. In refractory cases, immunosuppressive therapies such as rituximab or complement inhibitors like eculizumab may be considered [4]. Early diagnosis and aggressive therapy are essential for survival. Prevention through effective management of infections and minimizing anticoagulation interruption or dose reduction, particularly during the perioperative period, is recommended to avoid its occurrence [14].

Monitoring and Follow-Up

Regular monitoring of anticoagulation and assessment of cardiovascular risk factors is necessary. Patients on warfarin require routine INR checks. Those with recurrent thromboses despite therapeutic INR levels may be considered for intensified anticoagulation or switching to LMWH [25].

aPL levels are not routinely monitored after diagnosis, as they do not correlate well with disease activity. However, repeat testing may be useful in initially equivocal cases or when evaluating risk in asymptomatic individuals. In women with aPL but no prior thrombosis or pregnancy morbidity, prophylactic LDA may be considered on a case-by-case basis, especially in the presence of additional risk factors.

Clinical Cases: Use of Nailfold Capillaroscopy in a Lupus Patient

Clinical Case 1

Patient Mrs. L., 34 years old.

Medical History Diagnosed 6 years ago with SLE, positive ANA and anti-dsDNA, history of cutaneous flares and arthralgias. No prior organ involvement. Currently on hydroxychloroquine and low-dose steroids.

Reason for Consultation Over the past few months, the patient reports increasing episodes of *cold-induced color changes in the fingers*, evolving into painful white and blue discoloration, suggestive of *Raynaud's phenomenon*. She also reports occasional digital paresthesia and fatigue. There is no history of digital ulcers.

Clinical Findings

- Blood pressure and heart exam normal.
- No synovitis or active skin lesions.
- Nailfolds show periungual erythema but no infarcts or ulcers.

Investigations

Given the new-onset Raynaud's and the need to *stratify vascular risk*, an *NFC* is performed.

Capillaroscopic Findings (Fig. 7.1)

- Dilated capillaries.
- Occasional giant capillaries.
- Presence of hemorrhages.
- Overall disorganized architecture but *not a scleroderma pattern.*

These findings support *microangiopathy related to lupus* but *do not suggest systemic sclerosis* or a "scleroderma-like" vasculopathy.

Clinical Relevance

In this case, NFC was helpful to:

- Confirm the presence of microvascular damage consistent with lupus.

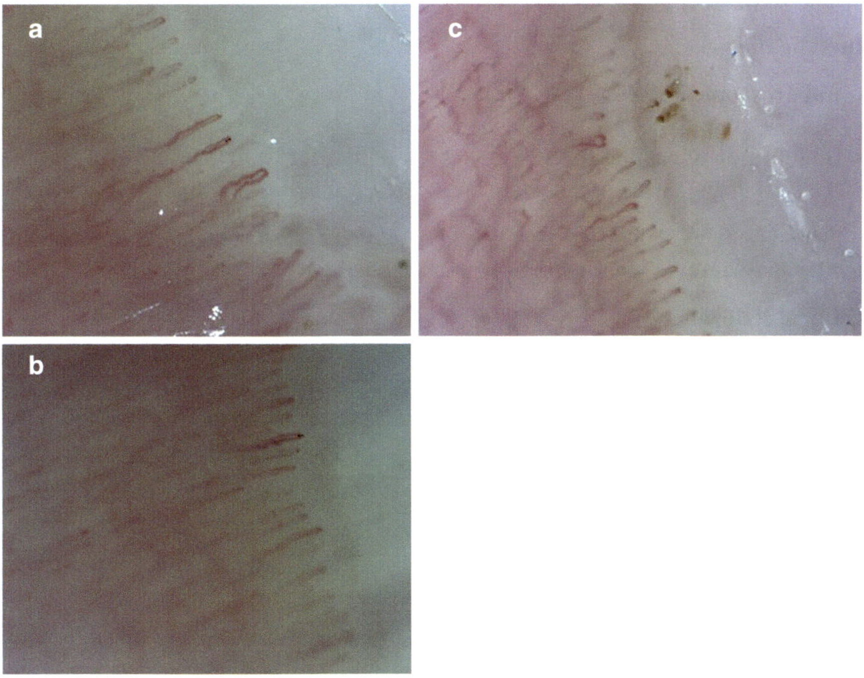

Fig. 7.1 Nailfold videocapillaroscopy classified as minor capillary abnormalities showing (**a**) and (**b**) Dilated capillaries; (**c**) hemorrhages

- Exclude capillaroscopic signs suggestive of an overlap with systemic sclerosis.
- Justify the use of vasodilators and close vascular monitoring without changing the diagnostic framework.

Clinical Case 2

Patient Mrs. D., 42 years old.

Medical History Diagnosed 5 years ago with SLE, positive ANA with anti-SSA, anti-RNP, anti-Sm, and anti-dsDNA, history of cutaneous flares, arthralgias with Jaccoud arthropathy and sclerodactyly. Currently on hydroxychloroquine and low-dose steroids. She is currently an active smoker.

Reason for Consultation Evaluate for possible evolution toward an overlap syndrome with systemic sclerosis.

Clinical Findings
- Blood pressure and heart exam normal.
- No synovitis or active skin lesions.
- Nailfolds show periungual erythema but no infarcts or ulcers.

Investigations

Capillaroscopic Findings (Fig. 7.2):
- Tortuous capillaries.
- Rarefaction of capillaritis.
- Overall disorganized architecture but *not a scleroderma pattern*.

These findings support *microangiopathy related to lupus* but *do not suggest systemic sclerosis* or a "scleroderma-like" vasculopathy.

Clinical Relevance
In this case, NFC was helpful to:

Confirm the presence of microvascular damage consistent with SLE.

Clinical Case 3

Patient Mrs. D., 45 years old.

Medical History Cutaneous and articular lupus and autoimmune hepatitis presented with a long-standing history of Raynaud's phenomenon, which worsened over the past winter. She reported biphasic color changes triggered by cold exposure but no digital ulcers or skin thickening.

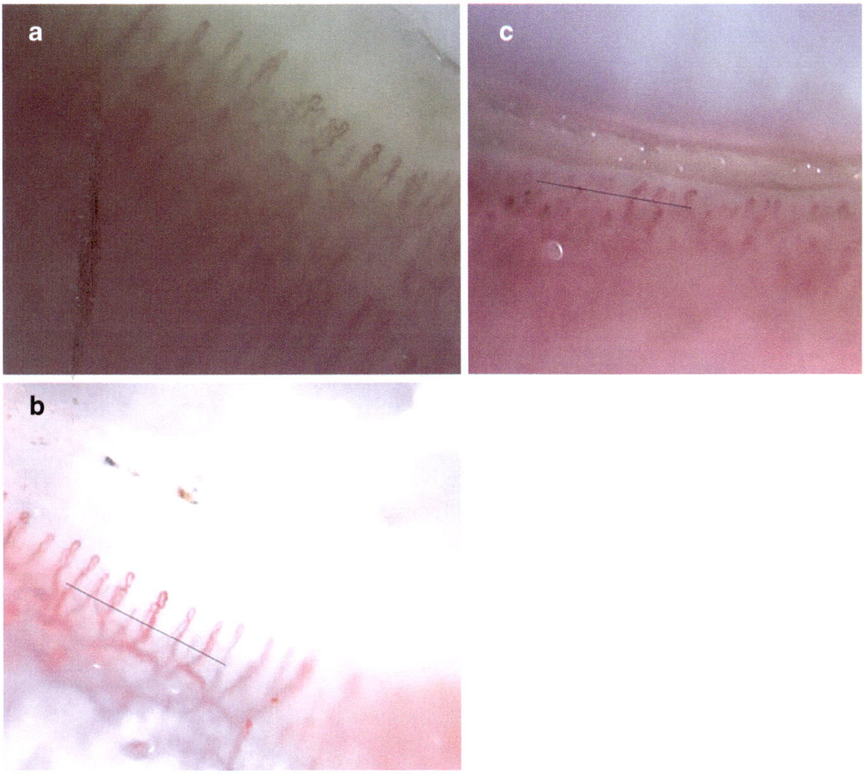

Fig. 7.2 Nailfold videocapillaroscopy classified as minor capillary abnormalities showing: (**a**) tortuous capillaries, (**b**) and (**c**) rarefaction of capillaritis

Reason for Consultation Assessment for an underlying SSc pattern.

Clinical Findings

- Blood pressure and heart exam normal.
- No synovitis or active skin lesions.
- Nailfolds show periungual erythema but no infarcts or ulcers.

Investigations

Capillaroscopic Findings (Fig. 7.3):

- Preserved capillary density.
- No giant capillaries.
- No architectural disorganization.
- Findings consistent with a normal non-scleroderma pattern.

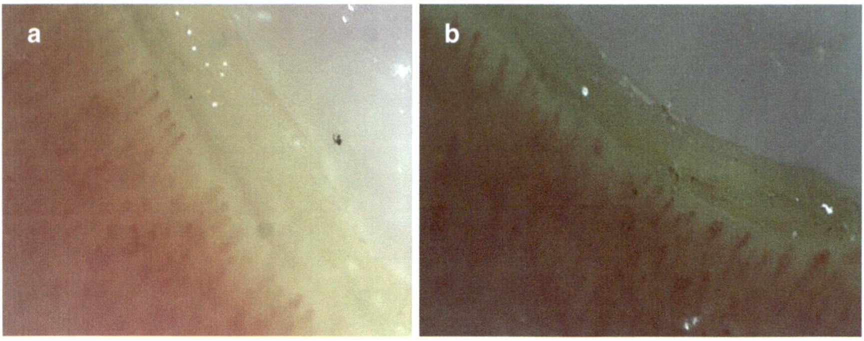

Fig. 7.3 (**a**) and (**b**) Nailfold videocapillaroscopy showing normal non-scleroderma pattern

Clinical Relevance

These results helped rule out a connective tissue disease overlap with SSc. The patient was reassured, and management focused on her primary autoimmune conditions and Raynaud's symptomatic treatment.

Clinical Case 4

Patient Mrs. B., 23 years old.

Medical History Recent diagnosis of SLE presented with newly developed Raynaud's phenomenon. There were no signs of sclerodactyly, digital ulcers, or telangiectasia.

Reason for Consultation Evaluate for possible evolution toward an overlap syndrome with systemic sclerosis, particularly in the setting of positive antinuclear antibodies.

Investigations

Capillaroscopic Findings (Fig. 7.4)
- Normal capillary architecture.
- No signs of microangiopathy.
- These findings excluded a scleroderma-spectrum disorder.

Clinical Relevance

The findings ruled out a scleroderma pattern and guided the clinical team to focus on lupus management without further workup for SSc. NFC thus played a valuable role in differential diagnosis.

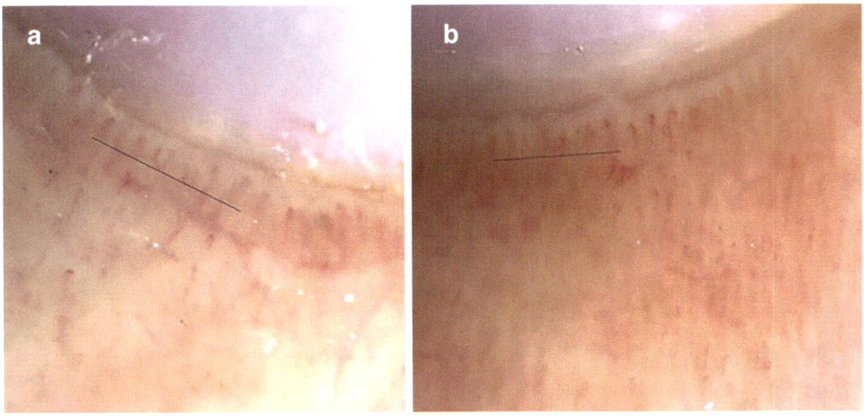

Fig. 7.4 (**a**) and (**b**) Nailfold videocapillaroscopy showing normal non-scleroderma pattern

Clinical Case 5

Patient Mrs. A., 22 years old.

Medical History Triple-positive antiphospholipid antibodies.

Reason for Consultation Evaluation after being diagnosed during a contraceptive workup by her midwife. She had no history of thrombosis or pregnancy complications but reported a mild Raynaud's phenomenon. Given the autoimmune background and risk of connective tissue disease development, an NFC was performed.

Investigations

Capillaroscopic Findings (Fig. 7.5):

- Normal capillary architecture.
- No evidence of capillary dropout, megacapillaries, or hemorrhages.
- These findings excluded a scleroderma-spectrum disorder.

Clinical Relevance

NFC provided useful reassurance in a complex immunological context.

Capillaroscopic Features in SLE and APS

NFC, a noninvasive and easily accessible technique, has become a valuable tool for assessing microvascular involvement in patients with autoimmune connective tissue diseases. It enables the direct visualization of capillary morphology and density at

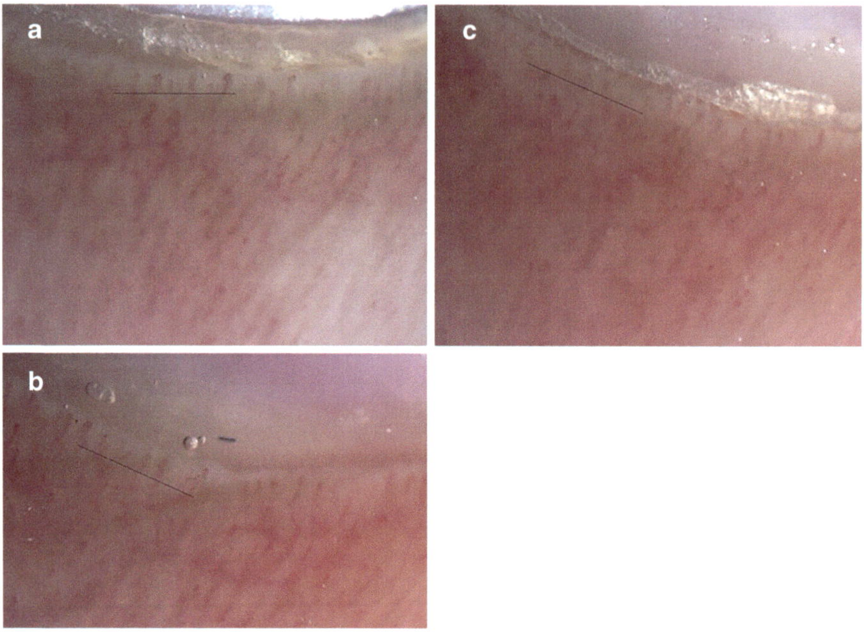

Fig. 7.5 (**a**, **b**, and **c**) Nailfold videocapillaroscopy showing a normal non-scleroderma pattern

the nailfold, providing insights into underlying microangiopathy often observed in SLE and other connective tissue diseases [6, 7].

While RP is a common symptom of autoimmune connective tissue diseases, including SLE and APS, NFC allows the detection of the morphological microvascular abnormalities, distinguishing it from systemic sclerosis (Fig. 7.6). Interestingly, a recent large-scale study involving 1181 patients with various connective tissue diseases revealed that a "scleroderma pattern" was present in approximately 2% among 108 SLE patients but was entirely absent among 22 patients with APS [12]. Similarly, Zhao et al. analyzed 85 patients with newly diagnosed SLE and found that the majority presented with nonspecific capillaroscopic abnormalities, followed by normal findings, and only a minority exhibited a scleroderma-like pattern [28]. This highlights the rarity of overt scleroderma-like microangiopathy and reinforces the importance of NFC in these conditions.

Regarding capillaroscopic abnormalities frequently observed in SLE and APS, they are typically nonspecific and do not follow the well-defined scleroderma pattern [12].

Typical capillaroscopic findings in SLE may include:

- Normal capillary morphology.
- Dilated or irregularly shaped capillaries.
- Occasional giant capillaries (less frequent than in SSc).
- Microhemorrhages.

- Capillary dropout (in a subset of patients).
- Disorganized architecture, often lacking the well-demarcated giant-capillary and avascular-area pattern characteristic of SSc.

The most reported alterations in APS patients are capillary tortuosity and microhemorrhages. Oral anticoagulants may represent a confounding factor for isolated microhemorrhages [10].

It is also noteworthy that many patients—particularly those with low disease activity—may present with normal or near-normal NFC patterns.

Despite its limited diagnostic specificity in SLE and APS, NFC remains useful in several clinical contexts (Fig. 7.6):

- Differentiating primary from secondary Raynaud's phenomenon.
- Identifying vascular overlap with systemic sclerosis.
- Guiding vascular management decisions, such as the use of vasodilators or antiplatelet agents.

Interestingly, a systematic review by Cutolo et al. highlighted the association between capillaroscopic changes and SLE disease activity [6]. These alterations were especially pronounced in patients with active lupus nephritis and cutaneous vasculitis, suggesting that microvascular damage may reflect broader systemic

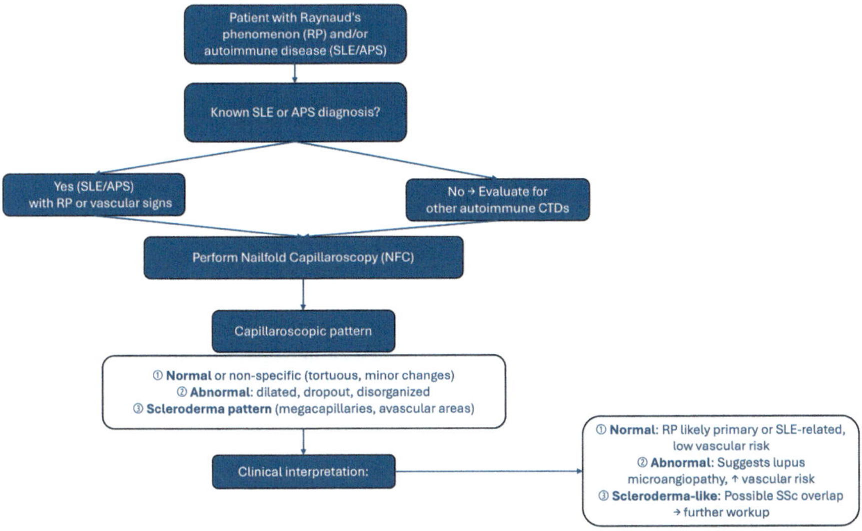

Fig. 7.6 Algorithm for the use of nailfold videocapillaroscopy in patients presenting with Raynaud's phenomenon and/or suspected autoimmune disease. The capillaroscopic pattern helps guide the diagnostic orientation: a normal pattern supports primary Raynaud's phenomenon; non-specific abnormalities may indicate low vascular risk in systemic lupus erythematosus; lupus-related microangiopathy suggests closer monitoring for organ involvement; and a scleroderma-type pattern strongly supports systemic sclerosis or possible overlap syndromes. RP Raynaud phenomenon, SLE systemic lupus erythematosus, APS antiphospholipid syndrome, CTDs connective tissue diseases, SSc systemic sclerosis

involvement. This association was also supported in juvenile-onset SLE, where similar capillaroscopic abnormalities correlated with disease manifestations [23]. Of note, Pimenta da Fonseca et al. found no significant differences in NFC patterns between SLE patients with and without Jaccoud's arthropathy, suggesting that joint deformities in this context may not reflect distinct microvascular involvement [19].

According to laboratory parameters, Makarem et al. reported a correlation between capillaroscopic abnormalities and the presence of anti-RNP antibodies, possibly indicating a subset of patients at higher risk for aggressive vascular manifestations [15]. The literature currently available does not allow for conclusions to be drawn about the correlation between markers of lupus activity and capillary abnormalities [6].

One of the most promising applications of NFC in SLE is its potential predictive value for severe vascular complications. Donnarumma et al., in a study of 65 SLE patients, demonstrated that the presence of avascular areas and significant capillary dropout was strongly associated with the subsequent development of pulmonary arterial hypertension (PAH), positioning NFC as a possible noninvasive screening tool for this life-threatening complication [8].

Finally, although several studies have demonstrated associations between microvascular abnormalities and markers of disease activity or high-risk clinical profiles, the primary role of nailfold NFC in SLE remains its capacity to help rule out scleroderma-spectrum disorders and assess vascular involvement in a broader clinical context.

Conclusion

NFC represents a useful and accessible tool in the clinical evaluation of Raynaud's phenomenon in the SLE or APS context. While the capillaroscopic patterns in SLE are most often nonspecific and lack the well-defined features of SSc, NFC plays a crucial role in ruling out scleroderma-spectrum disorders in patients with ambiguous or overlapping clinical signs. Recent studies also suggest potential correlations between capillaroscopic abnormalities and disease activity or vascular complications, such as pulmonary arterial hypertension. However, these findings remain exploratory, and further prospective studies are needed to clarify the prognostic value of NFC in SLE and APS. In current practice, its primary utility lies in enhancing clinical judgment, especially in the context of differential diagnosis and vascular risk assessment.

References

1. Aringer M, Costenbader K, Daikh D, et al. 2019 European league against rheumatism/American College of Rheumatology classification criteria for systemic lupus erythematosus. Ann Rheum Dis. 2019;78:1151–9. https://doi.org/10.1136/annrheumdis-2018-214819.
2. Barber MRW, Drenkard C, Falasinnu T, et al. Global epidemiology of systemic lupus erythematosus. Nat Rev Rheumatol. 2021;17:515–32. https://doi.org/10.1038/s41584-021-00668-1.
3. Barbhaiya M, Zuily S, Naden R, et al. 2023 ACR/EULAR antiphospholipid syndrome classification criteria. Ann Rheum Dis. 2023;82:1258–70. https://doi.org/10.1136/ard-2023-224609.
4. Bucciarelli S, Espinosa G, Cervera R, et al. Mortality in the catastrophic antiphospholipid syndrome: causes of death and prognostic factors in a series of 250 patients. Arthritis Rheum. 2006;54:2568–76. https://doi.org/10.1002/art.22018.
5. Cervera R, Piette J-C, Font J, et al. Antiphospholipid syndrome: clinical and immunologic manifestations and patterns of disease expression in a cohort of 1,000 patients. Arthritis Rheum. 2002;46:1019–27. https://doi.org/10.1002/art.10187.
6. Cutolo M, Melsens K, Wijnant S, et al. Nailfold capillaroscopy in systemic lupus erythematosus: a systematic review and critical appraisal. Autoimmun Rev. 2018;17:344–52. https://doi.org/10.1016/j.autrev.2017.11.025.
7. Dima A, Vonk MC, Garaiman A, et al. Clinical significance of the anti-Nucleolar Organizer Region 90 antibodies (NOR90) in systemic sclerosis: Analysis of the European Scleroderma Trials and Research (EUSTAR) cohort and a systematic literature review. Eur J Intern Med. 2024;125:104–10. https://doi.org/10.1016/j.ejim.2024.03.035.
8. Donnarumma JFS, Ferreira EVM, Ota-Arakaki J, Kayser C. Nailfold capillaroscopy as a risk factor for pulmonary arterial hypertension in systemic lupus erythematosus patients. Adv Rheumatol. 2019;59:1. https://doi.org/10.1186/s42358-018-0045-5.
9. Fanouriakis A, Kostopoulou M, Andersen J, et al. EULAR recommendations for the management of systemic lupus erythematosus: 2023 update. Ann Rheum Dis. 2024;83:15–29. https://doi.org/10.1136/ard-2023-224762.
10. Ferrari G, Gotelli E, Paolino S, et al. Antiphospholipid antibodies and anticoagulant therapy: capillaroscopic findings. Arthritis Res Ther. 2021;23:175. https://doi.org/10.1186/s13075-021-02551-6.
11. Girardi G, Berman J, Redecha P, et al. Complement C5a receptors and neutrophils mediate fetal injury in the antiphospholipid syndrome. J Clin Invest. 2003;112:1644–54. https://doi.org/10.1172/JCI18817.
12. Hysa E, Pizzorni C, Sammorì S, et al. Microvascular damage in autoimmune connective tissue diseases: a capillaroscopic analysis from 20 years of experience in a EULAR training and research referral centre for imaging. RMD Open. 2023;9:e003071. https://doi.org/10.1136/rmdopen-2023-003071.
13. Lee YH, Choi SJ, Ji JD, Song GG. Overall and cause-specific mortality in systemic lupus erythematosus: an updated meta-analysis. Lupus. 2016;25:727–34. https://doi.org/10.1177/0961203315627202.
14. Legault K, Schunemann H, Hillis C, et al. McMaster RARE-Bestpractices clinical practice guideline on diagnosis and management of the catastrophic antiphospholipid syndrome. J Thromb Haemost. 2018;16:1656–64. https://doi.org/10.1111/jth.14192.
15. Makarem YS, Selim ZI, Ismail S, et al. Nailfold capillaroscopy changes in systemic lupus erythematosus patients: correlation with disease activity and anti-uridin1-ribonucleoprotein antibodies. Reumatol Clin. 2025;21:501840. https://doi.org/10.1016/j.reumae.2025.501840.
16. Miyakis S, Lockshin MD, Atsumi T, et al. International consensus statement on an update of the classification criteria for definite antiphospholipid syndrome (APS). J Thromb Haemost. 2006;4:295–306. https://doi.org/10.1111/j.1538-7836.2006.01753.x.

17. Pengo V, Biasiolo A, Pegoraro C, et al. Antibody profiles for the diagnosis of antiphospholipid syndrome. Thromb Haemost. 2005;93:1147–52. https://doi.org/10.1160/TH04-12-0839.
18. Pengo V, Hoxha A, Andreoli L, et al. Trial of Rivaroxaban in AntiPhospholipid Syndrome (TRAPS): two-year outcomes after the study closure. J Thromb Haemost. 2021;19:531–5. https://doi.org/10.1111/jth.15158.
19. Pimenta da Fonseca E, Lins CF, de Sá Ribeiro DL, et al. Videocapillaroscopic findings in patients with systemic lupus erythematosus with or without Jaccoud Arthropathy. J Clin Rheumatol Pract Rep Rheum Musculoskelet Dis. 2021;27:S198–203. https://doi.org/10.1097/RHU.0000000000001617.
20. Rai R, Cohen H, Dave M, Regan L. Randomised controlled trial of aspirin and aspirin plus heparin in pregnant women with recurrent miscarriage associated with phospholipid antibodies (or antiphospholipid antibodies). BMJ. 1997;314:253–7. https://doi.org/10.1136/bmj.314.7076.253.
21. Rodríguez-Pintó I, Moitinho M, Santacreu I, et al. Catastrophic antiphospholipid syndrome (CAPS): descriptive analysis of 500 patients from the international CAPS registry. Autoimmun Rev. 2016;15:1120–4. https://doi.org/10.1016/j.autrev.2016.09.010.
22. Ruffatti A, Tonello M, Visentin MS, et al. Risk factors for pregnancy failure in patients with anti-phospholipid syndrome treated with conventional therapies: a multicentre, case–control study. Rheumatology. 2011;50:1684–9. https://doi.org/10.1093/rheumatology/ker139.
23. Schonenberg-Meinema D, Melsens K, Nassar-Sheikh Rashid A, et al. Capillaroscopy in childhood-onset systemic lupus erythematosus: a first systematic review. Clin Exp Rheumatol. 2020;38:350–4. https://doi.org/10.55563/clinexprheumatol/azl2bj.
24. Stammler R, Nguyen Y, Yelnik C, et al. Precipitating factors of catastrophic antiphospholipid syndrome: the role of anticoagulant treatment in a series of 112 patients. J Thromb Haemost. 2023;21:1258–65. https://doi.org/10.1016/j.jtha.2023.02.007.
25. Tektonidou MG, Andreoli L, Limper M, et al. EULAR recommendations for the management of antiphospholipid syndrome in adults. Ann Rheum Dis. 2019;78:1296–304. https://doi.org/10.1136/annrheumdis-2019-215213.
26. Tsokos GC, Lo MS, Costa Reis P, Sullivan KE. New insights into the immunopathogenesis of systemic lupus erythematosus. Nat Rev Rheumatol. 2016;12:716–30. https://doi.org/10.1038/nrrheum.2016.186.
27. Zen M, Salmaso L, Barbiellini Amidei C, et al. Mortality and causes of death in systemic lupus erythematosus over the last decade: data from a large population-based study. Eur J Intern Med. 2023;112:45–51. https://doi.org/10.1016/j.ejim.2023.02.004.
28. Zhao T, Lin F-A, Chen H-P. Pattern of nailfold capillaroscopy in patients with systemic lupus erythematosus. Arch Rheumatol. 2020;35:568–74. https://doi.org/10.46497/ArchRheumatol.2020.7763.

Chapter 8
Inflammatory Arthritis

Yasser El Miedany and Rahma A. Elziaty

Introduction

Nailfold capillaroscopy (NFC) is a noninvasive, in vivo technique used to visualize the microvasculature of the nailfold, providing insights into the morphology and density of capillaries at the dermal papillae. This valuable tool has gained significant traction in rheumatology, particularly in the assessment of systemic sclerosis (SSc), where specific capillaroscopic patterns are considered highly characteristic and even diagnostic [1, 2]. However, the utility of NFC extends beyond SSc, offering important diagnostic, prognostic, and monitoring capabilities in a range of inflammatory arthritis conditions.

The microvascular changes observed through NFC can reflect systemic microvascular damage that often accompanies chronic inflammatory processes. In inflammatory arthritis, such as rheumatoid arthritis (RA), psoriatic arthritis (PsA), and systemic lupus erythematosus (SLE) with arthritic manifestations, abnormal capillaroscopic patterns can provide clues about disease activity, severity, and potential for organ involvement [3, 4]. These patterns may include dilated capillaries, microhemorrhages, avascular areas, and disorganization of the capillary array, all indicative of microcirculatory disturbances [5].

Y. El Miedany (✉)
Canterbury Christ Church University, Canterbury, UK

Rheumatology and Rehabilitation, Ain Shams University, Cairo, Egypt

King's College, London, UK

R. A. Elziaty
Internal Medicine Department, Rheumatology Division, Faculty of Medicine,
Ain Shams University, Cairo, Egypt
e-mail: drrahmaelziaty@med.asu.edu.eg

Y. El Miedany, R. A. Elziaty (eds.), *Capillaroscopy*, Contemporary Rheumatology,
https://doi.org/10.1007/978-3-032-22966-3_8

While NFC is well-established in the context of connective tissue diseases, its role in pure inflammatory arthritis is still evolving and being increasingly recognized. Understanding the specific capillaroscopic alterations associated with different forms of inflammatory arthritis can aid in differential diagnosis, predict the risk of developing more severe systemic complications, and potentially guide therapeutic strategies [6–9]. This chapter will delve into the application of nailfold capillaroscopy in various inflammatory arthritis conditions, discussing its current utility, characteristic findings, and future prospects as a routine clinical assessment tool.

The Application of Nailfold Capillaroscopy in Various Inflammatory arthritis Conditions

- *The Unseen Battleground*: Pioneering the Role of Nailfold Capillaroscopy in Diverse Inflammatory Arthritis.

For decades, nailfold capillaroscopy (NFC) has been largely anchored to its foundational role in systemic sclerosis (SSc) and the differentiation of primary from secondary Raynaud's phenomenon. However, an innovative paradigm is emerging, positioning NFC not merely as a specific SSc biomarker but as a critical, accessible, and dynamic tool to unravel the nuanced microvascular pathology underlying the broader spectrum of inflammatory arthritis conditions. This expanding application moves beyond simply identifying "scleroderma patterns," embracing the subtler, yet equally significant, microvascular alterations that contribute to disease activity, prognosis, and therapeutic stratification across diverse arthritis.

While the dramatic architectural changes seen in SSc (e.g., giant capillaries, hemorrhages, avascularity) are pathognomonic, contemporary research and clinical experience are increasingly highlighting a more heterogeneous set of capillaroscopic abnormalities in other inflammatory arthritis. In rheumatoid arthritis (RA), for instance, while overt scleroderma-like patterns are rare, studies consistently report increased tortuosity, dilatation of capillaries, microhemorrhages, and sometimes reduced capillary density, particularly in patients with active disease or extra-articular manifestations [6, 9]. These subtle changes, often overlooked by traditional assessment, may reflect a chronic inflammatory burden on the microvasculature, potentially contributing to synovitis progression, joint damage, and even cardiovascular risk in RA [10]. The innovative use of NFC in RA is thus transitioning from a purely descriptive approach to exploring its potential as a noninvasive biomarker for microangiopathic burden, aiding in the early identification of patients at higher risk for severe outcomes or those who might benefit from more aggressive vascular protection strategies.

Similarly, in psoriatic arthritis (PsA), the microvascular landscape is distinct from SSc but equally informative. Beyond the often-cited "bushy" or "ramified" capillaries that are common in psoriasis itself, PsA patients can exhibit a spectrum of changes, including irregular capillary distribution, increased tortuosity, and occasionally subtle dilatations or hemorrhages that are more pronounced than in cutaneous psoriasis alone [6, 7, 11]. The innovation here lies in differentiating these specific patterns from those of undifferentiated arthritis or other connective tissue diseases, potentially aiding in early PsA diagnosis or subclassifying patients based on microvascular involvement, which could correlate with specific skin, nail, or joint manifestations, thereby contributing to precision medicine. NFC could potentially track the efficacy of biologic therapies on the microvasculature, offering a tangible visual biomarker of treatment response beyond clinical scores.

Even in *systemic lupus erythematosus (SLE)* without overt scleroderma features, NFC is proving to be a valuable adjunct. While the "lupus pattern" is less distinct than the "scleroderma pattern," observations include dilated capillaries, tortuosity, and occasional microhemorrhages, with some studies correlating these findings with disease activity, Raynaud's phenomenon, and even renal or neuropsychiatric involvement [12, 13]. The innovative application here is the use of NFC to *monitor microvascular inflammation and damage as an indicator of systemic disease activity*, particularly in patients where traditional inflammatory markers may be discordant with clinical presentation. This provides a direct, morphological assessment of small vessel pathology that complements serological and clinical assessments, offering a more holistic view of the systemic impact of lupus (for full details, please view the chapter on systemic lupus erythematosus).

- *Nailfold capillaroscopy in inflammatory arthritis*:

The innovation in applying NFC across this inflammatory arthritis extends beyond mere pattern recognition. It lies in:

Quantitative and Semi-quantitative Advancement: Moving beyond subjective visual assessment to objective measurements of capillary density, diameter, tortuosity index, and flow characteristics, often facilitated by advanced digital imaging and Artificial Intelligence (AI)-driven analysis, which can detect subtle changes imperceptible to the human eye [14].

Prognostic and Predictive Power: Investigating whether specific non-SSc capillaroscopic patterns can predict future disease flares, development of extra-articular manifestations (e.g., ILD, cardiovascular complications), or response to targeted therapies in different inflammatory arthritis.

Pathophysiological Insights: Utilizing NFC as a research tool to understand the commonalities and distinctions in microvascular damage pathways across diverse inflammatory conditions, shedding light on shared or distinct inflammatory mediators and cellular mechanisms [15].

Accessibility and Cost-Effectiveness: Reinforcing NFC as a relatively low-cost, noninvasive, and repeatable bedside procedure that can empower clinicians to gain valuable insights without resorting to more invasive or expensive techniques, particularly crucial in resource-limited settings.

In conclusion, the application of nailfold capillaroscopy in inflammatory arthritis is transcending its traditional confines. It is evolving into a versatile, dynamic imaging modality capable of providing unique, real-time insights into the microvascular battleground across RA, PsA, SLE, and other conditions. This innovative expansion promises to refine diagnostic pathways, enable more precise prognostic stratification, and guide personalized therapeutic strategies, ultimately improving outcomes for patients living with the complexities of inflammatory arthritis. The unseen battleground at the nailfold is indeed yielding profound revelations.

Current Utility and Characteristic Findings of Nailfold Capillaroscopy in Inflammatory Arthritis

The contemporary landscape of rheumatology demands increasingly refined diagnostic and prognostic tools. While the undisputed "gold standard" application of nailfold capillaroscopy (NFC) remains its pivotal role in differentiating primary from secondary Raynaud's phenomenon and confirming the characteristic "scleroderma pattern" in systemic sclerosis (SSc), an innovative shift is underway. This evolution recognizes NFC's broader utility as a noninvasive, accessible window into the systemic microvascular involvement that underpins various other inflammatory arthritis conditions. Beyond the dramatic hallmarks of SSc, the current utility of NFC in these diverse arthritis lies in detecting subtle yet significant microvascular aberrations, offering unique insights into disease activity, progression, and potential for organ involvement.

Current Utility and Characteristic Findings across Inflammatory Arthritis

1. *Rheumatoid Arthritis (RA)*:
    - *Current Utility*: NFC in RA is moving beyond simple presence/absence of scleroderma-like patterns to a more nuanced assessment of microangiopathic burden. It is increasingly utilized to identify subclinical microvascular damage, which can contribute to the severity of synovitis, joint erosion, and the heightened cardiovascular risk associated with RA [16, 17]. Furthermore, it may help distinguish RA from early SSc or undifferentiated connective tissue disease.
    - *Characteristic Findings*: Unlike SSc, a "scleroderma pattern" is generally absent in uncomplicated RA. Instead, characteristic findings often include:
        - *Increased capillary tortuosity*: A capillary limb curled but not crossing over itself [16, 18].
        - *Elongated capillaries*: Capillary loops may be abnormally long [18].
        - *Dilated capillaries*: Mild to moderate homogeneous dilatation can be observed, but typically without the "giant" morphology seen in SSc [18, 19].

- *Prominent subpapillary plexus*: The underlying venous plexus may be more visible [16].
- *Occasional microhemorrhages*: Small extravasations of blood can be present, reflecting capillary fragility or inflammatory damage [19].
- *Normal to slightly reduced capillary density*: While severe capillary loss is rare, some studies suggest a subtle reduction [18, 19] (Fig. 8.1).

2. *Psoriatic Arthritis (PsA)*:

- *Current Utility*: NFC in PsA offers critical insights into the interplay between skin and joint pathology. It serves as a valuable tool for early diagnosis, differentiating PsA from RA (especially in seronegative cases), and potentially correlating with disease severity, activity, and specific cutaneous or nail involvement [5, 6]. It may also aid in monitoring treatment response by observing changes in microvascular parameters.
- *Characteristic Findings*: PsA often presents a distinct set of microvascular patterns, often reflecting the coexistence of cutaneous psoriasis:
  - *"Bushy" or "Ramified" capillaries*: This is a hallmark feature, characterized by numerous, short, branching capillaries emerging from a single afferent limb [20, 21]. These are also seen in cutaneous psoriasis but are often more pronounced or widespread in PsA.
  - *Irregular capillary distribution*: The normal, orderly arrangement of capillaries can be disrupted [7].

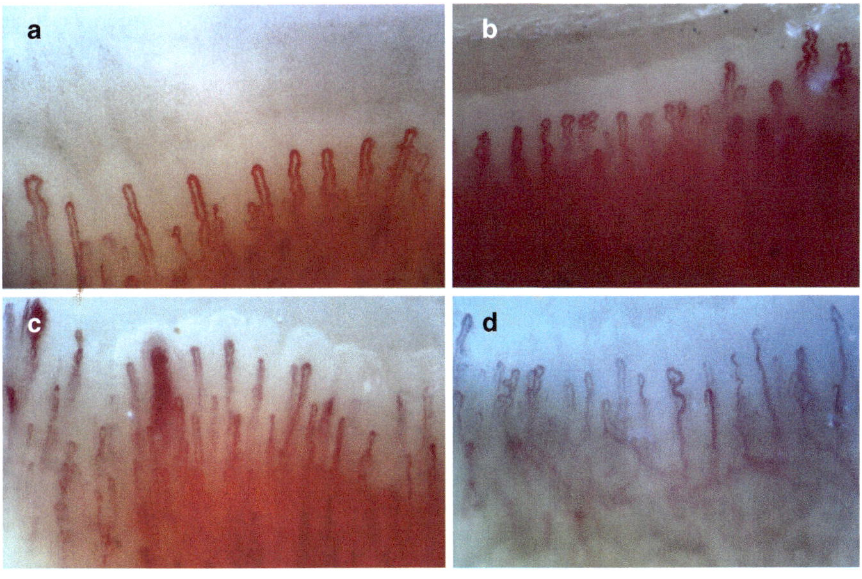

Fig. 8.1 (**a**): shows dilated, tortuous, and crossed capillaries. (**b**): Increased capillary tortuosity. (**c**): Dilated, tortuous capillaries and microhemorrhages. (**d**): tortuous capillaries and the A-V plexus

- *Increased tortuosity and disorganized architecture*: Capillaries may appear disarranged and convoluted [7, 20].
- *Dilated capillaries*: Capillary loops can be dilated, sometimes appearing enlarged [7, 21].
- *Occasional microhemorrhages*: Similar to RA, small hemorrhages may indicate microvascular fragility [7].
- *Reduced capillary density*: Some studies suggest a lower capillary density compared to healthy controls or even cutaneous psoriasis alone [7, 20, 21] (Fig. 8.2).

3. *Systemic Lupus Erythematosus (SLE)*:

- *Current Utility*: While the "scleroderma pattern" is less common and typically indicates overlap, NFC in SLE provides a direct visual assessment of microvascular inflammation and damage, which is integral to the disease's pathogenesis. It is increasingly used to assess overall disease activity, identify patients at risk of Raynaud's phenomenon, and potentially predict organ involvement, especially in cases where traditional inflammatory markers are not fully reflective of systemic inflammation [13, 22, 23].
- *Characteristic Findings*: SLE typically presents with a "nonspecific" pattern, although a "scleroderma-like" pattern can occur, particularly in overlap syndromes:
  - *Dilated capillaries*: Often homogeneous and mild to moderate in degree [13, 22].
  - *Increased tortuosity*: Capillaries appear winding [23].
  - *Microhemorrhages*: Frequent and often indicative of active microvascular inflammation [22].
  - *Erythrocyte aggregation ("sludging")*: Sluggish blood flow and clumping of red blood cells can be observed [13, 22, 23].
  - *Mildly disturbed architecture*: Overall organization may be less orderly than normal, but not as severe as in SSc.

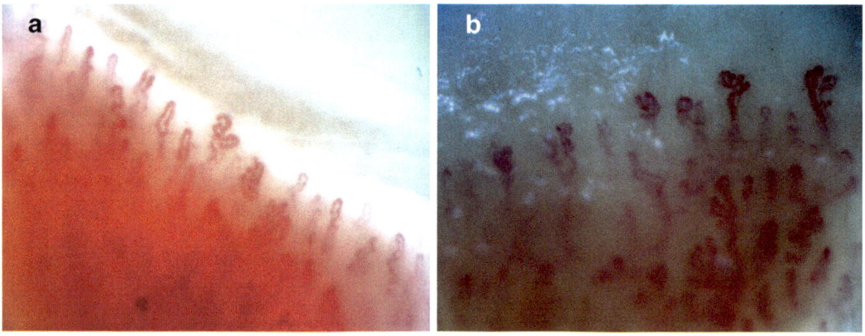

Fig. 8.2 (**a**): dilated, tortuous, and bushy capillaries. (**b**): decreased capillary density, bushy capillaries, and the A-V plexus

- *Pericapillary edema*: Swelling around the capillaries can sometimes be noted [23].
- *Absence of giant capillaries or significant avascularity*: These are typically not prominent unless there is an overlap with SSc [13].

4. *Juvenile Idiopathic Arthritis (JIA) and Other Inflammatory Arthritis (e.g., Ankylosing Spondylitis, Reactive Arthritis)*:

   - *Current Utility*: In JIA, NFC is gaining traction, especially in differentiating JIA-associated Raynaud's phenomenon from secondary causes and in potentially identifying subtypes with more pronounced microvascular involvement [24] (for further details, please go to our chapter on pediatric rheumatology). For other spondyloarthropathies like Ankylosing Spondylitis (AS) and Reactive Arthritis (ReA), NFC currently has a more limited, yet evolving, utility. While specific diagnostic patterns akin to SSc are not established, the presence of nonspecific microvascular changes might reflect systemic inflammation and could contribute to a broader understanding of disease burden, though more research is needed to establish clear clinical correlations and prognostic value [25, 26].
   - *Characteristic Findings (JIA)*:
     - Nonspecific changes are prevalent, including increased tortuosity, elongated capillaries, increased visibility of the subpapillary plexus, and occasional microhemorrhages [24].
     - Capillary dilatation has been observed, sometimes more frequently in oligoarticular and enthesitis-related JIA forms.
     - "Bushy" capillaries might be seen in psoriatic JIA subtypes [24] (Fig. 8.3).
   - *Characteristic Findings (AS, ReA)*:
     - Often show normal patterns or minor nonspecific abnormalities like mild tortuosity, slightly dilated capillaries, or minor structural changes. Significant "scleroderma-like" patterns are rare and usually point to an overlap syndrome. The presence of edema and nonspecific microangiopathy has been noted in AS, potentially linked to immune complex mechanisms [25, 26].

5. *In undifferentiated inflammatory arthritis*, where clinical features and serologic markers are insufficient to meet the criteria for a defined rheumatologic diagnosis, NFC may serve as a supplementary tool. The presence of abnormal capillaroscopic findings—such as dilated capillaries, irregular architecture, or early scleroderma-like changes—can raise suspicion for early connective tissue disease or impending overlap syndrome. In such cases, capillaroscopy contributes to risk stratification and closer follow-up strategies.

Overall, while NFC findings in these conditions are not diagnostic, they may assist in identifying subclinical vascular involvement, guiding further autoimmune work-up, and recognizing evolving disease patterns. As understanding of the vascular component of inflammatory arthritis expands, capillaroscopy may offer an additional layer of insight into complex or early-stage clinical presentations.

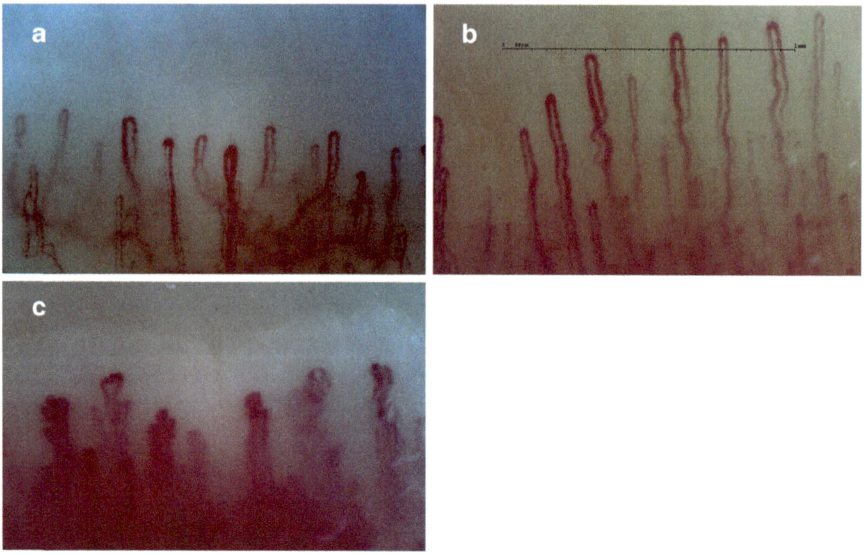

Fig. 8.3 (**a**): dilated, tortuous capillaries and A-V plexus. (**b**): elongated and tortuous capillaries. (**c**): elongated and bushy capillaries in psoriatic JIA subtype patients

The innovation in the current utility of NFC for inflammatory arthritis lies in its recognition as a *dynamic, "live biopsy" of systemic microvascular health*. It moves beyond a mere qualitative description to a quantitative and semi-quantitative analysis facilitated by modern videocapillaroscopes and emerging AI algorithms. This allows for the detection of subtle microcirculatory dysfunction, often preceding overt clinical symptoms or acting as a valuable marker of persistent inflammation. By offering a noninvasive, repeatable assessment of endothelial function and microvascular integrity, NFC is poised to become an increasingly integral component in the holistic assessment of inflammatory arthritis, contributing significantly to early risk stratification, personalized therapeutic strategies, and a deeper understanding of the systemic ramifications of chronic inflammation. Table 8.1 shows a comparison of microcirculation changes and nailfold capillaroscopy patterns in rheumatic diseases.

Table 8.1 Comparison of microcirculation changes and nailfold capillaroscopy patterns in rheumatic diseases

Feature/Disease category	Inflammatory arthritis (rheumatoid arthritis and psoriatic arthritis)	Systemic Sclerosis (SSc)	Other connective tissue diseases (e.g., SLE, MCTD, dermatomyositis)
Overall microcirculation changes	Generalized endothelial dysfunction, increased inflammatory mediators affecting microvessels, subtle microvascular remodeling, accelerated atherosclerosis risk	Severe, progressive microvascular damage leading to widespread structural abnormalities, obliteration of capillaries, and subsequent tissue ischemia. Endothelial cell activation and apoptosis	Diverse, often nonspecific microvascular inflammation and damage. Endothelial dysfunction is common. Varies based on specific overlap features (e.g., myositis features)
Characteristic NFC pattern	RA: Increased tortuosity, mild homogeneous dilatations, occasional microhemorrhages PsA: "Bushy" or "ramified" capillaries (often with psoriasis), irregular capillary distribution, increased tortuosity, occasional mild dilatations/hemorrhages	The "Scleroderma Pattern" is characterized by: *Giant capillaries* (markedly enlarged loops) *Microhemorrhages* *Avascular areas/capillary loss* *Architectural disorganization* (derangement of parallel alignment). Often categorized into Early, Active, and Late patterns based on severity	*SLE*: Nonspecific pattern with mild homogeneous capillary dilations, increased tortuosity, frequent microhemorrhages, and occasional erythrocyte aggregation ("sludging"). Severe avascularity or giant capillaries are present in overlap syndromes and in some cases with secondary vasculitis and/or severe activity *MCTD*: A "scleroderma-like" pattern (dilated loops, hemorrhages, some avascularity) is frequent but typically less severe or progressive than in SSc. Often combines features of its constituent diseases, potentially with prominent bushy capillaries *Dermatomyositis (DM)*: Highly characteristic pattern including bushy/ramified capillaries, enlarged/giant capillaries (often less uniform than SSc), microhemorrhages, and avascular areas/capillary loss

(continued)

Table 8.1 (continued)

Feature/Disease category	Inflammatory arthritis (rheumatoid arthritis and psoriatic arthritis)	Systemic Sclerosis (SSc)	Other connective tissue diseases (e.g., SLE, MCTD, dermatomyositis)
Key distinguishing NFC features	*Absence of true giant capillaries or extensive avascularity* (distinguishes from SSc, DM, and MCTD) *Less architectural disorganization* compared to SSc or severe DM PsA often has *bushy capillaries* linked to psoriasis	*Presence of giant capillaries (definitive hallmark)* Progressive and often severe *capillary loss/avascularity* Highly characteristic, evolving patterns (Early, Active, Late)	SLE: *Prominent microhemorrhages and erythrocyte aggregation*; generally less severe morphological changes than SSc/DM MCTD: Can have scleroderma features, but often *less pronounced avascularity and giant capillaries* than pure SSc, with varied features reflecting overlap DM: *Bushy capillaries* in conjunction with enlarged loops and avascular areas are a strong indicator A scleroderma-like pattern on nailfold capillaroscopy is considered a characteristic feature of dermatomyositis (DM) and mixed connective tissue disease (MCTD)
Clinical significance/ Utility of NFC	*Differentiating Raynaud's*: Helps rule out secondary Raynaud's from primary or points toward an underlying CTD *Diagnosis/classification*: Aids in differentiating RA/PsA from early CTD *Disease activity/Prognosis*: Microvascular changes may correlate with disease activity, joint damage progression, or increased cardiovascular risk *Monitoring therapy*: Potential to assess the impact of systemic therapy on microcirculation	*Early diagnosis of SSc*: Critical for identifying patients with a "scleroderma pattern" even before overt clinical features develop *Prognosis*: Patterns (Early, Active, and Late) correlate with the risk of future SSc-related complications (e.g., digital ulcers, organ involvement) and mortality *Monitoring disease progression*: Useful for tracking microvascular damage over time and guiding therapeutic decisions	*Diagnosis/Classification*: Helps in the diagnosis of specific CTDs and in identifying overlap syndromes. Particularly useful in distinguishing DM from polymyositis or other myopathies *Prognosis*: Capillaroscopic patterns in DM correlate with disease severity and organ involvement (e.g., ILD) *Disease Activity/Organ involvement*: Microvascular changes in SLE can correlate with disease activity and specific organ manifestations *Differentiating Raynaud's*: Essential in determining if Raynaud's is secondary to an underlying CTD

Evaluation of Microcirculation in Nailfold Capillaroscopy in Patients with Inflammatory Arthritis with Systemic Affection

The systemic nature of chronic inflammatory arthritis (IA), encompassing conditions such as rheumatoid arthritis (RA), psoriatic arthritis (PsA), and systemic lupus erythematosus (SLE), extends far beyond articular involvement. A critical and increasingly recognized aspect of this systemic impact is the heightened predisposition to *cardiovascular diseases (CVDs)*, including accelerated atherosclerosis, myocardial dysfunction, and increased cardiovascular mortality, often disproportionate to traditional risk factors [27]. Nailfold capillaroscopy (NFC), a noninvasive and accessible technique, offers a unique window into the microcirculation, providing a tangible reflection of widespread endothelial dysfunction and microvascular damage that underpins both the rheumatic disease itself and its associated CVD risk.

While the "scleroderma pattern" remains the hallmark NFC finding in systemic sclerosis, the evaluation of microcirculation in other IAs reveals distinct, albeit often subtler, abnormalities that are highly relevant to cardiovascular health. In *rheumatoid arthritis*, for instance, typical NFC findings include increased capillary tortuosity, homogeneous capillary dilatations, and occasional microhemorrhages, with a relative absence of giant capillaries or significant avascularity [9, 10]. These subtle structural changes in the nailfold capillaries are not merely local phenomena; they are increasingly recognized as surrogate markers of generalized microvascular pathology and endothelial dysfunction, which are crucial early events in the atherogenesis process. Studies suggest that specific capillaroscopic abnormalities in RA, such as reduced capillary density or increased tortuosity, may correlate with markers of subclinical atherosclerosis, including increased carotid intima-media thickness (cIMT) or impaired flow-mediated dilation (FMD) , pointing toward a shared pathway of microvascular and macrovascular damage [6, 8].

Similarly, in *psoriatic arthritis* and *systemic lupus erythematosus*, where CVD risk is also elevated, NFC provides valuable insights. PsA patients often exhibit characteristic "bushy" or "ramified" capillaries alongside irregular architecture, reflecting both cutaneous microvascular changes and systemic inflammatory processes [6, 22]. These findings can be indicative of a broader microvascular dysfunction that contributes to the pro-atherogenic environment in PsA. In *SLE*, NFC patterns are typically nonspecific, characterized by dilated loops, tortuosity, and microhemorrhages, without the severe destructive changes of SSc [13]. However, the presence and severity of these microvascular abnormalities in SLE have been linked to disease activity, chronic damage, and markers of subclinical CVD, including accelerated atherosclerosis and increased arterial stiffness [13, 22, 23]. The microvascular damage visualized via NFC serves as a direct, real-time indicator of the inflammatory burden's impact on small vessels, mirroring the systemic vascular insult.

The innovative utility of NFC in this context lies in its potential as a *noninvasive biomarker for cardiovascular risk stratification* in patients with inflammatory arthritis. By visually assessing the integrity and function of the microcirculation, NFC can identify patients with subclinical microvascular damage who may be at higher risk for future cardiovascular events, even before traditional CVD risk factors are overtly pathological or clinical symptoms emerge. This allows for earlier, more targeted interventions, including aggressive management of traditional CVD risk factors, optimization of anti-inflammatory therapies, and potentially, the initiation of specific vascular protective strategies [10]. Furthermore, NFC could potentially be used to *monitor the efficacy of immunomodulatory or cardiovascular-protective therapies* by observing changes in microvascular patterns over time, providing a tangible, morphological assessment of therapeutic impact on the systemic microcirculation.

In essence, the evaluation of microcirculation via nailfold capillaroscopy in inflammatory arthritis patients offers a critical bridge between rheumatic disease activity and cardiovascular comorbidity. By providing a direct, accessible, and repeatable assessment of small vessel health, NFC positions itself as an invaluable tool for comprehensive patient care, enabling earlier risk identification, more precise prognostic assessment, and ultimately, tailored management strategies aimed at mitigating the substantial cardiovascular burden in this vulnerable patient population. Table 8.2 shows the possible links between changes in nailfold capillaroscopy patterns and systemic/organ affections in rheumatic diseases, with a focus on cardiovascular links.

Table 8.2 Nailfold capillaroscopy patterns and possible link to systemic/organ affections in rheumatic diseases, with a focus on cardiovascular links

Feature/ Disease category	Inflammatory arthritis (rheumatoid arthritis and psoriatic arthritis)	Systemic sclerosis (SSc)	Other connective tissue diseases (e.g., SLE, MCTD, dermatomyositis)
Relation/Link to systemic/ organ affection (incl. CVD)	Cardiovascular Disease (CVD): Microvascular changes often correlate with markers of subclinical atherosclerosis (e.g., cIMT, impaired FMD) and increased long-term CVD risk, reflecting systemic endothelial dysfunction and inflammation Joint damage: Microvascular abnormalities in the synovium contribute to inflammatory processes and joint destruction Extra-articular manifestations: May correlate with conditions like rheumatoid vasculitis (RA) or psoriasis severity (PsA)	Cardiovascular Disease (CVD): SSc is strongly associated with high CVD risk, including pulmonary arterial hypertension (PAH), myocardial fibrosis, and accelerated atherosclerosis. The severity of the scleroderma pattern (e.g., "active" or "late") correlates with PAH risk and overall prognosis. Digital Ulcers/Ischemia: Direct link to severe microvascular obliteration Organ Fibrosis: The microvascular damage is central to the widespread fibrotic processes in skin, lungs (ILD), GI tract, and kidneys	Cardiovascular Disease (CVD): Microvascular changes, especially microhemorrhages and erythrocyte aggregation in SLE, reflect systemic inflammation and endothelial damage contributing to accelerated atherosclerosis, coronary microvascular dysfunction, and thrombosis Organ involvement: Capillaroscopic abnormalities in SLE can correlate with disease activity and specific organ manifestations (e.g., active skin involvement, though less consistently with renal involvement) ILD: Particularly in DM and MCTD, specific capillaroscopic patterns (e.g., bushy + avascular areas in DM) strongly correlate with the presence and severity of interstitial lung disease Myositis: Microvascular pathology is central to muscle damage in DM

(continued)

Table 8.2 (continued)

Feature/ Disease category	Inflammatory arthritis (rheumatoid arthritis and psoriatic arthritis)	Systemic sclerosis (SSc)	Other connective tissue diseases (e.g., SLE, MCTD, dermatomyositis)
Clinical significance/ Utility of NFC	CVD risk assessment: Potential to serve as a noninvasive tool for early identification and stratification of CVD risk, guiding more aggressive preventive strategies Disease activity/ Prognosis: Microvascular changes may reflect overall inflammatory burden and correlate with disease activity or severity Differential Diagnosis: Aids in distinguishing IA from early CTDs, especially in Raynaud's phenomenon	Early diagnosis and classification: Essential for identifying SSc, particularly in early stages or with isolated Raynaud's Prognosis and monitoring: Provides critical prognostic information (e.g., risk of digital ulcers, organ involvement like PAH) and monitors disease progression, guiding therapy	Diagnosis and classification: valuable for confirming specific CTDs (e.g., DM) or identifying overlap syndromes Prognosis and organ involvement: Patterns can correlate with severity and specific organ complications, particularly ILD in DM/MCTD, and general disease activity in SLE Raynaud's Evaluation: Helps determine if Raynaud's is secondary to an underlying CTD

Nailfold Capillaroscopy as a Future Routine Assessment Tool in Inflammatory Arthritis

The burgeoning era of precision medicine demands diagnostic tools that offer granular, real-time insights into disease pathology, enabling truly personalized care. While nailfold capillaroscopy (NFC) has proven indispensable in systemic sclerosis, its future prospects as a routine clinical assessment tool across the spectrum of inflammatory arthritis represent a significant paradigm shift, moving it from a specialized niche to an integrated, indispensable component of everyday rheumatological practice. This innovation hinges on advancements in technology, a deepening understanding of microvascular biomarkers, and the recognition of its unique capacity to visualize the dynamic interplay between inflammation and microvascular damage.

The current utility of NFC in inflammatory arthritis, like rheumatoid arthritis (RA), psoriatic arthritis (PsA), and systemic lupus erythematosus (SLE), already reveals characteristic, albeit often subtle, microvascular changes that correlate with disease activity and prognosis. The future routine integration will leverage several key innovations:

First, Artificial Intelligence (AI) and Machine Learning (ML) will revolutionize analysis and interpretation, democratizing expertise. Currently, interpretation requires significant training and carries a degree of inter-observer variability. AI algorithms, trained on vast datasets of capillaroscopic images from diverse inflammatory arthritis cohorts, will enable automated pattern recognition, quantitative measurements (e.g., capillary density, diameter, tortuosity index, blood flow velocity), and even predictive analytics with unprecedented speed and objectivity [14, 28]. This automated "capillaroscopist" will reduce the need for highly specialized training, making the technique accessible to a broader range of clinicians in various settings. Imagine an AI-powered system providing instant, standardized reports, flagging deviations from established norms for RA, PsA, or SLE patterns, thereby accelerating clinical decision-making (Fig. 8.4).

Second, the advent of affordable, user-friendly, and highly portable digital videocapillaroscopes will facilitate widespread adoption and tele-capillaroscopy. Current high-end devices can be cumbersome and costly. Future handheld or smartphone-integrated devices, paired with cloud-based AI analysis platforms, will enable seamless image acquisition and interpretation, even in general rheumatology clinics, satellite offices, or potentially even by trained nurses in primary care settings [11]. This democratization of access will make routine microvascular assessment feasible, particularly for early disease detection, timely referral, and continuous monitoring of chronic inflammatory conditions, bridging geographical gaps in expert care.

Third, the integration of capillaroscopic findings with multi-omics data (genomics, proteomics, and metabolomics) and advanced clinical metrics will unlock its true potential for precision monitoring and personalized treatment stratification. Beyond mere diagnosis, routine NFC will function as a dynamic "liquid biopsy"of the microcirculation, reflecting active inflammation, endothelial dysfunction, and subclinical damage in real-time [2]. For instance, longitudinal changes in specific capillaroscopic parameters in RA or PsA could predict flares, the onset of extra-articular manifestations (e.g., interstitial lung disease in PsA or vasculitis in RA), or inform therapeutic escalation/de-escalation before overt clinical signs manifest [6, 8]. This capability offers a powerful, noninvasive means to assess therapeutic response, tailoring treatment strategies based on visual evidence of microvascular amelioration or persistence of damage, moving beyond symptom-based assessments (Table 8.1).

Finally, as evidence accumulates on its prognostic value and cost-effectiveness (through preventing severe complications and guiding optimal therapy), NFC will increasingly justify its position in routine clinical guidelines for specific inflammatory arthritis. While current guidelines focus on SSc, future iterations will likely recommend NFC as a standard component of initial work-up and ongoing follow-up for patients with RA, PsA, and SLE, particularly those with Raynaud's phenomenon or suspected systemic involvement [6, 7, 29]. This will necessitate continued investment in large-scale, prospective, multicenter studies to solidify the evidence base for specific capillaroscopic biomarkers across these diverse conditions (Table 8.2).

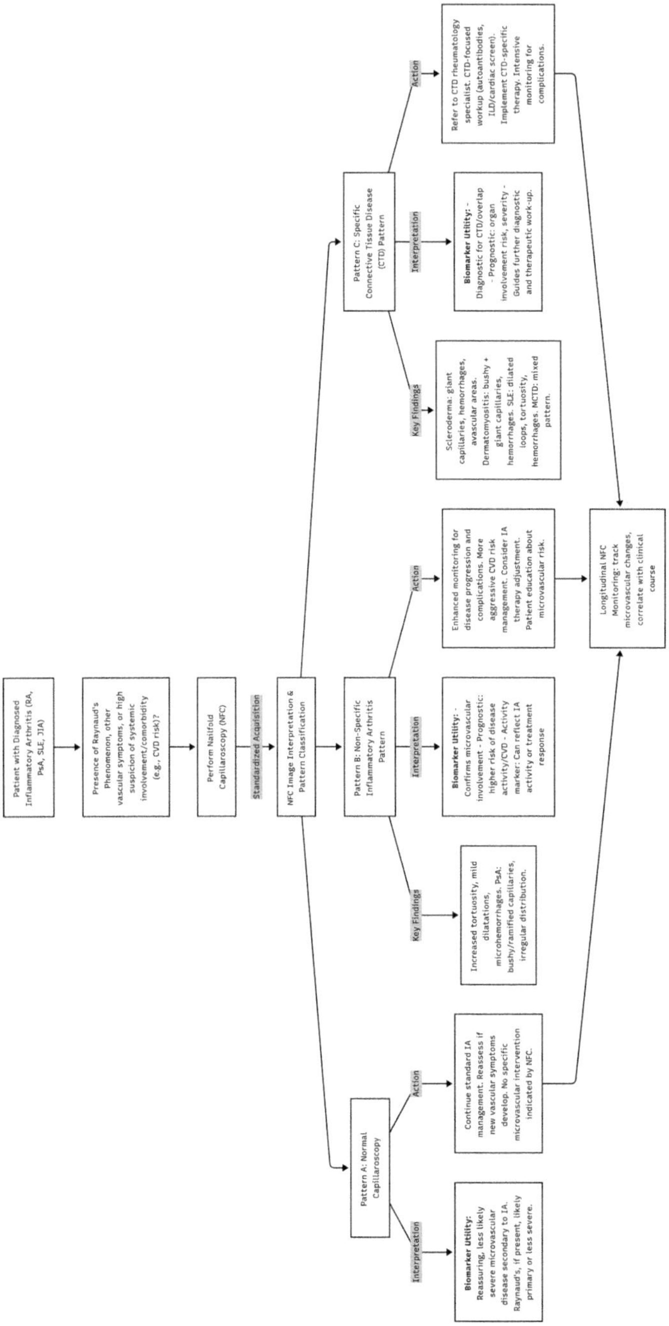

Fig. 8.4 Algorithmic approach to utilizing nailfold capillaroscopy as a microvascular biomarker in the management of inflammatory arthritis

In conclusion, the future of nailfold capillaroscopy in inflammatory arthritis is bright and transformative. It envisions a routine, accessible, AI-augmented assessment tool that provides unprecedented insights into the microvascular battleground, empowering clinicians with a visual, dynamic, and objective biomarker for disease activity, prognosis, and therapeutic optimization. This will usher in an era where microvascular health is routinely assessed and precisely managed, ultimately enhancing patient outcomes and advancing the frontiers of rheumatological care.

Case 1 A 30-year-old female with a 5-year history of seropositive rheumatoid arthritis (RA) presented to the rheumatology clinic with persistent pain, swelling, and stiffness in the metacarpophalangeal (MCP) and proximal interphalangeal (PIP) joints of both hands. Morning stiffness lasted for approximately 1 h, indicating ongoing inflammatory activity. She denied systemic features such as fever, weight loss, or fatigue. Importantly, she had no history of Raynaud's phenomenon, digital ulcers, or other signs suggestive of systemic sclerosis or connective tissue disease overlap

On examination, synovitis was evident in multiple small joints of the hands with no skin changes, nailfold infarcts, or sclerodactyly.

Investigations: elevated ESR and CRP, positive rheumatoid factor (RF) and anti-cyclic citrullinated peptide antibodies (anti-CCP), and renal and liver function tests were within normal limits.

Nailfold Capillaroscopy Examination Revealed dilated, tortuous capillary loops, A-V plexus, and microhemorrhages.

The patient was assessed as having active RA despite existing treatment. Management was escalated to address ongoing joint inflammation and microvascular risk; he continued on methotrexate, with dosage optimized to 25 mg/week, folic acid supplementation maintained, and a short course of low-dose corticosteroids (prednisolone 15 mg/day) was introduced to control flare. Initiation of biologic DMARD; TNF inhibitor (adalimumab 40 mg every 2 weeks) considered due to persistent disease activity.

Regular follow-up was arranged for clinical monitoring, joint assessment, treatment side-effect evaluation, and capillaroscopy if symptoms evolve.

Clinical Insight

While nailfold capillaroscopy is not routinely used in RA, its findings can reveal microangiopathic changes due to chronic inflammation and endothelial dysfunction. The presence of dilated loops and microhemorrhages without features like avascular areas or giant capillaries supports a pattern seen in chronic inflammatory arthritis rather than scleroderma spectrum disorders. In RA, these capillary abnormalities may correlate with disease activity and systemic inflammation. Thus, capillaroscopy can be a useful adjunct tool in RA patients, especially those with atypical symptoms or concerns for disease overlap (Fig. 8.5).

Case 2 A 35-year-old male with a 20-year history of *chronic plaque psoriasis* presented to the rheumatology clinic with complaints of new-onset *inflammatory low*

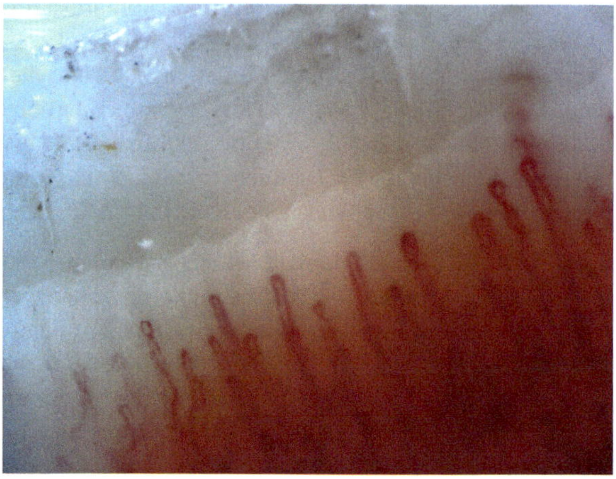

Fig. 8.5 Dilated, tortuous capillaries, A-V plexus with the presence of recent and old microhemorrhages

back pain of 6 months' duration. The back pain is characterized by insidious onset, morning stiffness lasting over 1 h, improvement with physical activity, and worsening with rest, consistent with an inflammatory pattern suggestive of axial involvement. Approximately 2 months prior to presentation, the patient began to develop *arthritis of the small joints of the hand, including DIP joints.* In addition, he noticed diffuse swelling of the left index finger, clinically consistent with *dactylitis.* He also reported pain and tenderness at the posterior aspect of his left heel, consistent with *Achilles tendinitis,* further indicating enthesitis, a hallmark feature of psoriatic arthritis (PsA)

Nailfold Capillaroscopy Examination Revealed reduced capillary density and bushy capillaries, suggesting microvascular involvement consistent with psoriatic arthritis-related microangiopathy.

Laboratory studies showed mildly elevated inflammatory markers (ESR and CRP). Rheumatoid factor (RF) and anti-cyclic citrullinated peptide antibodies (anti-CCP) were negative. HLA-B27 typing was positive.

Imaging Studies

- Hand X-rays demonstrated joint space narrowing and marginal erosions predominantly at the DIP joints, with early "pencil-in-cup" deformities suggestive of PsA.
- MRI sacroiliac joint imaging revealed bilateral sacroiliitis, supporting axial involvement.

The patient was started on *methotrexate* to manage peripheral arthritis and dactylitis, and due to the presence of axial involvement and enthesitis, a *biologic agent targeting IL-17* was added for better disease control. He also continued using *topical therapies for psoriasis* and was prescribed *NSAIDs* to relieve inflammatory back pain and Achilles tendinitis. The patient remains under regular follow-up in both rheumatology and dermatology outpatient clinics for ongoing assessment of joint and skin disease activity, monitoring of treatment response, and management of potential adverse effects.

Clinical Insight

The role of nailfold capillaroscopy in PsA is emerging. The observed reduced capillary density and bushy capillaries reflect microvascular involvement, which correlates with disease activity and systemic inflammation. These findings support the concept that PsA is not only a joint disease but also involves vascular pathology and microangiopathy.

The capillaroscopic abnormalities underscore the systemic nature of PsA and might be useful in monitoring disease progression or response to therapy in the future (Fig. 8.6).

Case 3 A 13-year-old female with a known history of juvenile idiopathic arthritis (JIA) since the age of 9 years presented to the pediatric rheumatology clinic with progressive joint pain and swelling over the past 3 months. Her symptoms were primarily localized to the right knee and left ankle, consistent with *oligoarticular involvement*. Morning stiffness lasting more than 60 min was reported. In addition to musculoskeletal symptoms, she also developed ocular discomfort, photophobia, and blurred vision, prompting an ophthalmological evaluation. Slit-lamp examination confirmed *anterior uveitis*, a known extra-articular manifestation of JIA

Nailfold Capillaroscopy Examination Revealed dilated capillary loops and microhemorrhages. There were no reported skin rashes, oral ulcers, or Raynaud's phenomenon. Laboratory investigations revealed ANA positive 1/160 speckled.

Clinical Insight

In juvenile idiopathic arthritis (JIA), especially the early-onset oligoarticular subtype, ANA positivity is strongly associated with an increased risk of chronic

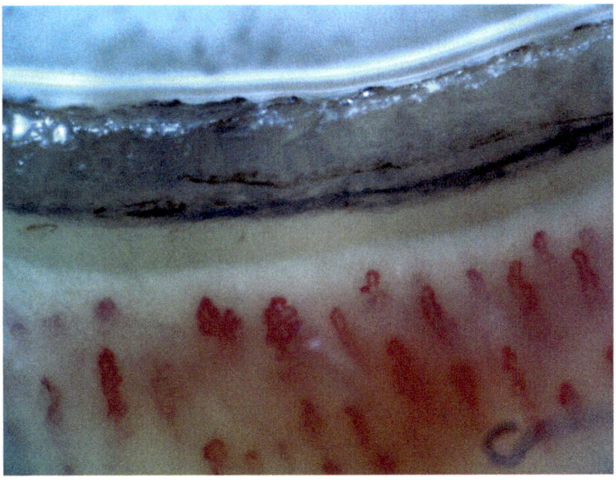

Fig. 8.6 Reduced capillary density, tortuous and bushy capillaries

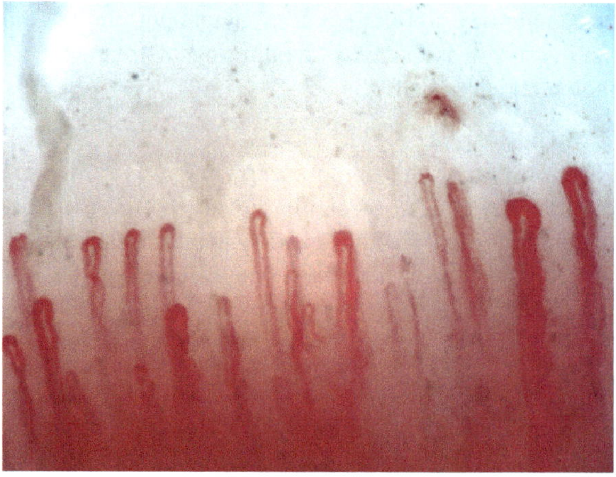

Fig. 8.7 Elongated, dilated capillaries and microhemorrhages

anterior uveitis. Although nailfold capillaroscopy is not routinely used in JIA, abnormal findings—such as dilated capillary loops and microhemorrhages—have been observed more frequently in ANA-positive patients and those with uveitis. These capillaroscopic changes may reflect underlying microvascular involvement and could suggest an evolving autoimmune process or potential overlap with other connective tissue diseases, highlighting the value of capillaroscopy as an adjunctive tool in selected cases (Fig. 8.7).

References

1. De Angelis R. A practical overview of the role of capillaroscopy in rheumatic diseases. J Autoimmune Dis Rheumatol. 2019;7:1–8.
2. Chojnowski MM, Felis-Giemza A, Olesińska M. Capillaroscopy - a role in modern rheumatology. Reumatologia. 2016;54(2):67–72. https://doi.org/10.5114/reum.2016.60215.
3. Etehad Tavakol M, Fatemi A, Karbalaie A, Emrani Z, Erlandsson BE. Nailfold capillaroscopy in rheumatic diseases: which parameters should be evaluated? Biomed Res Int. 2015;2015:974530. https://doi.org/10.1155/2015/974530.
4. Patil A, Sood I. Nailfold capillaroscopy in rheumatic diseases. Vascular biology - selection of mechanisms and clinical applications. IntechOpen; 2020. Available from: https://doi.org/10.5772/intechopen.92786.
5. Lambova SN, Müller-Ladner U. Nailfold capillaroscopy in systemic sclerosis - state of the art: the evolving knowledge about capillaroscopic abnormalities in systemic sclerosis. J Scleroderma Relat Disord. 2019;4(3):200–11. https://doi.org/10.1177/2397198319833486.
6. Graceffa D, Amorosi B, Maiani E, Bonifati C, Chimenti MS, Perricone R, Di Carlo A. Capillaroscopy in psoriatic and rheumatoid arthritis: a useful tool for differential diagnosis. Arthritis. 2013;2013:957480. https://doi.org/10.1155/2013/957480.
7. Prioteasă OG, Bobircă A, Anghel D, Groşeanu ML, Bojincă VC. Nailfold videocapillaroscopic changes in patients with psoriatic arthritis: a systematic review. Biomed Rep. 2025;23(2):130. https://doi.org/10.3892/br.2025.2008.
8. Anghel D, Sîrbu CA, Petrache OG, Opriş-Belinski D, Negru MM, Bojincă VC, Pleşa CF, Ioniţă Radu F. Nailfold videocapillaroscopy in patients with rheumatoid arthritis and psoriatic

arthropathy on ANTI-TNF-ALPHA therapy. Diagnostics (Basel). 2023;13(12):2079. https://doi.org/10.3390/diagnostics13122079.
9. Anyfanti P, Angeloudi E, Dara A, Arvanitaki A, Bekiari E, Kitas GD, Dimitroulas T. Nailfold videocapillaroscopy for the evaluation of peripheral microangiopathy in rheumatoid arthritis. Life. 2022;12:1167. https://doi.org/10.3390/life12081167.
10. Kęsiak A, Żuchowski P, Jeka S, et al. AB0592 evaluation of microcirculation in naifold capillaroscopy in patients with rheumatoid arthritis, considering the influence of cardiovascular diseases. Ann Rheum Dis. 2024;83:1579.
11. Cutolo M, Smith V. State of the art on nailfold capillaroscopy: a reliable diagnostic tool and putative biomarker in rheumatology? Rheumatology (Oxford). 2013;52(11):1933–40. https://doi.org/10.1093/rheumatology/ket153.
12. Cutolo M, Melsens K, Wijnant S, Ingegnoli F, Thevissen K, De Keyser F, Decuman S, Müller-Ladner U, Piette Y, Riccieri V, Ughi N, Vandecasteele E, Vanhaecke A, Smith V. Nailfold capillaroscopy in systemic lupus erythematosus: a systematic review and critical appraisal. Autoimmun Rev. 2018;17(4):344–52. https://doi.org/10.1016/j.autrev.2017.11.025.
13. Zhao T, Lin FA, Chen HP. Pattern of nailfold capillaroscopy in patients with systemic lupus erythematosus. Arch Rheumatol. 2020;35(4):568–74. https://doi.org/10.46497/ArchRheumatol.2020.7763.
14. Garaiman A, Nooralahzadeh F, Mihai C, Gonzalez NP, Gkikopoulos N, Becker MO, Distler O, Krauthammer M, Maurer B. Vision transformer assisting rheumatologists in screening for capillaroscopy changes in systemic sclerosis: an artificial intelligence model. Rheumatology (Oxford). 2023;62(7):2492–500. https://doi.org/10.1093/rheumatology/keac541. Erratum in: Rheumatology (Oxford) 2023;62(9):3221. https://doi.org/10.1093/rheumatology/kead156.
15. Cutolo M, Smith V. Detection of microvascular changes in systemic sclerosis and other rheumatic diseases. Nat Rev Rheumatol. 2021;17(11):665–77. https://doi.org/10.1038/s41584-021-00685-0.
16. van Eijk IC, Serné EH, Dijkmans BA, Smulders Y, Nurmohamed M. Microvascular function is preserved in newly diagnosed rheumatoid arthritis and low systemic inflammatory activity. Clin Rheumatol. 2011;30(8):1113–8. https://doi.org/10.1007/s10067-011-1750-1.
17. Cutolo M, Sulli A, Secchi ME, Olivieri M, Pizzorni C. The contribution of capillaroscopy to the differential diagnosis of connective autoimmune diseases. Best Pract Res Clin Rheumatol. 2007;21(6):1093–108. https://doi.org/10.1016/j.berh.2007.10.001.
18. Rajaei A, Dehghan P, Amiri A. Nailfold capillaroscopy in 430 patients with rheumatoid arthritis. Caspian. J Intern Med. 2017;8(4):269–74. https://doi.org/10.22088/cjim.8.4.269.
19. Angeloudi E, Anyfanti P, Dara A, Pagkopoulou E, Bekiari E, Sgouropoulou V, Garyfallos A, Doumas M, Kitas GD, Dimitroulas T. Peripheral nailfold capillary microscopic abnormalities in rheumatoid arthritis are associated with arterial stiffness: results from a cross-sectional study. Microvasc Res. 2023;150:104576. https://doi.org/10.1016/j.mvr.2023.104576.
20. Lazar LT, Guldberg-Møller J, Lazar BT, Mogensen M. Nailfold capillaroscopy as diagnostic test in patients with psoriasis and psoriatic arthritis: a systematic review. Microvasc Res. 2023;147:104476. https://doi.org/10.1016/j.mvr.2023.104476.
21. Sivasankari M, Arora S, Vasdev V, Mary EM. Nailfold capillaroscopy in psoriasis. Med J Armed Forces India. 2021;77(1):75–81. https://doi.org/10.1016/j.mjafi.2020.01.013.
22. Nasser M, Wadie M, Farid A, et al. Nailfold capillaroscopy in Egyptian systemic lupus erythematosus (SLE) patients: correlation with demographic features and serum levels of IL 17A and IFNs I. Egypt Rheumatol Rehabil. 2023;50:47. https://doi.org/10.1186/s43166-023-00215-8.
23. Marasco E, Duesing C, Keymel S, Zanframundo G, Codullo V, Sander O, Chehab G, Richter J, Fischer-Betz R, Bracaglia C, Sahin S, Triantafyllias K, Schwarting A, Keller L, Meyer A, Canuet M, Riou M, Cavazzana I, Fredi M, Franceschini F, Silvagni E, Bortoluzzi A, Scirè CA, Montecucco C, Cavagna L, Schneider M. P39 analysis of nailfold capillaroscopy findings and clinical features of patients with systemic lupus erythematosus and pulmonary arterial hypertension: lupus. Sci Med. 2024;11(Suppl 1):A68.1–A68.

24. Gerhold K, Becker MO. Nailfold capillaroscopy in juvenile rheumatic diseases: known measures, patterns and indications. Clin Exp Rheumatol. 2014;32(6 Suppl 86):S-183-8.
25. Batko B, Maga P, Urbanski K, Ryszawa-Mrozek N, Schramm-Luc A, Koziej M, Mikolajczyk T, McGinnigle E, Czesnikiewicz-Guzik M, Ceranowicz P, Guzik TJ. Microvascular dysfunction in ankylosing spondylitis is associated with disease activity and is improved by anti-TNF treatment. Sci Rep. 2018;8(1):13205. https://doi.org/10.1038/s41598-018-31550-y.
26. Lambova SN, Müller-Ladner U. Capillaroscopic pattern in inflammatory arthritis. Microvasc Res. 2012;83(3):318–22. https://doi.org/10.1016/j.mvr.2012.03.002.
27. Raadsen R, Hansildaar R, Pouw LC, Hooijberg F, Boekel L, Wolbink GJ, van Kuijk AW, Nurmohamed MT. Cardiovascular disease risk in patients with inflammatory arthritis nowadays still substantially elevated. RMD Open. 2023;9:e003485.
28. Lledó-Ibáñez GM, Sáez Comet L, Freire Dapena M, Mesa Navas M, Martín Cascón M, Guillén Del Castillo A, Simeon CP, Martinez Robles E, Todolí Parra J, Varela DC, Maldonado G, Marín A, Pérez Abad L, Aramburu J, Vela L, Ramos Ibáñez E, Del Gracia Tello BC. CAPI-detect: machine learning in capillaroscopy reveals new variables influencing diagnosis. Rheumatology (Oxford). 2025;64(6):3667–75. https://doi.org/10.1093/rheumatology/keaf073.
29. Smith V, Vanhaecke A, Herrick AL, Distler O, Guerra MG, Denton CP, Deschepper E, Foeldvari I, Gutierrez M, Hachulla E, Ingegnoli F, Kubo S, Müller-Ladner U, Riccieri V, Sulli A, van Laar JM, Vonk MC, Walker UA, Cutolo M. EULAR study group on microcirculation in rheumatic diseases. Fast track algorithm: how to differentiate a "scleroderma pattern" from a "non-scleroderma pattern". Autoimmun Rev. 2019;18(11):102394. https://doi.org/10.1016/j.autrev.2019.102394.

Chapter 9
Interstitial Lung Disease in Rheumatic Diseases

Giulio Forte, Antonio Ciancio, and Vasiliki Liakouli

Introduction

Among the extra-articular manifestations of rheumatic diseases, Interstitial Lung Disease (ILD) probably represents the most important complication in terms of morbidity, mortality, and challenges for therapeutic management. Despite the phenotypic similarities with primary ILDs, those associated with systemic autoimmune connective tissue diseases (CTD-ILDs) represent a clinically and biologically distinct subset, in which the coexistence of autoantibody production, chronic inflammation, and fibrotic remodeling necessitates a different conceptual framework, with notable implications for treatment strategies. Moreover, CTD-ILDs present with a variety of phenotypical patterns that, although sharing common concepts regarding clinical management, entail different screening and therapeutic approaches according to the underlying disease.

Knowledge of the variety of lung involvement throughout CTDs and prompt recognition of their clinical manifestations is essential for rheumatologists and trainees: even though a decrease in ILD-related mortality has been witnessed throughout the decades, thanks to consolidated screening strategies and the introduction of therapies able to tackle either the inflammatory process or the fibrotic progression, lung involvement is still the leading cause of death in Systemic sclerosis (SSc) and in Rheumatoid Arthritis (RA), it represents one of the main contributors to mortality beyond cardiovascular etiologies.

This chapter provides an overview of general aspects of CTD-ILDs, followed by an in-depth discussion of ILD manifestations and management across various CTDs.

G. Forte · A. Ciancio · V. Liakouli (✉)
Rheumatology Unit, Department of Precision Medicine, University of Campania "Luigi Vanvitelli", Naples, Italy
e-mail: giulio.forte@studenti.unicampania.it; antonio.ciancio@unicampania.it; vasiliki.liakouli@unicampania.it

Y. El Miedany, R. A. Elziaty (eds.), *Capillaroscopy*, Contemporary Rheumatology,
https://doi.org/10.1007/978-3-032-22966-3_9

Epidemiology

Prevalence and Risk Factors

The reported prevalence of ILD in CTDs is highly heterogeneous, influenced by disease subtype, diagnostic approach (clinical symptoms vs routine High-resolution computed tomography (HRCT) screening), and geographic or ethnic variation. For these reasons, studies across several CTDs are plagued by a high variability in the reported prevalence of ILD. As an example, according to a recent meta-analysis [1], in SSc, the reported prevalence ranges from 22% to 87% of patients, with an overall prevalence of 47%, while RA-ILD prevalence estimates range from 1% to 31%. Similar trends seem to affect studies in other rheumatic diseases, with idiopathic inflammatory myopathies (IIMs) reporting ILD prevalences around 41% (11–68%) and Sjögren's Disease-related ILD (SjD-ILD) accounting for nearly 16% of total SjD patients (6–49%). Mixed connective tissue disease (MCTD) and Systemic Lupus Erythematosus (SLE) seem to consistently show, respectively, the highest and lowest reported prevalence rates among all CTDs (MCTD: 56% overall, 25–78%; SLE: 6% overall, 2–14%).

Several risk factors have been identified for the development of ILD in patients with CTD. Among these, autoantibody profiles play a central role, reflecting both immunopathogenic and prognostic significance. In SSc, the presence of anti-topoisomerase I (Scl-70) antibodies has been consistently associated with a higher likelihood and severity of ILD, whereas anticentromere antibody positivity confers a relatively lower pulmonary risk profile [2–4]. Similarly, in RA, high-titer rheumatoid factor (RF) and anti-cyclic citrullinated peptide (anti-CCP) antibodies correlate with the occurrence of fibrotic lung involvement, suggesting that intense humoral autoimmunity may contribute to alveolar injury [5, 6]. In IIM, the detection of myositis-specific autoantibodies, such as anti-Jo-1, PL-7, and PL-12, is among the strongest predictors of ILD, and in some cases, the interstitial process may precede the appearance of overt muscular manifestations [1].

Environmental and host factors also modulate disease risk. A history of cigarette smoking, particularly in RA, acts as a potent cofactor, amplifying immune activation in the pulmonary microenvironment and synergizing with anti-citrulline autoimmunity to promote fibrosis [6]. Demographic characteristics, including older age and male sex, have been repeatedly linked to more severe or prevalent ILD across several cohorts, possibly reflecting both cumulative exposure and differential immune or fibrotic responses. Additionally, longer disease duration, high systemic inflammatory burden, and coexisting extrapulmonary organ involvement appear to predispose to pulmonary fibrosis, underscoring the systemic nature of tissue injury in these disorders [1].

Finally, accumulating evidence suggests a contribution from repeated alveolar and endothelial injury, potentially driven by microaspiration, inhalational exposure to pollutants, recurrent subclinical infections, or oxidative stress, all of which may act as chronic fibrogenic stimuli. Although less clearly defined than in idiopathic pulmonary fibrosis (IPF), genetic susceptibility likely modulates disease expression: polymorphisms in genes regulating fibrotic signaling, telomere maintenance, and innate immune pathways have been implicated in predisposing individuals to progressive fibrosing phenotypes, pointing to a shared genetic architecture between autoimmune and idiopathic interstitial lung disease [7].

Associations Between ILD Phenotypes and CTDs

The predominant patterns of lung injury differ according to the underlying autoimmune substrate. This variability reflects distinct pathobiological mechanisms, ranging from immune-mediated alveolitis and vascular injury to progressive fibroblast activation and extracellular matrix deposition, that converge on the shared outcome of interstitial fibrosis.

In SSc, for example, fibrosing Nonspecific Interstitial Pneumonia (NSIP) is the prototypical manifestation, mirroring the diffuse fibroproliferative vasculopathy that typifies the disease, whereas in RA, the pulmonary pathology often assumes a Usual Interstitial Pneumonia (UIP) morphology reminiscent of IPF, suggesting overlapping fibrotic pathways. Similarly, the antisynthetase syndrome (ASS) within the spectrum of IIMs are frequently characterized by rapidly progressive ILD (RP-ILD) dominated by NSIP or organizing pneumonia (OP) patterns, often presenting before overt myositis, underscoring the unique lung–muscle immunopathogenic axis in these conditions.

By contrast, in Sjogren Disease (SjD)D, MCTD, and SLE, lung involvement tends to be more variable, often encompassing NSIP, lymphoid interstitial pneumonia (LIP), or OP, sometimes with concomitant airway or pleural pathology.

Pathobiology

CTD-ILD is best conceptualized as an interplay of autoimmune injury, persistent alveolar–endothelial damage, and dysregulated fibrotic repair. While converging on a final common pathway of lung fibrosis, CTD-ILD diverges from idiopathic forms in the prominence of immune and inflammatory drivers.

In a susceptible host with systemic autoimmunity, repeated alveolar or capillary insults, due to microaspiration, low-grade infections, environmental exposures, oxidative stress, or mechanical strain, trigger release of danger-associated molecular patterns (DAMPs), chemokines, and proinflammatory mediators from injured epithelial or endothelial cells. The injured alveolar-capillary interface becomes a nidus for immune cell recruitment and activation.

Immune Drivers of Inflammation

From an immunopathogenic standpoint, fibrosis is initiated and propagated by both the innate and adaptive arms of the immune system. Within innate immunity, activated alveolar macrophages, dendritic cells, and neutrophils play pivotal roles in amplifying early inflammatory responses. Upon activation, these cells release a spectrum of mediators, including transforming growth factor-β (TGF-β), interleukin-1β (IL-1β), interleukin-6 (IL-6), platelet-derived growth factor (PDGF), and various chemokines, that not only recruit additional inflammatory cells but also directly stimulate fibroblast proliferation and differentiation. This local cytokine milieu establishes a permissive environment for extracellular matrix deposition and tissue remodeling [8].

The adaptive immune system further reinforces this process. Activated Th2 and Th17 lymphocytes secrete profibrotic cytokines such as IL-4, IL-13, and IL-17, which enhance fibroblast activation and collagen synthesis. In contrast, impaired function or reduced numbers of regulatory T-cells (Tregs) may fail to contain these inflammatory circuits, thereby permitting unrestrained fibrogenesis. In parallel, B-cell activation also plays a critical role in sustaining chronic injury: through the production of autoantibodies, B cells promote immune complex formation and complement activation within the alveolar interstitium, leading to recurrent cycles of epithelial and endothelial damage [8].

Importantly, several pleiotropic cytokines, notably IL-6, IL-17, and type I interferons, appear to serve as molecular bridges between inflammation and fibrosis, linking immune activation to fibroblast proliferation and extracellular matrix deposition [9].

Drivers of Fibrosis

The transition from inflammation to fibrosis is characterized by persistent fibroblast activation and maladaptive tissue repair. Following repetitive alveolar injury, both resident lung fibroblasts and bone-marrow–derived circulating fibrocytes are recruited to sites of damage, where they differentiate into myofibroblasts, the principal effector cells of fibrosis. These cells secrete large quantities of extracellular matrix (ECM) proteins, including collagens type I and III, fibronectin, and proteoglycans, which progressively replace the normal alveolar architecture with dense fibrotic tissue. TGF-β represents the master regulator of fibroblast proliferation, differentiation, and matrix synthesis through both canonical SMAD-dependent pathways and noncanonical signaling cascades, such as Wnt/β-catenin, p38 MAPK, and Hedgehog. These pathways act synergistically to amplify profibrotic transcriptional programs, leading to sustained ECM deposition. As matrix components accumulate, the mechanical stiffness of the interstitial environment increases, a change sensed by fibroblasts through integrin-mediated mechano-transduction. This biomechanical feedback loop promotes further myofibroblast activation and resistance to apoptosis, thereby establishing a self-perpetuating fibrotic circuit independent of the original inflammatory trigger [10, 11].

Progressively, this dysregulated repair culminates in structural remodeling of the lung parenchyma. Alveolar septa thicken, alveolar units collapse, and microvascular remodeling ensues, with loss of capillary networks and aberrant neovascularization. The architectural distortion manifests radiologically as reticulation, traction bronchiectasis, and, in advanced stages, subpleural honeycombing, reflecting cystic remodeling of the distal airspaces. Emerging evidence suggests that epithelial–mesenchymal transition (EMT), whereby injured alveolar epithelial cells acquire mesenchymal characteristics, may contribute additional myofibroblast precursors [12]. Ultimately, the crosstalk among epithelial, mesenchymal, and endothelial compartments, mediated by cytokines, growth factors, and extracellular vesicles, sustains the progression of fibrosis, driving the irreversible architectural damage that defines end-stage CTD-ILD.

Clinical and Radiological Phenotypes

ILD in rheumatic disorders displays a remarkably heterogeneous temporal relationship with the underlying systemic disease. Pulmonary involvement may arise at virtually any stage of the disease continuum, from the earliest phases of immune activation to the late sequelae of long-standing inflammation and tissue remodeling. However, distinct CTDs show characteristic temporal patterns of ILD development. In SSc and IIMs, particularly the antisynthetase syndromes, ILD often emerges within the first few years after diagnosis or even concurrently with systemic disease onset. In these settings, pulmonary manifestations frequently represent an early and prominent feature of disease activity, sometimes dominating the clinical picture and defining prognosis.

In contrast, in RA and certain overlap syndromes, ILD typically represents a late-stage complication, occurring after years of chronic synovial inflammation and cumulative immune activation. Here, the interstitial process likely reflects a combination of sustained systemic autoimmunity, long-term exposure to inflammatory mediators, and possibly additional environmental or pharmacologic insults (such as smoking), culminating in fibrotic remodeling of the lung parenchyma.

Intriguingly, in a subset of patients, ILD may precede any overt rheumatologic manifestations, serving as the initial or even sole clinical expression of an otherwise occult autoimmune disorder. In these individuals, the detection of interstitial pneumonia, particularly when accompanied by circulating autoantibodies or subtle extrapulmonary autoimmune features, often leads to classification under the entity known as "Interstitial Pneumonia with Autoimmune Features" (IPAF). This construct, introduced by the European Respiratory Society and American Thoracic Society in 2015, identifies patients who exhibit radiologic or histopathologic features of ILD in combination with serologic markers or clinical stigmata of systemic autoimmunity, yet do not meet formal classification criteria for a defined CTD. Clinically, IPAF is thought to represent an intermediate phenotype along the spectrum between idiopathic interstitial pneumonias and fully established CTD [13].

Clinical Phenotypes

In CTD-ILDs, the pathological landscape is governed primarily by two interconnected yet distinct processes: inflammation and fibrosis. These elements should not be viewed as mutually exclusive phenomena but rather as two poles of a dynamic spectrum that evolves and varies between patients and disease subsets. At one end of this continuum lie the inflammatory-dominant ILDs, in which alveolitis and immune-mediated injury of the alveolar-capillary interface predominate. These forms are typically characterized by cellular infiltration, ground-glass opacities on high-resolution CT, and relative preservation of lung architecture. Clinically, they are more likely to respond to immunosuppressive or immunomodulatory therapy, reflecting the reversibility of early inflammatory injury once immune activation is controlled.

At the opposite extreme are the fibrotic-dominant ILDs, in which chronic injury and aberrant tissue repair culminate in irreversible scarring of the lung interstitium. In these patients, fibroblast proliferation, myofibroblast persistence, and excessive extracellular matrix deposition lead to architectural distortion, traction bronchiectasis, and decreased pulmonary compliance. The resulting decline in lung function is largely refractory to anti-inflammatory therapy and instead requires the introduction of antifibrotic agents such as nintedanib or pirfenidone, which target profibrotic signaling pathways and attenuate the rate of functional deterioration.

Importantly, most patients with CTD-ILD exhibit mixed inflammatory and fibrotic features at varying degrees throughout the clinical course. This overlap underscores the need for individualized and dynamic therapeutic strategies, guided by careful longitudinal assessment of disease activity and progression through pulmonary function testing, imaging, and, where appropriate, biomarkers. The balance between inflammation and fibrosis may shift over time, either spontaneously or in response to therapy, making periodic reassessment crucial to optimize treatment.

Despite optimal management, a considerable proportion of both inflammatory and fibrotic ILDs eventually enter a progressive fibrosing phenotype (PF-ILD). This subset is defined by a relentless decline in lung function, worsening symptoms, and increasing fibrosis on imaging, regardless of underlying etiology, a behavior similar to IPF [14].

Radiologic Patterns

HRCT and histopathology provide complementary insights into the structural alterations underlying CTD-ILDs. Although the radiologic patterns observed in these disorders often resemble those described in idiopathic interstitial pneumonias, the distribution, degree of inflammation, and coexistence of multiple patterns within the same patient are typically more variable. The three most frequently recognized morphologic patterns are NSIP, UIP, and OP, with LIP representing a less common but distinctive variant.

The NSIP pattern is by far the most prevalent in CTD-ILDs. On HRCT, it appears as bilateral, symmetric ground-glass opacities accompanied by fine reticular lines and traction bronchiectasis, predominantly involving the basal and subpleural regions. Honeycombing is minimal or absent, and lung architecture remains relatively preserved. Histologically, NSIP is characterized by uniform interstitial thickening with variable degrees of inflammation and fibrosis, often displaying a temporally homogeneous appearance. This pattern typically corresponds to an inflammatory or mixed inflammatory-fibrotic process, which tends to respond favorably to immunosuppressive therapy and carries a relatively good prognosis.

The UIP pattern, in contrast, reflects more advanced and irreversible fibrotic remodeling. Radiologically, it is defined by coarse reticulation, architectural distortion, and subpleural honeycombing, predominantly in the lower lobes. HRCT frequently reveals a patchy, heterogeneous involvement with areas of normal parenchyma interspersed with fibrosis. Histopathologic examination confirms spatial and temporal heterogeneity, with alternating foci of fibroblast proliferation and dense collagen deposition adjacent to relatively preserved alveoli. Clinically, UIP correlates with reduced lung compliance and progressive decline in lung function, often with limited response to anti-inflammatory therapy; antifibrotic agents are generally indicated in this context.

The OP pattern is characterized by patchy airspace consolidations or ground-glass densities that may migrate over time. On HRCT, these lesions are typically peripheral or peribronchial and correspond histologically to intra-alveolar buds of granulation tissue (Masson bodies). OP represents an active reparative response to alveolar injury and is usually highly responsive to corticosteroid treatment, with potential for complete radiologic resolution. Finally, LIP, though rare, may be encountered in CTD-ILDs and manifests radiologically as diffuse ground-glass attenuation, thin-walled cysts, and small nodules, reflecting dense lymphoid infiltration of the interstitium.

When stratified by radiologic pattern, NSIP and UIP emerge as the two dominant morphologies across CTD-ILDs, while OP and LIP represent less frequent but pathognomonic entities in certain subgroups. NSIP accounts for most cases in SSc, IIM, and MCTD, with reported frequencies ranging between 27% and 76%, whereas the UIP pattern predominates in RA, representing nearly 46% of all RA-ILD cases.

The OP pattern is relatively more common in myositis-associated ILD (around 16%), while LIP occurs predominantly in Sjögren's disease (pooled prevalence around 7%), a finding consistent with the disease's lymphoproliferative pathology [1].

In recent years, increasing attention has been devoted to interstitial lung abnormalities (ILAs), radiologic findings of subtle, nondependent interstitial changes incidentally detected on HRCT in individuals without overt clinical or functional impairment. In the context of connective tissue diseases, ILAs are now recognized as a potential preclinical stage of ILD, representing early or subclinical manifestations of immune-mediated alveolar injury. Several longitudinal studies suggest that up to 15–30% of asymptomatic CTD patients, particularly those with SSc or RA, may exhibit ILAs at baseline imaging, and a subset of these cases progresses over time to clinically significant ILD [15].

Radiologically, ILAs may present as limited ground-glass opacities, reticulation, or minimal traction bronchiectasis involving less than 5–10% of the lung parenchyma. Although often indolent, their presence has been associated with impaired gas exchange, reduced DLCO, and a higher risk of progression to fibrosing disease, particularly when subpleural or basal in distribution. Early recognition of ILAs in at-risk autoimmune populations thus provides a unique window for timely surveillance and therapeutic intervention before irreversible fibrosis ensues [16].

Screening and Management

The management of CTD-ILD requires a long-term, dynamic approach that integrates structured monitoring, early detection of progression, and timely initiation or escalation of therapy. Current international recommendations emphasize that the trajectory of lung involvement is highly variable, ranging from stable, nonprogressive disease to relentless fibrosing forms, and therefore demands individualized surveillance and adaptive treatment strategies rather than a fixed, one-size-fits-all protocol. This section will focus on the general outlines of screening and management that apply to CTD-ILDs in general, with more detailed analysis being undertaken in the specific paragraphs.

Monitoring and Longitudinal Assessment

Pulmonary function testing (PFT), with relevance to forced vital capacity (FVC) and diffusing capacity for carbon monoxide (DLCO), is considered the most sensitive tool for detecting functional decline and should be performed at regular intervals, typically every 3–6 months during the first year after diagnosis, and subsequently every 6–12 months in clinically stable patients. Albeit essential, PFT cannot be used in substitution of HRCT, which is mandatory for screening in high-risk cases and provides complementary structural information. Serial HRCT is generally advised when functional decline, new respiratory symptoms, or auscultatory changes occur, but routine periodic re-scans in the absence of clinical progression are generally avoided to minimize radiation exposure [17].

In addition to PFT and HRCT, clinical assessment of symptoms, exercise tolerance, and oximetry remains an important adjunct evaluation in outpatient settings. Biomarkers such as serum KL-6, SP-D, or inflammatory indices are under investigation but are not yet standardized for routine monitoring [18]. Clinical cases must be subjected to a multidisciplinary evaluation, bringing together rheumatologists, pulmonologists, and radiologists, in order to guide management decisions [19]. Bronchoscopy and biopsy are generally not recommended for ILD diagnosis and are reserved for atypical or uncertain cases (e.g., consolidations that raise doubts about possible neoplasms) rather than for serial follow-up [20].

Treatment

The therapeutic strategy in CTD-ILD hinges on the balance between inflammatory activity and fibrotic remodeling. Inflammation-predominant disease, particularly early or cellular NSIP pattern, is usually approached with immunosuppressive or immunomodulatory therapy, aiming to control immune-mediated alveolar injury and prevent irreversible scarring. Agents such as mycophenolate mofetil, azathioprine, cyclophosphamide, rituximab, or calcineurin inhibitors are commonly employed, often in combination with short courses of corticosteroids (except in SSc, in which corticosteroid use is advised against), which should be tapered as soon as possible to reduce long-term toxicity [17].

In contrast, when fibrosis predominates, as in UIP or progressive fibrosing phenotypes, therapeutic emphasis shifts toward antifibrotic agents such as nintedanib or pirfenidone, which have been shown to slow the rate of FVC decline across various fibrosing ILDs. Increasingly, the two therapeutic domains are viewed not as mutually exclusive but as complementary, allowing a stepwise or combined approach based on the relative predominance of inflammation versus fibrosis and the pace of disease progression.

A new avenue for antifibrotic therapies has been opened with the FDA approval in October 2025 of nerandomilast, a phosphodiesterase 4B (PDE4B) inhibitor, for the treatment of idiopathic pulmonary fibrosis. While no data is available to date regarding its efficacy in CTD-ILD, there is growing interest in the potentialities of this novel therapeutic agent that, according to preclinical evidence, possesses both direct anti-inflammatory and antifibrotic effects [21].

Managing Progression

Despite optimal therapy, a subset of patients evolves into a PF-ILD, characterized by physiological decline, radiologic progression, or worsening symptoms within a defined timeframe. Recognition of this phenotype is critical, as it portends a poorer prognosis and warrants escalation of treatment, including the addition of antifibrotic therapy or transition to advanced interventions such as lung transplantation evaluation. Conversely, in RP-ILD, particularly in myositis and antisynthetase syndromes, a more aggressive, combination immunosuppressive regimen is often necessary, integrating high-dose corticosteroids with one or more cytotoxic or biologic agents to arrest fulminant inflammation.

Ultimately, the overarching principle across modern recommendations is that CTD-ILD management should be proactive, personalized, and continuously reevaluated. Early identification of progression, timely modification of therapy, and coordinated multidisciplinary care are key to improving long-term pulmonary and survival outcomes.

Interstitial Lung Disease in Idiopathic Inflammatory Myopathies

Introduction

IIMs, commonly referred to as myositis, represent a heterogeneous group of autoimmune disorders characterized primarily by inflammation and weakness of skeletal muscles [22]. Major subtypes of IIM include polymyositis (PM), dermatomyositis (DM), immune-mediated necrotizing myopathy (IMNM), antisynthetase syndrome (ASS), and inclusion body myositis (IBM). Each subtype presents distinct clinical and immunological features. Although the primary target of inflammation in IIM is the skeletal muscle, internal organ involvement is frequently observed. Interstitial lung disease (ILD) is notably the most common extramuscular manifestation and encompasses a heterogeneous group of diffuse parenchymal lung disorders characterized by inflammation and/or fibrosis of the lung interstitium [23]. ILD significantly impacts morbidity and mortality in patients with IIMs [23]. Typically, lung involvement in IIM is regarded as a complication that develops several years after the onset of muscle inflammation. However, in certain cases, as in clinically amyopathic dermatomyositis (CADM) and ASS-ILD, it may precede the muscular symptoms, while 16–65% of patients may even present isolated lung disease [24]. Recognizing the intersection of ILD and IIM is of utmost importance for clinical management, as their cooccurrence implies a more complex disease trajectory that requires a multidisciplinary approach. ILD occurring in the context of IIM (often termed *myositis-associated ILD*) significantly worsens patient outcomes. Pulmonary manifestations can range from subclinical forms, which are only detected by imaging, to RP-ILD that can quickly evolve to respiratory failure, which is among the major causes of death in IIM patients. Understanding this overlap is critical for early recognition and intervention. This chapter comprehensively explores ILD secondary to IIM, discussing epidemiology, pathogenesis, clinical presentation, diagnostic evaluation, imaging findings, histopathological features, differential diagnoses, therapeutic strategies, prognosis, and emerging research perspectives related to this overlap syndrome.

Epidemiology

ILD is a common complication of IIMs. Approximately 20–40% of adult IIM patients develop ILD, though estimates vary by population and myositis subtype. A 2021 meta-analysis reported a global prevalence of ILD in polymyositis/dermatomyositis of about 41% [25]. Notably, ILD risk is particularly high in certain subgroups; for example, ASS (characterized by anti-tRNA synthetase antibodies like anti-Jo-1) and CADM with anti-MDA5 antibodies have ILD prevalence rates reaching 70–95% in some cohorts [26]. In contrast, inclusion body myositis and pure necrotizing myopathy patients rarely develop ILD. Asian populations seem to have higher reported ILD prevalence in IIM (e.g., ~50% in some Asian DM cohorts) compared to European cohorts, due to a higher frequency of anti-MDA5 [26, 27]. This may reflect genetic and environmental factors or differences in clinical recognition.

IIMs themselves are rare diseases (estimated global prevalence of 2–25 per 100,000), and the incidence of IIM is estimated to range from 0.2 to 2 per 100,000 person-years [28]. Among IIM patients, the incidence of ILD varies by subtype, geographical area, age, and gender. ILD in IIM can present at any age, but most patients are adults in mid-life (40–60 years), with some studies noting a younger age of IIM onset in ILD-complicated cases. There is no conclusive data regarding sex predominance in IIM-ILD, but male sex seems to be associated with more aggressive disease and higher mortality [29].

ILD is a major determinant of prognosis in IIM. Population-based data demonstrate that IIM patients with ILD have higher mortality than those without [30]. For instance, the presence of ILD has been associated with early mortality in DM/PM, with 1-year survival dropping significantly in rapidly progressive cases. Causes of death in IIM often include respiratory failure due to ILD and infections related to immunosuppression. Recognizing the epidemiologic burden of ILD in IIM underscores the importance of timely diagnosis and treatment.

Pathogenesis

The pathogenesis of ILD in IIM is multifactorial, involving both the systemic autoimmune process of myositis and tissue-specific factors in the lung. Immune-mediated injury to muscle and lung likely shares pathogenic pathways. Inflammatory cell infiltrates (particularly CD4+ and CD8+ T-lymphocytes, B cells, macrophages, and plasmacytoid dendritic cells) have been found in affected muscle and lung tissue. Proinflammatory cytokines (e.g., IFN-α/β, TNF-α, IL-6) and type I interferon signatures are elevated in IIM and may contribute to lung inflammation. The concept of *"shared autoimmunity"* suggests that autoantibodies in IIM target antigens present in both muscle and lung, leading to parallel damage. For example, histidyl-tRNA synthetase (the Jo-1 antigen) is expressed in muscle, but anti-Jo-1 autoantibodies can form immune complexes that deposit in lung tissue, causing alveolitis. Additionally, some evidence indicates that myositis T-cells are cross-reactive to muscle and lung antigens, or that lung inflammation can trigger epitope spreading to muscle (perhaps explaining cases where ILD precedes myositis) [31] (Fig. 9.1).

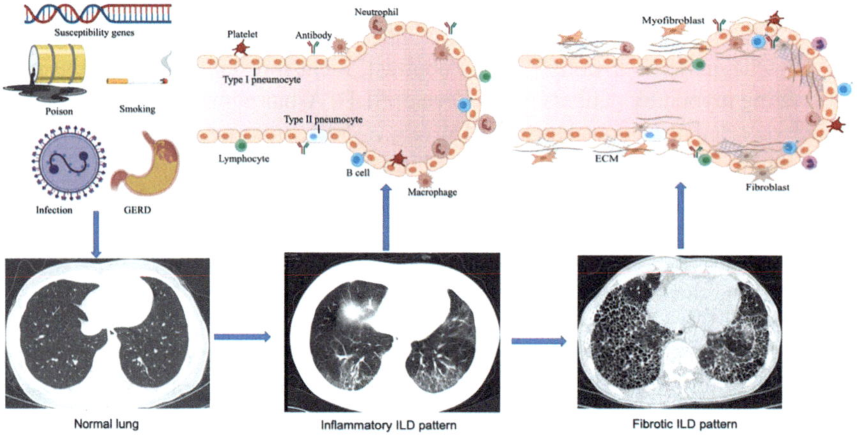

Fig. 9.1 Pathogenesis and progression of interstitial lung disease (ILD) in connective tissue diseaseSchematic representation of the multifactorial pathogenesis and radiologic progression of ILD. Genetic susceptibility and environmental exposures (e.g., smoking, gastroesophageal reflux, infections, toxins) initiate alveolar epithelial injury and immune activation. This triggers the recruitment of immune cells, including neutrophils, macrophages, lymphocytes, and B cells, resulting in the release of profibrotic mediators and the deposition of extracellular matrix (ECM). Over time, persistent injury and inflammation may progress from a reversible inflammatory ILD pattern to irreversible fibrosis. Representative high-resolution computed tomography (HRCT) images illustrate the transition from normal lung to inflammatory ILD (ground-glass opacities, reticulation) and advanced fibrotic ILD (traction bronchiectasis, honeycombing). (Reproduced from Shao et al. [7]. The original article is published under the Creative Commons Attribution (CC BY) license)

A feature of IIM pathogenesis is the presence of myositis-specific autoantibodies (MSAs) and myositis-associated autoantibodies (MAAs). These autoantibodies not only assist in diagnosis but also correlate with distinct clinical syndromes and ILD risk. Key MSAs include i. Anti-Jo-1 (anti-histidyl-tRNA synthetase): the most common anti-tRNA synthetases, present in 15–20% of IIM [32]. It defines the classic *antisynthetase syndrome* characterized by ILD, mechanic's hands, arthritis, Raynaud's, and myositis. Up to 70–80% of anti-Jo-1 positive patients develop ILD. Anti-Jo-1 is strongly associated with the HLA-DRB1*03:01 genotype* [33]; ii. Non-Jo-1 antisynthetase antibodies (e.g., anti-PL-7, PL-12, EJ, OJ, KS, Zo): Together with anti-Jo1, antisynthetase antibodies are present in up to 30% of IIM patients [34] and carry a high ILD risk. Cohorts indicate ILD occurs in the majority (often >70%) of patients with any anti-tRNA synthetase antibody. Notably, patients with anti-PL-7 or PL-12 may have a phenotype with more severe ILD and less myositis than anti-Jo-1 patients [32, 35]. For example, anti-PL-12 has been associated with OP pattern on imaging and more frequent "mechanic's hands" dermatologic findings; iii. Anti-MDA5 (anti-CADM-140): targets Melanoma Differentiation-Associated protein 5, an RNA-specific helicase involved in host defense against viruses. This MSA is found primarily in DM, especially the amyopathic form, and is highly associated with RP-ILD*)* [36]. Anti-MDA5 is more common in Asian populations (prevalence 30–50% in Asian DM/CADM cohorts). The estimated frequency in adults is 1–30%. Patients with anti-MDA5 often have minimal muscle inflammation but severe lung involvement; their ILD often manifests as an acute interstitial pneumonia or diffuse alveolar damage (DAD) pattern with high early mortality. The presence of MDA-5 antibodies in DM patients has been associated with a high frequency of ILD (90–95%) and, particularly, RP-ILD (50–80%) [37]. The presence of anti-MDA5 is a strong predictor of poor prognosis in IIM-ILD, with one study noting 90-day mortality significantly increased and 1-year survival only ~60–70%. These patients can develop a macrophage activation syndrome–like picture with very high serum ferritin, reflecting innate immune activation. Furthermore, ferritin levels correlate with anti-MDA5 ILD severity and outcomes [38]; iv. Anti-Mi-2, anti-TIF1γ, anti-NXP2, anti-SAE: These antibodies are associated with DM (often cancer-associated in the case of TIF1γ and NXP2). They have less frequent ILD involvement. For instance, anti-Mi-2 DM usually has prominent muscle and skin disease, but ILD is uncommon. Anti-TIF1γ and anti-NXP2 IIM patients are characterized by a high risk of developing cancer [39]; v. Anti-SRP, anti-HMGCR: These are seen in immune necrotizing myopathy; ILD is relatively rare in these subsets, as muscle necrosis predominates; vi. MAAs, such as anti-Ro52 (TRIM21), anti-PM/Scl, anti-Ku, and anti-U1 RNP, can be present in myositis, overlapping with other connective tissue diseases. Anti-Ro52 deserves special mention; while not specific to myositis, it often coexists with antisynthetase antibodies and has been linked to more severe ILD and a higher risk of developing progressive fibrosis [40]. Some experts consider the presence of anti-Ro52 in a myositis patient a "red flag" for aggressive ILD, and it may influence a decision to escalate therapy.

Associations with HLA haplotypes have been found, with the *HLA 8.1 haplotype* containing DRB1*03:01 and B*08:01 being strongly linked to anti-Jo1 ASS. Other genetic factors are also under investigation. Polymorphisms in genes like IFIH1 (which encodes MDA5), TNFAIP3 (A20, a negative regulator of NF-κB), and IRF5 have been studied in Chinese myositis cohorts [41]. One study in a Chinese population suggested that HLA-DRB1 variants, rather than IFIH1 polymorphisms, were associated with susceptibility to anti-MDA5-positive DM and ILD [42]. Additionally, genes related to lung fibrosis (such as TERT and TERC affecting telomere length, or the MUC5B promoter variant common in idiopathic pulmonary fibrosis) are being explored for contribution to CTD-ILD risk, although robust data in IIM-ILD are not yet available [43]. Short telomere syndromes have been noted as a risk factor for progressive pulmonary fibrosis in autoimmune ILD, raising the possibility that a subset of IIM-ILD patients might have an underlying genetic predisposition to fibrosis (e.g., occult familial pulmonary fibrosis) [44] (Fig. 9.2).

Various environmental exposures might precipitate or exacerbate IIM and associated ILD in genetically predisposed individuals [45]. Possible triggers include viral infections (a long-hypothesized trigger for DM/PM) and occupational or avocational inhalational exposures (silica, dust, mold), which have been linked to other autoimmune ILDs, and smoking. Additionally, statins have been associated with triggering immune necrotizing myopathy followed by anti-HMGCR antibodies,

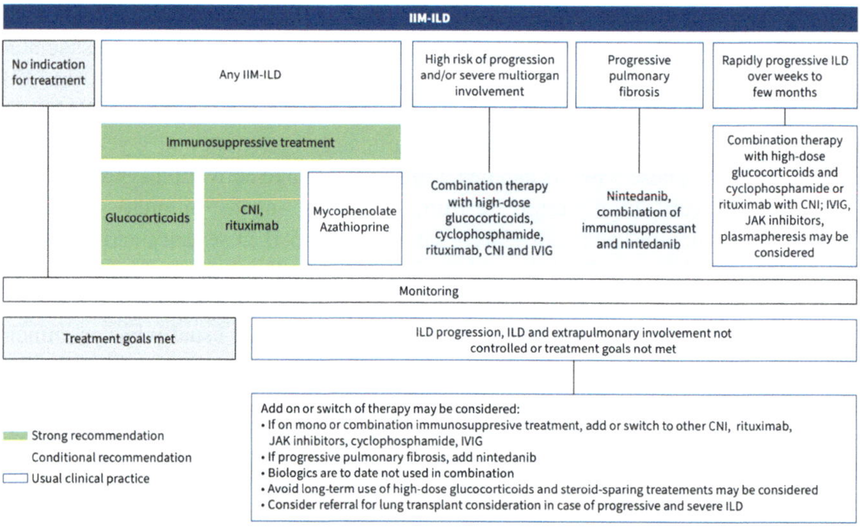

Fig. 9.2 Treatment of idiopathic inflammatory myopathy-associated interstitial lung disease (IIM-ILD) Algorithm outlining recommended therapeutic approaches in IIM-ILD according to ERS/EULAR guidelines. Glucocorticoids, calcineurin inhibitors, and rituximab are strongly recommended, while mycophenolate, azathioprine, and nintedanib receive conditional recommendations. (Reproduced from Antoniou et al. [121]. © The authors. Licensed under a Creative Commons Attribution 4.0 International License (CC BY 4.0))

though ILD is not common in this IIM subtype. Other drugs can cause both myositis and ILD (e.g., some checkpoint inhibitor immunotherapies), which need to be distinguished from idiopathic cases.

Clinical Presentation

Muscle Symptoms

Patients with IIM-ILD typically present with some combination of muscle and lung symptoms, though either may predominate. Muscle involvement in IIM classically causes symmetrical proximal muscle weakness (difficulty climbing stairs, rising from a chair, lifting arms), developing over weeks to months. Myalgias can occur but are often mild; true muscle pain is less prominent than weakness [23]. In DM, characteristic cutaneous findings may be a clue. The only two pathognomonic findings of DM include the following: i. Gottron papules: dorsal metacarpophalangeal and interphalangeal joints may show the presence of overlying erythematous or violaceous papules with or without scaling or ulceration; ii. Heliotrope rash: This is a characteristic skin finding of dermatomyositis and presents with a violaceous or erythematous rash affecting the upper eyelids with or without periorbital edema. This finding may not be apparent in patients with dark skin. Characteristic skin findings that are associated with DM are the following: i. Gottron sign: erythematous macules or patches over the elbows or knees; ii. Facial erythema: erythema over the cheeks and nasal bridge involving the nasolabial folds. The rash may extend up to the forehead and laterally up to the ears; iii. Shawl sign: erythema over the posterior aspect of the neck, upper back, and shoulders, at times, extending to the upper arms; iv. V sign: ill-defined erythematous macules involving the anterior aspect of the neck and the upper chest; v. Poikiloderma: atrophic skin with changes in pigmentation and telangiectasia in photo-exposed or nonexposed areas; vi. Holster sign: poikiloderma involving the lateral aspects of the thighs; vii. Periungual involvement: telangiectasias and cuticular overgrowth; viii. Mechanic's hands: hyperkeratotic, cracked horizontal lines on the palmar and lateral aspects of the fingers; ix. Hyker's feet: hyperkeratosis of the toes and/or plantar surfaces of the feet; x. Scalp involvement: diffuse poikiloderma, with scaling and pruritus; xi. Calcinosis cutis: calcium deposits in the skin [46].

Pulmonary Symptoms

The ILD component often manifests as respiratory complaints. The most common symptoms are progressive exertional dyspnea (shortness of breath on exertion) and persistent dry cough. Patients may initially attribute dyspnea to deconditioning from muscle weakness, but features like bibasilar "velcro" crackles on lung auscultation or hypoxemia on exertion point to ILD. In more acute or severe presentations (e.g.,

RP-ILD of anti-MDA5 DM), patients can develop acute respiratory failure with hypoxemia at rest, tachypnea, and rarely hemoptysis if diffuse alveolar damage or hemorrhage is present. Pleuritic chest pain is uncommon (unless there is concomitant organizing pneumonia involving the pleura or pneumothorax from cavitation, both relatively rare). Constitutional symptoms such as fever, weight loss, and fatigue may accompany active IIM and ILD, reflecting systemic inflammation.

The time of disease can vary significantly: i. Subacute presentation: Many IIM-ILD cases have an insidious onset over months. This is typical for ASS with NSIP/OP-pattern ILD. Such patients may already carry a myositis diagnosis when ILD is detected, or the two manifestations may be discovered around the same time; ii. Acute presentation: A subset, particularly anti-MDA5-positive DM patients, present with rapidly progressive ILD, often within weeks of the onset of systemic symptoms. Sometimes the lung disease dominates the initial presentation, and patients are hospitalized with what appears to be acute interstitial pneumonia or an acute respiratory distress syndrome (ARDS)-like picture before myositis is recognized. The presence of subtle DM skin findings or positive myositis antibodies can provide a clue in these cases of *"lung-predominant"* myositis; iii. ILD-first presentation: It is well documented that ILD can precede the classical muscle or skin manifestations of myositis by months or even years. For example, an individual might be under evaluation for "idiopathic NSIP" when later they develop muscle weakness or a myositis-specific antibody is found, clinching the diagnosis of an underlying IIM. Thus, multidisciplinary evaluation is key—clinicians should consider occult IIM in any "idiopathic" ILD case that has positive myositis antibodies or extrapulmonary signs (e.g., unexplained mild CPK elevation, mechanic's hands, rash). Early rheumatologic input and myositis antibody testing can reveal the diagnosis [47].

Extrapulmonary Manifestations

Because IIMs are systemic, patients may also have arthralgia or inflammatory arthritis (especially in ASS) [48], dysphagia from esophageal muscle involvement [49], or cardiac involvement (arrhythmias, cardiomyopathy) [50], all of which may influence management but are beyond this chapter's primary focus. These features, if present, reinforce the systemic autoimmune nature of the illness and often coexist with ILD in ASS.

Diagnostic Evaluation

Diagnosing ILD in the context of IIM requires integrating laboratory, imaging, and functional tests, often via a multidisciplinary approach (rheumatology, pulmonology, radiology, and pathology) [51].

Laboratory Tests

All patients with suspected IIM-ILD should undergo testing for muscle enzymes and autoantibodies. Creatine kinase (CK) and aldolase are often elevated in polymyositis and classic dermatomyositis, sometimes to thousands of U/L, but can be normal in amyopathic cases or after muscle damage has progressed to fibrosis. Other muscle-related labs include AST/ALT (which can be elevated from muscle injury) and LDH [52]. In the context of ILD, autoantibody testing is crucial. A myositis antibody panel (available in many labs) can detect MSAs (e.g., Jo-1, PL-7, PL-12, EJ, OJ, KS, ZO, Mi-2, MDA5, TIF1γ, SRP, SAE) and MAAs (Ro52, Ku, PM/Scl, U1 RNP, etc.) [53]. If the specific myositis panel is not available, at least test for ANA (often positive in IIM), extractable nuclear antigens (to catch overlap antibodies like U1 RNP or Ro/La), and possibly RF/CCP to check for RA overlap [54]. Additionally, inflammatory markers (ESR, C-reactive protein (CRP)) may be elevated but are nonspecific. Lastly, ferritin levels can be extremely high in anti-MDA5 DM and serve as a marker of macrophage activation and ILD severity [38].

Pulmonary Function Tests (PFTs)

PFTs should be performed to assess lung function and quantify impairment. A restrictive pattern is typical, with reduced FVC and total lung capacity (TLC). The DLCO is often reduced out of proportion to volume loss, reflecting impaired gas exchange from interstitial thickening. Baseline PFTs help stage the ILD. Restrictive syndromes of different entities are typical of lung involvement in IIM. Serial PFTs are equally important for follow-up; a drop in FVC or DLCO by >10% is generally considered potential ILD progression and may prompt therapy escalation. In recent years, different definitions have been developed to identify a "progressive phenotype" in ILD, including IIM-ILD. In 2022 the American Thoracic Society developed a widely used definition: two of the following criteria must be satisfied: (i) deterioration of respiratory symptoms; (ii) an absolute decline in either FVC >5% predicted within 1 year follow-up or DLCO decline of >10% within 1 year follow-up; (iii) progression of at least one HRCT sign (increase in severity and extent of traction bronchiectasis; increase or appearance of new honeycomb; new ground-glass opacities (GGO) with traction bronchiectasis; new fine reticulations; greater extent or irregularity of reticulations; increase in lung volume loss) [14].

Notably, PFTs in IIM-ILD can be confounded by muscle weakness (affecting maximal effort) or concomitant respiratory muscle involvement [22].

Imaging

A chest X-ray is often the first imaging obtained, but can be normal or only subtly abnormal in early ILD (e.g., minor basal reticulations). HRCT of the chest is the gold standard imaging test for ILD diagnosis and characterization. HRCT can detect

ILD changes even when the chest X-ray is normal [55]. Common findings in myositis-associated ILD on HRCT include GGO, irregular linear opacities, patchy consolidation, traction bronchiectasis, and sometimes honeycombing. Specific HRCT patterns are discussed in detail in section "Imaging of ILD in IIMs".

Blood Gas and Exercise Testing

Resting arterial blood gas may show mild hypoxemia in advanced cases. More often, exercise desaturation (e.g., on a 6-min walk test) is an early indicator of ILD before resting hypoxemia occurs. This can be a useful baseline metric for monitoring response to treatment [56].

Electromyography (EMG) and Muscle Biopsy

If the myositis diagnosis is uncertain, an EMG can show irritative myopathic changes, and a muscle biopsy can confirm inflammation (lymphocytic infiltrates, fiber necrosis). However, in many cases of IIM-ILD, the clinical presentation plus autoantibody tests obviate the need for muscle biopsy. Muscle biopsy is rarely needed if classic skin findings or antibodies are present [57].

Lung Biopsy

A lung biopsy is also usually not indicated primarily due to risk: an invasive procedure can trigger a flare of myositis or cause a pneumothorax in already compromised lungs. Most diagnoses can be established by less invasive means. In cases where ILD is atypical or rapidly progressive, and diagnosis is unclear, a bronchoalveolar lavage (BAL) may be considered to exclude infection and look for lymphocytic inflammation (BAL lymphocytosis can support an inflammatory ILD). A surgical lung biopsy or cryobiopsy might be reserved for patients where other differentials like malignancy or alternative ILD are strongly suspected, but typically, the presence of a myositis-specific antibody and compatible HRCT obviates the need for lung biopsy [58].

Imaging of ILD in IIMs

Role of HRCT

Chest HRCT is the cornerstone for identifying and typing ILD in myositis. Typical HRCT patterns seen in IIM-associated ILD include nonspecific interstitial pneumonia (NSIP), considered the most common type, with an estimated prevalence up to

41%. UIP, OP, and diffuse alveolar damage (DAD) were seen in 24%, 19%, and 14.5% of patients, respectively. Desquamative interstitial pneumonia (DIP), respiratory bronchiolitis, and LIP each were reported in <6% of patients [59–61]. Below, we detail each major pattern: NSIP (Nonspecific Interstitial Pneumonia): This is the most common HRCT pattern in IIM-ILD. NSIP on HRCT is characterized by ground-glass opacities (reflecting cellular inflammation) and fine reticular markings that are usually bilateral and symmetric, often with a basilar and subpleural distribution. Unlike UIP, NSIP usually has no general honeycombing and often has subpleural sparing. There may be volume loss in affected areas and traction bronchiectasis if fibrosis is present (fibrotic NSIP). Pathologically, NSIP in IIM is often a cellular NSIP (inflammatory) but can evolve to fibrotic NSIP, making it difficult to distinguish from the UIP pattern. In IIM patients, NSIP often coexists with organizing pneumonia elements (giving a mixed pattern). NSIP is commonly associated with ASS (e.g., anti-Jo1). It typically indicates a steroid-responsive process; thus, low-to-medium steroid doses are often indicated. OP (Organizing Pneumonia): OP can be seen in myositis-ILD either as the primary pattern or mixed with NSIP. On HRCT, OP is suggested by patchy consolidations often in a peripheral or peribronchovascular distribution. Ground-glass opacity can overlay areas of consolidation (sometimes called "atoll" or reversed halo sign in OP). OP lesions may migrate or change over time. In IIM, an OP or NSIP/OP overlap pattern is especially common in certain antibody subgroups like anti-PL-12 or anti-EJ antisynthetase syndrome. OP often corresponds pathologically to organizing fibroblastic plugs in airways (bronchiolitis obliterans organizing pneumonia). It usually responds well to corticosteroids. One study noted OP (including mixed patterns) in up to ~30–40% of anti-MDA5 ILD cases. UIP (Usual Interstitial Pneumonia): UIP is less common in IIM-ILD but can occur, especially in chronic, long-standing cases or certain autoantibody groups (e.g., anti-OJ synthetase or overlap with RA). On HRCT, UIP is characterized by basal predominant, subpleural reticulations, honeycombing, and traction bronchiectasis, with an apico-basilar gradient. Honeycombing (subpleural cystic changes) is the hallmark of UIP. In IIM, overt UIP changes (honeycomb lung) may represent an end-stage fibrotic transformation of prior NSIP/OP disease. Some evidence suggests anti-OJ antibody patients have a higher chance of UIP changes (one cohort found honeycombing in ~60% of anti-OJ cases, versus <5% in anti-Jo1). Importantly, the presence of a UIP pattern in myositis has prognostic implications: it is associated with more progressive pulmonary fibrosis and worse outcomes. AIP/DAD (Acute Interstitial Pneumonia/Diffuse Alveolar Damage): This pattern corresponds to rapidly progressive, acute lung injury. On HRCT, features include diffuse bilateral ground-glass opacities often with dependent consolidation (similar to an ARDS picture). Sometimes an "unclassifiable" pattern is reported, consisting of diffuse mixed ground-glass and consolidation that does not fit neatly into NSIP or UIP categories. In IIM, this pattern is most commonly seen in anti-MDA5 dermatomyositis. It indicates an aggressive course, often reflecting DAD pathologically (hyaline membranes, fibrin in alveoli). Hozumi et al. described that anti-MDA5 ILD often defies classic categorization, with HRCT showing diffuse GGO, consolidation, and mild reticulations, effectively a mixed pattern leaning toward OP/DAD [62, 63].

Treatment

Management of ILD associated with IIMs is challenging and must be individualized. While no large randomized trials exist specifically for IIM-ILD, treatment strategies are guided by retrospective studies, case series, and general principles in managing connective tissue disease–associated ILD. Immunosuppression is the cornerstone of therapy, with the goals of controlling lung inflammation, halting fibrosis, and treating the underlying myositis. Close collaboration between rheumatologists and pulmonologists is necessary. Key elements of treatment include:

Glucocorticoids (GCs): High-dose corticosteroids are typically first-line therapy for IIM-ILD. A common regimen is prednisone 0.75–1 mg/kg/day (e.g., 60 mg daily for an average adult). In severe or rapidly progressive cases, IV pulse methylprednisolone (e.g., 1 gram daily for 3 days) may be given initially. Steroids have broad anti-inflammatory effects and often produce symptomatic improvement in both muscle and lung within weeks. However, steroid monotherapy achieves a complete response in only ~40–50% of IIM-ILD patients. Given the significant side effects of prolonged high-dose steroids (infection risk, hyperglycemia, osteoporosis, etc.), most patients are started on additional steroid-sparing immunosuppressants early, rather than using steroids alone long-term [64].

Calcineurin Inhibitors (CNIs): *Tacrolimus* and *cyclosporine* are frequently used, especially in antisynthetase syndrome and anti-MDA5 ILD. These agents inhibit T-cell activation. Tacrolimus, in particular, has shown efficacy in retrospective studies: for example, adding tacrolimus led to pulmonary function improvement in 94% of refractory myositis-ILD patients in one series. Tacrolimus is often started at 0.5–1 mg twice daily, adjusting to trough levels of 5–10 ng/mL. Cyclosporine (dose range ~ 100–150 ng/mL) has also been reported to be effective in anti-Jo1 ILD. Many Japanese centers use tacrolimus as a first-line adjunct to steroids, especially for anti-MDA5 DM, given the high fatality of that condition. Side effects: CNIs can cause nephrotoxicity (hence, monitoring renal function and drug levels closely is essential), hypertension, neurotoxicity (tremor), and gum hypertrophy. They may be combined with other agents if needed [65].

Mycophenolate Mofetil (MMF): MMF is a purine synthesis inhibitor that has become a favored steroid-sparing agent for ILD in connective tissue diseases. In IIM-ILD, studies show MMF (2–3 g/day) helps stabilize or improve lung function while allowing steroid taper. It has been observed that IIM-ILD patients on MMF maintained stable FVC with a reduced prednisone dose. MMF is generally well-tolerated; GI upset and cytopenias are the main side effects [66].

Azathioprine (AZA): AZA (1.5–2.5 mg/kg/day) is another conventional immunosuppressant used in myositis and ILD. It can be particularly useful in ASS. Studies have shown that over half of anti-Jo1 ILD patients respond to AZA with clinical improvement. AZA may be chosen for those who cannot tolerate MMF or in combination with low-dose steroids for maintenance. Its side effect profile overlaps with MMF (cytopenias, liver enzyme elevation, GI intolerance).

Cyclophosphamide (CYC): CYC (usually IV pulse cyclophosphamide, e.g., 500–1000 mg/m^2 monthly) has been used for severe ILD or cases refractory to initial therapy, and especially for RP-ILD (like anti-MDA5). It is borrowed from scleroderma ILD experience and has shown benefit in case series of myositis-ILD. Combined regimens of high-dose steroids + CYC + tacrolimus have been advocated for anti-MDA5-positive DM with RP-ILD, aiming to suppress inflammation aggressively within the first critical months. CYC is typically given for 6 months, then transitioned to another maintenance agent (AZA or MMF). The side effects include cytopenia, hemorrhagic cystitis, infection risk, and gonadal toxicity. CYC has significant toxicity, so it is reserved for life-threatening diseases.

Rituximab (RTX): RTX, an anti-CD20 B-cell depleting monoclonal antibody, has emerged as an important therapy for refractory myositis and ILD. It is often considered when patients do not adequately respond to steroids + conventional immunosuppressants. RTX appears particularly useful in antisynthetase syndrome and severe ILD (some experts even use it early in anti-Jo1 cases with progressive ILD). The usual dosing is the RA protocol: 1 gram IV twice, 2 weeks apart, repeated every 6 months. In one study of anti-Jo1 ILD, adding RTX enabled steroid taper and lung function stabilization [67]. RTX's B-cell suppression is likely to reduce autoantibody production (e.g., lowering anti-Jo1 and anti-Ro52 levels). The side effects include infusion reactions, risk of infections (especially if combined with other immunosuppressants), progressive multifocal leukoencephalopathy (rare), neutropenia, and lymphopenia. Immunoglobulin levels should be monitored with long-term use (IVIG supplementation is considered if IgG drops significantly, especially <400 mg/dl).

Intravenous Immunoglobulin (IVIG): IVIG (2 g/kg given over 2–5 days every 4 weeks) is widely used for DM muscle disease and has been used as adjunct therapy in refractory cases of IIM-ILD. While robust data on ILD outcomes are limited, IVIG may help by modulating the immune system. One series noted ~40% of patients had ≥10% FVC improvement when IVIG was added to ongoing therapy, along with the ability to reduce steroid dose. IVIG is often considered *salvage therapy* for patients who have failed multiple other agents or have contraindications to further immunosuppression [68]. The high costs associated with therapy, alongside the need for repeated infusions, represent significant limitations to large-scale use, but it may be particularly useful in patients who also have active muscle and/or skin disease that is refractory to other treatments, given its known benefits in DM rash and strength. Furthermore, it may represent the elective choice in patients with cancer-related DM/PM [69].

Other Biologics and Novel Therapies

Janus Kinase Inhibitors (JAK Inhibitors) Small studies suggest JAK inhibitors like tofacitinib can be beneficial in anti-MDA5 dermatomyositis with ILD. Kurasawa et al. reported improved survival in a retrospective series using tofacitinib in severe anti-MDA5 ILD. JAK inhibitors target the interferon and cytokine pathways (e.g., IL-6, which is implicated in MDA5 ILD). They are emerging as a potential therapy in refractory cases, although safety (infection risk) is a concern when combined with other immunosuppressants. Some case reports have shown dramatic improvement of RP-ILD with tofacitinib after failure of standard therapy. As of 2025, clinical trials are underway to better define their role [70].

Antifibrotic Therapy Recognizing that some IIM-ILD patients develop a progressive pulmonary fibrosis (PPF) phenotype, antifibrotic drugs such as nintedanib or pirfenidone (approved for IPF) are being explored. The INBUILD trial demonstrated nintedanib slows FVC decline in progressive fibrosing ILDs (which included some CTD-ILD) [71]. While not specific to myositis, if a patient's ILD behaves like IPF (progressive despite immunosuppression), adding nintedanib may be considered off-label. There are case reports of using pirfenidone in refractory antisynthetase fibrosis. Ongoing studies like the TRAIL1 trial (for RA-ILD) and others in SSc-ILD may inform this practice for IIM-ILD.

Other Treatments Experimental use of other agents like abatacept (CTLA4-Ig, T-cell costimulation blocker) or tocilizumab (anti-IL6 receptor) in myositis might indirectly benefit ILD, but data are sparse. Abatacept showed some efficacy in refractory polymyositis in a trial and might help ILD if T-cell driven. Anti-IL-1 or anti-TNF are generally not used unless overlapping with another condition. Plasma exchange therapy has been tried in severe anti-SRP myopathy or anti-MDA5 ILD with mixed results; it might help rapidly clear circulating antibodies in a fulminant case [72]. Figure 9.3 is a flow chart showing the treatment pathway for SSc-ILD.

Prognosis and Follow-Up

While it is difficult to delineate a clear general prognostic trajectory given the high heterogeneity of presentations within the same disease category, some studies may help provide context. Broadly speaking, IIM patients with ILD have a 10-year survival that is significantly lower than those without ILD, with one cohort reporting a 5-year survival of ~70% in ILD-positive myositis versus >90% in ILD-negative. Rapidly progressive ILD cases (mostly anti-MDA5) have a 6-month mortality of ~30–50% even with aggressive immunosuppression. ASS-associated ILD, on the other hand, often responds to therapy, and many patients have chronic courses with 5-year survival reaching 80–85%. Progressive fibrotic cases may succumb over 5–10 years due to respiratory failure akin to IPF. Infection is also a significant cause

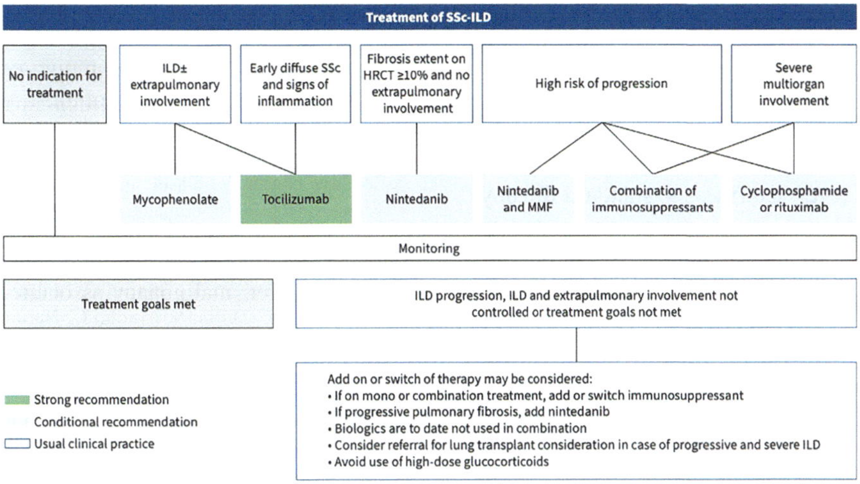

Fig. 9.3 Treatment of systemic sclerosis-associated interstitial lung disease (SSc-ILD)Algorithm summarizing the ERS/EULAR evidence-based recommendations for the management of SSc-ILD. Mycophenolate and tocilizumab are strongly recommended, while nintedanib and other immunosuppressive combinations are conditionally recommended depending on disease severity, progression risk, and extrapulmonary involvement. (Reproduced from Antoniou et al. [121]. © The authors. Licensed under a Creative Commons Attribution 4.0 International License (CC BY 4.0))

of death, given long-term immunosuppression [73]. Key factors associated with worse outcomes include:

Demographic factors: Older age at IIM onset portends worse ILD outcomes (less physiological reserve, more fibrosis). In the Japanese cohort, older age adversely affected ILD risk in DM, and interestingly, male sex was not as clearly a risk as in IPF, but in PM, female sex had a higher ILD risk, which might reflect a selection bias of which PM patients get ILD. African American patients with IIM in some US cohorts have shown more severe myositis and possibly worse ILD outcomes (mirroring the trend seen in SSc-ILD).

Anti-MDA5 positivity: This is among the strongest predictors of poor prognosis. As noted, 1-year survival in anti-MDA5 ILD can be ~60–70%, with most deaths in the first 6 months due to rapidly progressive ILD. Even with aggressive therapy, mortality is high. Conversely, patients without anti-MDA5 (e.g., anti-Jo1) generally have a better prognosis if promptly treated.

Other autoantibody profiles: Besides MDA5, some studies suggest non-Jo1 synthetase antibodies (PL-7, PL-12) might have worse outcomes than Jo1, though data are mixed. The presence of overlapping anti-Ro52 is associated with more severe, treatment-resistant ILD [40].

Rapidly progressive ILD: Regardless of the antibody, a fulminant ILD course (respiratory failure developing over weeks) carries a high mortality risk. The need for mechanical ventilation in myositis-ILD is a grave prognostic sign.

Extent of fibrosis on HRCT: Baseline imaging showing extensive fibrosis (honeycombing, traction bronchiectasis) indicates an established irreversible component and is linked to progressive pulmonary fibrosis (PPF). Honeycombing on initial CT in DM was found to predict subsequent pulmonary deterioration.

Pulmonary function impairment: A low baseline FVC or DLCO, or a significant decline (>10% FVC) over 6–12 months, signals a worse prognosis and possible refractoriness to standard therapy.

Malignancy: In cancer-associated dermatomyositis, the presence of an active malignancy can worsen overall prognosis and complicate treatment decisions (immunosuppression vs. cancer therapy priorities). However, malignancy-associated myositis typically carries less ILD risk.

Response to initial therapy: Patients who stabilize or improve within the first 3–6 months of therapy (symptoms, PFTs, imaging) tend to have a much better long-term prognosis than those with continually worsening lung function despite therapy. Lack of response might prompt experimental approaches or transplant evaluation.

Special Considerations

Certain subgroups and clinical scenarios in IIM-ILD merit special discussion due to their unique features and management:

Rapidly Progressive ILD (RP-ILD) in IIM This refers to ILD that worsens precipitously over weeks to a few months, leading to acute respiratory failure. In the context of myositis, RP-ILD is most classically associated with anti-MDA5-positive dermatomyositis (clinically amyopathic DM). However, a subset of antisynthetase syndrome patients can also have accelerated ILD, and rarely, even "classic" DM/PM can present this way. RP-ILD typically manifests as an acute interstitial pneumonia (DAD) pattern with diffuse alveolar damage, and clinically can be indistinguishable from acute respiratory distress syndrome (ARDS). Patients may present with rapidly escalating oxygen needs, high-resolution CT showing new bilateral consolidations on top of ground-glass, and often systemic inflammatory signs (fever, high ferritin).

Management of RP-ILD requires urgent, aggressive therapy. A common approach (particularly for anti-MDA5 DM) is the combination of high-dose corticosteroids + calcineurin inhibitor (tacrolimus or cyclosporine) + cyclophosphamide from the outset. Some regimens also add IVIG or plasmapheresis. For example, a patient might receive pulse methylprednisolone (1 g daily × 3), start tacrolimus, and IV cyclophosphamide 500–1000 mg every 2–4 weeks, altogether. If there is no improvement, rituximab or tofacitinib can be considered in salvage. Despite these measures, mortality is high. These cases are usually managed in ICU settings, often with mechanical ventilation or high-flow oxygen support. It is crucial to exclude infection (via BAL if possible) before attributing everything to ILD flare, as infection can mimic an RP-ILD flare and requires antibiotics instead.

One special syndrome is acute respiratory failure in anti-MDA5 DM, where patients can also develop features of macrophage activation syndrome (MAS) or hemophagocytic lymphohistiocytosis (HLH), an extremely high ferritin, cytopenias, and coagulopathy. In these scenarios, therapies like JAK inhibitors (tofacitinib) or even etanercept (as used in MAS for Still's disease) have been tried. Some Japanese protocols use plasma exchange in anti-MDA5 RP-ILD to remove cytokines and autoantibodies, with anecdotal success. ECMO (extracorporeal membrane oxygenation) has been used as a bridge in fulminant cases if recovery is deemed possible with therapy.

Anti-MDA5-Positive Disease

Phenotype Patients may have the classic skin findings of dermatomyositis (Gottron's papules, heliotrope rash) or only subtle signs like cutaneous ulcers or a palmar papule rash. They often have little muscle weakness (thus "amyopathic"). The ILD tends to be aggressive. Nearly all anti-MDA5 patients have some ILD, and about half develop the rapidly progressive form.

Laboratory Exams Beyond positive anti-MDA5 antibody, they often have high ferritin (reflecting macrophage activation) and IL-18 and IL-6 elevations.

Prognosis As mentioned, very guarded. Even with optimal therapy, reported mortality rates range from 30% to 50%. However, those who survive the initial 6–12 months often stabilize and can have a more chronic course. There is a subset of anti-MDA5 DM (especially outside East Asia) that is not fulminant and responds to therapy, so outcomes are not universally dismal.

Management Nuances Early combination therapy is standard. Additionally, prophylaxis for pneumocystis pneumonia is critical here due to the intense immunosuppression. If the patient improves, immunosuppression is maintained for a long duration, given the high relapse risk. JAK inhibitors (like tofacitinib or baricitinib) have shown promise in case series for anti-MDA5 ILD, they may help the interferon-driven inflammation. For example, tofacitinib 5 mg twice daily was added to standard therapy in one series with a 60% response. This is now a subject of clinical trials.

Anti-MDA5 Double-Positive with Other Antibodies Sometimes anti-MDA5 coexists with another antibody, e.g., anti-Ro52 or anti-TIF1γ. Coexistence of anti-Ro52 can make ILD even more severe (two high-risk antibodies). These cases might justify extremely aggressive therapy upfront (some experts would add rituximab earlier).

Monitoring In anti-MDA5 ILD, monitoring ferritin can be useful; declining ferritin often parallels clinical improvement, whereas rising ferritin may herald a flare or macrophage activation recurrence.

Antisynthetase Syndrome (ASS) While often a more "chronic" ILD, certain antisynthetase patients (especially anti-PL7 or PL12) can have severe ILD. ASS as a whole is important to recognize because it has multisystem features (myositis, ILD, arthritis, Raynaud's, and mechanic's hands). These patients need a comprehensive approach: rheumatologic medications as discussed, plus symptomatic relief for Raynaud's (calcium channel blockers) or arthritis (NSAIDs or hydroxychloroquine if mild, though HCQ might not be used if significant myositis is active). The presence of ASS also raises the question of cancer screening (though cancer is more strongly associated with TIF1γ or NXP2 antibodies in dermatomyositis than with antisynthetase). A peculiarity: Anti-Jo1 vs. non-Jo1 antisynthetase antibodiessome studies show worse survival in non-Jo1 (like PL7 and PL12), perhaps due to more ILD and less muscle symptoms delaying diagnosis. So clinicians should not underestimate ILD risk in those lesser-known synthetase antibodies.

Overlap Syndromes Occasionally, patients have features of multiple autoimmune diseases (e.g., an overlap of systemic sclerosis and antisynthetase syndrome). These cases might have additional considerations, like a higher risk of pulmonary hypertension (from scleroderma) or different malignancy risks. Treatment usually needs to cover all bases (e.g., if scleroderma overlaps, one might also consider therapies for skin thickening like IV cyclophosphamide, which incidentally also treats ILD).

Interstitial Lung Disease in Systemic Sclerosis

Introduction

SSc, also known as scleroderma, is a rare, complex, autoimmune connective tissue disease characterized by immune dysregulation, vasculopathy, and progressive fibrosis of the skin and internal organs. The disease manifests with a wide clinical spectrum, ranging from limited cutaneous involvement to diffuse skin thickening and severe organ fibrosis. Major organ systems typically affected include the lungs, heart, gastrointestinal tract, and kidneys. Among these, pulmonary involvement, particularly ILD and pulmonary arterial hypertension (PAH), represents a leading cause of morbidity and mortality in SSc patients. ILD in SSc significantly impacts patients' functional status and survival. While skin fibrosis remains the hallmark of SSc, internal organ complications often define the disease prognosis and guide therapeutic decisions. Early recognition and management of pulmonary complications in SSc are critical, as ILD can progress insidiously and lead to respiratory failure [74]. This chapter provides a comprehensive overview of SSc-associated ILD, covering its epidemiology, pathogenesis, clinical features, diagnostic work-up, imaging, and histopathological patterns, differential diagnoses, treatment approaches, and prognosis. Understanding the interplay between immune dysregulation and fibrosis in SSc is essential to improving patient outcomes through timely diagnosis and multidisciplinary care.

Epidemiology

SSc is a rare autoimmune disease with an estimated worldwide prevalence ranging from 50 to 300 cases per million individuals, though rates vary based on geographic region and ethnicity. It predominantly affects middle-aged adults, with a higher incidence observed in females, who represent approximately 80% of cases. Limited cutaneous SSc is more common than the diffuse form, accounting for about two-thirds of patients. Lung fibrosis occurs in more than 90% of patients with SSc. The prevalence of SSc-ILD varies depending on the assessment method (radiography or HRCT), the screening strategy (systematic HRCT versus selection of patients based on the results ofPFTs), the targeted populations (dcSSc versus lcSSc), and the differences in geographic location or expertise of the medical center. ILD develops more frequently and progresses more aggressively in patients with diffuse cutaneous involvement and those positive for specific autoantibodies such as anti-topoisomerase I (Scl-70). Pulmonary complications are a leading cause of mortality in SSc, underscoring the importance of early detection and monitoring in at-risk populations.

Pathogenesis

The pathogenesis of systemic sclerosis-associated interstitial lung disease (SSc-ILD) is a complex process involving both immune and nonimmune cells. The initial pathogenic event likely involves repetitive injury to the pulmonary vascular tree, triggered by environmental factors and infections in genetically predisposed individuals, leading to loss of self-tolerance and production of autoantibodies against vascular molecules. This promotes local inflammation through chemokine production and activation of both innate and adaptive immune systems. Transforming growth factor-β (TGF-β) strongly induces endothelial-to-mesenchymal transition, a process highly activated in SSc. Vascular injury results in thrombin production, contributing to local hypercoagulation and fibroblast activation and differentiation into myofibroblasts, which deposit extracellular matrix proteins, causing fibrosis. Thrombin also enhances the release of profibrotic cytokines, including TGF-β, connective tissue growth factor (CTGF), platelet-derived growth factor (PDGF), and monocyte chemoattractant protein 1 (MCP1) by various lung cells and induces endothelial apoptosis. Activation of B cells, autoantibody production, and Toll-like receptor stimulation lead to type I interferon production and plasmacytoid dendritic cell activation, further boosting interferon and interleukin-6 release. These cytokines stimulate T helper 2 cells and macrophages to produce profibrotic factors, perpetuating fibrosis. The combined effects of TGF-β, CTGF, and PDGF-BB drive fibroblast collagen and matrix protein synthesis, resulting in irreversible lung fibrosis [75].

Classification

SSc-ILD can be classified by distinct histopathological patterns, such as NSIP, UIP, OP, LIP, and diffuse alveolar damage. These subtypes differ in the degree of inflammation and fibrosis present. NSIP, the predominant histological form, typically appears on HRCT as ground-glass opacities predominantly in the peripheral, subpleural, and basal lung regions, with preservation of the lung's overall structure. Fibrotic NSIP manifests additional features, including reticulations and traction bronchiectasis. The UIP pattern shows disrupted lung architecture with patchy fibrosis and cystic honeycomb changes, and it is linked to poorer outcomes compared to NSIP. There are cases where advanced fibrosis does not align with these defined patterns. Diagnosis of SSc-ILD relies primarily on HRCT imaging, which correlates well with histopathology, making lung biopsy unnecessary unless clinical and imaging findings are inconsistent or raise suspicion for other diseases like malignancy or infection. This classification aids prognosis and guides management decisions in SSc-ILD patients.

Screening and Early Diagnosis

Early detection of interstitial lung disease in systemic sclerosis is crucial for improving patient outcomes, yet standardized screening guidelines remain elusive. While HRCT remains the most sensitive method to identify ILD, its use as a routine screening tool is weighed against concerns about radiation exposure. PFTs, including FVC and DLCO, are commonly utilized but may lack sensitivity in detecting early or subclinical ILD when abnormalities are subtle or absent. Clinical symptoms such as exertional dyspnea and dry cough often manifest late and lack specificity, complicating early clinical recognition. Current recommendations emphasize baseline HRCT coupled with PFTs at initial diagnosis of systemic sclerosis, particularly in high-risk subgroups (e.g., diffuse cutaneous subtype, presence of anti-Scl-70 antibodies). Regular monitoring with serial PFTs every 3–6 months is advised to capture clinically meaningful changes that warrant repeat imaging. Emerging modalities such as lung ultrasound and lung MRI offer potential as non-invasive adjunctive tools for screening but require further validation. Integrative screening strategies combining imaging, functional testing, and biomarkers are likely to enhance early ILD identification and facilitate timely intervention to alter disease trajectory [76–79].

Stratification of ILD

Stratification of ILD in SSc is essential for tailored clinical management and prediction of disease progression. Patients can be categorized based on the extent of pulmonary fibrosis observed on HRCT alongside PFT results, such as FVC. Limited ILD is defined when fibrosis involves less than 20% of the lung parenchyma or when FVC is 70% or above of the predicted value. Extensive disease refers to fibrosis affecting 20% or more of the lung or an FVC below 70% of predicted [80]. Stratification of SSc-ILD patients by risk, progression rate, and disease severity is essential for guiding clinical management and improving prognosis. Risk factors linked to ILD progression include older age at disease onset, male sex, diffuse cutaneous systemic sclerosis subtype, shorter disease duration, positivity for anti-topoisomerase I antibodies (Scl-70), reduced baseline FVC) and DLCO, extensive disease on HRCT, and elevated acute phase reactants. The clinical course of SSc-ILD varies widely, with some patients experiencing slow or nonprogressive disease, while others have a rapid decline in lung function marked by worsening fibrosis and respiratory symptoms. Severity stratification differentiates subclinical ILD, characterized by minimal radiological involvement, absence of symptoms, and normal pulmonary function, from clinical ILD, which presents with more extensive fibrosis, functional impairment, and symptomatic burden. Early identification of high-risk and progressive phenotypes enables timely initiation of therapy and appropriate monitoring intervals, which is crucial given the potential for irreversible lung damage [81–83]. Biomarkers such as serum KL-6 and C-reactive protein, alongside clinical and imaging parameters, are increasingly being integrated into stratification models to enhance prediction accuracy and personalize patient care [84, 85].

Candidate Patients for Treatment, Appropriate Treatment Regimens, and Response to Therapy

Selecting patients for treatment in SSc-ILD involves identifying those with clinical or subclinical disease who are at risk of progression or have already demonstrated functional decline. Candidates typically include individuals with clinical ILD defined by abnormal HRCT findings and PFT impairments such as FVC below 80% of predicted. Additionally, patients with mild or subclinical ILD but high-risk features, such as diffuse cutaneous systemic sclerosis subtype (dcSSc), positivity for anti-Scl-70 antibodies, short disease duration, or radiological ground-glass opacities, may benefit from early therapeutic intervention. Patients presenting with progressive fibrotic phenotypes, rapid lung function decline, or significant symptom burden also require prompt treatment to alter disease trajectory and improve quality of life [86].

Treatment

Immunosuppressive therapies constitute the mainstay of SSc-ILD treatment, with MMF favored due to its demonstrated efficacy and safety profile in randomized controlled trials. Cyclophosphamide remains an option, particularly in severe or refractory cases. More recently, antifibrotic agents, notably nintedanib, have been approved for progressive fibrotic SSc-ILD, either as monotherapy or in combination with immunosuppressants, to slow pulmonary function decline [87, 88]. Biologic agents such as tocilizumab and rituximab have shown promise in targeting immune pathways, especially early in the disease course [89, 90]. Autologous hematopoietic stem cell transplantation (AHSCT) is an option for patients with early rapidly progressive diffuse cutaneous systemic sclerosis who are at high risk of organ failure and refractory to conventional therapies; it has demonstrated potential to improve survival and skin involvement and stabilize or improve lung function, although it is reserved for use in specialized centers due to risks related to treatment-related mortality and toxicity [91–93]. Treatment choice should be individualized based on disease severity, progression risk, comorbidities, and patient preference, while balancing efficacy and potential adverse effects.

Regular monitoring of SSc-ILD treatment response is crucial to adjust therapeutic strategies and optimize outcomes. Clinical evaluation complemented by serial PFT, including FVC and diffusing capacity for DLCO, every 3–6 months, is recommended to detect meaningful functional changes. Repeat HRCT imaging may be performed periodically or if clinical or functional deterioration occurs to assess radiological progression. Patient-reported outcomes related to respiratory symptoms and quality of life are valuable adjuncts to objective measures. Integration of biomarkers and advanced imaging modalities may further refine the assessment of treatment efficacy and facilitate early intervention to prevent irreversible lung damage [94–96].

Interstitial Lung Disease in Rheumatoid Arthritis

Rheumatoid arthritis-associated interstitial lung disease (RA-ILD) is the most common and serious extra-articular manifestation of RA, contributing significantly to patient morbidity and mortality [97, 98]. Lung involvement occurs in up to 60% of

RA patients when sensitive imaging is used, though clinically apparent ILD develops in a smaller subset, approximately 5–10% [99, 100]. RA-ILD typically arises in patients with established RA, usually within 5–10 years of articular disease, although in a minority of cases, pulmonary manifestations can precede joint symptoms [99, 101]. Risk factors include male sex, older age, cigarette smoking, and high autoantibody titers (rheumatoid factor and anti-citrullinated protein antibody), as well as high disease activity [99, 102, 103]. Seropositive RA is especially prone to ILD, though even seronegative RA carries an elevated risk compared with the general population [98, 103]. Clinically, RA-ILD is heterogeneous: some patients remain stable, while others experience relentlessly progressive fibrosis, resembling idiopathic pulmonary fibrosis (IPF) [103] (Fig. 9.4).

Pathogenesis reflects an interplay of autoimmunity and fibrotic remodeling. Genetic susceptibility overlaps with IPF, particularly the MUC5B promoter variant, which has been associated with RA-ILD [104]. Environmental triggers such as cigarette smoking may drive posttranslational modifications like citrullination in the lung, breaking tolerance and promoting autoantibody production (9,10). Local immune-fibrotic interactions, including upregulation of IL-17A and TGF-β pathways, contribute to fibroblast activation and collagen deposition [99]. Histopathologic studies frequently reveal lymphoid aggregates, rheumatoid nodules, and features of follicular bronchiolitis, highlighting the autoimmune imprint in addition to fibrotic remodeling [99, 102].

Radiologically, the most common pattern is UIP, identified in nearly half of cases, followed by NSIP. UIP carries a poor prognosis with a median survival of 3–5 years, comparable to IPF, while NSIP generally has a more indolent course and better therapeutic response [99, 103]. HRCT shows basal, subpleural fibrosis with honeycombing and traction bronchiectasis in UIP, versus GGO in NSIP [102].

Management of RA-ILD is multidisciplinary. Glucocorticoids are frequently used in acute or severe presentations, often with immunosuppressants such as mycophenolate mofetil or azathioprine and cyclophosphamide in more aggressive disease [101, 102]. Rituximab and abatacept are increasingly favored because of dual efficacy in articular and pulmonary disease, with growing observational evidence of stabilization of lung function [101–103]. Tocilizumab has also been conditionally recommended for progressive RA-ILD despite first-line therapy [101]. More recently, antifibrotic agents such as nintedanib and pirfenidone, originally developed for IPF, have shown promise in slowing functional decline in RA-ILD with progressive fibrosing features, particularly those with UIP pattern, as demonstrated in the INBUILD trial [104]. Guidelines now suggest a case-by-case approach to antifibrotics, balancing benefits against tolerability and cost [101]. Ultimately, management requires close collaboration between rheumatologists and pulmonologists, with supportive care and referral for lung transplantation in advanced cases.

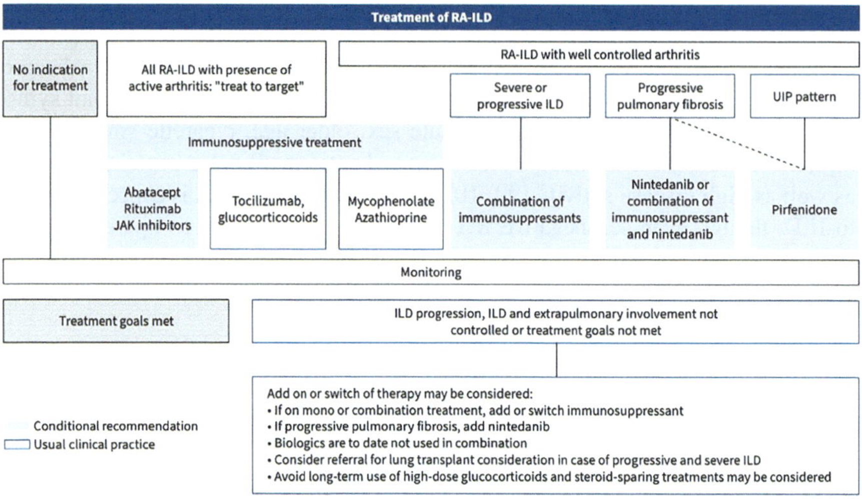

Fig. 9.4 Treatment of rheumatoid arthritis-associated interstitial lung disease (RA-ILD)ERS/EULAR treatment algorithm for RA-ILD based on the presence of arthritis activity and ILD severity. Immunosuppressive agents (abatacept, rituximab, JAK inhibitors) are recommended in active arthritis, while antifibrotic therapy (nintedanib, pirfenidone) may be considered in progressive fibrosing or UIP-pattern ILD. (Reproduced from Antoniou et al. [121].)

Interstitial Lung Disease in Sjögren's Disease

SjD is a chronic systemic autoimmune disease classically defined by lymphocytic infiltration of exocrine glands, resulting in sicca symptoms such as xerostomia and xerophthalmia. However, SjD extends well beyond glandular involvement, with a wide array of extraglandular manifestations affecting multiple organ systems, including the lungs [105]. The estimated prevalence of SjD in the general population ranges from 0.5% to 4%, making it one of the more common systemic autoimmune diseases after RA [105]. Pulmonary involvement represents a clinically significant, though frequently under-recognized, extraglandular feature of SjD. While overt respiratory disease is reported in approximately 9–20% of patients, subclinical abnormalities detected by HRCT or PFTs can be identified in up to 65% of cases [105–107]. These findings highlight the often-occult nature of lung disease in SjD and underscore the importance of systematic respiratory assessment, even in the absence of symptoms.

Among pulmonary complications, ILD is the most significant, contributing substantially to both morbidity and mortality [105–108]. The prevalence of ILD in SjD varies depending on the studied population and diagnostic criteria, with estimates generally ranging from 10% to 20% [108, 109]. A large multicenter Korean cohort of 1306 patients found ILD in approximately 6%, with NSIP and UIP identified as the main radiological patterns, accounting for 54% and 22% of ILD cases, respectively [108]. Prognosis varies: in one longitudinal cohort, 1-, 3-, and 5-year survival rates were 93.5%, 85.8%, and 81.1%, respectively, with older age, elevated C-reactive protein (CRP), lower forced vital capacity (FVC), and UIP pattern on HRCT acting as independent predictors of mortality [110]. Ten-year survival estimates for SjD-ILD generally range between 79% and 82%, with respiratory failure being a leading cause of death [109].

NSIP is the most frequently reported histopathological and radiological pattern in SjD-ILD across multiple series [108, 111]. Other less common subtypes include UIP (10–22%), OP, and LIP [105, 109, 110]. The prognostic implications of these subtypes are significant: NSIP and OP typically show better responses to corticosteroids and immunosuppressive therapies, while UIP is associated with a more fibrosing course and poorer outcomes [105, 111].

LIP deserves particular attention in the context of SjD due to its unique immunopathologic features and radiological profile. Histologically, LIP is characterized by diffuse infiltration of alveolar septa and peribronchiolar interstitium with polyclonal lymphocytes and plasma cells, often forming germinal centers and lymphoid follicles [112]. Unlike fibrotic ILD patterns, LIP reflects a primarily lymphoproliferative process, with less architectural distortion. On HRCT, LIP is commonly associated with ground-glass opacities, interlobular septal thickening, centrilobular nodules, and most distinctively, thin-walled cysts (<30 mm), sometimes containing internal septations or nodular components [105, 113, 114]. The pathogenesis of cyst formation is attributed to bronchiolar obstruction or peribronchiolar lymphoid proliferation leading to air trapping and alveolar remodeling. Notably, radiological overlap with NSIP or other ground-glass dominant patterns may complicate diagnostic classification [105]. Clinically, LIP tends to follow an indolent course and may respond well to corticosteroids or immunosuppressants, although progression to fibrosis or transformation into B-cell lymphomas, particularly mucosa-associated lymphoid tissue (MALT) lymphomas, has been documented [112].

The clinical trajectory of SjD-ILD is heterogeneous. While NSIP and OP subtypes often respond favorably to immunosuppression, fibrosing patterns such as UIP are more likely to exhibit chronic progression and reduced survival [105, 110, 111]. Acute exacerbations, progressive PFT decline, and significant mortality are not uncommon. In one study, 19% of patients experienced acute exacerbations, 29% showed meaningful declines in PFTs, and 9% died over a median follow-up of 4 years [107]. Radiologic progression, manifested by increased reticulation, traction bronchiectasis, and honeycombing, correlates with clinical deterioration [111]. Given the potential discordance between clinical symptoms, functional measures, and imaging findings, regular monitoring through serial HRCT, DLCO, and FVC is advocated to guide timely intervention [111].

In the absence of robust randomized controlled trials, treatment of SjD-ILD remains largely empirical. Observation may be appropriate for mild or stable disease, while progressive or symptomatic cases often warrant corticosteroids in combination with immunosuppressive agents such as mycophenolate mofetil, azathioprine, or cyclophosphamide [105, 106]. Rituximab has shown promise in refractory cases, particularly in the context of lymphoid-predominant pathology

[106]. For patients with fibrosing phenotypes, antifibrotic agents like nintedanib are under active investigation as adjunctive therapy [108]. Importantly, due to the potential for lymphoproliferative transformation, particularly in LIP, vigilant surveillance and a multidisciplinary approach are essential [112].

Interstitial Lung Disease in Systemic Lupus Erythematosus

SLE is a chronic autoimmune disease characterized by marked clinical heterogeneity and multiorgan involvement, driven by immune complex deposition, autoantibody production, and systemic inflammation [115]. Pulmonary involvement is one of the most frequent extrarenal complications, occurring in up to 20–90% of patients during the disease course [116, 117]. The spectrum of lung manifestations is broad, encompassing both acute and chronic forms that may involve the pleura, interstitium, vasculature, and airways.

Pleuritis is the most common pulmonary manifestation, often presenting with pleuritic chest pain and small, bilateral, exudative effusions [116]. Though frequently benign, recurrent pleural involvement can contribute to significant discomfort and impaired respiratory mechanics. Less common but clinically severe manifestations include acute lupus pneumonitis and diffuse alveolar hemorrhage (DAH). These present acutely with dyspnea, fever, hypoxemia, and diffuse alveolar infiltrates, often mimicking infection or ARDS. DAH carries high mortality and requires immediate immunosuppressive therapy [120]. SLE also confers increased thrombotic risk, particularly in the presence of antiphospholipid antibodies. Pulmonary embolism may be an early or late complication and requires prompt recognition and anticoagulation. In some patients, especially those with overlap syndromes or long-standing disease, PAH may develop, either as an isolated manifestation or secondary to vasculopathy, thromboembolic disease, or chronic hypoxia. While less common than in SSc, PAH in SLE is associated with significant morbidity and may be asymptomatic until advanced [118]. Among chronic pulmonary manifestations, ILD, though less prevalent than in other connective tissue diseases, represents a clinically significant complication. Its reported prevalence ranges from 3% to 9% (1, 3), though higher rates of subclinical involvement have been observed in HRCT-based studies (4, 5). Risk factors for SLE-ILD include older age, long disease duration, Raynaud's phenomenon, sclerodactyly, and the presence of anti-RNP antibodies, features that may overlap with MCTD or SSc [115, 116, 119].

Clinically, ILD may be silent or manifest with exertional dyspnea, nonproductive cough, and reduced exercise tolerance. On auscultation, fine bibasilar crackles may be heard, but their absence does not exclude parenchymal disease [117]. PFTs typically reveal a restrictive ventilatory defect with reduced diffusing capacity for DLCO, even in early stages. HRCT is the gold standard for detection, often showing ground-glass opacities, reticular infiltrates, and in advanced cases, traction bronchiectasis or honeycombing [116, 118]. Histologically, NSIP is the most common pattern in SLE-ILD, marked by lymphocytic and mononuclear infiltrates without prominent fibrosis [115, 118]. Less frequent patterns include OP, LIP, follicular bronchiolitis, and, rarely, UIP, the latter associated with more fibrosing behavior and poorer outcomes [115, 116].

Management of SLE-associated pulmonary disease depends on the clinical context. In pleural or inflammatory parenchymal disease, corticosteroids remain first-line, often in combination with immunosuppressants such as mycophenolate mofetil, azathioprine, cyclophosphamide, or rituximab, tailored to disease severity and patient comorbidities [115, 116]. For severe or fibrosing ILD, rituximab and cyclophosphamide are frequently employed as steroid-sparing agents [116]. The potential role of antifibrotic therapy is increasingly recognized: nintedanib, shown in the INBUILD trial to reduce FVC decline in progressive fibrosing ILDs, is being considered off-label for selected SLE patients with a fibrosing phenotype [120]. Prognosis varies according to the type and severity of lung involvement. Patients with NSIP or OP may remain stable with appropriate treatment, while those with UIP, PAH, or DAH carry a higher risk of deterioration and mortality (2, 4) [116]. In one Japanese multicenter study, 5-year survival for SLE-ILD was approximately 85%, with smoking, thrombocytopenia, and radiologic fibrosis emerging as negative prognostic factors [116]. Longitudinal monitoring using HRCT, DLCO, and FVC is essential for early detection of progression and timely therapeutic adjustment.

Clinical Cases

Case 1: MDA5-Positive Dermatomyositis Mimicking Adult-Onset Still's Disease with Rapidly Progressive Interstitial Lung Disease

Clinical History

A 45-year-old male presented in June 2022 with symmetric inflammatory arthralgia involving the wrists, hands, and shoulders; low-grade fever (up to 38 °C); morning stiffness (~30 min); a malar erythematous rash; and pruritic erythematous lesions on the elbows and hands, along with unintentional weight loss of 20 kg. The combination of systemic and articular symptoms, fever, and rash led to a presumptive diagnosis of adult-onset Still's disease (AOSD). Treatment was initiated with methotrexate (7.5 mg/week), hydroxychloroquine, and low-dose prednisone. Methotrexate was temporarily discontinued due to hepatotoxicity. The AOSD diagnosis was reaffirmed in October 2022, and immunosuppressive therapy was intensified with methotrexate 10 mg/week and methylprednisolone 8 mg/day.

By March 2023, the patient experienced clinical relapse with recurrent inflammatory arthralgias, oral aphthosis, and febrile episodes following corticosteroid tapering.

In May 2023, chest HRCT revealed ILD with an OP pattern and mediastinal/axillary lymphadenopathy—an atypical finding for AOSD. This prompted a reassessment of the diagnosis.

Despite the initiation of canakinumab in June 2023, the clinical response was inadequate. In December 2023, the appearance of Raynaud's phenomenon, digital ulcers, worsening dyspnea, and dysphagia further supported an alternative diagnosis. Notably, nailfold videocapillaroscopy demonstrated a scleroderma pattern (active subtype), which is not characteristic of AOSD.

In February 2024, a repeat HRCT revealed pneumomediastinum with subcutaneous emphysema and interstitial thickening. Serological testing identified anti-MDA5 and anti-Ro52 autoantibodies, supporting the diagnosis of CADM. The presence of rapidly progressive ILD, MDA5 positivity, and a scleroderma-type capillaroscopic pattern clearly distinguished this case from AOSD.

Laboratory and Clinical Findings
- Autoantibodies: ANA and ENA negative; myositis blot positive for anti-MDA5 and anti-Ro52.
- Capillaroscopy: scleroderma pattern, active subtype.
- Muscle strength: mild proximal weakness (MRC 3–4/5); no significant CK elevation.
- ECG: supraventricular bigeminy and transient T-wave inversions.
- Inflammatory markers: elevated during flares; anemia of chronic disease.

Imaging
- Chest HRCT (May 2023): OP-pattern ILD with mediastinal/axillary lymphadenopathy.
- Chest HRCT (February 2024): pneumomediastinum with interstitial thickening and post-inflammatory fibrotic areas.
- Chest HRCT (July 2024): bilateral subpleural fibrotic consolidations, traction bronchiectasis, interlobular and intralobular septal thickening.

These imaging findings, particularly the rapidly progressive ILD, were key to distinguishing the case from AOSD and supporting a diagnosis of MDA5-positive dermatomyositis.

Diagnosis
CADM, anti-MDA5 and anti-Ro52 positive, complicated by RP-ILD disease, initially misdiagnosed as adult-onset Still's disease.

Treatment
The patient received multiple immunosuppressive therapies:

- Methotrexate (June–September 2022)—discontinued due to hepatotoxicity.
- Canakinumab (June–December 2023)—inadequate disease control.

- Systemic corticosteroids—oral prednisone (up to 25 mg/day) and intravenous methylprednisolone pulses (500 mg/day for 3 days) during flares.
- Cyclophosphamide—V monthly (500 mg/month, February–September 2024).
- Mycophenolate mofetil—maintenance therapy.
- Cyclosporine—attempted during early disease stage.
- Nintedanib—initiated July 2024 for fibrosing ILD, later dose-reduced due to gastrointestinal intolerance.
- Rituximab—off-label biosimilar therapy under approval process for long-term immunosuppression.

Case 2: Inflammatory Myopathy with Severe ILD and Respiratory Failure in a Patient with Multi-Autoantibody Positivity

Clinical History

A patient with a history of systemic autoimmune disease presented in early 2023 with inflammatory arthralgia involving the shoulders (with marked functional impairment), elbows, wrists, hands, knees, and ankles, along with joint swelling (notably of the hands and knees) and diffuse myalgia in all four limbs.

By October 2023, the patient developed progressive dyspnea on mild exertion and dysphagia for solids. Pulmonary function tests revealed a mixed ventilatory defect with severe restrictive impairment. Chest HRCT confirmed ILD. Laboratory findings included ANA 1:160 (fine speckled), high-titer anti-SSA (Ro52) positivity, low-titer rheumatoid factor, elevated inflammatory markers (ESR 76 mm/h, CRP 4.26 mg/dL), and mildly increased creatine phosphokinase (CPK 544 U/L).

Based on arthritis, myalgia, dysphagia, systemic inflammation, and ILD, a presumptive diagnosis of inflammatory myopathy with secondary ILD was made. Prednisone 12.5 mg/day was initiated with symptomatic improvement.

Immunological Profile

- Ro-52 antibodies: high titer.
- Th/To antibodies: low titer.
- Mi-2 antibodies: low titer.
- ANA: 1:640, fine speckled (AC-4), cytoplasmic, and dense fine speckled (AC-19) patterns.

Imaging

Serial Chest HRCT scans (2023–2025) demonstrated progressive fibrosing ILD with the following findings:

- January 2024: diffuse inter- and intralobular septal thickening, superimposed ground-glass and consolidative opacities (more prominent in upper lobes), mantellar and centrilobular distribution in lower lobes, and multiple subcentimetric lymph nodes in Barety's space and subcarinal region.

- July 2024: marked interstitial thickening with reticular changes, traction bronchiectasis, and cystic changes in posterior basal regions bilaterally; cardiomegaly with mild pericardial effusion; mediastinal lymphadenopathies up to 15 mm.
- January 2025: subpleural and peripheral interlobular thickening, parasubpleural and centrilobular emphysematous bullae, and mantellar ground-glass opacities, consistent with peripheral fibrotic remodeling.

The radiological progression toward fibrosing ILD, with traction bronchiectasis, peripheral ground-glass opacities, consolidations with an OP pattern, and worsening respiratory failure, suggested severe chronic lung involvement requiring aggressive management.

Diagnosis
Inflammatory myopathy associated with progressive fibrosing interstitial lung disease and respiratory failure, positive for anti-Ro52, Th/To, and Mi-2 antibodies.

Treatment
The patient was treated with a combination of immunosuppressive and antifibrotic therapies:

- Corticosteroids: tapered oral prednisone, currently 5 mg daily.
- Rituximab: initiated in late 2024 (ongoing).
- Intravenous immunoglobulins (IVIG): administered during hospitalization in November 2024.
- Mycophenolate mofetil: 1 g BID.
- Nintedanib: 150 mg BID.

Clinical Insight
This case represents a typical presentation of progressive fibrosing ILD and respiratory failure in the context of inflammatory myopathy. The presence of high-titer anti-Ro52 antibodies, in combination with MSA such as Mi-2 and Th/To, has been increasingly recognized as a marker of severe and rapidly progressive pulmonary involvement.

Case 3: Progressive Fibrosing NSIP in a Patient with Autoimmune Features Consistent with IPAF

Clinical History
A female patient with a complex medical history, including Hashimoto's thyroiditis, endometriosis, allergic asthma, laparoscopic cholecystectomy with adhesiolysis (2024), and right breast cancer (2019) treated with mastectomy and ongoing endocrine therapy, presented in late 2020 with exertional dyspnea.

Initial imaging in November 2020 revealed reticular abnormalities. By March 2022, subpleural ground-glass opacities and septal thickening, predominantly in basal areas, were evident. Rheumatologic evaluation revealed ANA positivity

(1:160, nucleolar pattern), low-titer ACPA and rheumatoid factor, and anti-Ro52 antibody detection in September 2023. Videocapillaroscopy in 2025 demonstrated an early scleroderma pattern.

Despite lacking a defined connective tissue disease, the coexistence of autoimmune serologies, ILD on imaging, and capillaroscopic abnormalities led to a diagnosis of interstitial pneumonia with autoimmune features (IPAF) in 2023.

Pulmonary Imaging

Serial Chest HRCT scans over 18 months revealed a progressive fibrosing pattern consistent with fibrosing NSIP:

- September 2023: vascular-stromal thickening, peribronchial fibrotic striae, and honeycombing in lower lobes; basal emphysematous bullae.
- March 2024: progression of lower-lobe fibrosis, honeycombing, and reticular changes.
- September 2024: persistent reticulations, increased vasculo-stromal markings, and emphysematous changes.
- February 2025: bibasal GGO, subpleural reticulations, and cranio-caudal fibrotic progression, consistent with fibrosing NSIP.

Diagnosis

IPAF with a fibrosing NSIP pattern, associated with ANA and anti-Ro52 antibody positivity, and early scleroderma-pattern capillaroscopic abnormalities.

Treatment

- Nintedanib 150 mg BID (since December 2022).
- Mycophenolate mofetil 2 g/day (initiated May 2024).
- Low-dose corticosteroids (prednisone 5 mg/day).

Clinical Insight

This case illustrates a progressive fibrosing ILD with autoimmune features fulfilling IPAF criteria in a patient with subtle but suggestive signs of systemic autoimmunity. The presence of anti-Ro52 antibodies, frequently associated with inflammatory myopathies, along with radiologic and capillaroscopic findings, supports the hypothesis of an early or incomplete form of inflammatory myopathy with secondary ILD, currently presenting as an IPAF phenotype. Accurate phenotyping and longitudinal reassessment are essential for timely reclassification and treatment adaptation.

References

1. Joy GM, Arbiv OA, Wong CK, Lok SD, Adderley NA, Dobosz KM, Johannson KA, Ryerson CJ. Prevalence, imaging patterns and risk factors of interstitial lung disease in connective tissue disease: a systematic review and meta-analysis. Eur Respir Rev. 2023;32(167):220210. https://doi.org/10.1183/16000617.0210-2022.

2. Khanna D, Tashkin DP, Denton CP, Renzoni EA, Desai SR, Varga J. Etiology, risk factors, and biomarkers in systemic sclerosis with interstitial lung disease. Am J Respir Crit Care Med. 2020;201(6):650–60. https://doi.org/10.1164/rccm.201903-0563CI.
3. Ramahi A, Lescoat A, Roofeh D, Nagaraja V, Namas R, Huang S, Varga J, O'Dwyer D, Wang B, Flaherty K, Kazerooni E, Khanna D. Risk factors for lung function decline in systemic sclerosis-associated interstitial lung disease in a large single-centre cohort. Rheumatology (Oxford). 2023;62(7):2501–9. https://doi.org/10.1093/rheumatology/keac639.
4. Distler O, Assassi S, Cottin V, Cutolo M, Danoff SK, Denton CP, Distler JHW, Hoffmann-Vold AM, Johnson SR, Müller Ladner U, Smith V, Volkmann ER, Maher TM. Predictors of progression in systemic sclerosis patients with interstitial lung disease. Eur Respir J. 2020;55(5):1902026. https://doi.org/10.1183/13993003.02026-2019.
5. Kelly C, et al. Current issues in rheumatoid arthritis-associated interstitial lung disease. Lancet Rheumatol. 2021;3(11):e798–807. https://doi.org/10.1016/S2665-9913(21)00250-2.
6. Koduri G, Solomon JJ. Identification, monitoring, and management of rheumatoid arthritis-associated interstitial lung disease. Arthritis Rheumatol. 2023;75(12):2067–77. https://doi.org/10.1002/art.42640.
7. Shao T, Shi X, Yang S, Zhang W, Li X, Shu J, Alqalyoobi S, Zeki AA, Leung PS, Shuai Z. Interstitial lung disease in connective tissue disease: a common lesion with heterogeneous mechanisms and treatment considerations. Front Immunol. 2021;12:684699. https://doi.org/10.3389/fimmu.2021.684699.
8. Kamiya M, Carter H, Espindola MS, Doyle TJ, Lee JS, Merriam LT, Zhang F, Kawano-Dourado L, Sparks JA, Hogaboam CM, Moore BB, Oldham WM, Kim EY. Immune mechanisms in fibrotic interstitial lung disease. Cell. 2024;187(14):3506–30. https://doi.org/10.1016/j.cell.2024.05.015.
9. She YX, Yu QY, Tang XX. Role of interleukins in the pathogenesis of pulmonary fibrosis. Cell Death Discov. 2021;7:52. https://doi.org/10.1038/s41420-021-00437-9.
10. Hinz B. Mechanical aspects of lung fibrosis: a spotlight on the myofibroblast. Proc Am Thorac Soc. 2012;9(3):137–47. https://doi.org/10.1513/pats.201202-017AW.
11. Deng Z, Fan T, Xiao C, Tian H, Zheng Y, Li C, He J. TGF-β signaling in health, disease, and therapeutics. Signal Transduct Target Ther. 2024;9(1):61. https://doi.org/10.1038/s41392-024-01764-w.
12. Li W, Xie Y, Chen Z, Cao D, Wang Y. Epithelial-mesenchymal transition in pulmonary fibrosis: molecular mechanisms and emerging therapeutic strategies. Front Med (Lausanne). 2025;12:1658001. https://doi.org/10.3389/fmed.2025.1658001.
13. Fischer A, Antoniou KM, Brown KK, Cadranel J, Corte TJ, du Bois RM, Lee JS, Leslie KO, Lynch DA, Matteson EL, Mosca M, Noth I, Richeldi L, Strek ME, Swigris JJ, Wells AU, West SG, Collard HR, Cottin V, ERS/ATS Task Force on Undifferentiated Forms of CTD-ILD. An official European Respiratory Society/American Thoracic Society research statement: interstitial pneumonia with autoimmune features. Eur Respir J. 2015;46(4):976–87. https://doi.org/10.1183/13993003.00150-2015.
14. Raghu G, Remy-Jardin M, Richeldi L, Thomson CC, Inoue Y, Johkoh T, Kreuter M, Lynch DA, Maher TM, Martinez FJ, Molina-Molina M, Myers JL, Nicholson AG, Ryerson CJ, Strek ME, Troy LK, Wijsenbeek M, Mammen MJ, Hossain T, Bissell BD, Herman DD, Hon SM, Kheir F, Khor YH, Macrea M, Antoniou KM, Bouros D, Buendia-Roldan I, Caro F, Crestani B, Ho L, Morisset J, Olson AL, Podolanczuk A, Poletti V, Selman M, Ewing T, Jones S, Knight SL, Ghazipura M, Wilson KC. Idiopathic pulmonary fibrosis (an update) and progressive pulmonary fibrosis in adults: an official ATS/ERS/JRS/ALAT clinical practice guideline. Am J Respir Crit Care Med. 2022;205(9):e18–47. https://doi.org/10.1164/rccm.202202-0399ST.
15. Moodley Y. Interstitial lung abnormalities: challenges and opportunity. Lancet Respir Med. 2025;13(9):776–8. https://doi.org/10.1016/S2213-2600(25)00214-0.
16. Moodley Y, Mackintosh JA. A comprehensive review of interstitial lung abnormalities. Respirology. 2025;30(5):385–97. https://doi.org/10.1111/resp.70026.

17. Antoniou KM, Distler O, Gheorghiu AM, Moor CC, Vikse J, Bizymi N, Galetti I, Brown G, Bargagli E, Allanore Y, Corte TJ, Dieudé P, Cottin V, Fisher BA, Fabre A, Giles JT, Kreuter M, Lundberg IE, Poletti V, Maurer B, Renzoni EA, Müller-Ladner U, Strek ME, Sverzellati N, Studenic P, Mohammed J, Nagavci B, Stamm T, Tonia T, Crestani B, Hoffmann-Vold AM. ERS/EULAR clinical practice guidelines for connective tissue diseases associated interstitial lung disease. Ann Rheum Dis. 2025;S0003-4967(25):04320–1. https://doi.org/10.1016/j.ard.2025.08.021.
18. Elhai M, Avouac J, Allanore Y. Circulating lung biomarkers in idiopathic lung fibrosis and interstitial lung diseases associated with connective tissue diseases: where do we stand? Semin Arthritis Rheum. 2020;50(3):480–91. https://doi.org/10.1016/j.semarthrit.2020.01.006.
19. De Lorenzis E, Bosello SL, Varone F, Sgalla G, Calandriello L, Natalello G, Iovene B, Cicchetti G, Gigante L, Verardi L, Gremese E, Richeldi L, Larici AR. Multidisciplinary evaluation of interstitial lung diseases: new opportunities linked to rheumatologist involvement. Diagnostics (Basel). 2020;10(9):664. https://doi.org/10.3390/diagnostics10090664.
20. Tomassetti S, Ravaglia C, Puglisi S, Ryu JH, Colby TV, Cavazza A, Wells AU, Pavone M, Vancheri C, Lavorini F, Matucci-Cerinic M, Rosi E, Luzzi V, Gori L, Rossi G, Donati L, Dubini A, Piciucchi S, Poletti V. Impact of lung biopsy information on treatment strategy of patients with interstitial lung diseases. Ann Am Thorac Soc. 2022;19(5):737–45. https://doi.org/10.1513/AnnalsATS.202104-466OC.
21. Maher TM, Assassi S, Azuma A, Cottin V, Hoffmann-Vold AM, Kreuter M, Oldham JM, Richeldi L, Valenzuela C, Wijsenbeek MS, Clerisme-Beaty E, Coeck C, Gu H, Ritter I, Schlosser A, Stowasser S, Voss F, Weimann G, Zoz DF, Martinez FJ, FIBRONEER-ILD Trial Investigators. Nerandomilast in patients with progressive pulmonary fibrosis. N Engl J Med. 2025;392(22):2203–14. https://doi.org/10.1056/NEJMoa2503643.
22. Lundberg IE, Fujimoto M, Vencovsky J, Aggarwal R, Holmqvist M, Christopher-Stine L, Mammen AL, Miller FW. Idiopathic inflammatory myopathies. Nat Rev Dis Primers. 2021;7(1):86. https://doi.org/10.1038/s41572-021-00321-x.
23. Saketkoo LA, Ascherman DP, Cottin V, Christopher-Stine L, Danoff SK, Oddis CV. Interstitial lung disease in idiopathic inflammatory myopathy. Curr Rheumatol Rev. 2010;6(2):108–19. https://doi.org/10.2174/157339710791330740.
24. Sehgal S, Patel A, Chatterjee S, Fernandez AP, Farver C, Yadav R, Li Y, Danoff SK, Saygin D, Huapaya JA, Wilfong EM, Highland KB. Idiopathic inflammatory myopathies related lung disease in adults. Lancet Respir Med. 2025;13(3):272–88. https://doi.org/10.1016/S2213-2600(24)00267-4. Epub 2024 Nov 29.
25. Sun KY, Fan Y, Wang YX, Zhong YJ, Wang GF. Prevalence of interstitial lung disease in polymyositis and dermatomyositis: a meta-analysis from 2000 to 2020. Semin Arthritis Rheum. 2021;51(1):175–91.
26. Kurtzman DJB, Vleugels RA. Anti-melanoma differentiation-associated gene 5 (MDA5) dermatomyositis: a concise review with an emphasis on distinctive clinical features. J Am Acad Dermatol. 2018;78(4):776–85. https://doi.org/10.1016/j.jaad.2017.12.010.
27. Betteridge Z, McHugh N. Myositis-specific autoantibodies: an important tool to support diagnosis of myositis. J Intern Med. 2016;280(1):8–23. https://doi.org/10.1111/joim.12451.
28. Khoo T, Lilleker JB, Thong BY, Leclair V, Lamb JA, Chinoy H. Epidemiology of the idiopathic inflammatory myopathies. Nat Rev Rheumatol. 2023;19(11):695–712. https://doi.org/10.1038/s41584-023-01033-0.
29. Hallowell RW, Paik JJ. Myositis-associated interstitial lung disease: a comprehensive approach to diagnosis and management. Clin Exp Rheumatol. 2022;40(2):373–83. https://doi.org/10.55563/clinexprheumatol/brvl1v.
30. Bai Z, Shen G, Dong L. Analysis of risk factors of interstitial lung disease and mortality rates in Chinese patients with idiopathic inflammatory myopathy. Int J Rheum Dis. 2021;24(6):815–27. https://doi.org/10.1111/1756-185X.14128.
31. Yanagihara T, Inoue Y. Insights into pathogenesis and clinical implications in myositis-associated interstitial lung diseases. Curr Opin Pulm Med. 2020;26(5):507–17. https://doi.org/10.1097/MCP.0000000000000698.

32. Huang K, Aggarwal R. Antisynthetase syndrome: a distinct disease spectrum. J Scleroderma Relat Disord. 2020;5(3):178–91. https://doi.org/10.1177/2397198320902667.
33. O'Hanlon TP, Carrick DM, Arnett FC, Reveille JD, Carrington M, Gao X, Oddis CV, Morel PA, Malley JD, Malley K, Dreyfuss J, Shamim EA, Rider LG, Chanock SJ, Foster CB, Bunch T, Plotz PH, Love LA, Miller FW. Immunogenetic risk and protective factors for the idiopathic inflammatory myopathies: distinct HLA-A, -B, -Cw, -DRB1 and -DQA1 allelic profiles and motifs define clinicopathologic groups in caucasians. Medicine (Baltimore). 2005;84(6):338–49. https://doi.org/10.1097/01.md.0000189818.63141.8c.
34. McHugh N, Tansley S. Autoantibodies in myositis. Nat Rev Rheumatol. 2018;14:290–302. https://doi.org/10.1038/nrrheum.2018.56.
35. Marie I, Josse S, Decaux O, Dominique S, Diot E, Landron C, Roblot P, Jouneau S, Hatron PY, Tiev KP, Vittecoq O, Noel D, Mouthon L, Menard JF, Jouen F. Comparison of long-term outcome between anti-Jo1- and anti-PL7/PL12 positive patients with antisynthetase syndrome. Autoimmun Rev. 2012;11(10):739–45. https://doi.org/10.1016/j.autrev.2012.01.006.
36. González-Moreno J, Raya-Cruz M, Losada-Lopez I, Cacheda AP, Oliver C, Colom B. Rapidly progressive interstitial lung disease due to anti-MDA5 antibodies without skin involvement: a case report and literature review. Rheumatol Int. 2018;38(7):1293–6. https://doi.org/10.1007/s00296-018-3991-7.
37. McPherson M, Economidou S, Liampas A, Zis P, Parperis K. Management of MDA-5 antibody positive clinically amyopathic dermatomyositis associated interstitial lung disease: a systematic review. Semin Arthritis Rheum. 2022;53:151959. https://doi.org/10.1016/j.semarthrit.2022.151959.
38. Ding Y, Ge Y. Anti-melanoma differentiation-associated gene 5 antibody-positive dermatomyositis complicated with macrophage activation syndrome. Ther Adv Chronic Dis. 2022;13:20406223221098128. https://doi.org/10.1177/20406223221098128.
39. Trallero-Araguás E, Gil-Vila A, Martínez-Gómez X, Pinal-Fernández I, Alvarado-Cardenas M, Simó-Perdigó M, Selva-O'Callaghan A. Cancer screening in idiopathic inflammatory myopathies: ten years experience from a single center. Semin Arthritis Rheum. 2022;53:151940. https://doi.org/10.1016/j.semarthrit.2021.12.008.
40. Sabbagh S, Pinal-Fernandez I, Kishi T, Targoff IN, Miller FW, Rider LG, Mammen AL, Childhood Myositis Heterogeneity Collaborative Study Group. Anti-Ro52 autoantibodies are associated with interstitial lung disease and more severe disease in patients with juvenile myositis. Ann Rheum Dis. 2019;78(7):988–95. https://doi.org/10.1136/annrheumdis-2018-215004.
41. Chen S, Wang Q, Wu Z, Li Y, Li P, Sun F, Zheng W, Wu Q, Wu C, Deng C, Zhang F, Li Y. Genetic association study of TNFAIP3, IFIH1, IRF5 polymorphisms with polymyositis/dermatomyositis in Chinese Han population. PLoS One. 2014;9(10):e110044. https://doi.org/10.1371/journal.pone.0110044.
42. Gono T, Kawaguchi Y, Kuwana M, Sugiura T, Furuya T, Takagi K, Ichida H, Katsumata Y, Hanaoka M, Ota Y, Yamanaka H. Brief report: association of HLA-DRB1*0101/*0405 with susceptibility to anti-melanoma differentiation-associated gene 5 antibody-positive dermatomyositis in the Japanese population. Arthritis Rheum. 2012;64(11):3736–40. https://doi.org/10.1002/art.34657.
43. Alder JK, Chen JJ, Lancaster L, Danoff S, Su SC, Cogan JD, Vulto I, Xie M, Qi X, Tuder RM, Phillips JA 3rd, Lansdorp PM, Loyd JE, Armanios MY. Short telomeres are a risk factor for idiopathic pulmonary fibrosis. Proc Natl Acad Sci USA. 2008;105(35):13051–6. https://doi.org/10.1073/pnas.0804280105.
44. Remuzgo-Martínez S, Atienza-Mateo B, Ocejo-Vinyals JG, Pulito-Cueto V, Prieto-Peña D, Genre F, Marquez A, Llorca J, Mora Cuesta VM, Fernández DI, Riesco L, Ortego-Centeno N, Gómez NP, Mera A, Martínez-Barrio J, López-Longo FJ, Lera-Gómez L, Moriano C, Díez E, Tomero E, Calvo-Alén J, Romero-Bueno F, Sanchez-Pernaute O, Nuño L, Bonilla G, Grafia I, Prieto-González S, Narvaez J, Trallero-Araguas E, Selva-O'Callaghan A, Gualillo O, Martín J, Cavagna L, Castañeda S, Cifrian JM, Renzoni EA, López-Mejías R, González-

Gay MA. HLA association with the susceptibility to anti-synthetase syndrome. Joint Bone Spine. 2021;88(3):105115. https://doi.org/10.1016/j.jbspin.2020.105115.
45. Bax CE, Maddukuri S, Ravishankar A, Pappas-Taffer L, Werth VP. Environmental triggers of dermatomyositis: a narrative review. Ann Transl Med. 2021;9(5):434. https://doi.org/10.21037/atm-20-3719.
46. Mainetti C, Terziroli Beretta-Piccoli B, Selmi C. Cutaneous manifestations of dermatomyositis: a comprehensive review. Clin Rev Allergy Immunol. 2017;53:337–56. https://doi.org/10.1007/s12016-017-8652-1.
47. Hallowell RW, Danoff SK. Diagnosis and management of myositis-associated lung disease. Chest. 2023;163(6):1476–91. https://doi.org/10.1016/j.chest.2023.01.031.
48. Patel P, Marinock JM, Ajmeri A, Brent LH. A review of antisynthetase syndrome-associated interstitial lung disease. Int J Mol Sci. 2024;25(8):4453. https://doi.org/10.3390/ijms25084453.
49. Labeit B, Pawlitzki M, Ruck T, Muhle P, Claus I, Suntrup-Krueger S, Warnecke T, Meuth SG, Wiendl H, Dziewas R. The impact of dysphagia in myositis: a systematic review and meta-analysis. J Clin Med. 2020;9(7):2150. https://doi.org/10.3390/jcm9072150.
50. Zhu H, Li R, Tan H, Ding T, Yuan Y, Wen Z, Zhao J, Liu M, Shi Q, Li L. Cardiac involvement in idiopathic inflammatory myopathies. J Inflamm Res. 2025;18:3879–88. https://doi.org/10.2147/JIR.S503928.
51. Furini F, Carnevale A, Casoni GL, Guerrini G, Cavagna L, Govoni M, Sciré CA. The role of the multidisciplinary evaluation of interstitial lung diseases: systematic literature review of the current evidence and future perspectives. Front Med (Lausanne). 2019;6:246. https://doi.org/10.3389/fmed.2019.00246.
52. Dourado E, Bottazzi F, Cardelli C, Conticini E, Schmidt J, Cavagna L, Barsotti S. Idiopathic inflammatory myopathies: one year in review 2022. Clin Exp Rheumatol. 2023;41(2):199–213. https://doi.org/10.55563/clinexprheumatol/jof6qn.
53. Chaudhry S, Christopher-Stine L. Myositis interstitial lung disease and autoantibodies. Front Med (Lausanne). 2023;10:1117071. https://doi.org/10.3389/fmed.2023.1117071.
54. Bahmer T, Romagnoli M, Girelli F, Claussen M, Rabe KF. The use of auto-antibody testing in the evaluation of interstitial lung disease (ILD)--A practical approach for the pulmonologist. Respir Med. 2016;113:80–92. https://doi.org/10.1016/j.rmed.2016.01.019.
55. Ghodrati S, Pugashetti JV, Kadoch MA, Ghasemiesfe A, Oldham JM. Diagnostic accuracy of chest radiography for detecting fibrotic interstitial lung disease. Ann Am Thorac Soc. 2022;19(11):1934–7. https://doi.org/10.1513/AnnalsATS.202112-1377RL.
56. Otake K, Misu S, Fujikawa T, Sakai H, Tomioka H. Exertional desaturation is more severe in idiopathic pulmonary fibrosis than in other interstitial lung diseases. Phys Ther Res. 2023;26(1):32–7. https://doi.org/10.1298/ptr.E10218.
57. Lundberg IE, Fujimoto M, Vencovsky J, Aggarwal R, Holmqvist M, Christopher-Stine L, Mammen AL, Miller FW. Idiopathic inflammatory myopathies. Nat Rev Dis Primers. 2021;7(1):87. https://doi.org/10.1038/s41572-021-00325-7.
58. Kannappan R, Kumar R, Cichelli K, Brent LH. A review of myositis-associated interstitial lung disease. J Clin Med. 2024;13(14):4055. https://doi.org/10.3390/jcm13144055.
59. Flashner BM, VanderLaan PA, Nurhussien L, Rice MB, Hallowell RW. Pulmonary histopathology of interstitial lung disease associated with antisynthetase antibodies. Respir Med. 2022;191:106697. https://doi.org/10.1016/j.rmed.2021.106697.
60. Fujisawa T, Hozumi H, Kono M, Enomoto N, Hashimoto D, Nakamura Y, et al. Prognostic factors for myositis-associated interstitial lung disease. PLoS One. 2014;9(6):e98824. https://doi.org/10.1371/journal.pone.0098824.
61. Douglas WW, Tazelaar HD, Hartman TE, Hartman RP, Decker PA, Schroeder DR, Ryu JH. Polymyositis-dermatomyositis-associated interstitial lung disease. Am J Respir Crit Care Med. 2001;164(7):1182–5. https://doi.org/10.1164/ajrccm.164.7.2103110.
62. Bryson T, Sundaram B, Khanna D, Kazerooni EA. Connective tissue disease-associated interstitial pneumonia and idiopathic interstitial pneumonia: similarity and difference. Semin Ultrasound CT MR. 2014;35(1):29–38. https://doi.org/10.1053/j.sult.2013.10.010.

63. Hozumi H, Fujisawa T, Nakashima R, Johkoh T, Sumikawa H, Murakami A, Enomoto N, Inui N, Nakamura Y, Hosono Y, Imura Y, Mimori T, Suda T. Comprehensive assessment of myositis-specific autoantibodies in polymyositis/dermatomyositis-associated interstitial lung disease. Respir Med. 2016;121:91–9. https://doi.org/10.1016/j.rmed.2016.10.019.
64. Iaccarino L, Bartoloni E, Gerli R, Alunno A, Barsotti S, Cafaro G, Gatto M, Talarico R, Tripoli A, Zen M, Neri R, Doria A. Drugs in induction and treatment of idiopathic inflammatory myopathies. Autoimmun Highlights. 2014;5(3):95–100. https://doi.org/10.1007/s13317-014-0065-z.
65. Go DJ, Park JK, Kang EH, et al. Survival benefit associated with early cyclosporine treatment for dermatomyositis-associated interstitial lung disease. Rheumatol Int. 2016;36:125–31. https://doi.org/10.1007/s00296-015-3328-8.
66. Fischer A, Brown KK, Du Bois RM, Frankel SK, Cosgrove GP, Fernandez-Perez ER, Huie TJ, Krishnamoorthy M, Meehan RT, Olson AL, Solomon JJ, Swigris JJ. Mycophenolate mofetil improves lung function in connective tissue disease-associated interstitial lung disease. J Rheumatol. 2013;40(5):640–6. https://doi.org/10.3899/jrheum.121043.
67. Narváez J, Cañadillas E, Castellví I, Alegre JJ, Vicens-Zygmunt V, Bermudo G, Vidal-Montal P, Molina Molina M, Nolla JM. Rituximab in the treatment of progressive interstitial lung disease associated with the antisynthetase syndrome. Arthritis Res Ther. 2024;26(1):122. https://doi.org/10.1186/s13075-024-03353-2. Erratum in: Arthritis Res Ther. 2024;26(1):128. 10.1186/s13075-024-03357-y.
68. Wang DX, Shu XM, Tian XL, Chen F, Zu N, Ma L, Wang GC. Intravenous immunoglobulin therapy in adult patients with polymyositis/dermatomyositis: a systematic literature review. Clin Rheumatol. 2012;31(5):801–6. https://doi.org/10.1007/s10067-012-1940-5.
69. Aggarwal R, Charles-Schoeman C, Schessl J, Bata-Csörgő Z, Dimachkie MM, Griger Z, Moiseev S, Oddis C, Schiopu E, Vencovský J, Beckmann I, Clodi E, Bugrova O, Dankó K, Ernste F, Goyal NA, Heuer M, Hudson M, Hussain YM, Karam C, Magnolo N, Nelson R, Pozur N, Prystupa L, Sárdy M, Valenzuela G, van der Kooi AJ, Vu T, Worm M, Levine T, ProDERM Trial Group. Trial of intravenous immune globulin in dermatomyositis. N Engl J Med. 2022;387(14):1264–78. https://doi.org/10.1056/NEJMoa2117912.
70. Kurasawa K, Arai S, Namiki Y, et al. Tofacitinib for refractory interstitial lung diseases in anti-melanoma differentiation-associated 5 gene antibody-positive dermatomyositis. Rheumatology (Oxford). 2018;57:2114–9.
71. Ceribelli A, Tonutti A, Isailovic N, De Santis M, Selmi C. Interstitial lung disease associated with inflammatory myositis: autoantibodies, clinical phenotypes, and progressive fibrosis. Front Med (Lausanne). 2023;10:1068402. https://doi.org/10.3389/fmed.2023.1068402.
72. Moghadam-Kia S, Oddis CV. Current and new targets for treating myositis. Curr Opin Pharmacol. 2022;65:102257. https://doi.org/10.1016/j.coph.2022.102257.
73. Murray SG, Schmajuk G, Trupin L, Lawson E, Cascino M, Barton J, Margaretten M, Katz PP, Yelin EH, Yazdany J. A population-based study of infection-related hospital mortality in patients with dermatomyositis/polymyositis. Arthritis Care Res (Hoboken). 2015;67(5):673–80. https://doi.org/10.1002/acr.2250.
74. Volkmann ER, Andréasson K, Smith V. Systemic sclerosis. Lancet. 2023;401:304–18.
75. Liakouli V, Ciancio A, Del Galdo F, Giacomelli R, Ciccia F. Systemic sclerosis interstitial lung disease: unmet needs and potential solutions. Nat Rev Rheumatol. 2024;20(1):21–32. https://doi.org/10.1038/s41584-023-01044-x.
76. Frauenfelder T, et al. Screening for interstitial lung disease in systemic sclerosis: performance of high-resolution CT with limited number of slices: a prospective study. Ann Rheum Dis. 2014;73:2069–73.
77. Rahaghi FF, et al. Expert consensus on the management of systemic sclerosis-associated interstitial lung disease. Respir Res. 2023;24:6.
78. Gargani L, et al. Prognostic value of lung ultrasound B-lines in systemic sclerosis. Chest. 2020;158:1515–25.
79. Gargani L, et al. Lung magnetic resonance imaging in systemic sclerosis: a new promising approach to evaluate pulmonary involvement and progression. Clin Rheumatol. 2021;40:1903–12.

80. Goh NSL, et al. Interstitial lung disease in systemic sclerosis: a simple staging system. Am J Respir Crit Care Med. 2008;177:1248–54.
81. Denton CP, et al. Extent of fibrosis and lung function decline in patients with systemic sclerosis and interstitial lung disease: data from the SENSCIS trial. Rheumatology. 2023;62:1870–6.
82. Hoffmann-Vold AM, et al. Progressive interstitial lung disease in patients with systemic sclerosis-associated interstitial lung disease in the EUSTAR database. Ann Rheum Dis. 2021;80:219–27.
83. Raghu G, et al. Idiopathic pulmonary fibrosis (an update) and progressive pulmonary fibrosis in adults: an official ATS/ERS/JRS/ALAT clinical practice guideline. Am J Respir Crit Care Med. 2022;205:e18–47.
84. Cole A, Denton CP. Biomarkers in systemic sclerosis associated interstitial lung disease (SSc-ILD). Curr Treat Options Rheumatol. 2022;8:152–70.
85. Ishikawa N, Hattori N, Yokoyama A, Kohno N. Utility of KL-6/MUC1 in the clinical management of interstitial lung diseases. Respir Investig. 2012;50:3–13.
86. Giacomelli R, et al. Interstitial lung disease in systemic sclerosis: current and future treatment. Rheumatol Int. 2017;37:853–63.
87. Tashkin DP, et al. Cyclophosphamide versus placebo in scleroderma lung disease. N Engl J Med. 2006;354:2655–66.
88. Tashkin DP, et al. Mycophenolate mofetil versus oral cyclophosphamide in scleroderma-related interstitial lung disease (SLS 2): a randomised controlled, double-blind, parallel group trial. Lancet Respir Med. 2016;4:708–19.
89. Khanna D, et al. Safety and efficacy of subcutaneous tocilizumab in systemic sclerosis: results from the open-label period of a phase II randomised controlled trial (faSScinate). Ann Rheum Dis. 2018;77:212–20.
90. Maher TM, RECITAL Investigators, et al. Rituximab versus intravenous cyclophosphamide in patients with connective tissue disease-associated interstitial lung disease in the UK (RECITAL): a double-blind, double-dummy, randomised, controlled, phase 2b trial. Lancet Respir Med. 2023;11:45–54.
91. Burt RK, et al. Autologous non-myeloablative haemopoietic stem-cell transplantation compared with pulse cyclophosphamide once per month for systemic sclerosis (ASSIST): an open-label, randomised phase 2 trial. Lancet. 2011;378:498–506.
92. Van Laar JM, et al. Autologous hematopoietic stem cell transplantation vs intravenous pulse cyclophosphamide in diffuse cutaneous systemic sclerosis: a randomized clinical trial. JAMA. 2014;311:2490–8.
93. Sullivan KM, et al. Myeloablative autologous stem-cell transplantation for severe scleroderma. N Engl J Med. 2018;378:35–47.
94. Volkmann ER, et al. Changes in plasma CXCL4 levels are associated with improvements in lung function in patients receiving immunosuppressive therapy for systemic sclerosis-related interstitial lung disease. Arthritis Res Ther. 2016;18:305.
95. Assassi S, et al. Predictive significance of serum interferon-inducible protein score for response to treatment in systemic sclerosis-related interstitial lung disease. Arthritis Rheumatol. 2021;73:1005–13.
96. Assassi S, et al. Peripheral blood gene expression profiling shows predictive significance for response to mycophenolate in systemic sclerosis-related interstitial lung disease. Ann Rheum Dis. 2022;81:854–60.
97. Kelly CA, Saravanan V, Nisar M, et al. Rheumatoid arthritis–related interstitial lung disease: associations, prognostic factors and physiological and radiological characteristics—a large multicentre UK study. Rheumatology (Oxford). 2014;53(9):1676–82.
98. Bongartz T, Nannini C, Medina-Velasquez YF, et al. Incidence and mortality of interstitial lung disease in rheumatoid arthritis: a population-based study. Arthritis Rheum. 2010;62(6):1583–91.
99. Spagnolo P, Lee JS, Sverzellati N, Rossi G, Cottin V. The lung in rheumatoid arthritis: focus on interstitial lung disease. Arthritis Rheumatol. 2018;70(10):1544–54.

100. Olson AL, Swigris JJ, Sprunger DB, et al. Rheumatoid arthritis–interstitial lung disease–associated mortality. Am J Respir Crit Care Med. 2011;183(3):372–37.
101. Johnson SR, Bernstein EJ, Bolster MB, et al. 2023 American College of Rheumatology/American College of Chest Physicians guideline for the treatment of interstitial lung disease in people with systemic autoimmune rheumatic diseases. Arthritis Rheumatol. 2024;76(8):1182–200.
102. Solomon JJ, Danoff SK, Gibbons MA, et al. Lung disease in rheumatoid arthritis. Chest. 2023;163(1):22–38.
103. Kelly CA, Nikiphorou E, Giles JT, et al. Rheumatoid arthritis-related interstitial lung disease: state of the art and future perspectives. Lancet Rheumatol. 2021;3(12):e906–18.
104. Flaherty KR, Wells AU, Cottin V, et al. Nintedanib in progressive fibrosing interstitial lung diseases. N Engl J Med. 2019;381(18):1718–27.
105. Negrini S, et al. Sjögren's syndrome: a systemic autoimmune disease. Clin Exp Med. 2022;22(1):9–25.
106. Parambil JG, et al. Interstitial lung disease in primary Sjögren's syndrome. Chest. 2006;130(5):1489–95.
107. Palm O, et al. Clinical pulmonary involvement in primary Sjogren's syndrome: prevalence, quality of life and mortality—a retrospective study based on registry data. Rheumatology (Oxford). 2013;52(1):173–9.
108. Lin W, et al. Interstitial lung disease in primary Sjögren's syndrome. BMC Pulm Med. 2022;22(1):73.
109. Luppi F, Sebastiani M, Silva M, Sverzellati N, Cavazza A, Salvarani C, Manfredi A. Interstitial lung disease in Sjögren's syndrome: a clinical review. Clin Exp Rheumatol. 2020;38 Suppl 126(4):291–300. Epub 2020 Oct 23.
110. Alhamad EH, et al. Clinical characteristics and outcomes in patients with primary Sjogren's syndrome-associated interstitial lung disease. Ann Thorac Med. 2021;16(2):156–64.
111. Oliveira RP, et al. Connective tissue disease-associated interstitial lung disease. Pulmonology. 2022;28(2):113–8.
112. Cha SI, et al. Lymphoid interstitial pneumonia: clinical features, associations and prognosis. Eur Respir J. 2006;28(2):364–9.
113. Johkoh T, et al. Lymphocytic interstitial pneumonia: thin-section CT findings in 22 patients. Radiology. 1999;212(2):567–72.
114. Swigris JJ, et al. Lymphocytic interstitial pneumonia: a narrative review. Chest. 2002;122(6):2150–64.
115. De Pascale R, et al. Diagnosis and management of lung involvement in systemic lupus erythematosus and Sjögren's syndrome: a literature review. Ther Adv Musculoskelet Dis. 2021;13:1–15.
116. Shin JI, et al. Systemic lupus erythematosus and lung involvement: a comprehensive review. J Clin Med. 2022;11:6714.
117. Amarnani R, et al. Lupus and the lungs: the assessment and management of pulmonary manifestations of systemic lupus erythematosus. Front Med (Lausanne). 2021;7:610257.
118. Hao YJ, et al. Connective tissue disease-associated pulmonary arterial hypertension in Chinese patients. Eur Respir J. 2014;43(3):862–72.
119. Senkal N, et al. Interstitial lung disease in patients with systemic lupus erythematosus: a cohort study. Turk J Med Sci. 2021;52(1):76–82.
120. Flaherty KR, et al. Nintedanib in progressive fibrosing interstitial lung diseases. N Engl J Med. 2019;381(18):1718–27.
121. Antoniou KM, Distler O, Gheorghiu AM, et al. ERS/EULAR clinical practice guidelines for connective tissue disease-associated interstitial lung disease. Eur Respir J. 2025;67(1):2402533. https://doi.org/10.1183/13993003.02533-2024.

Chapter 10
Pediatric Capilloroscopy

Ivan Foeldvari and Zeynep Özcan

Role of Nailfold Capillaroscopy in Children with Rheumatic Diseases

How to conduct nailfold capillaroscopy (NF) was discussed in previous chapters. In pediatric patients, we prefer to use a handheld capillaroscope; this can be used even in small children if they sit on the lap of their parents.

Pediatric patients have different norm values for NF findings from adults, which was first shown by Terrerie et al. [1], where her group assessed normal findings in healthy children and adolescents. The sample comprised 329 individuals with a mean age of 8.2 years. It was found that the number of capillaries increases, but even in the youngest, it is around 6/mm. A unique feature is that around 30% have abnormal capillaries, and even 10% have enlarged capillaries. Piotto et al. [2] from the same Brazilian group reviewed 100 healthy children with video NF and assessed capillary dimensions (capillary loop length, capillary width, and intercapillary distance), and the number of capillaries/mm was evaluated in 900 capillaries using a stereomicroscope under 100× magnification. Intra- and interobserver agreements were tested.

The capillary dimensions (mean ± SD) were capillary loop length 278.6 ± 60.3 μm, intercapillary distance 124.1 ± 28.1 μm, and capillary width 15.0 ± 2.6 μm. Teenagers between 15 and 18 years old had longer and more enlarged capillaries than the other age groups ($p < 0.001$ and $p = 0.012$, respectively).

They also found a significant increase in the number of capillaries/mm with age ($p < 0.001$). There was a positive correlation between age and number of capillaries/mm, capillary length, and capillary width ($p < 0.001, R = 0.796$; $p < 0.001, R = 0.368$; $p = 0.004$, $R = 0.285$, respectively). There was a good intra- and interobserver

I. Foeldvari (✉) · Z. Özcan
Hamburg Centre for Pediatric and Adolescent Rheumatology, Hamburg, Germany

Y. El Miedany, R. A. Elziaty (eds.), *Capillaroscopy*, Contemporary Rheumatology,
https://doi.org/10.1007/978-3-032-22966-3_10

concordance. Enlarged capillaries were defined as >2 *times the normal diameter* (20–50 um loops). Avascular areas were present in 11% and 10% of capillaries, respectively. A weak negative correlation was found between the intercapillary distance and the number of capillaries/mm ($p = 0.05$; $R = -0.20$). There was a positive correlation between age and number of capillaries/mm, capillary length, and capillary width.

The next step was done by the EULAR Study Group on Microcirculation in Rheumatic Diseases. They started an international collaboration to collect nailfold capillaroscopic data from children and adolescents with and without juvenile rheumatic and musculoskeletal diseases (jRMD) [3].

In consecutive jRMD children and matched HCs from 13 centers worldwide, 16 NVC images per patient were acquired locally and read centrally per the international consensus standard evaluation of the EULAR Study Group on Microcirculation in Rheumatic Diseases [4]. A total of 95 patients with juvenile idiopathic arthritis (JIA), 22 with juvenile Dermatomyositis (jDM), 20 with childhood-onset systemic Lupus Erythematoses (cSLE), 13 with juvenile SSc (jSSc), 21 with localized scleroderma (lSc),18 with MCTD, and 20 with primary RP (PRP) were included. NVC differences between juvenile subgroups and HCs were calculated through multivariable regression analysis.

A total of 6474 images were assessed from 413 subjects (mean age 12.1 years, 70.9% female). The quantitative NVC characteristics were significantly lower or higher in the following subgroups compared with HCs: for density, lower in jSSc, JDM, MCTD, cSLE, and lSc; for dilations, higher in jSSc, MCTD, and JDM; for abnormal shapes, higher in JDM and MCTD; for hemorrhages, higher in jSSc, MCTD, JDM, and cSLE. The qualitative NVC assessment of JIA, lSc, and PRP did not differ from HCs, whereas the cSLE and jSSc, MCTD, JDM, and cSLE subgroups showed more nonspecific and scleroderma patterns, respectively. This study showed that cSLE, jSSc, and JDM patients have, as expected from adult data, a pathologic NF pattern. It also showed that primary Raynaud patients showed a normal NF pattern. This project is ongoing with more patients and longitudinal observation.

To assess the association between NF abnormalities and pediatric autoimmune diseases, a systematic search of PubMed, EMBASE, and Scopus was performed in a publication [5] to identify all studies published before March 17, 2021. Observational studies reporting NFC outcomes in children with autoimmune disease and healthy controls (HC) were eligible for inclusion. Odds ratios (OR) and 95% confidence intervals (CI) were pooled using a random-effects meta-analytical model [5]. Nine of 3665 studies reporting on 641 patients (398 subjects, 243 controls) were included. Pediatric patients with autoimmune disease were 9.88 (95% CI 3.16–30.87, I2 = 80.1%) times more likely to have abnormal nailfold capillaries than HC. Of the capillaroscopic features, dilated capillaries (OR 27.90, 95% CI 2.17–349.05, I2 = 59.9%) were the most likely abnormality observed on NFC. This was followed by the likelihood of reduced capillary density (<7 capillaries/mm) (OR 19.91, 95% CI 3.79–105.52, I2 = 0%), giant capillaries (OR 12.87, 95% CI 2.38–69.45, I2 = 0%), hemorrhages (OR 13.89, 95% CI, 5.34–36.16, I2 = 0%), and avascularity (OR 10.38, 95% CI 2.20–49.04, I2 = 0%). Patients with pathologic findings had the diagnosis of jSLE, jMCTD, jDM, or secondary Raynaud phenomenon, but interestingly, primary Raynaud phenomenon too. Patients with JIA and Kawasaki disease had normal NF findings.

Primary and Secondary Raynaud's Syndrome (RP) in Children

Raynaud's Phenomenon (RP) is already described in Chap. 3. In the pediatric population, we differentiate primary and secondary Raynaud's phenomenon as in adults. We have sparse data regarding the prevalence of RP in children. In a cross-sectional survey in the UK interviewing 720 schoolchildren aged 12 to 15, the prevalence of 15% of RP was found [6]. Which is close to the expected prevalence in adults. Data regarding prevalence in children under the age of 12 years is very rare. A multicenter report found RP in 2.2% of children aged 0 to 10 and in 20% of those aged 10 to 20; however, there was a very wide range in the documented rate of onset among centers and between boys and girls [7].

In the primary RP, we expect normal (NF) findings [1, 3] and no antibody pattern suggestive of connective tissue disease, like positive ANA or antiphospholipid antibodies. In the secondary RP, we expect pathologic NF changes [3] and an antibody pattern suggestive of an evolving connective tissue disease.

Is a Positive NF Finding Prognostic of the Evolvement of a Connective Tissue Disease?

The highest positive predictive value to predict the evolvement of a connective tissue disease has an ANA positivity (OR 11.13), followed by capillary loss, defined by less than 6/mm capillary density in a recent nested case control study [8]. In this study, 83 patients diagnosed with RP and having undergone NC in childhood were retrospectively included. Based on whether they were diagnosed with a connective tissue disease (CTD) during follow-up, patients were classified as PRP or SRP.

To assess the prognostic value of capillaroscopy findings for the development of connective tissue disease, Pavlov-Dolijanovic [9] followed a group of 250 children and adolescents (mean age 15 years) with Raynaud phenomenon for 1 to 6 years after the first capillaroscopy. Every 6 months, they were screened for signs and symptoms of connective tissue disease. Analysis was performed on capillary changes registered 6 months before the development of connective tissue disease. Capillary changes were classified into three types: normal, nonspecific, and sclerodermatous. At the end of the follow-up period, 191 (76%) subjects had primary Raynaud phenomenon, 27 (10.8) were diagnosed as having undifferentiated connective tissue disease, and 32 (12.8%) fulfilled the criteria for a diagnosis of a specific connective tissue disease. Systemic lupus erythematosus was found in nine (3.6%) patients, rheumatoid arthritis in 10 (4%) patients (six of them with juvenile-onset rheumatoid arthritis), and scleroderma spectrum disorders in 13 (5.2%). The mean time for the evolution of Raynaud phenomenon into undifferentiated connective tissue disease or a definite connective tissue disease was 2 years. Of all the subjects, only 10 (4%) showed scleroderma pattern capillary changes 6 months before the expression of a particular disease: eight (62%) of these developed scleroderma spectrum disorders, one expressed systemic lupus erythematosus, and one had undifferentiated connective tissue disease.

In another retrospective study [10] of 123 patients with RP associated with ANA positivity and positive NF findings turned out to be at risk of developing a connective tissue disease. 8 of the 123 (10%) developed over two years a connective tissue disease. In another retrospective study [11] of 94 patients with RP over 3 years, 8.5% developed a connective tissue disease with the same risk factors.

Guidance on How to Follow Patients with Raynaud's Phenomenon

The consensus meeting in Hamburg developed guidance [12] on how to follow patients with RP depending on their ANA and NF findings. This was later adopted from the SHARE group [13]. (Fig. 10.1). Patients with ANA positivity and NF-positive findings should be followed every 3 months. These recommendations were never prospectively validated.

Childhood SLE (jSLE)

Recent studies, with the use of definitions from the EULAR microcirculation group [4], have shown that the majority of cSLE patients show many capillary changes when compared to age-matched healthy controls, but this has to be confirmed by larger multicenter cohorts [3, 14]. The number of capillary hemorrhages was observed to correlate with SLEDAI, a disease activity marker [14]. A capillary leakage was also prescribed in the study of Schonenberg-Meinema et al., the so-called "pericapillary extravasation." The pattern described in jSLE is a "nonspecific" pattern [4]. We need long-term data on how this pattern evolves in jSLE. In 15% to 19% of jSLE patients, a scleroderma pattern was seen [3, 14, 15], but the presence of the scleroderma pattern does not seem to correlate with disease activity [15].

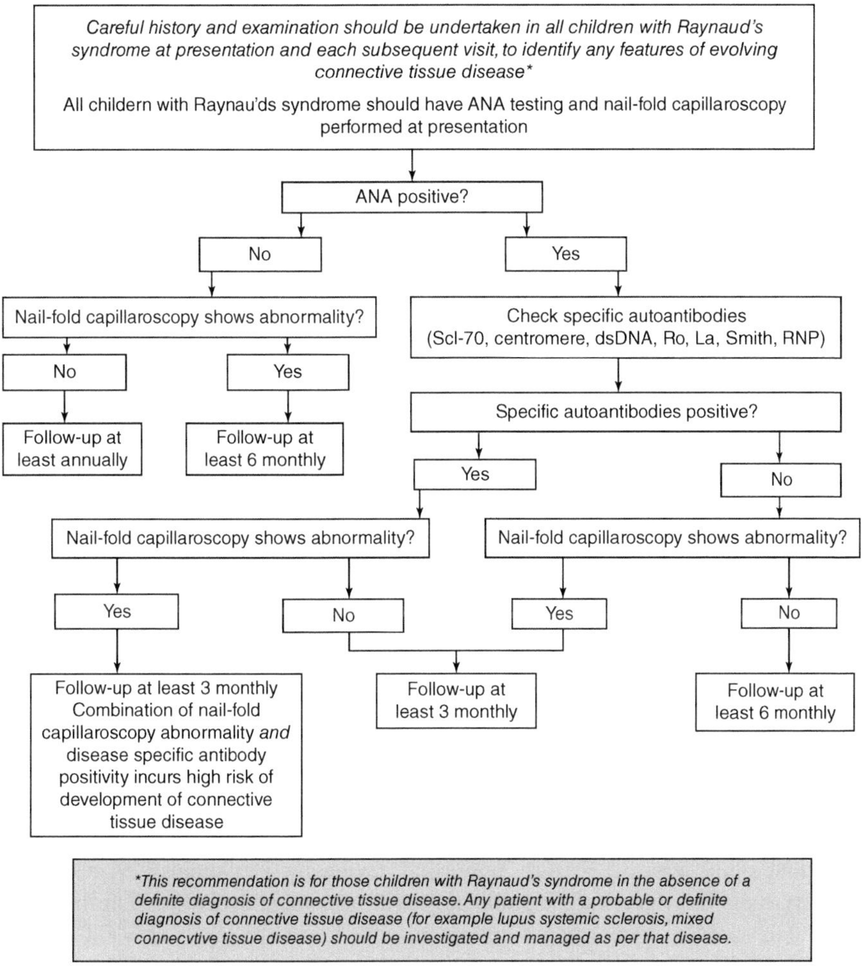

Fig. 10.1 Recommendation of investigation RP according ANA positivity and NF findings [12]

Juvenile Dermatomyositis (jDM)

Recent studies, with the use of definitions from the EULAR microcirculation group [4], have shown that the majority of jDM patients show many capillary changes [3]. In a larger study [16], including 58 patients with a median disease duration of 16.8 (range 2–38), years were clinically examined and compared with matched controls. Compared to controls, patients had a decreased number of capillaries (mean SD 6.4 /mm versus 7.6/mm; $P = 0.001$) and showed more abnormality in all other NF parameters; 36% of patients versus 4% of controls had a number of nailfolds <6/mm ($P < 0.001$).

Giant capillaries, scleroderma, and neovascular patterns were found in 9%, 84%, and 41% of patients, respectively. Patients with active disease (n = 30) presented more frequently with a neovascular pattern than patients with inactive disease (n = 28) (P = 0.041). Decreased numbers of capillaries and neovascular patterns were associated with higher levels of disease activity and impaired muscle function.

The same group assessed the correlation of NF findings and pulmonary and cardiac findings [17]. Patients with a low number of capillaries (<6 capillaries/mm) (n = 21), compared to patients with a normal number of nailfold capillaries (>/=6 capillaries/mm) (n = 37), had lower forced vital capacity (89.7% versus 98.5% predicted), total lung capacity (87.8% versus 94.5% predicted), and more often had low DLco values (15 [71%] of 21 patients versus 14 [38%] of 37 controls) (all $P < 0.05$). Use of HRCT to assess airway disease was more frequent in the group with a low number of nailfold capillaries (6 [30%] of 20 patients versus 3 [8%] of 36 patients in the normal number of nailfold capillaries group; P = 0.034). No associations between the number of nailfold capillaries and cardiac parameters or between neovascular patterns and pulmonary or cardiac parameters were observed.

In jDM, the number of capillaries increases if patients reach remission.

Juvenile Mixed Connective Tissue Disease (jMCTD)

Raynaud's phenomenon was the most reported sign at onset in 69.7% of cases (n = 150) [18]. jMCTD patients show a capillary scleroderma(-like) pattern; the published number of cases is very low [3, 15].

Juvenile Sjögren Syndrome

The first study was just recently published, reviewing 11 patients [19]. Capillary density reduction correlated significantly with articular involvement (arthralgias) (p = 0.024). Microhemorrhages correlated with lower C3 levels (p = 0.034). No specific NVC pattern for jSjD was identified, whereas abnormal capillary shapes were significantly higher in jSjD patients than HCs (p = 0.005). NF abnormalities were not associated with SjD-specific instrumental tests (biopsy, imaging, Schirmer's test). RP was present in 8% of jSjD patients. We need more data on this patient group to know the clinical relevance of these findings.

Juvenile Systemic Sclerosis

RP is the first sign of the disease in 60% of the patients [20], and in the juvenile scleroderma inception cohort (www.juvenile-scleroderma.com), 90% of the patients have RP with a mean disease duration of 2.4 years [21, 22].

Reviewing 237 patients in the juvenile scleroderma inceptions cohort and comparing patients with and without positive NF findings, it could be shown that the 183 patients with positive NF findings were significantly more commonly ANA positive and had more common RP, history of ulcerations, positive HRCT findings for interstitial lung disease, esophageal reflux, muscle weakness, elevated CK value, and presence of contractures. A positive NF finding was defined by the examiner (only published as an abstract, Annual EULAR meeting 2024).

Case Vignettes

Case 1: Juvenile Systemic Sclerosis (Male, 16 Years)

Presentation: Raynaud's phenomenon, digital skin ulcers, cutaneous thickening, MRSS score of 16, Gottron papules on the fingers, rash, subjective muscle weakness, and arthralgia. Serology: ANA 1:3200 (positive), ENA screen positive, anti-Scl-70 negative, anti-β2-glycoprotein positive.

Capillaroscopy: giant capillaries, frequent microhemorrhages, reduced capillary density with evident dropout, avascular areas, and prominent bushy/tortuous neoangiogenesis with architectural disorganization—constituting a late scleroderma pattern. The extent of avascularity and neoangiogenesis paralleled the severity of cutaneous involvement and ischemic complications (ulcers).

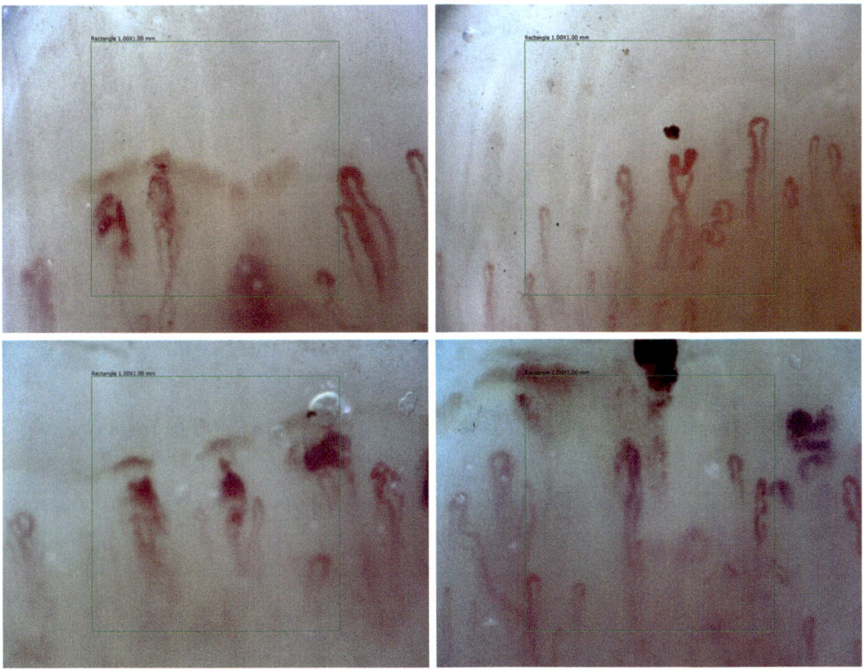

Case 2: Juvenile Dermatomyositis (Female, 7 Years)

Presentation: subfebrile temperatures, facial and acral rash, constipation, proximal muscle weakness; MMT8: 36; MRI confirmed myositis of the lower extremities. Serology: ANA 1:800 (positive), creatine kinase elevated, C-reactive protein negative, PM-Scl-100 positive.

Capillaroscopy: decreased capillary density with clear dropout and avascular areas and scattered microhemorrhages (with fissured periungual skin). No giant capillaries or bushy/tortuous loops were observed. The pattern is compatible with active inflammatory microangiopathy in JDM.

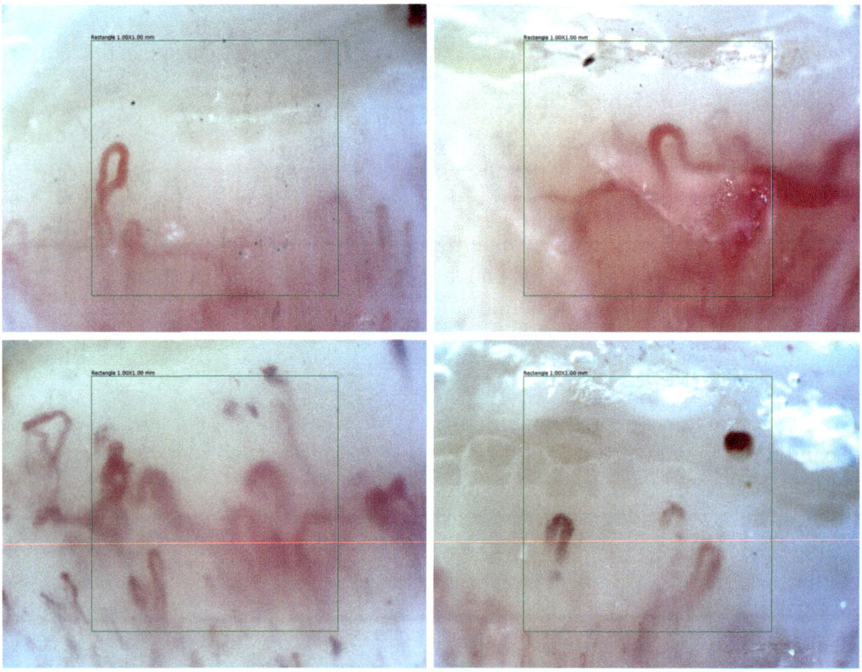

Case 3: Mixed Connective Tissue Disease (Female, 15 Years)

Presentation: Raynaud's phenomenon and digital calcinosis; no muscle weakness, no skin thickening (MRRS:0), or inflammatory rash. Serology: ANA 1:3200 (positive), ENA screen positive, anti-RNP positive, anti-β2-glycoprotein positive, borderline anticardiolipin antibodies.

Capillaroscopy: reduced capillary density without significant avascular fields, absence of giant capillaries or hemorrhages, and abundant bushy/tortuous loops with neoangiogenesis—yielding an early scleroderma-like pattern. These findings support microvascular involvement.

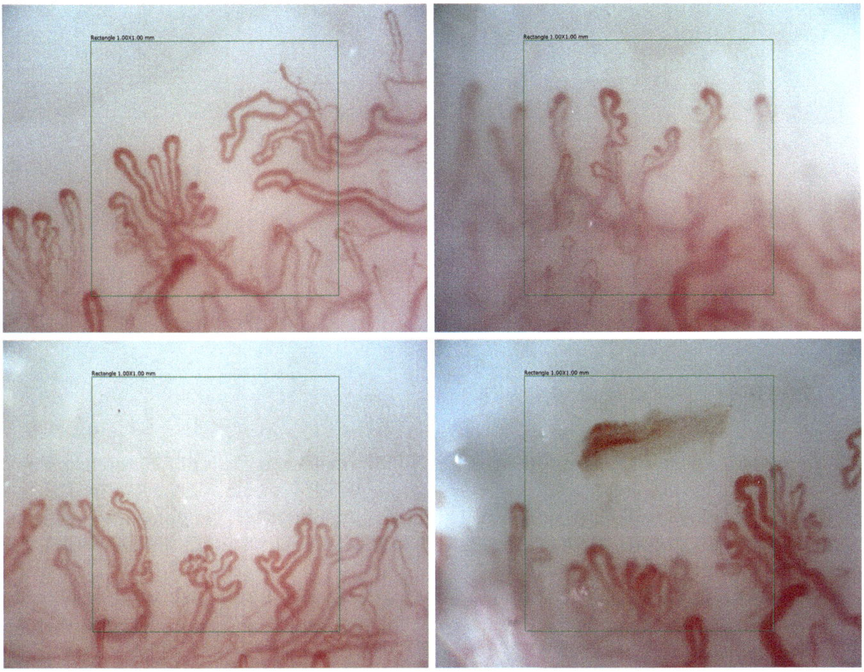

Case 4: Primary Raynaud's Phenomenon (Female, 15 Years)

The patient presented with a nine-year history of recurrent color changes of the hands upon cold exposure, characterized by alternating red and blue discoloration extending from the fingers to the wrists. No digital ulcers, arthralgia, or systemic symptoms were reported. Physical examination revealed bluish discoloration of the fingers without cutaneous thickening, telangiectasias, or other trophic changes.

Serological testing showed a negative ANA (1:50) and no other laboratory abnormalities. *Capillaroscopy* demonstrated a normal distribution of approximately eight capillaries per millimeter, without giant capillaries, hemorrhages, or morphological abnormalities. The overall findings were consistent with a normal capillaroscopic pattern.

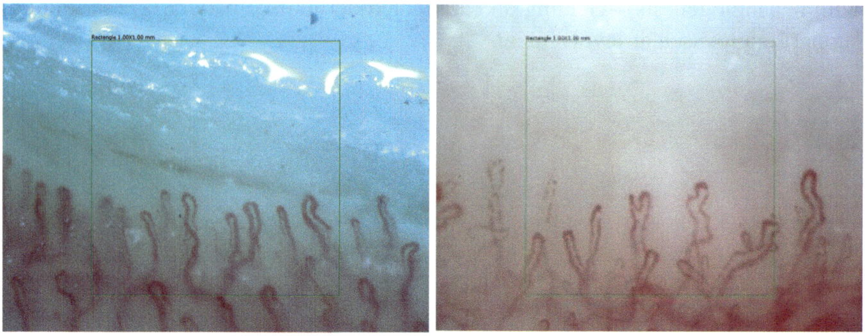

References

1. Terreri MT, Andrade LE, Puccinelli ML, Hilario MO, Goldenberg J. Nail fold capillaroscopy: normal findings in children and adolescents. Semin Arthritis Rheum. 1999;29(1):36–42.
2. Piotto DP, Sekiyama J, Kayser C, Yamada M, Len CA, Terreri MT. Nailfold videocapillaroscopy in healthy children and adolescents: description of normal patterns. Clin Exp Rheumatol. 2016;34 Suppl 100(5):193–9.
3. Melsens K, Cutolo M, Schonenberg-Meinema D, Foeldvari I, Leone MC, Mostmans Y, et al. Standardised nailfold capillaroscopy in children with rheumatic diseases: a worldwide study. Rheumatology (Oxford). 2023;62(4):1605–15.
4. Smith V, Herrick AL, Ingegnoli F, Damjanov N, De Angelis R, Denton CP, et al. Standardisation of nailfold capillaroscopy for the assessment of patients with Raynaud's phenomenon and systemic sclerosis. Autoimmun Rev. 2020;19:102458.
5. Li AR, Burke CD, Purvis CS, Lee LW. Association between nailfold capillaroscopy abnormalities and autoimmune disease in pediatric populations. Pediatr Dermatol. 2022;39:197.
6. Jones GT, Herrick AL, Woodham SE, Baildam EM, Macfarlane GJ, Silman AJ. Occurrence of Raynaud's phenomenon in children ages 12-15 years: prevalence and association with other common symptoms. Arthritis Rheum. 2003;48(12):3518–21.
7. Planchon B, Pistorius MA, Beurrier P, De Faucal P. Primary Raynaud's phenomenon. Age of onset and pathogenesis in a prospective study of 424 patients. Angiology. 1994;45(8):677–86.
8. Farenhorst CA, Roon AM, Gessel AI, Stel AJ, Bootsma H, Armbrust W, et al. Capillary microscopy is a potential screening method for connective tissue disease in children with Raynaud's phenomenon. Pediatr Rheumatol Online J. 2022;20(1):11.
9. Pavlov-Dolijanovic S, Damjanov N, Ostojic P, Susic G, Stojanovic R, Gacic D, et al. The prognostic value of nailfold capillary changes for the development of connective tissue disease in children and adolescents with primary raynaud phenomenon: a follow-up study of 250 patients. Pediatr Dermatol. 2006;23(5):437–42.
10. Nigrovic PA, Fuhlbrigge RC, Sundel RP. Raynaud's phenomenon in children: a retrospective review of 123 patients. Pediatrics. 2003;111(4 Pt 1):715–21.
11. Falcini F, Rigante D, Candelli M, Martini G, Corona F, Petaccia A, et al. Anti-nuclear antibodies as predictor of outcome in a multi-center cohort of Italian children and adolescents with Raynaud's phenomenon. Clin Rheumatol. 2015;34(1):167–9.
12. Pain CE, Constantin T, Toplak N, Moll M, Iking-Konert C, Piotto DP, et al. Raynaud's syndrome in children: systematic review and development of recommendations for assessment and monitoring. Clin Exp Rheumatol. 2016;34 Suppl 100(5):200–6.

13. Zulian F, Culpo R, Sperotto F, Anton J, Avcin T, Baildam EM, et al. Consensus-based recommendations for the management of juvenile localised scleroderma. Ann Rheum Dis. 2019;78:1019–24.
14. Schonenberg-Meinema D, Bergkamp SC, Nassar-Sheikh Rashid A, van der Aa LB, de Bree GJ, Ten Cate R, et al. Nailfold capillary abnormalities in childhood-onset systemic lupus erythematosus: a cross-sectional study compared with healthy controls. Lupus. 2021;30(5):818–27.
15. Schonenberg-Meinema D, Bergkamp SC, Nassar-Sheikh Rashid A, Gruppen MP, Middelkamp-Hup MA, Armbrust W, et al. Nailfold capillary scleroderma pattern may be associated with disease damage in childhood-onset systemic lupus erythematosus: important lessons from longitudinal follow-up. Lupus Sci Med. 2022;9(1):e000572.
16. Barth Z, Witczak BN, Flato B, Koller A, Sjaastad I, Sanner H. Assessment of microvascular abnormalities by nailfold capillaroscopy in juvenile dermatomyositis after medium- to long-term followup. Arthritis Care Res (Hoboken). 2018;70(5):768–76.
17. Barth Z, Schwartz T, Flato B, Aalokken TM, Koller A, Lund MB, et al. Association between nailfold capillary density and pulmonary and cardiac involvement in medium to longstanding juvenile dermatomyositis. Arthritis Care Res (Hoboken). 2019;71(4):492–7.
18. Terminiello A, Marrani E, Pagnini I, Maccora I, Maniscalco V, Rumeileh SA, et al. Childhood mixed connective tissue disease at disease onset: evidence from a systematic review. Autoimmun Rev. 2024;23(4):103513.
19. Lercara A, Malattia C, Hysa E, Gattorno M, Cere A, Lavarello C, et al. Microvascular status in juvenile Sjogren's disease: the first nailfold videocapillaroscopy investigation. Clin Rheumatol. 2024;43(2):733–41.
20. Martini G, Foeldvari I, Russo R, Cuttica R, Eberhard A, Ravelli A, et al. Systemic sclerosis in childhood: clinical and immunologic features of 153 patients in an international database. Arthritis Rheum. 2006;54(12):3971–8.
21. Foeldvari I, Klotsche J, Torok KS, Kasapcopur O, Adrovic A, Stanevica V, et al. Characteristics of the first 80 patients at timepoint of first assessment included in the juvenile systemic sclerosis inception cohort. www.juvenilescleroderma.com. J Scleroderma Relat Disord. 2018;4:1–13.
22. Foeldvari I, Klotsche J, Kasapcopur O, Adrovic A, Terreri MT, Sakamoto AP, et al. Differences sustained between diffuse and limited forms of juvenile systemic sclerosis in an expanded international cohort. Arthritis Care Res (Hoboken). 2022;74(10):1575–84.

Chapter 11
The Expanding Diagnostic Horizon of Nailfold Capillaroscopy in Non-Rheumatic Disease

Yasser El Miedany and Rahma A. Elziaty

Introduction

Nailfold capillaroscopy (NFC) has historically been synonymous with the assessment and classification of Systemic Sclerosis (SSc) and related connective tissue diseases, where its capacity to visualize microvascular damage aids in early diagnosis and prognostication of the "scleroderma pattern" [1]. However, the utility of this noninvasive, cost-effective, and reproducible technique extends far beyond the confines of rheumatology. As an accessible "window to the microcirculation, " NFC offers a unique in vivo view of endothelial function and microangiopathy, reflecting systemic vascular health with remarkable precision [2].

The microcirculation is the ultimate target of numerous systemic pathologies, serving as the essential interface for oxygen, nutrient, and waste exchange. The detection of capillary architectural derangements, microhemorrhages, reduced capillary density, and altered flow dynamics via NFC is increasingly recognized as a sensitive biomarker for generalized vascular dysfunction [3]. This might represent a shared pathway of the disease and its impact on the microcirculation. This chapter focuses on the accumulating evidence that links specific NFC abnormalities to a broad spectrum of non-rheumatic illnesses, suggesting a shared microvascular component in their pathogenesis and progression.

Y. El Miedany (✉)
Canterbury Christ Church University, Canterbury, UK

Rheumatology and Rehabilitation, Ain Shams University, Cairo, Egypt

King's College, London, UK

R. A. Elziaty
Internal Medicine Department, Rheumatology Division, Faculty of Medicine, Ain Shams University, Cairo, Egypt
e-mail: drrahmaelziaty@med.asu.edu.eg

Y. El Miedany, R. A. Elziaty (eds.), *Capillaroscopy*, Contemporary Rheumatology,
https://doi.org/10.1007/978-3-032-22966-3_11

The following sections will systematically explore the compelling evidence supporting the integration of NFC into the diagnostic and prognostic frameworks of major disease categories. This expands the clinical application of NFC and its role in systemic diseases, including: 1. Cardiovascular and Cardiometabolic Conditions, where NFC provides a novel avenue for risk stratification. Capillaroscopic changes, such as reduced density and architectural distortion, are increasingly correlated with conventional cardiovascular risk factors, including hypertension, and with the extent of subclinical vascular damage, such as carotid intima-media thickness (IMT) and coronary artery disease risk [4]. 2. Diabetes Mellitus: Microangiopathy is a hallmark of diabetes. NFC allows for the detailed assessment of diabetic microvascular pathology, offering insights into the early stages of the disease that precede clinical complications, thereby facilitating timely intervention [5]. 3. Infectious Diseases: The microvascular consequences of severe systemic infections will be discussed, exemplified by the study of COVID-related microclots, which are currently being actively investigated. NFC provides real-time visualization of microthrombotic and inflammatory events, underscoring its potential role in understanding long-term sequelae [6]. 4. Dermatologic Conditions: In conditions like psoriasis, NFC reveals microvascular changes (e.g., increased tortuosity and architectural disorganization) that may reflect the systemic inflammatory burden and predict associated comorbidities, including elevated carotid IMT [7]. 5. Hematologic and Renal Disorders: The chapter will examine how hematological dyscrasias, such as sickle cell disease, and microvascular stress from Chronic Kidney Disease (CKD) manifest specific and quantifiable alterations in the nailfold capillary bed, offering a surrogate marker for disease severity and organ damage progression [8]. 6. Oncology and Paraneoplastic Syndromes: Emerging evidence suggests that distinct capillaroscopic patterns may be associated with malignancy, either through paraneoplastic microangiopathy or chemotherapy-induced toxicity, positioning NFC as a potentially valuable tool in the rapidly evolving field of onco-rheumatology [9].

In summary, by aggregating and critically analyzing these findings, this chapter aims to establish NFC as a powerful, generalizable tool for the assessment of systemic microvascular health, positioning it to become a vital, accessible component of non-rheumatic clinical evaluation and personalized medicine.

Nailfold Capillaroscopy in Cardiovascular and Cardiometabolic Conditions

Nailfold capillaroscopy (NFC) provides a noninvasive opportunity to observe the microcirculatory changes that often precede or accompany macrovascular disease, positioning it as a powerful tool for early risk stratification in cardiovascular and cardiometabolic conditions. The fundamental principle is that microvascular damage observed in the nailfold reflects generalized systemic microangiopathy.

Hypertension (HTN)

Hypertension is characterized by chronic vascular stress leading to structural and functional microvascular changes. NFC findings are recognized as a sensitive, early indicator of this generalized damage, often correlating with target organ damage [10–12].

Capillary Density Reduction A key finding in hypertensive patients is a reduction in functional capillary density, which reflects early arteriolar remodeling and rarefaction. This loss of capillaries is a powerful independent predictor of adverse cardiovascular outcomes and is linked to elevated peripheral vascular resistance (Fig. 11.1).

Morphological Changes NFC in HTN frequently reveals capillary tortuosity and dilatation as a compensatory response to altered blood flow dynamics. The most severe changes, including capillary dropout and microhemorrhages, are typically seen in patients with uncontrolled or severe hypertension and may resemble the nonspecific changes seen in early connective tissue diseases (Fig. 11.1).

Prognostic Value Studies have correlated specific NFC abnormalities (e.g., lower capillary density) with the severity of hypertensive retinopathy and the progression of left ventricular hypertrophy (LVH), establishing the technique as a complementary tool for assessing HTN-related end-organ damage.

Idiopathic Pulmonary Arterial Hypertension (IPAH)

While the microvascular changes in SSc-associated PAH are well-documented (SSc pattern), NFC provides critical insights into the pathogenesis of Idiopathic Pulmonary Arterial Hypertension (IPAH), suggesting a systemic vasculopathy beyond the pulmonary circulation [13, 14].

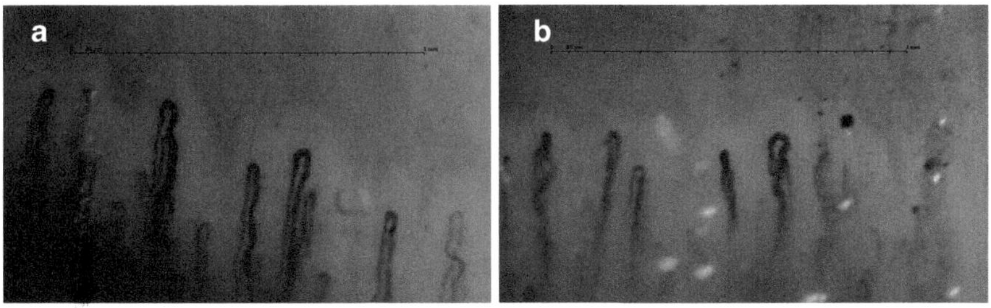

Fig. 11.1 NFC images in a patient with chronic HTN showing decreased capillary density, dilated capillaries (**a**, **b**), and microhemorrhages (**b**)

Capillary Pattern: A significant subset of IPAH patients exhibit abnormal NFC findings, even in the absence of a defined connective tissue disease. These findings include nonspecific microvascular abnormalities such as increased tortuosity, slightly dilated loops, and focal capillary loss.

Endothelial Dysfunction: The presence of these abnormalities is thought to reflect generalized endothelial dysfunction, which is central to the pathobiology of PAH. NFC findings, particularly a reduction in capillary density, can correlate with the severity of pulmonary hemodynamics and exercise capacity, suggesting that systemic microvascular stress contributes to the overall clinical picture (Fig. 11.2).

Differential Diagnosis: NFC serves a vital role in the initial workup of suspected PAH by helping to distinguish between IPAH and connective tissue disease-associated PAH, guiding subsequent management and prognostic assessment.

Atherosclerosis, Carotid Intima-Media Thickness (IMT), and Coronary Risk

NFC offers a unique opportunity to bridge the gap between microscopic vascular change and macroscopic atherosclerotic burden.

Atherosclerotic Microangiopathy: NFC patterns, particularly architectural disorganization and reduced capillary density, have been found to correlate with traditional markers of systemic atherosclerosis. The microvascular rarefaction is hypothesized to reflect the general state of the arteriolar bed supplying the vasa vasorum, contributing to the atherosclerotic process (Fig. 11.3).

Correlation with Carotid IMT: Several high-level studies have demonstrated a significant association between specific NFC abnormalities and increased carotid intima-media thickness (CIMT), an established surrogate marker for subclinical atherosclerosis and cardiovascular event risk. Capillary dropout and reduced capillary density appear to be particularly strong correlates of increased CIMT, suggesting that NFC can be used as a simple screening tool to identify individuals requiring more intensive cardiovascular risk management (Fig. 11.3).

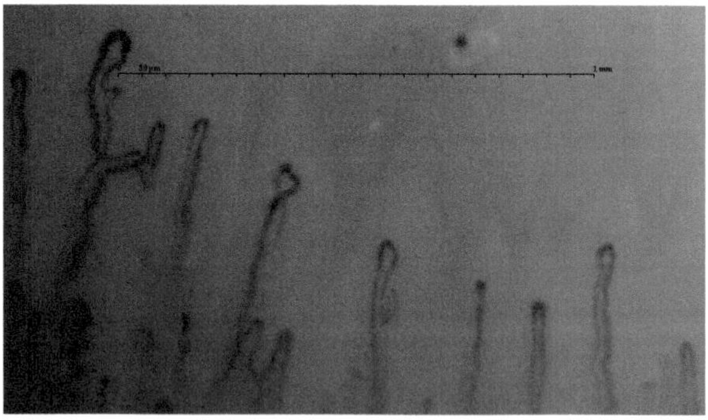

Fig. 11.2 Decreased density and dilated and abnormally shaped capillaries in a patient with IPAH; PAP: 34 mmHg

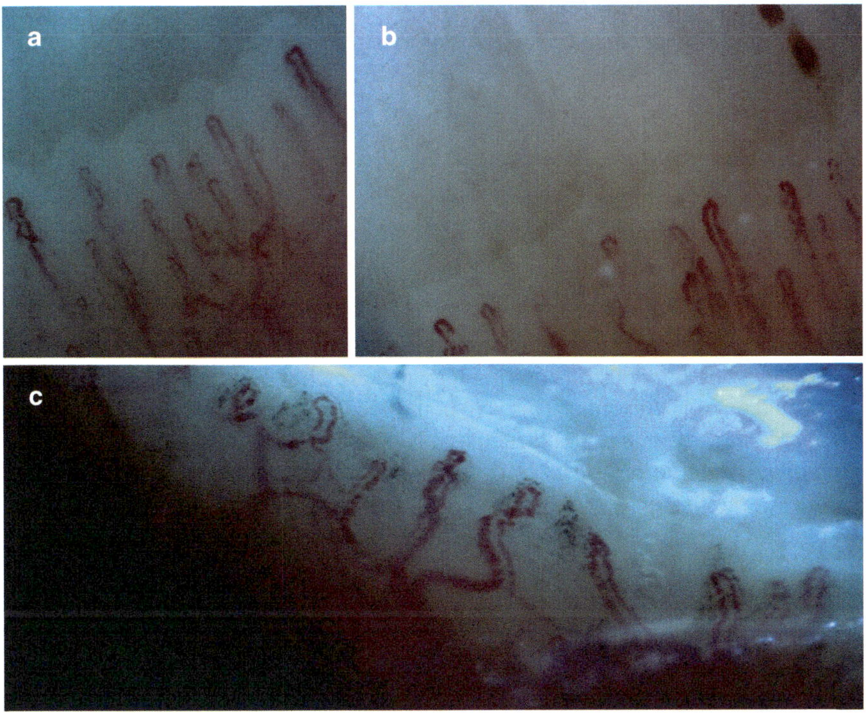

Fig. 11.3 NFC in a patient with increased carotid IMT and atherosclerotic plaque in the right carotid. Capillary dropout and microhemorrhages (**b**, **c**). Granular appearance with sluggish flow (**a**–**c**) and architectural disorganization (**c**)

Coronary Artery Disease (CAD) Risk: NFC metrics have shown prognostic value in predicting major adverse cardiovascular events. Capillary abnormalities have been independently associated with the extent and severity of CAD, providing evidence that the microcirculation is an active participant, not just a passive recipient, of the atherosclerotic process. The noninvasive nature of NFC makes it highly attractive for integrating into primary care risk assessment protocols alongside standard metrics like the Framingham Risk Score [15].

Diabetes Mellitus

Nailfold capillaroscopy (NFC) serves as a valuable, noninvasive tool for visualizing and quantifying microvascular damage associated with Diabetes Mellitus (DM), particularly diabetic microangiopathy. Since DM is fundamentally a systemic disorder affecting the microvasculature, NFC findings often reflect the severity and duration of the disease and can potentially predict the onset of later complications. The changes observed are typically nonspecific but are collectively indicative of chronic endothelial dysfunction and microcirculatory stress.

Key Capillaroscopic Findings in Diabetes

The most common abnormalities identified by NFC in patients with Type 1 and Type 2 DM, often increasing in prevalence with disease duration and poor glycemic control, include:

- *Increased Tortuosity and Dilatation*: Capillary loops frequently display excessive twisting or corkscrew morphology and are often significantly dilated (ectasia and microaneurysms). This is hypothesized to be a compensatory response to altered flow dynamics and local tissue hypoxia [16] (Fig. 11.4).
- *Reduced Capillary Density (Rarefaction)*: A critical finding is the *loss of capillaries* (rarefaction or dropout), which reflects chronic vascular damage and reduced peripheral blood supply. Reduced functional capillary density is considered a key morphological sign of diabetic microangiopathy and correlates with increased systemic vascular resistance and cardiovascular risk [5] (Fig. 11.4).
- *Atypical Morphology*: The presence of bushy or disorganized capillaries, often associated with microhemorrhages (small blood dots due to leakage), is more common in DM patients than in healthy controls, reflecting increased capillary fragility and permeability [17] (Fig. 11.4).
- *Altered Flow*: Functional assessment using videocapillaroscopy frequently shows slowing of capillary blood flow and impaired vasomotion responses, indicating functional endothelial dysfunction, which precedes frank structural damage [18].

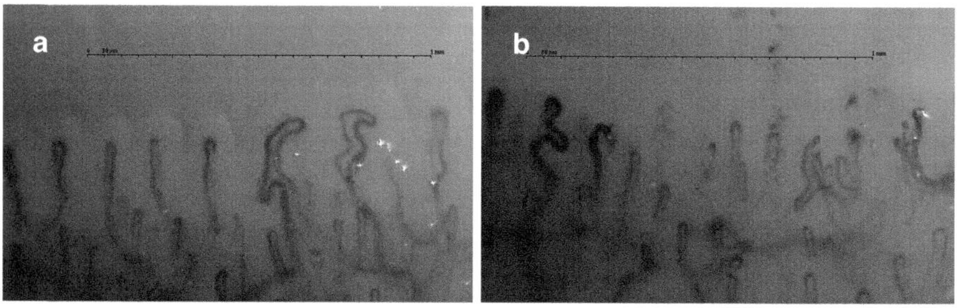

Fig. 11.4 NFC of a patient with diabetic nephropathy. Presence of ectasia and tortuous capillaries (**a**, **b**). Presence of ramified capillaries and small dots of microhemorrhages (**b**)

Clinical and Prognostic Significance

The microvascular changes detected by NFC in DM hold significant clinical and prognostic value:

- *Correlation with Microvascular Complications*: NFC findings have been shown to correlate significantly with established diabetic microvascular complications, including retinopathy (the severity of capillary changes often mirrors the severity of retinal changes) and nephropathy (microalbuminuria) [5, 19].
- *Predictive Potential*: Quantifiable metrics, such as capillary density and loop diameter, are being investigated as potential predictors of adverse outcomes and the development of overt complications, allowing for earlier identification of patients who require tighter glucose and blood pressure control [20, 21].
- *Distinction from Connective Tissue Disease*: While the changes are generally nonspecific (unlike the "scleroderma pattern"), NFC is crucial for differentiating typical diabetic microangiopathy from the capillary abnormalities induced by coexisting connective tissue diseases, which may present with secondary Raynaud's phenomenon in DM patients.

Nailfold Capillaroscopy in Infectious Diseases: Focus on COVID-19 Microangiopathy

The utility of Nailfold Capillaroscopy (NFC) is gaining traction in the field of infectious disease, particularly in visualizing the systemic microvascular sequelae of acute and chronic infections. This is highly relevant in understanding conditions where widespread endothelial dysfunction and microthrombosis are key pathophysiological drivers, most notably in the context of COVID-19 and related viral syndromes [22].

Viral Infections and Endothelial Damage

Viral infections, including influenza, HIV, and especially SARS-CoV-2, are known to directly or indirectly induce systemic inflammation and damage to the endothelium. The microvasculature, being a major site of endothelial activity, provides a vulnerable target. NFC can capture these changes, revealing a functional and structural microangiopathy that reflects the overall severity of the systemic inflammatory response [22].

COVID-19-Related Microclots and Microangiopathy

The SARS-CoV-2 virus is recognized for inducing a pro-thrombotic state and widespread endotheliitis (inflammation of the endothelium), leading to both macro- and microvascular complications [23]. NFC has proven to be a particularly insightful tool in assessing this COVID-19-related microangiopathy:

- *Microthrombosis and Sludging*: A hallmark finding in both acute and long COVID patients is the observation of sludging of blood flow and evidence of microclots within the nailfold capillaries. This phenomenon is indicative of impaired fibrinolysis and generalized microvascular obstruction, leading to localized tissue hypoxia [24] (Fig. 11.5).
- *Capillary Dropout and Atypical Architecture*: Patients with severe COVID-19 or those with persistent vascular symptoms often exhibit a significant reduction in functional capillary density (capillary dropout) and architectural disorganization. This structural damage is thought to contribute to long-term symptoms, including fatigue and persistent tissue ischemia [4] (Fig. 11.5).
- *Correlation with Clinical Severity*: NFC abnormalities have been shown to correlate with the severity of acute COVID-19 infection, particularly in patients requiring intensive care. This suggests that the extent of peripheral microvascular damage mirrors the severity of pulmonary and other organ microvascular compromise [6].
- *Persistent Microvascular Dysfunction (Long COVID)*: Crucially, NFC findings provide an objective, visual marker for ongoing pathology in Long COVID. The persistence of microvascular abnormalities (microclots, reduced flow) in symptomatic patients weeks or months after viral clearance suggests chronic microvascular dysfunction is a core mechanism of the post-acute COVID-19 syndrome [25].

In this context, NFC transitions from a diagnostic aid to a *potential functional biomarker*, offering a noninvasive means to monitor the efficacy of anti-thrombotic

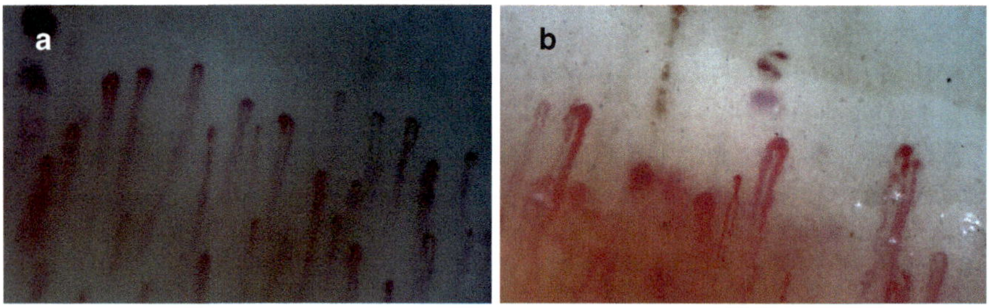

Fig. 11.5 NFC of a patient presented with post-COVID bluish discoloration of toes. Microthrombosis and sludging of blood flow and evidence of microclots within the nailfold capillaries (**a**, **b**). Presence of small dots of microhemorrhages (recent and old) (**a**, **b**). Significant capillary dropout (**b**)

or anti-inflammatory therapies targeting the microcirculation in post-viral syndromes.

Nailfold Capillaroscopy in Dermatologic Conditions

Nailfold capillaroscopy (NFC) offers a unique perspective into the systemic microvascular involvement of primary dermatologic diseases. Beyond the skin, these conditions, driven by chronic inflammation and immune dysregulation, often exhibit microcirculatory changes visible at the nailfold, which may reflect the overall disease burden and predict associated cardiovascular comorbidities [26].

Psoriasis

Psoriasis is a common, chronic inflammatory skin disorder often associated with systemic inflammation and increased cardiovascular risk. NFC is increasingly utilized to visualize the microvascular component of this systemic inflammatory state.

- *Capillary Morphology and Ramifications*: The most characteristic finding in psoriasis is the presence *of "bushy" or "ramified" capillary loops* [27]. These represent an intense proliferative and angiogenic response, resulting in highly enlarged and disorganized capillary formations. The extent of these bushy loops often correlates with the severity of skin lesions (e.g., PASI score) and the inflammatory activity of the disease (Fig. 11.6).
- *Tortuosity and Dilatation*: Psoriatic patients commonly show increased capillary tortuosity and marked dilatation [28, 29]. This is interpreted as a manifestation of chronic inflammation leading to endothelial proliferation and altered blood flow dynamics in the dermal papillary loops (Fig. 11.6).
- *Link to Atherosclerosis (IMT)*: Crucially, NFC findings in psoriasis help bridge the gap between skin inflammation and macrovascular risk. The presence and severity of capillaroscopic abnormalities (e.g., capillary density reduction or severe ramification) have been independently associated with increased carotid intima-media thickness (CIMT) [22]. This correlation suggests that the microvascular damage visualized at the nailfold is a valuable, noninvasive biomarker for subclinical atherosclerosis and heightened coronary risk in psoriatic patients.

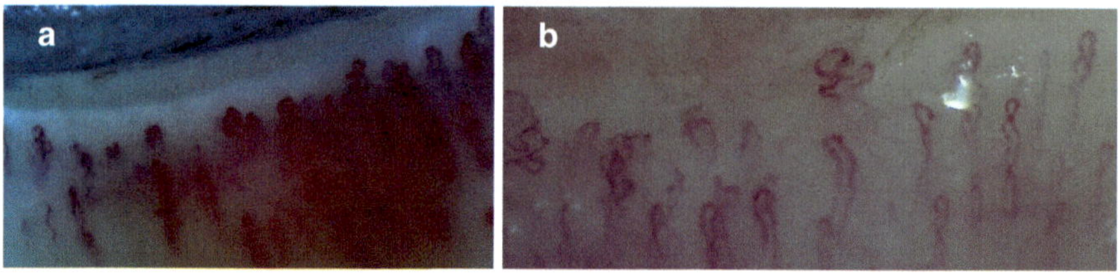

Fig. 11.6 (**a**) Presence of bushy capillaries, ramification, increased tortuosity, and pericapillary edema in a patient with active skin psoriasis. (**b**) Follow-up NFC of the same case after treatment and marked improvement of psoriatic rash; decreased number of bushy capillaries and disappearance of pericapillary edema

Alopecia Areata and Chronic Dermatitis

While the evidence is less extensive than in psoriasis, NFC studies in other inflammatory dermatoses support the idea that microvascular changes reflect the underlying immune-mediated process.

- *Alopecia Areata (AA)*: This autoimmune condition targeting hair follicles has been associated with microvascular alterations, including increased capillary tortuosity and nonspecific dilatation [31]. These changes suggest a degree of systemic microcirculatory dysfunction, potentially reflecting the autoimmune or inflammatory burden.
- *Chronic Dermatitis (e.g., Atopic Dermatitis)*: In chronic, inflammatory skin conditions, NFC often reveals nonspecific microvascular abnormalities, such as increased tortuosity, mild dilatation, and occasional microhemorrhages [32]. These findings are indicative of local and potentially systemic endothelial activation secondary to the persistent inflammatory state. While these changes are not unique to dermatitis, their presence confirms the participation of the microcirculation in the inflammatory cascade, emphasizing that the skin condition is not purely localized.

Nailfold Capillaroscopy in Hematologic Disorders

Nailfold capillaroscopy (NFC) is a valuable, noninvasive tool for evaluating the systemic microvascular consequences of hematologic disorders. Changes observed at the nailfold often reflect alterations in blood viscosity, red blood cell (RBC) function, and local oxygen delivery, making NFC an important surrogate marker for microcirculatory integrity and disease severity [33].

Sickle Cell Disease and Hemoglobinopathies

Sickle cell disease (SCD) and related hemoglobinopathies are characterized by chronic hemolysis, endothelial activation, and episodic vaso-occlusion, leading to widespread microvascular damage. NFC offers a direct visualization of these processes.

- *Flow Abnormalities (Sludging)*: The most characteristic finding in SCD, particularly during or leading up to vaso-occlusive crises (VOCs), is impaired blood flow or sludging within the capillaries. The abnormal, rigid shape of sickled erythrocytes leads to increased blood viscosity and mechanical obstruction of the small vessels, which is directly observable in real-time by videocapillaroscopy [8, 34] (Fig. 11.7).
- *Capillary Dropout and Avascular Areas*: Chronic microvascular injury from recurrent VOCs results in permanent structural damage, manifested as reduced capillary density (rarefaction) and the presence of avascular areas [35]. This loss of functional capillaries contributes to chronic tissue ischemia and is associated with overall disease severity and end-organ damage (Fig. 11.7).
- *Morphological Changes*: Patients often exhibit tortuous, elongated, or irregularly shaped loops as a result of chronic endothelial stress and compensatory mechanisms [8, 35].

Anemia and Myeloproliferative Disorders

NFC provides insight into how extreme variations in RBC count, viscosity, and cell function affect the microcirculation in other hematologic conditions.

- *Anemia*: In cases of severe chronic anemia, NFC may reveal increased capillary flow velocity and dilated capillary loops [33]. These findings are generally considered a physiological compensatory mechanism reflecting increased cardiac output and reduced blood viscosity, aimed at maintaining adequate tissue oxygen delivery. The changes are typically reversed upon correction of the anemia.

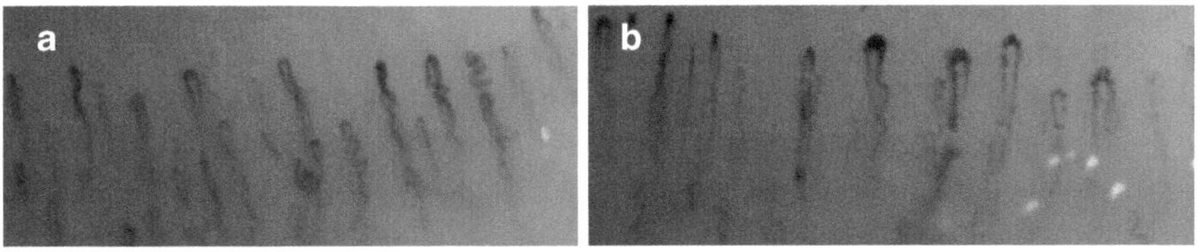

Fig. 11.7 Tortuous, elongated, and abnormally shaped capillaries (**a**). Impaired blood flow or sludging within the capillaries and presence of avascular areas (**b**)

- *Myeloproliferative Disorders (MPDs)*: MPDs, such as polycythemia vera (PV) and essential thrombocythemia (ET), are associated with altered blood rheology, hyperviscosity, and a high risk of both thrombotic and hemorrhagic events.
  - *Polycythemia Vera (PV)*: Due to the increased RBC mass, NFC often demonstrates markedly slowed blood flow (sludging) and sometimes dilated, congested loops due to hyperviscosity. These findings correlate with the increased risk of microvascular complications typical of PV, such as erythromelalgia and digital ischemia [36, 37].
  - *Essential Thrombocythemia (ET)*: While less pronounced, flow abnormalities related to platelet aggregation can sometimes be detected. The key clinical utility is in ruling out an underlying connective tissue disease in patients presenting with Raynaud's phenomenon, which can be an initial symptom of MPDs [36].

Nailfold Capillaroscopy in Renal Disease and Chronic Kidney Disease (CKD)

Nailfold Capillaroscopy (NFC) is a critical noninvasive tool for evaluating the microvascular damage inherent to Chronic Kidney Disease (CKD). The microcirculation acts as a vital bridge between the circulatory system and the kidney's filtration units, the glomeruli. Consequently, microvascular changes observed at the nailfold are highly relevant, mirroring the systemic vascular remodeling and endothelial dysfunction that drive both renal failure and cardiovascular comorbidity in CKD patients [38].

Microvascular Alterations in CKD and End-Stage Renal Disease (ESRD)

NFC studies consistently reveal significant microvascular abnormalities in CKD patients, particularly those progressing to End-Stage Renal Disease (ESRD) and those undergoing hemodialysis:

- *Capillary Dropout (Rarefaction)*: The most prevalent and clinically significant finding is a marked reduction in functional capillary density (rarefaction), characterized by fewer capillary loops per millimeter [38, 39]. This microvascular loss is considered a structural manifestation of chronic endothelial injury and widespread arteriolar remodeling.
- *Morphological Changes*: Other common findings include capillary dilatation and increased tortuosity. These changes are thought to be compensatory efforts to maintain blood flow against increased peripheral resistance and arterial stiffness, which are accelerated in CKD [40].
- *Atypical Patterns*: The microcirculation in CKD often exhibits nonspecific abnormal patterns that include bizarre loop shapes, microhemorrhages, and

structural disorganization. These abnormalities are more pronounced in patients with advanced disease (lower Glomerular Filtration Rate—GFR) and those with coexisting risk factors like hypertension and diabetes [41].

Clinical Significance and Prognostic Value

The microvascular damage observed via NFC is more than a correlative finding; it holds significant prognostic potential in the management of renal patients:

- *Association with Cardiovascular Risk*: The same mechanisms (endothelial dysfunction, arterial stiffness, microvascular loss) drive both renal progression and Cardiovascular Disease (CVD), which is the leading cause of mortality in CKD patients. Reduced capillary density, as measured by NFC, has been independently linked to markers of advanced atherosclerosis and increased cardiovascular event risk in this population [42, 43].
- *Renal Function Correlation*: The severity of NFC abnormalities, especially the degree of capillary rarefaction, often correlates inversely with the residual renal function (i.e., directly with the severity of CKD) [41]. This suggests NFC could serve as a noninvasive tool for tracking disease severity or the efficacy of nephroprotective treatments.
- *Dialysis-Related Changes*: Microvascular integrity is particularly compromised in patients on hemodialysis, potentially due to repeated inflammation and volume shifts. NFC can be used to monitor changes in microcirculation before and after dialysis sessions or over long-term treatment [44].

Nailfold Capillaroscopy in Oncology and Paraneoplastic Syndromes

The intersection of cancer and microvascular disease is an area of emerging research for Nailfold Capillaroscopy (NFC). Malignancy is fundamentally a disease of uncontrolled angiogenesis and systemic inflammation, both of which severely impact the microcirculation. NFC can provide a unique, noninvasive window into these systemic effects, particularly in the context of paraneoplastic phenomena and chemotherapy-induced damage [9, 45].

Paraneoplastic Microangiopathy

In some cases, cancer can induce systemic microvascular changes—known as paraneoplastic syndromes—before or alongside the primary tumor presentation. NFC findings can reflect this underlying process:

- *Atypical Vascular Patterns*: Specific, though nondiagnostic, capillaroscopic abnormalities have been observed in patients with various solid and hematological malignancies, often resembling a nonspecific inflammatory pattern [46]. These may include moderate capillary dilatation, increased tortuosity, and occasional microhemorrhages.
- *Raynaud's Phenomenon*: The presence of secondary Raynaud's phenomenon (RP) in an older adult without typical autoimmune markers should raise suspicion for a paraneoplastic etiology. NFC helps in this differential diagnosis by showing a microangiopathic pattern that is distinct from the classic "scleroderma pattern" but still indicates underlying systemic vascular dysfunction [47].
- *Predictive Potential*: The identification of a pronounced microangiopathy by NFC in an individual with otherwise unexplained systemic symptoms (e.g., severe fatigue, weight loss) may prompt a more extensive search for an occult malignancy, highlighting the technique's potential role as a flagging biomarker [46].

Chemotherapy-Induced Microvascular Damage

A separate, critical application of NFC in oncology involves monitoring the microvascular toxicity of cancer treatments, especially those targeting vascular growth or inducing systemic vasoconstriction.

- *Angiogenesis Inhibitors*: Therapies targeting the Vascular Endothelial Growth Factor (VEGF) pathway (VEGF inhibitors), such as bevacizumab, often induce systemic microvascular effects, including hypertension and microthrombosis. NFC can visualize the impact of these drugs on capillary morphology and blood flow, with some studies noting changes like capillary rarefaction and microaneurysms that may be dose-limiting or predictive of adverse effects [2].
- *Cytotoxic Agents*: Certain traditional chemotherapeutic agents can also directly or indirectly damage the microvasculature. NFC has been used to assess the prevalence of digital microangiopathy in survivors of childhood cancers who received specific cytotoxic treatments, linking the damage to long-term vascular morbidity [49].

To summarize, in oncology, NFC acts as a surrogate marker for systemic inflammation and a tool for pharmacovigilance, providing valuable noninvasive data on the vascular effects of powerful modern cancer therapeutics. *Some paraneoplastic cases will be discussed in detail in the chapter Clinical Case Scenarios, "Case Number 12 and Case Number 26."*

The evidence presented throughout this chapter decisively confirms that Nailfold Capillaroscopy (NFC) is no longer an ancillary technique confined primarily to rheumatology. Rather, it has emerged as a generalizable, noninvasive biomarker for systemic microvascular health and endothelial integrity across a broad spectrum of non-rheumatic diseases.

Unifying the Microvascular Component

Our systematic review of NFC findings highlights a common thread across seemingly disparate pathologies:

- *Cardiovascular and Cardiometabolic Risk*: In hypertension and atherosclerosis, NFC abnormalities like capillary rarefaction and reduced density serve as critical in vivo correlates of subclinical vascular damage (e.g., increased carotid IMT). This positions NFC as a viable tool for stratifying cardiovascular risk and monitoring therapeutic efficacy in primary care settings.
- *Systemic Vascular Stress*: In Chronic Kidney Disease (CKD) and Idiopathic Pulmonary Arterial Hypertension (IPAH), the observed microvascular loss and disorganization reflect generalized endothelial dysfunction that transcends the primary organ pathology. Similarly, in diabetes mellitus, NFC provides a direct visual link between glycemic control and the extent of microangiopathy, correlating with the risk of complications like retinopathy and nephropathy.
- *Inflammation and Rheology*: In inflammatory dermatoses like psoriasis, specific morphological changes (e.g., bushy loops) reflect the systemic inflammatory burden, correlating with accelerated cardiovascular risk. In hematologic disorders such as sickle cell disease, NFC provides a real-time, functional assessment of blood flow and micro-occlusion, serving as a dynamic marker for disease activity.
- *Emerging Applications*: The ability of NFC to visualize COVID-19-related microclots and monitor chemotherapy-induced microvascular toxicity in oncology underscores its utility as a powerful tool for pharmacovigilance and understanding novel microthrombotic pathologies.

Future Directions

The future integration of NFC into non-rheumatic practice hinges on two key advancements:

1. *Standardization and Quantification*: Establishing universal, quantitative scoring systems for non-scleroderma patterns will enhance reproducibility and integrate NFC metrics into large-scale, prospective clinical trials.
2. *Clinical Implementation*: Future research must focus on the cost-effectiveness and predictive superiority of NFC when used alongside conventional markers. Demonstrating that NFC can non-invasively identify high-risk individuals earlier than current methods will secure its definitive place as a *standard component of systemic vascular assessment* outside of the rheumatology clinic.

In conclusion, NFC provides a compelling and accessible window into the human microcirculation, offering physicians across multiple specialties a vital, functional biomarker for advancing early diagnosis, prognostic stratification, and truly personalized patient management (Table 11.1).

Case 1: Hypertension with Increased Carotid Intima-Media Thickness and Plaque—Capillaroscopic Correlation

A 58-year-old male with a 10-year history of essential hypertension presented for vascular risk assessment. He complained of occasional headaches and mild dizziness but denied chest pain, visual disturbance, or limb weakness. He had no history of diabetes, smoking, or connective tissue disease.

Examination: Vital signs: BP 150/95 mmHg, pulse 78/min, regular. Cardiovascular: Normal heart sounds, no murmurs or bruits. Carotid examination: No audible bruit. Peripheral pulses: Palpable and symmetrical. Skin and extremities: No cyanosis, ulceration, or Raynaud's phenomenon.

Laboratory Results: Fasting blood glucose: 96 mg/dL. Lipid profile: Total cholesterol 228 mg/dL, LDL 155 mg/dL, HDL 42 mg/dL, triglycerides 180 mg/dL. Serum creatinine: 1.1 mg/dL. ESR: 18 mm/hr. CRP: Mildly elevated (6 mg/L). ANA: Negative.

Carotid Duplex Ultrasound Findings Bilateral increased IMT and early atherosclerotic plaque formation, indicating hypertensive vascular remodeling and subclinical atherosclerosis.

- Right common carotid artery (CCA): Intima-media thickness (IMT) = 1.1 mm (increased).
- Left CCA: IMT = 1.2 mm with a small hyperechoic plaque at the carotid bulb.
- Flow: No significant stenosis.

Capillaroscopy Findings Mildly disorganized, with irregular distribution of loops. Dilated and tortuous capillaries, especially in the distal rows. Capillary density: Slightly decreased. Microhemorrhages: Occasional. Granular appearance with sluggish flow (Fig. 11.8).

Capillaroscopic findings reflect hypertensive microangiopathy due to chronic endothelial stress and vascular remodeling, correlating with the macrocirculatory changes seen in carotid arteries.

The patient kept on Amlodipine 5 mg daily plus an ACE inhibitor to optimize blood pressure control: Target <130/80 mmHg. Start statin therapy for atherosclerotic risk reduction. Lifestyle modification: Salt restriction, weight control, and regular exercise. Low-dose aspirin (75 mg/day) for secondary prevention.

Follow-up: Repeat carotid duplex and nailfold capillaroscopy in 6–12 months to assess vascular improvement or stabilization.

Table 11.1 Nailfold capillaroscopy findings in non-rheumatic diseases

Disease category	Specific condition	Primary NFC findings	Underlying pathophysiology reflected
Microvascular rarefaction (capillary loss)	Chronic Kidney Disease (CKD)	Severe capillary dropout (rarefaction) and structural disorganization	Systemic endothelial dysfunction; chronic microvascular injury mirroring renal disease progression and cardiovascular risk
	Hypertension (HTN)	Reduced functional capillary density (rarefaction)	Arteriolar remodeling and reduced peripheral microvascular density; indicator of end-organ damage
Flow abnormalities (sludging and obstruction)	Sickle cell disease	Sludging (slowed/stopped flow), micro-occlusions, and chronic capillary dropout	Vaso-occlusion caused by rigid, sickled red blood cells; predictor of vaso-occlusive crises
	COVID-19	Persistence of microclots and marked sludging of blood flow	Chronic endothelial activation and fibrinolytic impairment, contributing to post-viral syndrome symptoms
Compensatory/ Angiogenic changes	Psoriasis	Bushy or ramified loops, increased tortuosity, and prominent dilatation	Intense chronic inflammation and compensatory angiogenesis; linked to accelerated subclinical atherosclerosis (IMT)
	Diabetes Mellitus (DM)	Increased tortuosity, dilatation (ectasia), and nonspecific loop morphology (e.g., corkscrew)	Endothelial cell damage and compensatory efforts against altered blood rheology; correlates with the severity of retinopathy
Nonspecific systemic vasculopathy	Idiopathic PAH (IPAH)	Nonspecific capillary dilatation and mild rarefaction	Generalized, non-autoimmune-driven systemic endothelial dysfunction parallel to pulmonary vascular remodeling
	Oncology (paraneoplastic)	Nonspecific dilatation, microhemorrhages, or patterns resembling mild microangiopathy	Systemic effects of occult malignancy or monitoring of chemotherapy-induced vascular toxicity (e.g., anti-VEGF effects)

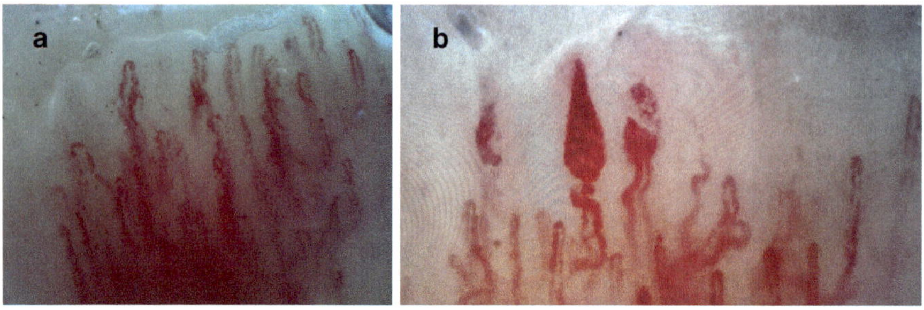

Fig. 11.8 Decreased capillary density and presence of microhemorrhages (**a**, **b**). Disorganized and irregularly arranged capillaries (**b**). Granular appearance with sluggish flow (**a**)

Case 2: Diabetes Mellitus with Diabetic Retinopathy—Capillaroscopic Correlation

A 55-year-old man with type 2 diabetes mellitus for 12 years presented for evaluation of visual blurring in both eyes for the past 6 months. He denied Raynaud's phenomenon, digital ulcers, or other connective tissue disease symptoms. His diabetes was suboptimally controlled despite oral hypoglycemic agents.

Examination: He was obese with a BMI of 31, no pallor or cyanosis, warm extremities, and no digital ulcers or gangrene. He had mild distal sensory neuropathy.

Fundus Examination: Background diabetic retinopathy: multiple microaneurysms, dot and blot hemorrhages, and hard exudates in both eyes. No proliferative changes or macular edema.

Laboratory Results: Fasting blood glucose: 178 mg/dL. HbA1c: 8.6%. Lipid profile: Elevated triglycerides (240 mg/dL), LDL 165 mg/dL. Serum creatinine: 1.0 mg/dL. Urine microalbumin: Positive (125 mg/day). ANA: Negative.

Capillaroscopy Findings: Capillary density: Slightly reduced compared to normal. Capillary morphology: Presence of dilated, elongated, and tortuous capillaries with ectasia and occasional microhemorrhages (Fig. 11.9).

Findings indicate microangiopathy secondary to long-standing diabetes, reflecting endothelial damage and capillary remodeling similar to that seen in retinal microcirculation.

Both retinal and nailfold microcirculations showed features of microvascular damage—capillary dilatation, hemorrhages, and mild rarefaction—suggesting a systemic microangiopathic process affecting multiple vascular beds. The degree of capillaroscopic alteration correlated with the severity of retinopathy.

We arrange for optimizing glycemic control (target HbA1c <7%). Start statins for dyslipidemia. Maintain blood pressure <130/80 mmHg. Encourage smoking cessation and exercise.

Repeat capillaroscopy and fundus examination after 6–12 months to assess vascular progression or improvement.

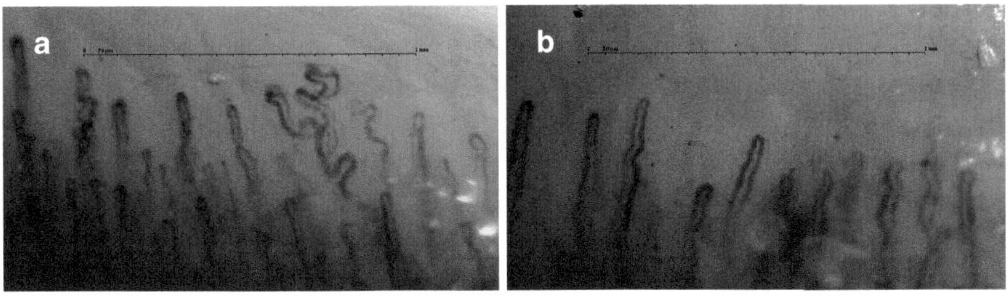

Fig. 11.9 Presence of tortuous, elongated capillaries and microhemorrhages (**a**, **b**). Presence of ectasia and abnormally shaped capillaries (**a**)

Case 3: Idiopathic Pulmonary Arterial Hypertension—Capillaroscopic Changes and Disease Progression

A 35-year-old woman presented with progressive exertional dyspnea and occasional dizziness for 1 year. She denied Raynaud's phenomenon, arthralgia, or skin thickening. There was no history of connective tissue disease, congenital heart disease, or thromboembolic events.

Examination Blood pressure 110/70 mmHg, pulse 86/min, SpO_2 93% on room air. Cardiovascular: Accentuated P_2 but no murmur over the pulmonary area. Chest examination: normal. Mild cyanosis and cool extremities, but no digital ulcers. Skin was of normal texture, with no sclerodactyly or telangiectasia.

Laboratory Results: ANA, ENA: Negative. ESR: 12 mm/hr. CRP: 5 mg/L. BNP: Elevated (580 pg/mL). Liver and renal functions: Normal.

Echocardiography and Right Heart Catheterization Right ventricular systolic pressure: 68 mmHg. Mean pulmonary arterial pressure (PAP): 40 mmHg. Pulmonary vascular resistance: Elevated. Normal left heart function.

The diagnosis of Idiopathic Pulmonary Arterial Hypertension (IPAH) was made. The patient was advised to avoid cold exposure and vasoconstrictive drugs. She was maintained on a phosphodiesterase-5 inhibitor (Sildenafil 50 mg BID).

Initial Capillaroscopy Findings Capillary architecture: Generally preserved, with mild disorganization in distal rows. Capillary density: Slightly reduced. Capillary morphology: Few dilated capillaries with mild tortuosity. Microhemorrhages: Occasional. Background: Mild pallor. Early microvascular dysfunction reflecting endothelial involvement secondary to pulmonary hypertension (Fig. 11.10).

Follow-Up (After 12 Months—Worsening Pulmonary Hypertension)

The patient's dyspnea worsened (NYHA Class III). Echocardiography revealed right ventricular systolic pressure increased to 75 mmHg with mild right ventricular dilation.

Repeat Capillaroscopy Findings Capillary density: Further reduction with avascular areas. Capillary morphology: Increased tortuosity and dilatation, presence of meandering and bushy-appearing capillaries. Background: Pale with sluggish blood flow. Architecture: Moderately to severely disorganized. Progression from mild to moderate–severe microangiopathy, reflecting systemic endothelial dysfunction parallel to the worsening pulmonary vascular disease (Fig. 11.11).

The patient started an endothelin receptor antagonist (Bosentan 125 mg BID), diuretics for right heart failure symptoms, Supplemental oxygen, and supervised exercise. Follow-up capillaroscopy every 6–12 months to monitor peripheral microvascular involvement and to detect worsening systemic microangiopathy, which may parallel disease progression and predict prognosis.

Capillaroscopy in idiopathic pulmonary hypertension initially shows mild capillary dilatation and rarefaction, which progresses over time to significant capillary loss, increased tortuosity, abnormal shape of capillaries, and disorganization as pulmonary vascular disease advances. These findings may reflect generalized endothelial dysfunction in systemic and pulmonary microcirculations.

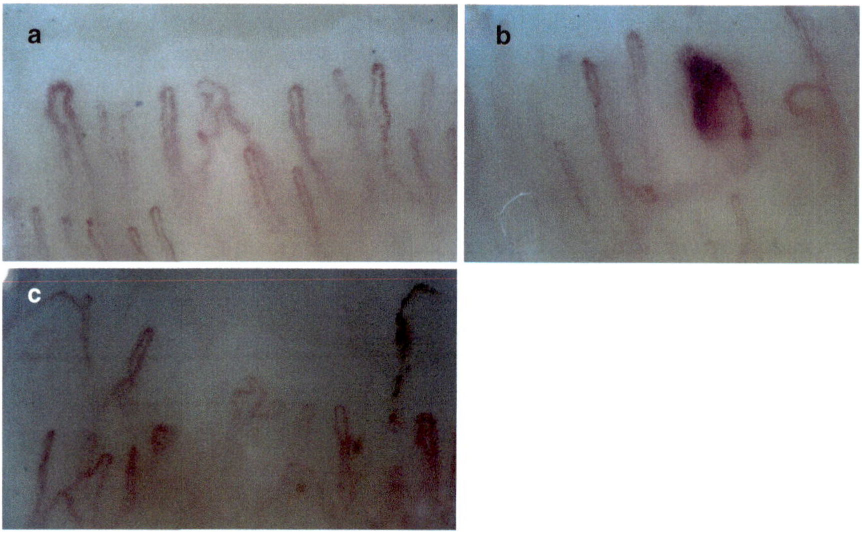

Fig. 11.10 Initial NFC shows reduced capillary density. Mild capillary dilatation, tortuous capillaries with some abnormally shaped capillaries (**a**, **c**). Presence of recent (**b**) and old microhemorrhages (**c**)

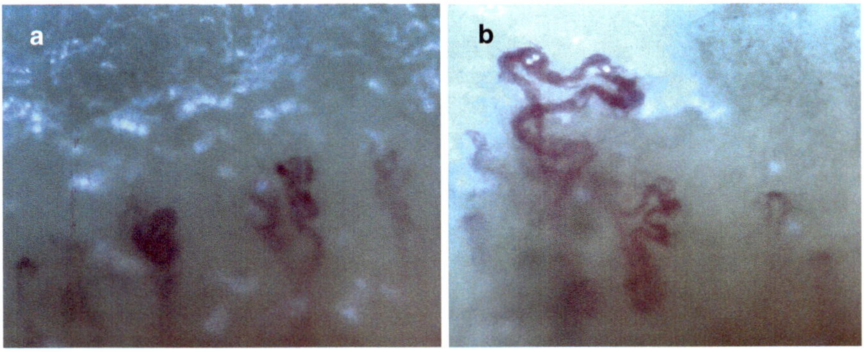

Fig. 11.11 Follow-up NFC after 12 months: Marked decrease in capillary density and pale background (**a**, **b**). Presence of abnormally shaped capillaries like bushy capillaries (**a**, **b**) and meandering capillaries (**b**)

Case 4: COVID-19 Patient with Acral Cyanosis

A 42-year-old woman, previously healthy, presented 4 weeks after a mild COVID-19 infection (confirmed by PCR) with bluish discoloration of her fingers and toes (Fig. 11.12). She reported mild tingling and coldness but no digital ulcers or gangrene. There was no history of Raynaud's phenomenon, smoking, or autoimmune disease.

Examination: Vital signs: Stable, oxygen saturation 97% on room air. Peripheral pulses: Palpable bilaterally. Bluish discoloration over the distal phalanges of fingers and toes, no necrosis or ulceration. No joint swelling, sclerodactyly, or skin thickening.

Capillaroscopy Findings: Dilated capillary loops and areas of microhemorrhages. Occasional areas of capillary rarefaction. No giant capillaries or avascular areas. Findings consistent with microangiopathic changes secondary to endothelial dysfunction post-COVID-19 (Fig. 11.13).

Laboratory Results: CBC: Mild lymphopenia. ESR: 35 mm/hr., CRP: 18 mg/L. D-dimer: Elevated (2.1 μg/mL). ANA, ENA, and antiphospholipid antibodies: Negative. Ferritin: Elevated. Coagulation profile: Normal PT, aPTT.

Plan of Management: Warm protection and avoidance of cold exposure. Low-dose aspirin (75 mg/day). Short course of vasodilator (diltiazem 30 mg BID) for symptomatic relief. Monitor for thrombotic complications or progression to digital ischemia. Follow-up capillaroscopy in 3 months to assess endothelial recovery.

The patient reported gradual improvement in finger and toe discoloration. No new ischemic lesions or ulcers appeared. The tingling sensation subsided, and the digits regained normal temperature and color.

Follow-Up After 3 Months

Follow-up capillaroscopy (3 months post-COVID-19): Improvement in microvascular pattern: Previously noted dilated capillaries were mostly resolved.

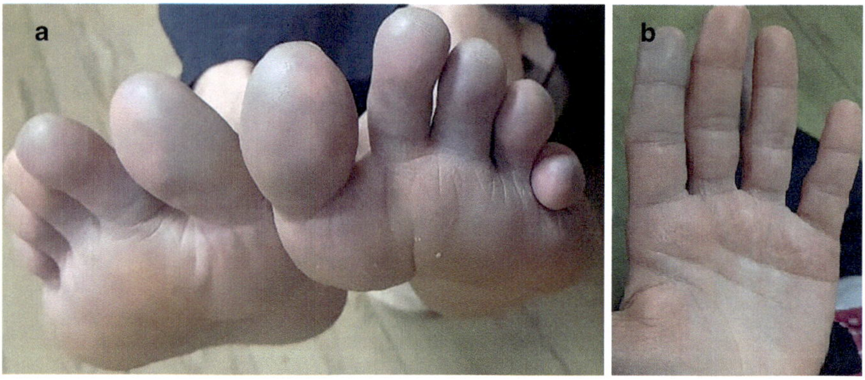

Fig. 11.12 Bluish discoloration of the fingers (**b**) and toes (**a**)

Disappearance of microhemorrhages. Capillary density: Restored to near-normal levels with no significant avascular areas. Architecture: Homogeneous, regular capillary distribution; no giant capillaries or neoangiogenesis observed. Findings consistent with partial to near-complete endothelial recovery after post-COVID microangiopathy (Fig. 11.14).

Follow-up Laboratory Results (at 3 months): ESR: 15 mm/hr. CRP: 3 mg/L. D-dimer: Normalized (0.4 μg/mL). ANA, antiphospholipid antibodies: Negative.

We advised our patient to continue warm protection and avoidance of cold exposure, discontinue Altiazem (no recurrence of vasospasm), continue low-dose aspirin for another 3 months as prophylaxis, and routine follow-up at 6 months and 12 months to ensure full vascular recovery.

COVID-19–related endothelial dysfunction led to transient microangiopathic changes visible on capillaroscopy (dilated loops, hemorrhages, and focal rarefaction). Over 3 months, these changes largely reversed, highlighting the reversible nature of COVID-related microvascular injury in the absence of underlying connective tissue disease.

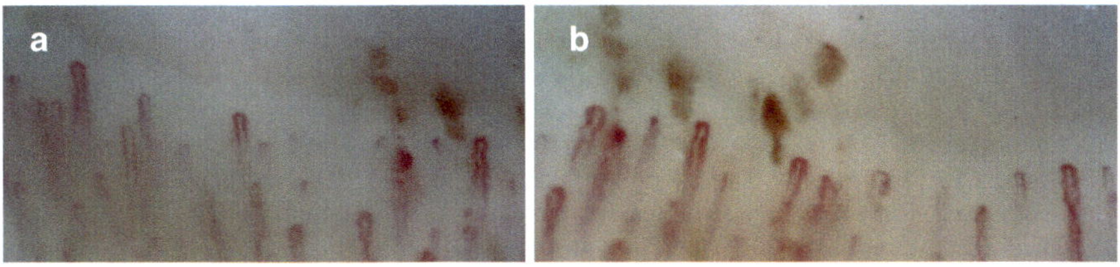

Fig. 11.13 NFC after 4 weeks post COVID infection: dilated capillaries, microhemorrhages (recent and old), and decreased capillary density (**a**, **b**). Occasional areas of capillary rarefaction (**b**)

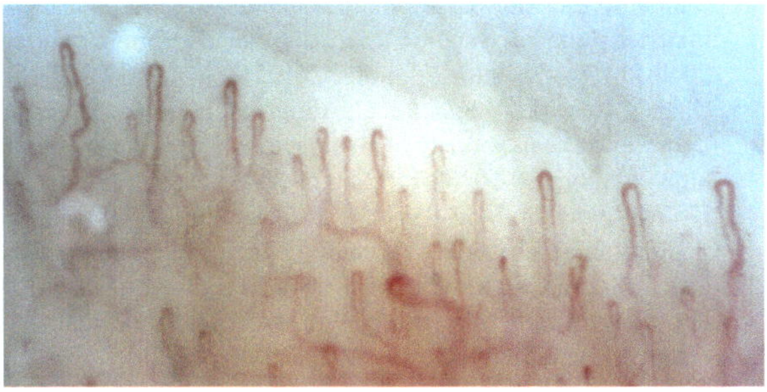

Fig. 11.14 Follow-up NFC after 3 months: Improvement in microvascular pattern; capillary density is back to normal; previously noted dilated capillaries started to resolve with the disappearance of microhemorrhages

References

1. Cutolo M, Smith V. Detection of microvascular changes in systemic sclerosis and other rheumatic diseases. Nat Rev Rheumatol. 2021;17(11):665–77. https://doi.org/10.1038/s41584-021-00685-0.
2. Chojnowski MM, Felis-Giemza A, Olesińska M. Capillaroscopy - a role in modern rheumatology. Reumatologia. 2016;54(2):67–72. https://doi.org/10.5114/reum.2016.60215.
3. Lambova SN. Nailfold capillaroscopy - practical implications for rheumatology practice. Curr Rheumatol Rev. 2020;16(2):79–83. https://doi.org/10.2174/157339711602200415083444.
4. Mishra A, Grover C, Singal A, Narang S, Das GK. Nailfold capillary changes in newly diagnosed hypertensive patients: an observational analytical study. Microvasc Res. 2021;136:104173. https://doi.org/10.1016/j.mvr.2021.104173.
5. Maldonado G, Guerrero R, Paredes C, Ríos C. Nailfold capillaroscopy in diabetes mellitus. Microvasc Res. 2017;112:41–6. https://doi.org/10.1016/j.mvr.2017.03.001.
6. Natalello G, De Luca G, Gigante L, Campochiaro C, De Lorenzis E, Verardi L, Paglionico A, Petricca L, Martone AM, Calvisi S, Ripa M, Cavalli G, Della-Torre E, Tresoldi M, Landi F, Bosello SL, Gremese E, Dagna L. Nailfold capillaroscopy findings in patients with coronavirus disease 2019: broadening the spectrum of COVID-19 microvascular involvement. Microvasc Res. 2021;133:104071. https://doi.org/10.1016/j.mvr.2020.104071.
7. Orlando G, Molon B, Viola A, Alaibac M, Angioni R, Piaserico S. Psoriasis and cardiovascular diseases: an immune-mediated cross talk? Front Immunol. 2022;13:868277. https://doi.org/10.3389/fimmu.2022.868277.
8. Sapozhnikov M, Rehman M, Johnson C, Daich J, Salciccioli L, Gillette P, Lazar JM. Characterization of microvascular disease in patients with sickle cell disease using nailfold capillaroscopy. Microvasc Res. 2019;125:103877. https://doi.org/10.1016/j.mvr.2019.04.007.
9. Lambova SN, Muller-Ladner U. Nailfold capillaroscopy within and beyond the scope of connective tissue diseases. Curr Rheumatol Rev. 2018;14(1):12–21. https://doi.org/10.2174/1573397113666170615093600.

10. Lim MWS, Setjiadi D, Dobbin SJH, Lang NN, Delles C, Connelly PJ. Nailfold videocapillaroscopy in the study of cardiovascular disease: a systematic review. Blood Press Monit. 2023;28(1):24–32. https://doi.org/10.1097/MBP.0000000000000624.
11. Tibiriçá E, Lorenzo A, Oliveira GMM. Microcirculation and cardiovascular diseases. Arq Bras Cardiol. 2018;111(2):120–1. https://doi.org/10.5935/abc.20180149.
12. Bonacci E, Santacroce N, D'Amico N, Mattace R. Nail-fold capillaroscopy in the study of microcirculation in elderly hypertensive patients. Arch Gerontol Geriatr. 1996;22(Suppl 1):79–83. https://doi.org/10.1016/0167-4943(96)86918-4.
13. Smits AJ, Isebia K, Combee-Duffy C, et al. Low nailfold capillary density in patients with pulmonary arterial hypertension and chronic thromboembolic pulmonary hypertension: biomarker of clinical outcome? Sci Rep. 2024;14:19467. https://doi.org/10.1038/s41598-024-69017-y.
14. Corrado A, Correale M, Mansueto N, Monaco I, Carriero A, Mele A, Colia R, Di Biase M, Cantatore FP. Nailfold capillaroscopic changes in patients with idiopathic pulmonary arterial hypertension and systemic sclerosis-related pulmonary arterial hypertension. Microvasc Res. 2017;114:46–51. https://doi.org/10.1016/j.mvr.2017.06.005.
15. Chen Y, Ren M, Wang C, et al. Abnormal peripheral microcirculation by nailfold videocapillaroscopy reveals severity of atherosclerosis in coronary heart disease. Sci Rep. 2025;15:22283. https://doi.org/10.1038/s41598-025-03471-0.
16. He W, Zhang M, Mao R, Han C, Shi L, Wu H. Association between nailfold capillaroscopic findings and diabetes: a systematic review and meta-analysis. Acta Diabetol. 2025;62:983.
17. Pazos-Moura CC, Moura EG, Bouskela E, Torres-Filho IP, Breitenbach MM. Nailfold capillaroscopy in diabetes mellitus: morphological abnormalities and relationship with microangiopathy. Braz J Med Biol Res. 1987;20(6):777–80.
18. Okabe T, Kunikata H, Yasuda M, Kodama S, Maeda Y, Nakano J, Takeno D, Fuse N, Nakazawa T. Relationship between nailfold capillaroscopy parameters and the severity of diabetic retinopathy. Graefes Arch Clin Exp Ophthalmol. 2024;262(3):759–68. https://doi.org/10.1007/s00417-023-06220-z.
19. Rohit R, Neha C, Shruti B, Shivani V, Kumar KN, Ravi K. Correlation of nailfold capillaroscopic changes using handheld dermatoscope with varying grades and severity of diabetic retinopathy in patients with type 2 diabetes mellitus: a pilot observational cross-sectional analytical study. J Clin Ophthalmol Res. 2025;13(1):48–56. https://doi.org/10.4103/jcor.jcor_91_24.
20. Abd El-Khalik DM, Hafez EA, Hassan HE, Mahmoud AE, Ashour DM, Morshedy NA. Nail folds capillaries abnormalities associated with type 2 diabetes mellitus progression and correlation with diabetic retinopathy. Clin Med Insights Endocrinol Diabetes. 2022;15:11795514221122828. https://doi.org/10.1177/11795514221122828.
21. Maldonado G, Paredes C, Roberto G, Ríos C. Nailfold Capillaroscopy a non-invasive tool for direct observation of microvascular damage in diabetes mellitus: review. JSM Atheroscler. 2017;2(4):1037.
22. Gotelli E, Campitiello R, Pizzorni C, Sammorì S, Aitella E, Ginaldi L, De Martinis M, Carubbi F, Di Ruscio E, Cuomo G, Martinelli E, Marrone S, De Angelis R, Giuggioli D, Guiducci S, Ingegnoli F, Riccieri V, Sebastiani M, Sulli A, Smith V, Cutolo M, Study Group on Capillaroscopy and Microcirculation in Rheumatic Diseases of the Italian Society of Rheumatology (CAPSIR). Multicentre retrospective detection of nailfold videocapillaroscopy abnormalities in long covid patients. RMD Open. 2025;11(2):e005469. https://doi.org/10.1136/rmdopen-2025-005469.
23. Ackermann M, Verleden SE, Kuehnel M, Haverich A, Welte T, Laenger F, Vanstapel A, Werlein C, Stark H, Tzankov A, Li WW, Li VW, Mentzer SJ, Jonigk D. Pulmonary vascular endothelialitis, thrombosis, and angiogenesis in Covid-19. N Engl J Med. 2020;383(2):120–8. https://doi.org/10.1056/NEJMoa2015432.
24. Pretorius E, Vlok M, Venter C, Bezuidenhout JA, Laubscher GJ, Steenkamp J, Kell DB. Persistent clotting protein pathology in Long COVID/Post-Acute Sequelae of

COVID-19 (PASC) is accompanied by increased levels of antiplasmin. Cardiovasc Diabetol. 2021;20(1):172. https://doi.org/10.1186/s12933-021-01359-7.
25. Mondini L, Confalonieri P, Pozzan R, Ruggero L, Trotta L, Lerda S, Hughes M, Bellan M, Confalonieri M, Ruaro B, Salton F, Tavano S. Microvascular alteration in COVID-19 documented by Nailfold Capillaroscopy. Diagnostics (Basel). 2023;13(11):1905. https://doi.org/10.3390/diagnostics13111905.
26. Senet P, Fichel F, Baudot N, Gaitz JP, Tribout L, Frances C. La capillaroscopie péri-unguéale en dermatologie [Nail-fold capillaroscopy in dermatology]. Ann Dermatol Venereol. 2014;141(6–7):429–37. French. https://doi.org/10.1016/j.annder.2014.04.120.
27. Bardehle F, Sies K, Enk A, Rosenberger A, Fink C, Haenssle H. Nailfold videocapillaroscopy identifies microvascular pathologies in psoriasis vulgaris: results of a prospective controlled study. J Dtsch Dermatol Ges. 2021;19(12):1736–44. https://doi.org/10.1111/ddg.14606.
28. Prioteasă OG, Bobircă A, Anghel D, Groşeanu ML, Bojincă VC. Nailfold videocapillaroscopic changes in patients with psoriatic arthritis: a systematic review. Biomed Rep. 2025;23(2):130. https://doi.org/10.3892/br.2025.2008.
29. Khafagy NH, EL-Khateeb EA, Aidaros MA. Correlation of nail capillary morphology with metabolic syndrome and disease severity in psoriatic patients. QJM Int J Med. 2024;117(Sup plement_2):hcae175.217. https://doi.org/10.1093/qjmed/hcae175.217.
30. Elmesiry AM, Mahmoud SA, Mohamed MS, Aly H, Elmotaleb YA, Ghit MM, Ibrahim AS, Elazab SA, Mokhtar M, Rageh EA, Moussa MA, Ismail S, El Zokm SM, Hamoud H. Nailfold capillaroscopy findings in patients with psoriasis vulgaris and different domains of psoriatic arthritis. J Psoriasis Psoriatic Arthritis. 2024;9(3):89–97. https://doi.org/10.1177/24755303241238988.
31. Gerkowicz A, Krasowska D, Pietrzak A, Michalak-Stoma A, Bartosińska J, Juszkiewicz-Borowiec M, Chodorowska G. Videocapillaroscopic alterations in alopecia areata. Biomed Res Int. 2013;2013:160203. https://doi.org/10.1155/2013/160203.
32. Dong LB, Wei YZ, Lan GP, Chen JT, Xu JJ, Qin J, An L, Tan HS, Huang YP. High resolution imaging and quantification of the nailfold microvasculature using optical coherence tomography angiography (OCTA) and capillaroscopy: a preliminary study in healthy subjects. Quant Imaging Med Surg. 2022;12(3):1844–58. https://doi.org/10.21037/qims-21-672.
33. Smith V, Ickinger C, Hysa E, Snow M, Frech T, Sulli A, Cutolo M. Nailfold capillaroscopy. Best Pract Res Clin Rheumatol. 2023;37(1):101849. https://doi.org/10.1016/j.berh.2023.101849.
34. Cheung AT, Chen PC, Larkin EC, Duong PL, Ramanujam S, Tablin F, Wun T. Microvascular abnormalities in sickle cell disease: a computer-assisted intravital microscopy study. Blood. 2002;99(11):3999–4005. https://doi.org/10.1182/blood.v99.11.3999.
35. Bharara R, Browne R, Seydafkan S, Salciccioli L, Rehman M, Zhang Y, Tena M, Malhi P, Hanono M, Chen SX, Daich J, Lazar JM. Characterization of microvascular disease in pediatric sickle cell disease using nailfold capillaroscopy. Microvasc Res. 2021;136:104150. https://doi.org/10.1016/j.mvr.2021.104150.
36. Ersozlu ED, Bakirci S, Sunu C, Ertürk Z, Açıkgöz SB, Tamer A. Use of nailfold video capillaroscopy in polycythemia vera. Arch Rheumatol. 2021;37(3):404–10. https://doi.org/10.46497/ArchRheumatol.2022.9271.
37. Nigro A. Reversibility of acrocyanosis and improvement of capillaroscopic pattern in a patient with polycythemia vera treated with ruxolitinib: a case report. Blood Res. 2025;60:8. https://doi.org/10.1007/s44313-024-00053-3.
38. Adel H, Eldeeb AA, Hamdy F. Nailfold capillaroscopic changes in patients with glomerular diseases. Reumatol Clin (Engl Ed). 2025;21(1):101803. https://doi.org/10.1016/j.reumae.2025.101803.
39. Jangid S, Madke B, Balwani M. A cross-sectional case-control study of nailfold capillaroscopy changes in patients with chronic kidney disease in tertiary care hospital in Central India [version 1; peer review: awaiting peer review]. F1000Res. 2024;13:322. https://doi.org/10.12688/f1000research.147712.1.

40. Schoina M, Loutradis C, Memmos E, Dimitroulas T, Pagkopoulou E, Doumas M, Karagiannis A, Garyfallos A, Papagianni A, Sarafidis P. Microcirculatory function deteriorates with advancing stages of chronic kidney disease independently of arterial stiffness and atherosclerosis. Hypertens Res. 2021;44(2):179–87. https://doi.org/10.1038/s41440-020-0525-y.
41. Querfeld U, Mak RH, Pries AR. Microvascular disease in chronic kidney disease: the base of the iceberg in cardiovascular comorbidity. Clin Sci (Lond). 2020;134(12):1333–56. https://doi.org/10.1042/CS20200279.
42. Theodorakopoulou MP, Dipla K, Zafeiridis A, Sarafidis P. Endothelial and microvascular function in CKD: evaluation methods and associations with outcomes. Eur J Clin Investig. 2021;51(8):e13557. https://doi.org/10.1111/eci.13557.
43. Theodorakopoulou MP, Schoina M, Sarafidis P. Assessment of endothelial and microvascular function in CKD: older and newer techniques, associated risk factors, and relations with outcomes. Am J Nephrol. 2020;51(12):931–49. https://doi.org/10.1159/000512263.
44. Suzuki H, Nagano H, Kawagoe K, Miura I, Masamoto K. A non-invasive approach to monitoring microcirculatory health before and after hemodialysis in renal patients using nailfold video capillaroscopy with optical reflectance analysis. GeroScience. 2025;47:6473–86. https://doi.org/10.1007/s11357-025-01700-y.
45. Mansueto N, Rotondo C, Corrado A, Cantatore FP. Nailfold capillaroscopy: a comprehensive review on common findings and clinical usefulness in non-rheumatic disease. J Med Investig. 2021;68(1.2):6–14. https://doi.org/10.2152/jmi.68.6.
46. Ingegnoli F, Sciascera A, D'Ingianna E, Fantini F. Systemic sclerosis, capillary leak syndrome and nasopharyngeal carcinoma: an unusual association or paraneoplastic manifestations? Rheumatology (Oxford). 2009;48(2):201–2. https://doi.org/10.1093/rheumatology/ken422.
47. Lambova S, Müller-Ladner U. Capillaroscopic pattern in paraneoplastic Raynaud's phenomenon. Rheumatol Int. 2013;33(6):1597–9. https://doi.org/10.1007/s00296-010-1715-8.
48. Coschignano MA, De Ciuceis C, Agabiti-Rosei C, Brami V, Rossini C, Chiarini G, Malerba P, Famà F, Cosentini D, Muiesan ML, Salvetti M, Petelca A, Capellini S, Arnoldi C, Nardin M, Grisanti S, Rizzoni D, Berruti A, Paini A. Microvascular structural alterations in cancer patients treated with antiangiogenic drugs. Front Cardiovasc Med. 2021;8:651594. https://doi.org/10.3389/fcvm.2021.651594.
49. Steeghs N, Rabelink TJ, Op't Roodt J, Batman E, Cluitmans FH, Weijl NI, de Koning E, Gelderblom H. Reversibility of capillary density after discontinuation of bevacizumab treatment. Ann Oncol. 2010;21(5):1100–5. https://doi.org/10.1093/annonc/mdp417.

Chapter 12
Interpretation of Findings

Francesca Motta, Antonio Tonutti, and Maria De Santis

Introduction

Nailfold videocapillaroscopy (NVC) is a noninvasive, highly informative imaging technique that allows clinicians and researchers to visualize and assess the microvascular architecture at the nailfold bed. This standardized method is capable of providing detailed, high-resolution images of the capillary network, as shown in the previous chapters.

The microcirculation, comprising the smallest blood vessels such as capillaries, arterioles, and venules, plays a crucial role in tissue perfusion, nutrient exchange, and immune response. Alterations in microvascular structure and function are fundamental to the pathogenesis of numerous diseases, particularly connective tissue disorders. In these conditions, microvascular damage often precedes overt clinical manifestations, making early detection and monitoring of microvascular changes crucial for diagnosis, prognosis, and therapeutic decision-making.

NVC has emerged as an indispensable tool in the evaluation of patients with Raynaud's phenomenon and suspected or established scleroderma spectrum disorder diseases, where characteristic microvascular abnormalities serve as early hallmarks of the disease and correlate with clinical severity. Beyond systemic sclerosis, NVC findings have been documented in other connective tissue diseases, such as dermatomyositis and mixed connective tissue disease, reflecting the commonality of microvascular involvement across these conditions, despite differences suggesting divergent features in disease pathogenesis. Its non-invasive nature, coupled with

F. Motta · A. Tonutti · M. De Santis (✉)
Rheumatology and Clinical Immunology, IRCCS Humanitas Research Hospital, Rozzano, Milan, Italy

Department of Biomedical Sciences, Humanitas University, Pieve Emanuele, Milan, Italy
e-mail: francesca.motta2@humanitas.it; antonio.tonutti@humanitas.it; maria.de_santis@hunimed.eu

Y. El Miedany, R. A. Elziaty (eds.), *Capillaroscopy*, Contemporary Rheumatology,
https://doi.org/10.1007/978-3-032-22966-3_12

the ability to repeat assessments over time, makes NVC particularly valuable for longitudinal disease monitoring.

The technique involves the use of digital videocapillaroscopes to magnify the nailfold capillaries, enabling detailed evaluation of their morphology, density, and blood flow. Standardized scoring systems have been developed to categorize patterns observed, aiding in clinical interpretation and research consistency. NVC findings have both diagnostic and prognostic relevance, as certain capillaroscopic patterns and lesions are associated with disease progression, organ involvement, and response to therapy.

Despite many advantages, the interpretation of NVC images requires expertise and experience, since variability in findings can occur due to technical factors, environmental conditions, and individual patient characteristics, underscoring the need for standardized procedures and training. Nonetheless, the growing body of literature supports the utility of NVC as a window into the microvascular alterations underlying various connective tissue diseases.

This chapter aims to provide a comprehensive overview of the findings obtainable through NVC, their clinical significance, and the interpretive frameworks that help clinicians utilize this technique effectively. By understanding the microvascular patterns and their implications, healthcare providers can improve disease diagnosis, monitor progression, and tailor therapeutic strategies more precisely, ultimately enhancing patient care.

Technical Aspects of NVC

To ensure accurate, reproducible, and clinically meaningful results, it is essential to understand the technical components and standardized procedures involved in performing NVC.

Modern NVC employs digital videocapillaroscopes equipped with high-resolution cameras capable of magnifications ranging from 200× to 600×. These devices utilize optical zoom and focus adjustments to optimize image clarity. Some systems are integrated with computer software that facilitates image capture, storage, and analysis. Light sources, often LED-based, provide uniform illumination to enhance capillary visualization without causing discomfort or heat effects.

Prior to examination, the patient should be seated comfortably in a warm room (around 20–25 °C) to promote vasodilation and improve capillary visibility. The examined hand (typically the second to fifth fingers) is positioned palm-up, with the fingers slightly abducted and extended. The examiner ensures that the nailfolds are clean and free from nail polish or lotions, as these can interfere with image clarity. A drop of immersion oil or mineral oil is applied to the nailfold to reduce light refraction and improve optical clarity.

The procedure involves selecting the distal row of nailfold capillaries, which are the most superficial and accessible. The examiner focuses the camera on the proximal nail fold of each finger, capturing multiple images (usually 3–5 per finger) to account for within-site variability. Consistency in imaging location, magnification, and lighting conditions is crucial across sessions to allow reliable comparisons over time.

Captured images are analyzed visually or via specialized software to assess capillary morphology (e.g., shape, size, and architecture), density (number of capillaries per millimeter), and blood flow. Standardized scoring systems, such as the Cutolo or Maricq classifications or the EULAR fast-track algorithm, categorize patterns as normal, nonspecific, or abnormal [1–4]. Quantitative measures, including capillary density, giant capillary count, and hemorrhage frequency, are often recorded to facilitate objective assessment.

Inter- and intra-observer variability can influence NVC results. Thus, rigorous training and adherence to standardized protocols are vital for clinicians and technicians. Recent advances, including automated image analysis and machine learning algorithms, will aim to reduce subjectivity and improve consistency.

In summary, meticulous attention to equipment setup, patient preparation, imaging protocol, and analysis methodology ensures that NVC provides reliable, reproducible, and clinically valuable data about microvascular health.

All the images presented in this chapter belong to the personal archive of Professor Maria De Santis.

Normal NVC Findings

In healthy individuals, NVC reveals a characteristic and highly organized microvascular architecture that reflects normal physiological microcirculation. Understanding these baseline features is essential for distinguishing between normal variations and pathological changes observed in disease states.

The typical capillary net in healthy subjects exhibits a uniform, hairpin-shaped, or looped structure (Fig. 12.1). These capillaries are elongated, with a diameter generally ranging from 7 to 9 mm, and feature a well-defined, narrow lumen with minimal variation in shape or size. The capillary loops are arranged in an ordered and parallel fashion, radiating from the nailfold bed, with a density ranging from approximately 7 to 15 capillaries per millimeter, with an average of about 8–12 per mm. Minimal or absent pericapillary edema can be observed; blood flow is

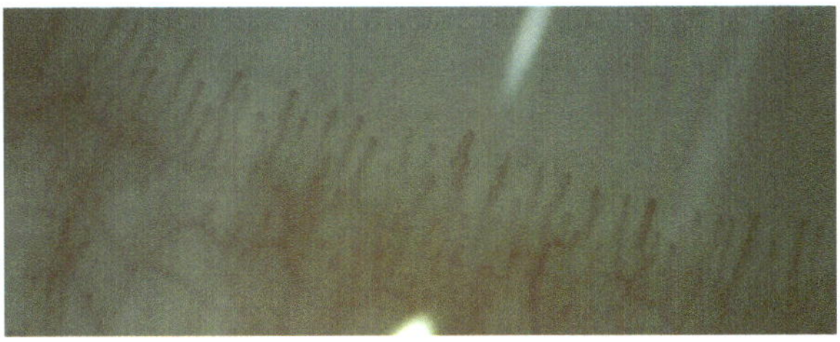

Fig. 12.1 Normal NVC pattern

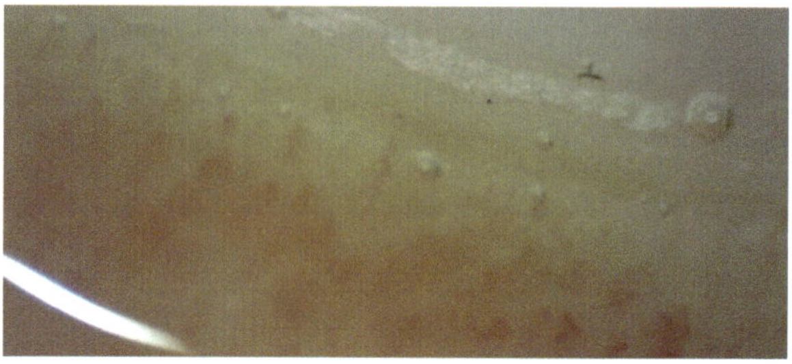

Fig. 12.2 Apparently reduced capillary density in a patient undergoing repeated manicures; the capillaries are shortened and tortuous, but findings are overall still suggestive of normality

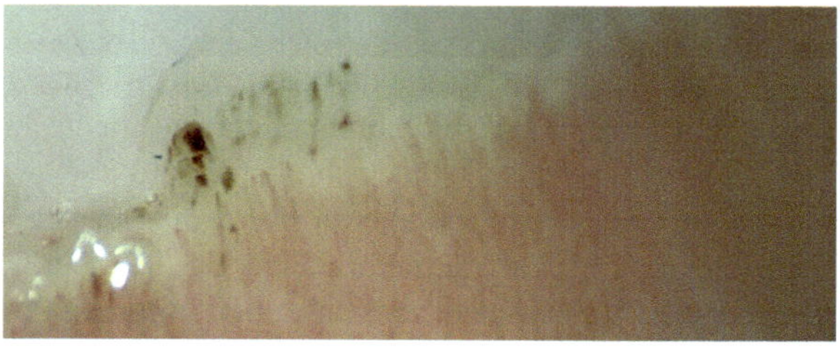

Fig. 12.3 Meta-traumatic microhemorrhages; the reader should note their occurrence within a normal NVC picture in the absence of suspicious elements

continuous. The subpapillary venous plexus, from which the capillaries originate or terminate, is visible in 10–30% of healthy subjects.

A hallmark of normal microvascular architecture is the consistent and adequate capillary density, supporting sufficient tissue perfusion and reflecting the intact, functional microvascular network. A decrease below 7 capillaries per millimeter is a pathologic feature suggesting microvascular compromise; nevertheless, some variation can be observed in normal individuals, depending on age, skin pigmentation, and environmental factors, such as repeated manicures (Fig. 12.2) or manual occupations.

Normal capillaries exhibit continuous and unobstructed blood flow, with no evidence of stasis or sluggish circulation. The flow appears smooth and uniform within each loop, and capillaries are well perfused during the examination. Capillary loops are typically evenly spaced, with no prominent hemorrhages or microbleeds, indicating vessel integrity and absence of fragility. Meta-traumatic microhemorrhages can be found (Fig. 12.3).

While the above features represent the typical normal findings, minor variations can occur. Occasionally, morphologic deviations such as slight tortuosity, mild irregularity, or enlargement are considered within normal limits, especially in children and older adults or in certain ethnic groups. In particular, these variations are considered within the spectrum of normality when not accompanied by other pathological features. In some cases, diffuse and homogeneous minor aspecific alterations can be found in normal subjects, such as diffuse tortuosity and enlargement (Fig. 12.4) and capillaries diffusely shortened (Fig. 12.5) or elongated (Fig. 12.6). Generally, diffuse and homogeneous minor aspecific alterations can be considered normal.

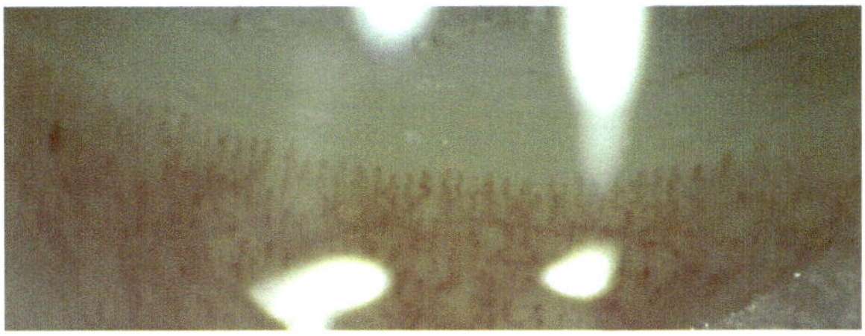

Fig. 12.4 Diffuse tortuosity and homogeneous ectasias. Please note that the subpapillary venous plexus is visible herein

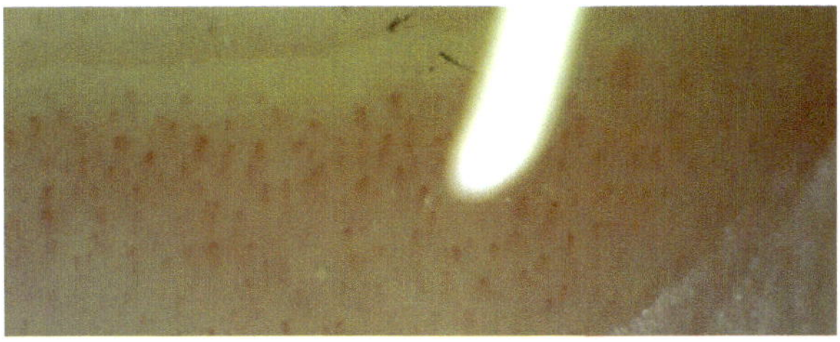

Fig. 12.5 Diffuse shortened capillaries

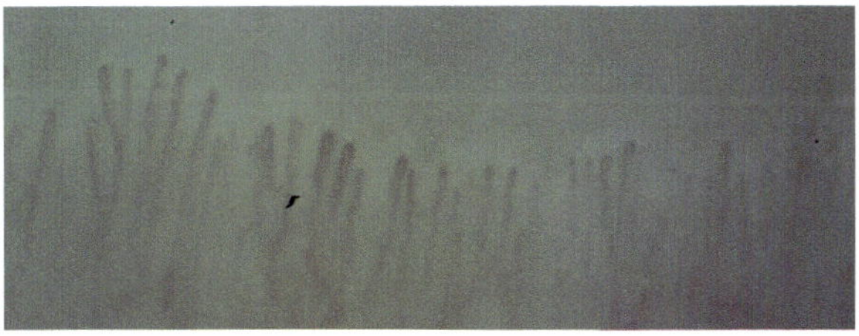

Fig. 12.6 Diffuse elongated capillaries

It is crucial for the clinician to recognize normal features in order to provide a baseline against which pathological changes can be identified, aiding early diagnosis and monitoring of microvascular involvement in various diseases [5–7].

Pathological Capillaroscopic Findings

By providing a window into the microvascular architecture, NVC reveals not only normal features but also a range of pathological alterations that reflect underlying disease processes. Recognizing these abnormalities is crucial for disease diagnosis, staging, and monitoring. In the context of systemic sclerosis, these findings often follow characteristic specific patterns, but similar alterations and patterns can also be present in other connective tissue diseases and inflammatory conditions. This section provides an in-depth overview of the key pathological features, their classifications, and their clinical significance.

Edema and Flow Alterations

Both reversible endothelial damage and inflammation lead to capillary leakage with consequent pericapillary edema. Edema is an aspecific finding, common in both primary and secondary Raynaud's phenomenon (Figs. 12.7 and 12.8). A granular blood flow appearance, reflecting slow microcirculation, is also frequently found in these contexts (Fig. 12.9). Rarely, the flow may even appear interrupted, with images similar to stationary microthrombi being observable in the capillary bed (Fig. 12.10).

Fig. 12.7 Peripapillary edema in a patient with primary Raynaud's phenomenon

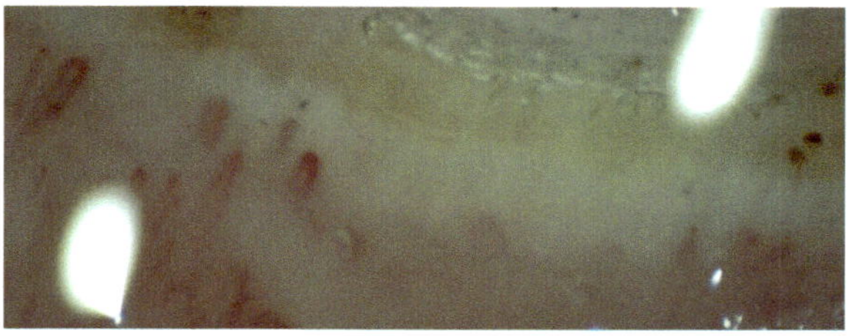

Fig. 12.8 Severe edema in a patient with NVC findings of a scleroderma pattern

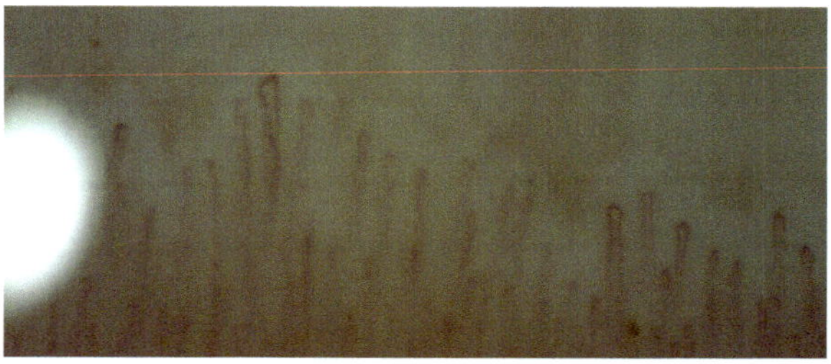

Fig. 12.9 Granular blood flow appearance

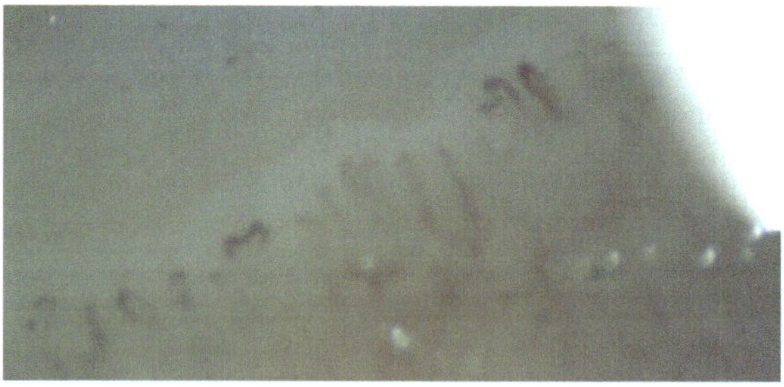

Fig. 12.10 Microthrombi-like appearance

Fig. 12.11 Bizarre capillary shapes and irregular tortuosities in a patient with anti-Ku autoantibodies

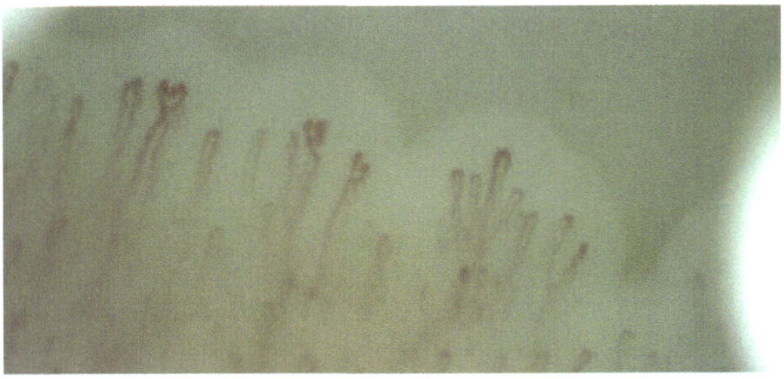

Morphological Abnormalities and Architectural Disorganization

Beyond different individual features, the overall architecture of the capillary bed can be disrupted, leading to irregular arrangements and loss of normal patterning, such as tortuosity (increased vessel twisting and curling) and disorganized capillary loops (loss of orderly distribution, with overlapping or irregular branching). These alterations reflect ongoing microvascular damage and repair, but even if they are often seen in active phases of connective tissue diseases, they do not refer to a specific disease pattern (Fig. 12.11). As previously shown, in some cases, a single alteration can be observed diffusely across all fields; for example, broadly tortuous, dilated, shortened, or elongated capillaries. The regularity in these cases argues against a pathological condition.

Capillary Dilation

Capillary dilation refers to the enlargement of the capillary lumen beyond normal size. Capillary dilation results from endothelial cell activation, inflammation, or structural damage, leading to increased vessel permeability and remodeling. It reflects compensatory angiogenesis or microvascular injury.

Ectasia is a dilation exceeding 20 μm (but less than 50 μm) in diameter and can be focal or diffuse. It can be considered a minor aspecific alteration in the absence of other more specific features (Fig. 12.12). An enlargement of more than 50 μm in diameter is referred to as a microaneurysm if it is focal within the capillary hairpin (Fig. 12.12), while it is defined as a giant capillary if it homogeneously involves all the afferent, loop, and efferent branches of the capillary (Fig. 12.13).

Giant capillaries are characteristic of early and active phases of systemic sclerosis, can be observed prior to tissue ischemia or ulceration, and define the early or active scleroderma pattern, depending on whether they are associated with evidence of capillary loss. Giants are also seen in other diseases belonging to the scleroderma spectrum, mainly dermatomyositis and allied inflammatory myopathies (Fig. 12.14),

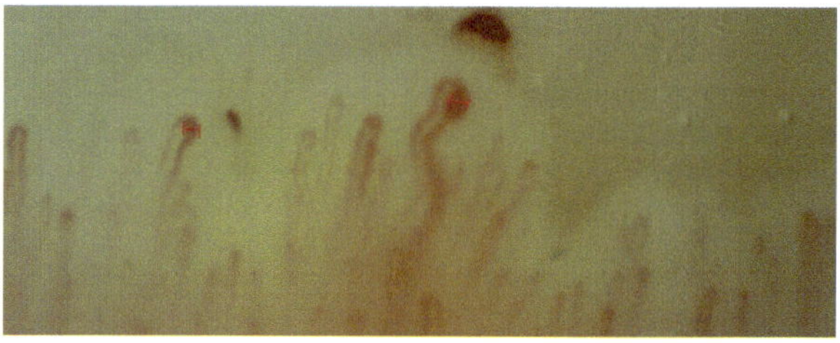

Fig. 12.12 Ectasias and microaneurysms

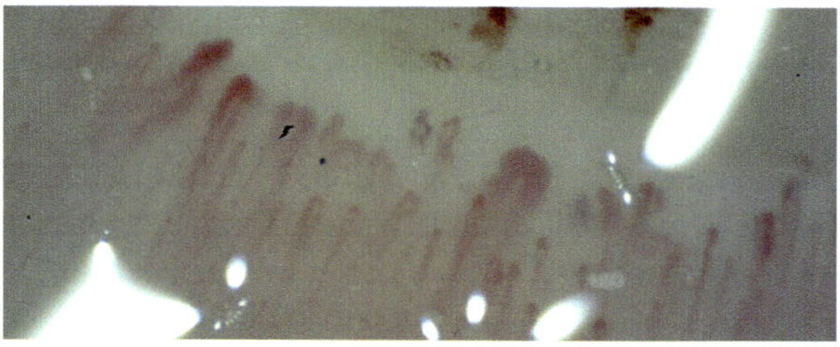

Fig. 12.13 Giant capillaries in the context of an early scleroderma pattern

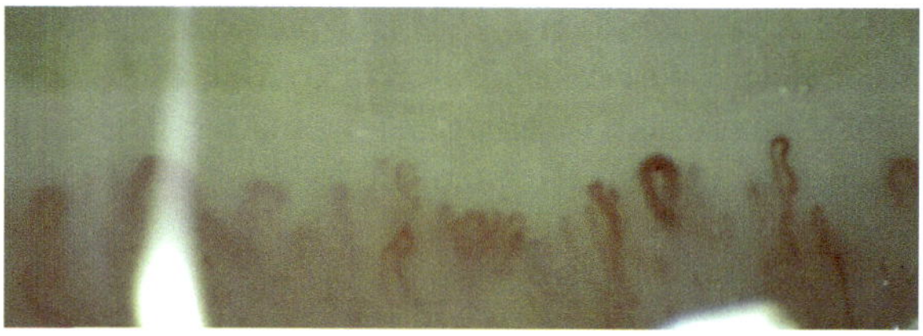

Fig. 12.14 Giant capillaries, reduced capillary density, and neoangiogenesis in a patient with anti-Pm/Scl-positive dermatomyositis

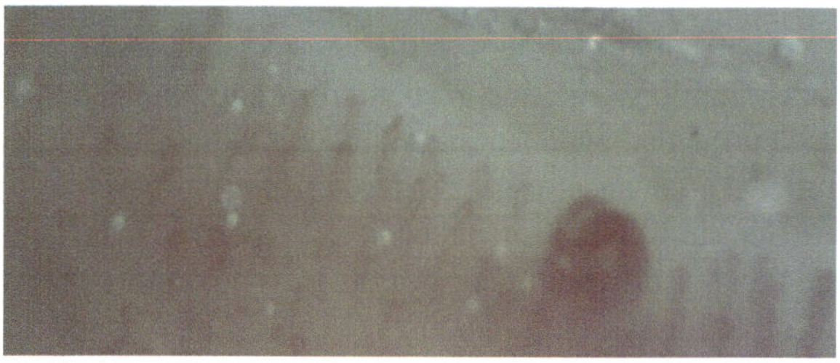

Fig. 12.15 An isolated giant capillary in a patient with primary Raynaud's phenomenon (i.e., persistently negative clinical evolution and absence of antinuclear and specific autoantibodies)

mixed connective tissue disease, and overlapping conditions. Nevertheless, anecdotally, isolated giant capillaries can be observed in usually unrelated conditions, as is the case with primary Raynaud's phenomenon (Fig. 12.15) or morphea (Fig. 12.16). While evidence of giants should prompt further investigation in these contexts, their evolutionary potential is poorly defined.

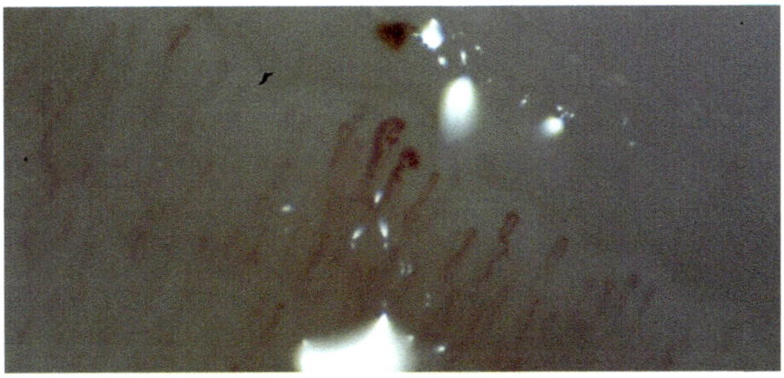

Fig. 12.16 A giant capillary and a microaneurysm in a patient with morphea and negative serum autoantibodies

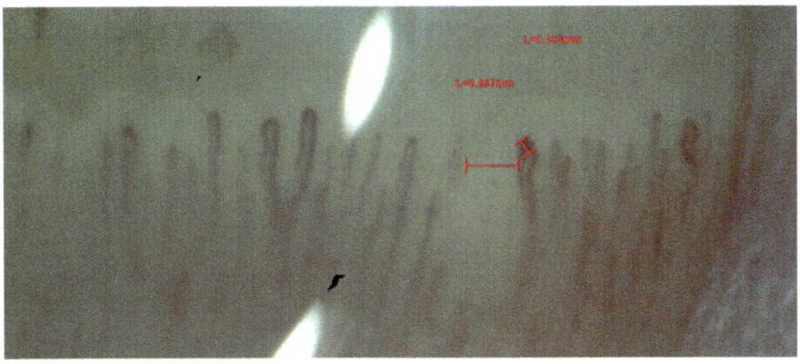

Fig. 12.17 An empty papilla and a microaneurysm

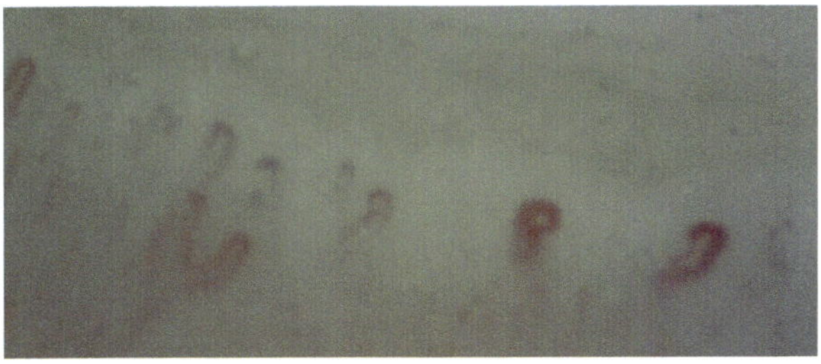

Fig. 12.18 Avascular areas that, together with giant capillaries, define an active scleroderma pattern

Capillary Dropout

Capillary dropout refers to the loss of capillaries, leading to areas devoid of visible microvessels. Empty papillae are areas less than 500 μm with missing capillaries (i.e., generally less than 2 missing "hairpins" within the expected normal architecture; Fig. 12.17) and can also be found in nonpathological contexts. If they are not associated with other major alterations and do not lead to reduced capillary density, empty papillae are aspecific findings. On the other hand, avascular areas are defined if capillary dropout exceeds 500 μm in extent (2 or more missing capillaries; Fig. 12.18). These regions appear as large, empty spaces on capillaroscopic images and represent a highly suspicious finding.

Repeated injury, endothelial apoptosis, or fibrosis causes capillary destruction. The loss of capillaries impairs tissue perfusion, resulting in ischemia. Avascular areas correlate with disease progression, tissue ulceration, and organ involvement in systemic sclerosis. They are a hallmark of systemic sclerosis progressing from active to late stage and indicate irreversible microvascular damage.

Neoangiogenesis

Neoangiogenesis describes the formation of new, often abnormal, blood vessels arising to replace preexisting capillaries that have undergone apoptosis. These new vessels appear as ramified, bushy, or bushy-like formations with multiple branches and irregular shapes, often arising directly from the subpapillary venous plexus. They result from endothelial activation and hypoxia, which in turn stimulate angiogenic pathways (e.g., VEGF expression). However, such neo-vessels are structurally abnormal, fragile, and inefficient. Neoangiogenesis indicates ongoing microvascular repair and active disease. They can be seen in the late scleroderma pattern but more frequently in dermatomyositis patients, where they tend to reflect active cutaneous and vascular inflammation (Fig. 12.19). Neoangiogenesis can also be found in nonpathological contexts, particularly if not associated with major alterations or when present as single lesions (Fig. 12.20).

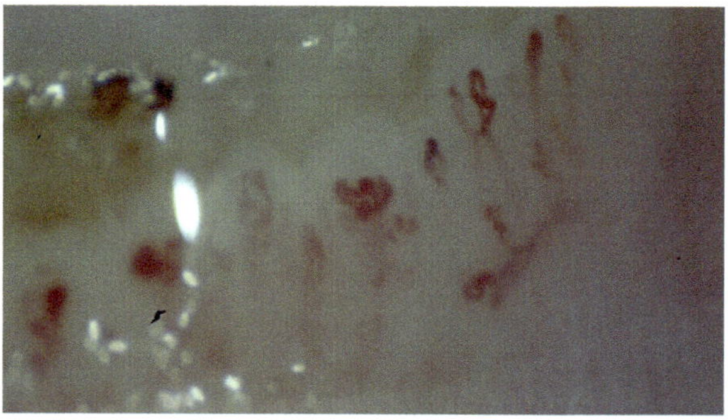

Fig. 12.19 Neoangiogenesis in a dermatomyositis patient

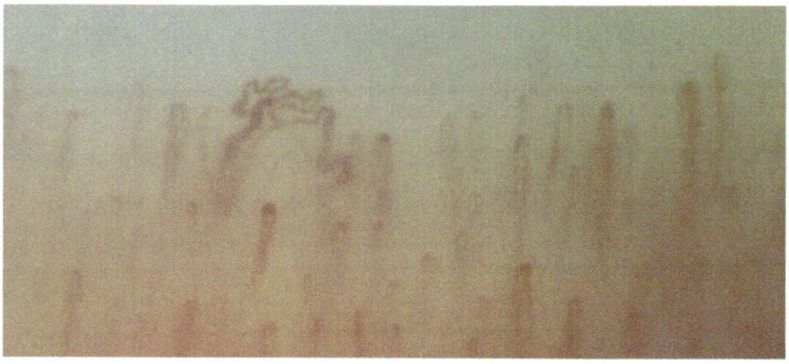

Fig. 12.20 An isolated neoangiogenesis in a patient with an otherwise normal NVC pattern

Hemorrhages and Microbleeds

Microhemorrhages appear as punctate or linear dark spots on NVC images, reflecting extravasation of blood from fragile or damaged capillaries. They are often associated with dilated or tortuous vessels.

Fragile vessel walls due to endothelial damage or inflammation lead to leakage. Capillary rupture can also occur in areas of neoangiogenesis. The presence of hemorrhages indicates capillary fragility and active vascular injury and correlates with disease activity. Microhemorrhages are common in systemic sclerosis and dermatomyositis but can also be observed in association with other microangiopathies, as in the case of systemic lupus erythematosus, particularly when associated with the presence of antiphospholipid antibodies (Fig. 12.21). Less often, microhemorrhages are found as aspecific findings in patients with Raynaud's phenomenon or undifferentiated connective tissue disease (Fig. 12.22).

Fig. 12.21 Microhemorrhages in a lupus patient with antiphospholipid antibodies

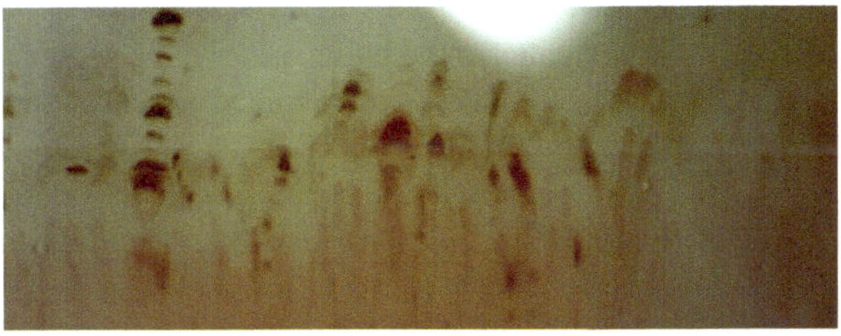

Fig. 12.22 Microhemorrhages in a patient with Raynaud's phenomenon and positive ANA

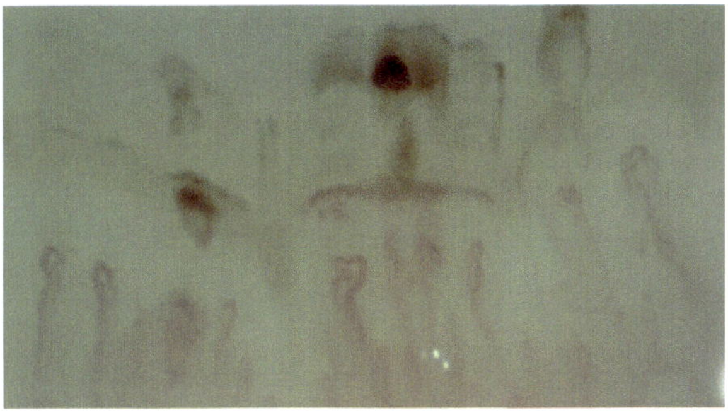

Classification of Pathological Patterns

Based on the combination and severity of these findings, capillaroscopic abnormalities are classified into distinct patterns:

(a) Normal pattern: uniform, hairpin-shaped, or elongated capillaries with a diameter of 7–9 μm.

Dense, evenly spaced loops with a density of 7–15 capillaries per millimeter. No significant hemorrhages (none-rare), papillary loss (none-rare), dilations (none-rare), tortuosities (none-rare), or architectural disorganization. Blood flow appears smooth and unobstructed; absent edema.

(b) Minor aspecific changes: minimal edema, irregular flow, capillaries with irregular shapes, such as tortuosity, dilated loops, minimal capillary loss (<2), and microhemorrhages, but generally preserved architecture.

(c) Major aspecific changes: altered architecture with presence of microaneurysms (but not giant capillaries), empty papillae (but not avascular areas), and diffuse microhemorrhages (Fig. 12.23);

(d) Scleroderma pattern: the hallmarks are the presence of giant capillaries (in the distal row) and evidence of reduced vascular density (<7 capillaries/mm) or avascular areas (Fig. 12.24). These findings are not specific to systemic sclerosis and can be easily found in the so-called "scleroderma spectrum disorders," such as dermatomyositis, anti-synthetase syndrome, anti-MDA5 and anti-Ku positive connective tissue diseases, mixed connective tissue disease, and overlapping diseases. In systemic sclerosis, a temporal variation can be observed

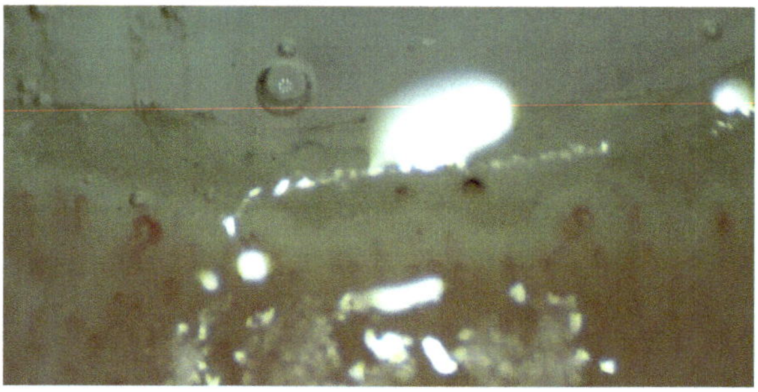

Fig. 12.23 An empty papilla and a microaneurysm in a patient with Raynaud's phenomenon and positive ANA

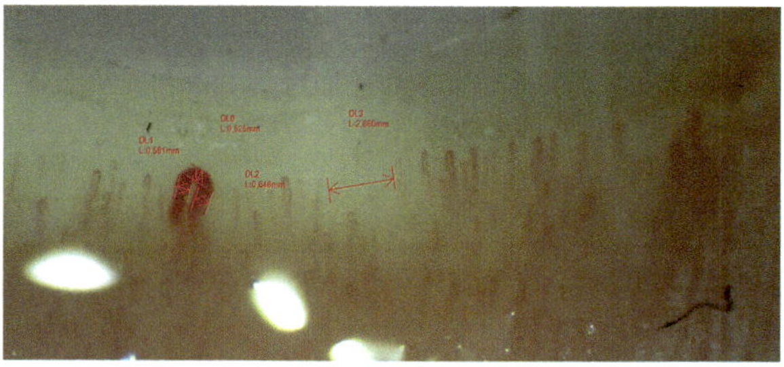

Fig. 12.24 A giant capillary and an avascular area in a scleroderma patient

with few giant capillaries but preserved capillary density characterizing the early scleroderma pattern, while the coexistence of giant capillaries and avascular areas is seen in the active pattern, and extensive capillary loss with no residual giant capillaries characterizes the late scleroderma pattern.

Clinical Implications of NVC Findings

NVC has emerged as a crucial tool in the management of autoimmune and connective tissue diseases, owing to its ability to visualize microvascular alterations directly. The clinical relevance of capillaroscopic findings extends beyond mere morphological descriptions, impacting diagnosis, prognostication, and therapeutic monitoring.

One of the primary applications of NVC is its role in early and differential diagnosis of systemic sclerosis and related disorders. In the appropriate clinical context, the evidence of a scleroderma pattern, along with the presence of a significant number of microaneurysms, microhemorrhages, empty papillae, and neoangiogenesis, are highly suggestive of scleroderma spectrum disorders and can aid in intercepting patients in preclinical phases, such as before the manifestation of puffy hands, skin thickening, digital vasculopathy, or organ involvement. For instance, this is the case of patients complaining of Raynaud's phenomenon (or equivalent symptoms) associated with antinuclear or specific autoantibody findings.

Moreover, NVC aids in differentiating primary Raynaud's phenomenon (a benign condition) from secondary Raynaud's, which is associated with underlying (or high risk of developing) connective tissue disease. The absence of major aspecific lesions and scleroderma patterns in primary Raynaud's makes NVC a valuable screening and diagnostic adjunct, reducing the need for invasive or costly investigations.

The microvascular abnormalities observed via NVC are not static but often reflect a transient state in the disease progression. For instance, the progression from an early to late capillaroscopic pattern in systemic sclerosis correlates with increasing disease severity and risk of internal organ involvement. In particular, the presence of an active scleroderma pattern indicates ongoing vascular injury, often associated with inflammatory activity, and extensive capillary dropout and neoangiogenesis have been reported to predict the occurrence of pulmonary arterial hypertension. Furthermore, NVC is revealed as an important prognostic tool. The extent of capillary loss and the development of avascular zones strongly correlate with the risk of digital ulcers, tissue ischemia, and pulmonary arterial hypertension. Several longitudinal studies have shown that capillaroscopic progression across different patterns predicts worse clinical outcomes.

NVC also plays a pivotal role in monitoring therapeutic efficacy, since microvascular abnormalities can improve, stabilize, or deteriorate over time, providing real-time feedback on the impact of treatment. For example, vasodilator therapies, immunosuppressants, or targeted treatments aimed at reducing vascular injury can lead to a reduction in hemorrhages and neoangiogenesis, or even partial restoration of capillary architecture. Serial NVC examinations can allow clinicians to detect early signs of microvascular response or failure, enabling timely therapeutic adjustments. A decrease in the number of giant capillaries or microhemorrhages may indicate decreased disease activity, while worsening vascular changes could prompt escalation or modification of treatment. Such dynamic assessment is invaluable, especially in early-stage disease, where intervention can prevent irreversible tissue damage.

Furthermore, NVC can help identify patients at higher risk of complications, guiding preventive measures such as vasodilator therapy to reduce digital ischemia or ulcers. It also provides objective endpoints in clinical trials evaluating new therapies targeting microvascular damage.

In conclusion, capillaroscopic findings have clinical implications in terms of diagnosis and staging of connective tissue diseases. They facilitate early diagnosis and differentiation of connective tissue diseases, serve as biomarkers of disease activity and prognosis, and enable clinicians to monitor treatment responses objectively. As technology advances and standardized scoring systems become more widespread, the integration of NVC into routine clinical practice promises to improve patient outcomes through personalized, timely, and targeted management strategies.

Limitations and Challenges

Despite its role in assessing microvascular involvement in connective tissue diseases, NVC has several limitations that can impact its clinical utility and reproducibility. Addressing these challenges is essential for optimizing its application in both research and routine practice.

One of the primary concerns with NVC is inter- and intra-observer variability. Differences in image acquisition, interpretation, and classification can lead to inconsistent results. Variability may stem from subtle differences in magnification, focus, lighting, and patient positioning. Furthermore, the dynamic nature of microvascular changes, which can fluctuate over time due to environmental factors (temperature, stress) or disease activity, complicates longitudinal assessments. To mitigate this, standardized protocols and classification criteria have been developed, but variability still persists, especially across different centers and operators.

NVC requires trained operators with expertise in capturing high-quality images and interpreting subtle morphological features. The technique's success hinges on the operator's skill in selecting appropriate fingers, positioning the hand, and maintaining consistent imaging conditions. Inexperienced operators may produce suboptimal images, leading to misclassification or oversight of important findings. This dependence on operator skill highlights the need for comprehensive training programs and certification to improve consistency.

Interpreting capillaroscopic images can be challenging due to overlapping features among different diseases or nonspecific findings. For example, minor tortuosity or dilation may be seen in healthy individuals or in aging, making it difficult to distinguish pathological from physiological changes. Additionally, certain features, such as neoangiogenesis or microhemorrhages, may appear in various conditions, reducing specificity. The lack of universally accepted, quantitative scoring systems further complicates interpretation. Advanced image analysis tools and standardized classification schemes aim to address this, but their widespread adoption remains limited.

While high-resolution digital videocapillaroscopes have improved image quality, limitations such as inadequate focus, insufficient magnification, or artifacts from patient movement can affect image clarity. Environmental factors, such as room temperature, can influence microvascular appearance, necessitating controlled conditions during examination.

Some diseases exhibit overlapping capillaroscopic features, making differential diagnosis difficult solely based on morphology. Moreover, early or mild disease may produce subtle changes that are hard to detect, potentially delaying diagnosis.

While NVC is a powerful, noninvasive tool, these limitations highlight the importance of standardized protocols, operator training, and complementary diagnostic approaches. Ongoing technological advances and consensus guidelines are expected to improve reproducibility and interpretation, enhancing their role in clinical practice.

Future Directions in Nailfold Videocapillaroscopy

As the field of microvascular imaging advances, several promising developments are poised to enhance the diagnostic and prognostic utility of NVC. These innovations aim to improve image quality, objectivity, and integration with other diagnostic tools, ultimately broadening their clinical applications.

Emerging imaging modalities, such as high-definition optical coherence tomography (OCT) and super-resolution microscopy, are being explored to achieve even greater detail and deeper tissue visualization. Digital videocapillaroscopes with higher magnification, improved illumination, and real-time image stabilization are helping reduce artifacts and operator dependence. Additionally, the integration of artificial intelligence is enabling automated image acquisition, feature recognition, and classification, reducing subjective variability and increasing reproducibility.

Currently, many capillaroscopic assessments rely on qualitative or semi-quantitative scoring systems, which can be subjective. Future developments focus on fully quantitative analysis, measuring parameters such as capillary density, loop dimensions, tortuosity indices, and hemorrhage counts using computer-aided tools. Such objective metrics facilitate precise disease staging, monitoring progression, and evaluating therapeutic responses. Advanced image processing algorithms capable of automatically extracting these parameters are being developed and validated, paving the way for standardized, reproducible assessments.

Combining NVC with other noninvasive techniques can provide a more comprehensive picture of vascular health. For example, integrating capillaroscopy with laser Doppler flowmetry or optical spectroscopy enables simultaneous assessment of microvascular structure and blood flow dynamics. Additionally, correlating NVC findings with serological markers, high-resolution imaging of internal organs (like echocardiography or pulmonary function tests), and clinical scores can enhance diagnostic accuracy and prognostic predictions. Such multimodal approaches are particularly valuable in complex autoimmune diseases, where microvascular damage is a key feature.

Future research aims to leverage big data and machine learning to identify patterns predictive of disease progression or response to therapy. Longitudinal studies utilizing automated, quantitative NVC metrics could enable personalized treatment strategies and early interventions before irreversible tissue damage occurs.

Efforts are underway to develop universally accepted standards, guidelines, and scoring systems, supported by international collaborations. These initiatives will facilitate multicenter studies, comparison of results, and broader clinical adoption. Incorporating telemedicine and remote image analysis can also expand access to expert assessment in resource-limited settings.

Technological innovations, combined with quantitative, integrated, and standardized approaches, promise to elevate NVC from a mainly descriptive tool to a precise, predictive, and universally applicable modality in vascular and autoimmune disease management [8].

Conclusion

NVC has established itself as a useful, noninvasive tool in the assessment of microvascular health, particularly in connective tissue diseases such as systemic sclerosis. The key findings from NVC include detailed visualization of capillary morphology, density, and blood flow, revealing characteristic patterns such as normal architecture, nonspecific abnormalities, and disease-specific patterns like the scleroderma pattern. These patterns encompass features such as giant capillaries, microhemorrhages, capillary dropout, neoangiogenesis, and architectural disorganization, which reflect different stages and activity levels of microvascular damage.

The ability to distinguish between these patterns provides critical insights into disease diagnosis, staging, and progression. For example, the presence of giant capillaries and microhemorrhages in early systemic sclerosis can facilitate prompt diagnosis, while extensive capillary loss and neoangiogenesis in late stages correlate with tissue ischemia and increased risk of digital ulcers. Similarly, in dermatomyositis, NVC reveals distinctive features that help differentiate these conditions from other diseases with overlapping clinical features like polymyositis.

Clinically, NVC offers significant advantages: it is a quick, noninvasive, and reproducible technique that allows for serial assessments, enabling clinicians to monitor disease activity, evaluate response to therapy, and predict outcomes. Its findings guide management decisions, improve early diagnosis, and can even serve as a biomarker for disease severity and prognosis. Furthermore, ongoing technological advances, including automated image analysis and integration with other diagnostic modalities, promise to enhance its precision and applicability.

In summary, NVC is a powerful tool that bridges microvascular pathology with clinical practice, providing valuable diagnostic, prognostic, and monitoring information. Its continued evolution and standardization are expected to expand its role, ultimately improving patient care and outcomes in vascular and autoimmune diseases.

References

1. Cutolo M, Sulli A, Pizzorni C, Seriolo B. Nailfold videocapillaroscopy assessment of microvascular damage in systemic sclerosis. Rheumatology. 2000;39(6):744–7.
2. Maricq HR, LeRoy EC. The significance of capillary abnormalities in systemic sclerosis. Arthritis Rheum. 1980;23(3):319–27.
3. Sulli A, Secchi ME, Pizzorni C, et al. Nailfold videocapillaroscopy assessment of microvascular damage in systemic sclerosis. Rheumatology. 2010;49(1):67–74.
4. Smith V, Herrick AL, Ingegnoli F, et al. Standardisation of nailfold capillaroscopy for the assessment of patients with Raynaud's phenomenon and systemic sclerosis. Autoimmun Rev. 2020;19(3):102458.
5. Smith V, Vanhaecke A, Vacca A, et al. New perspectives in nailfold capillaroscopy: advances and future directions. Clin Exp Rheumatol. 2021;39(4):701–11.
6. Tavori H, Levy Y, Kivity S. Nailfold videocapillaroscopy in connective tissue diseases. Autoimmun Rev. 2018;17(4):372–8.
7. Herrick AL. Microvascular imaging in systemic sclerosis: the role of capillaroscopy. Curr Opin Rheumatol. 2014;26(6):674–80.
8. Tiev KP, Amor B, Fardet L, et al. Capillaroscopy in connective tissue diseases: advances and clinical implications. Autoimmun Rev. 2019;18(11):102370.

Chapter 13
Clinical Application of Capillaroscopy

Marco Matucci Cerinic and Veronica Batani

This chapter focuses on the clinical application of nailfold video capillaroscopy (NVC), providing an evidence-based overview of its role in everyday rheumatology practice.

By allowing direct structural assessment of the microcirculation, NVC enables both qualitative (pattern recognition) and quantitative (measurement of capillary abnormalities such as reduced density, giant capillaries, and aberrant morphology) evaluations. These two levels of analysis are applied in clinical practice primarily in two settings (Fig. 13.1):

1. In the assessment and differential diagnosis of Raynaud's phenomenon (RP), mainly to investigate the presence or monitor the possible evolution into a connective tissue disease, particularly disorders within the scleroderma spectrum, which includes systemic sclerosis (SSc), idiopathic inflammatory myopathies (IIMs), and mixed connective tissue disease (MCTD);
2. In patients with an established diagnosis of systemic sclerosis, to support disease staging and to predict the risk of internal organ involvement.

M. M. Cerinic
Vita-Salute San Raffaele University, Milan, Italy

Unit of Immunology, Rheumatology, Allergy and Rare Diseases (UnIRAR), Inflammation, Fibrosis and Ageing Initiative (INFLAGE), IRCCS Ospedale San Raffaele, Milan, Italy
e-mail: matuccicerinic.marco@hsr.it

V. Batani (✉)
Vita-Salute San Raffaele University, Milan, Italy

Unit of Immunology, Rheumatology, Allergy and Rare Diseases (UnIRAR), Inflammation, Fibrosis and Ageing Initiative (INFLAGE), IRCCS Ospedale San Raffaele, Milan, Italy

Leeds Institute of Rheumatology and Muscoloskeletal Medicine, University of Leeds, Leeds, Regno Unito, UK

Department of Medical and Surgical Sciences for Children and Adults, University of Modena and Reggio Emilia, Modena, Italy

Y. El Miedany, R. A. Elziaty (eds.), *Capillaroscopy*, Contemporary Rheumatology,
https://doi.org/10.1007/978-3-032-22966-3_13

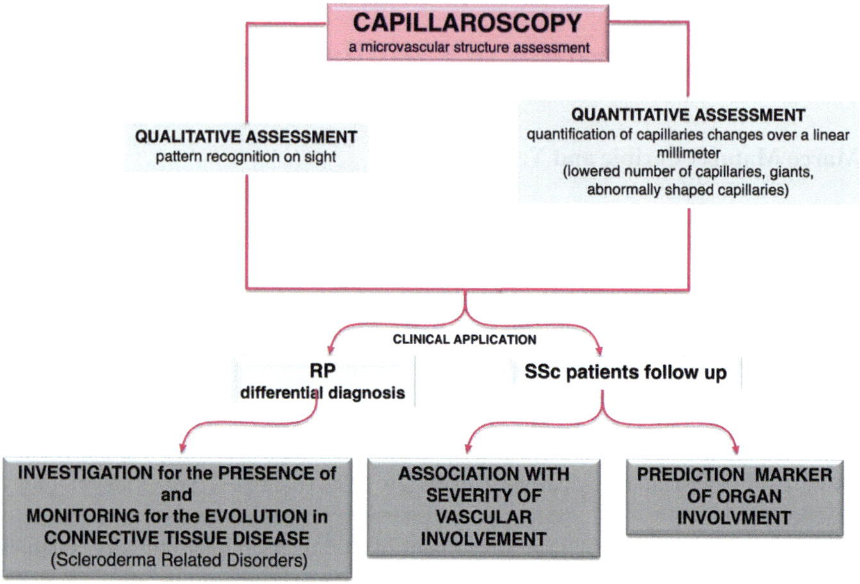

Fig. 13.1 Clinical application of capillaroscopy. RP Raynaud's phenomenon, SSc Systemic sclerosis

Technique, Normal Findings, and How to Distinguish Capillaroscopic Patterns

Technique

Before exploring the clinical applications of capillaroscopy, it is essential to define the most widely used device, how the examination is performed in clinical practice, and what are the normal and abnormal features of the nailfold microvasculature. These parameters were initially described in the 1970s by Maricq and later expanded upon by LeRoy and Medsger [1] and then by Cutolo and Smith [2].

Among the various devices used for nailfold examination, such as conventional optical microscopes, dermatoscopes, and other magnification tools, only the dermatoscope and the videocapillaroscope have demonstrated sufficient inter- and intra-observer reliability in comparative studies. This makes them the preferred instruments in both everyday rheumatologic evaluation and research environments [3].

In clinical practice, nailfold videocapillaroscopy (NVC) is the most reliable and standardized method for the assessment of microvascular alterations, particularly in patients with Raynaud's phenomenon or suspected connective tissue diseases. According to the EULAR and Scleroderma Clinical Trials Consortium (SCTC) consensus, the gold standard device is the digital videocapillaroscope, which combines a high-resolution optical system (usually ×200 magnification) with a digital video camera and LED illumination, integrated into a handheld probe. This configuration allows for consistent and high-quality imaging across different clinical settings [4].

The videocapillaroscope offers several practical advantages: it is easy to use, even by nonexperts, thanks to its ergonomic design and portability. It is suitable for use in patients with limited joint mobility or contractures, where traditional microscopy may be impractical. The device also supports digital image storage and can be integrated with specialized software for image analysis and semi-automated quantification, which is essential when evaluating morphological and structural capillary changes. By saving the images, clinicians can more easily perform side-by-side comparisons during follow-up visits, allowing for the detection of temporal changes and disease progression or stabilization.

Normal Findings

Despite the higher cost, which often limits access to specialized centers, videocapillaroscopy is nowadays a cornerstone in the clinical setting. Therefore, as nailfold capillaroscopy becomes more routinely used across diverse healthcare settings, establishing a uniform method for describing and documenting its findings has become essential. Recognizing this need, experts from both the SCTC and the EULAR microcirculation working group have collaborated to define a shared set of criteria. This collaborative effort resulted in the development of standardized guidelines to ensure consistent interpretation of videocapillaroscopic images acquired at 200× magnification [4–7].

According to this framework, four key quantitative parameters should be assessed when analyzing a nailfold capillaroscopic image:

1. *Capillary density* (number of loops per linear millimeter)
2. *Capillary morphology* (shape and structure of individual capillaries)
3. *Capillary dimensions* (most commonly the width of the apical limb)
4. *Presence or absence of microhemorrhages*

Once these quantitative characteristics have been evaluated, a qualitative judgment can be made by interpreting the overall image and recognizing patterns.

Normal reference values have been defined for each of the main capillaroscopic parameters, providing the basis for identifying physiological findings and recognizing deviations suggestive of pathology. These criteria allow clinicians to distinguish a normal capillaroscopic pattern, which reflects an intact and healthy microvascular architecture.

As shown in Table 13.1 below, a *normal pattern* is characterized by a capillary density of at least seven loops per linear millimeter, apical diameters not exceeding 20 μm, and the absence of microhemorrhages. Regarding morphology, loops are considered normal when they display a single convex apex, which may present in one of three typical configurations: hairpin, tortuous, or crossing. All these forms represent physiological variations within a normal structural framework [4–7] (Fig. 13.2).

Table 13.1 Characteristics of normal capillaroscopy findings

Capillaroscopic characteristic	Normal description	
Capillary density (/mm)	≥ 7 capillaries per linear millimeter	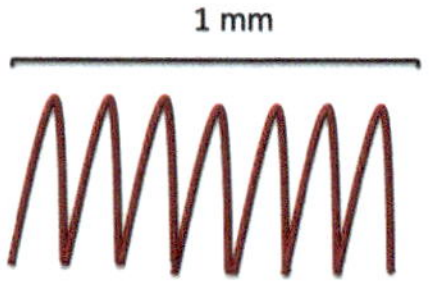
Capillary dimension (μm)	Apical diameter ≤ 20 μm, measured at the apex of the loop	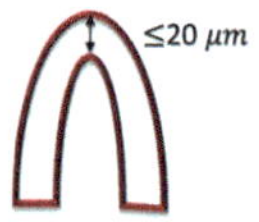
Capillary morphology	Normal morphology includes loops with a single convex apex, which may appear in one of three shapes: Hairpin Tortuous Crossing	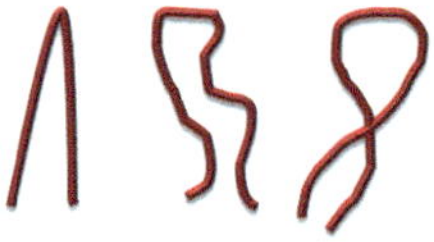
Microhemorrhages	Absent	

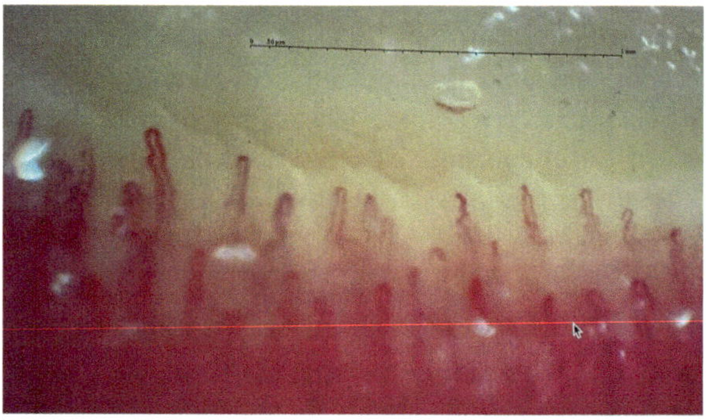

Fig. 13.2 Normal capillaroscopic picture at NVC

How to Distinguish Capillaroscopic Patterns

Anything that deviates from these normal characteristics is considered a *capillaroscopic abnormality*, which can be classified into two main categories: specific abnormalities (the scleroderma pattern) and nonspecific abnormalities [5–10].

1. *Specific abnormalities—defining the "scleroderma pattern"*

   According to the EULAR/SCTC consensus, only two capillaroscopic abnormalities are considered specific enough to define the presence of a *scleroderma pattern*: giant capillaries and severely reduced capillary density. These will be detailed below.

   - *The presence of giant capillaries*, defined as homogeneously enlarged loops with an apical diameter equal to or greater than 50 μm.

- *Severe capillary loss,* quantified as a density of fewer than four capillaries per linear millimeter.
- Based on the combination and evolution of these findings, three progressive scleroderma patterns have been described by Cutolo and internationally validated:
- Early pattern: Presence of a few giant capillaries with a normal or near-normal capillary density (≥7/mm); hemorrhages may be observed, but abnormal shapes are absent.
- Active pattern: Coexistence of frequent giant capillaries and moderate capillary loss (<7/mm), often accompanied by microhemorrhages and early architectural disorganization.
- Late pattern: Marked capillary loss (<4/mm) with disorganized architecture and the emergence of abnormal shapes (neo-angiogenesis); giant capillaries are typically no longer observed.

These alterations, visualized through 200× magnification videocapillaroscopy, are highly informative for the diagnosis, staging, and prognostication of systemic sclerosis and other scleroderma-spectrum diseases, as will be discussed in the following section.

2. *Nonspecific abnormalities:*
   These refer to alterations that *do not meet the criteria for a scleroderma pattern* but may still be observed in other connective tissue diseases or even in non-rheumatic conditions and healthy subjects [9]. They include:
   - *Shape abnormalities*, such as capillaries with multiple convexities or morphologies that differ from the typical normal forms, for example, arborized loops
   - *Dimension abnormalities*, usually capillary dilations with an apical diameter greater than 20 μm but less than 50 μm
   - *Mild reduction in capillary density*, without the presence of avascular areas
   - *Presence of microhemorrhages*

A simplified and pragmatic approach to interpreting nailfold capillaroscopic images has been proposed by the EULAR Study Group on Microcirculation in Rheumatic Diseases, known as the *Fast Track algorithm* (Fig. 13.3). This model allows clinicians to quickly classify capillaroscopic findings using three essential decision rules, making it particularly effective in routine clinical settings. The flowchart below summarizes its application [8].

- Rule 1—Normal density and no giant capillaries:
  If the capillary density is ≥7 per millimeter and giant capillaries are absent, the image is classified as a non-scleroderma pattern (Category 1).
- Rule 2—Severely reduced density or presence of giants:
  If the density is ≤3 capillaries per millimeter, or if giant capillaries are present (regardless of density), the image is considered consistent with a scleroderma pattern (Category 2). This also includes images showing advanced morphological abnormalities, such as those seen in the late phase of the disease.

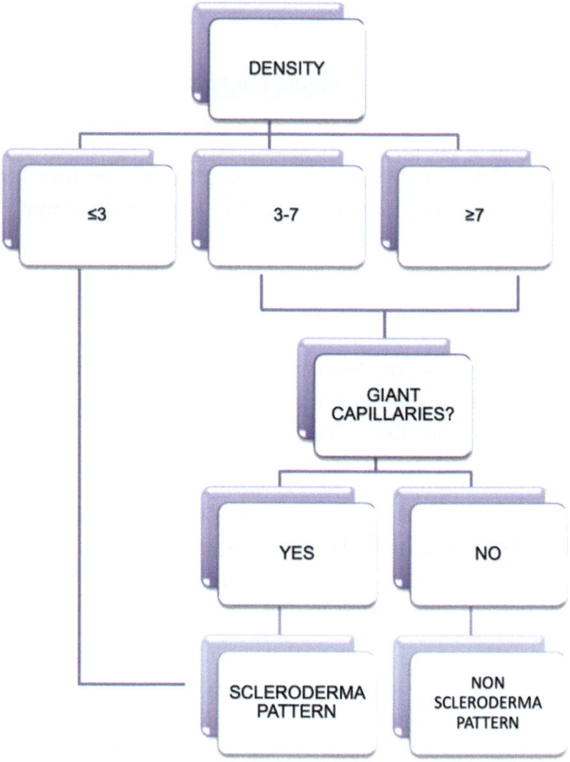

Fig. 13.3 Schematic representation of the Fast Track Algorithm

- Rule 3—Intermediate cases:
  If the findings do not clearly meet the criteria in Rule 1 or Rule 2 (i.e., density between 4 and 6 capillaries/mm and no giant capillaries), the image is again classified as a non-scleroderma pattern (Category 1) by exclusion.

This streamlined algorithm, by focusing on capillary density and the presence of giant capillaries, provides a fast, reliable, and reproducible method to categorize capillaroscopic findings into either category 1 (non-scleroderma pattern) or category 2 (scleroderma pattern). Its simplicity and strong clinical applicability make it especially valuable for both experienced rheumatologists and clinicians working in high-throughput settings or with limited expertise in capillaroscopy.

While the Fast Track algorithm was developed for use with nailfold videocapillaroscopy (NVC), its core principles can also be applied using dermatoscopy, a lower-cost and more widely available tool, particularly common in clinical practice in the United Kingdom and the United States.

Although dermatoscopes offer lower magnification and resolution compared to videocapillaroscopes, an international consensus, led by experts from the EULAR Study Group, has recently proposed a preliminary algorithm for the structured evaluation of nailfold capillaries using dermoscopy. This approach mirrors the main capillaroscopic parameters used in NVC-based assessments.

When the Fast Track algorithm is applied via dermoscopy, clinicians can often still determine whether the findings are compatible with a scleroderma pattern (category 2) or a non-scleroderma pattern (category 1). In situations where the dermatoscopic image is unclear or the findings are nonspecific, a follow-up evaluation with videocapillaroscopy is recommended to confirm the classification [8].

Clinical Application of Capillaroscopy

The identification of capillaroscopic nonspecific abnormalities and the scleroderma pattern has led to the development of numerous studies exploring their clinical significance. These investigations have demonstrated associations between capillaroscopic findings and:

- The presence of specific connective tissue diseases in patients with Raynaud's phenomenon;
- Disease severity, risk of internal organ involvement, and related complications.

These insights have highlighted the clinical value of capillaroscopy across different disease stages and patient populations [6].

Investigation and Follow-Up of Raynaud's Phenomenon (RP)

As discussed in the previous chapters of this book, Raynaud's phenomenon (RP) can occur as a primary condition or as a secondary manifestation of various underlying causes. Among the secondary forms, autoimmune diseases are the most common (10–20% of RP cases), and systemic sclerosis (SSc) and scleroderma-related diseases are the conditions most frequently associated with RP [10]. For instance, Raynaud's phenomenon occurs in more than 95% of patients with systemic sclerosis (SSc) and in approximately 75% of those with mixed connective tissue disease (MCTD) [11]. However, primary RP, which is not related to any underlying disease, is also observed in about 5% of the general population as a benign functional condition [12, 13]. This overlap highlights the importance of having reliable tools to support the etiological assessment of RP and guide clinical decision-making. In this context, capillaroscopy can serve as a valuable aid in the diagnostic evaluation of patients presenting with RP. Indeed, nailfold capillaroscopy provides valuable insight into the microvascular architecture of the nailfold capillary bed. When integrated with clinical and serological findings, capillaroscopic features help guide the differential diagnosis and may suggest one etiology over another [14, 15]. In particular, capillaroscopy plays a key role in raising the suspicion of an underlying autoimmune connective tissue disease. However, it is important to emphasize that capillaroscopic findings alone are not sufficient for a definitive diagnosis of the cause of RP; they should always be interpreted within the broader clinical context.

The clinical correlation between nailfold capillaroscopy (NVC) findings and the underlying etiology of Raynaud's phenomenon is summarized in Fig. 13.4, which outlines how different capillaroscopic patterns distribute across primary RP, non-rheumatologic secondary causes, and rheumatologic diseases, including the scleroderma spectrum.

The clinical relevance of capillaroscopy in the evaluation of Raynaud's phenomenon has progressively evolved over the last few decades. Maricq was among the first to demonstrate that nailfold capillaroscopy could reveal characteristic microvascular changes in patients with scleroderma-related disorders. Through wide-field microscopy, he identified a distinct capillaroscopic profile, which is now known as the "scleroderma pattern," that was strongly associated with connective tissue diseases, particularly systemic sclerosis [9, 16, 17].

Later, capillaroscopy also gained significance when used to exclude disease. In 1992, LeRoy and Medsger included the presence of normal capillaries as one of the criteria for the classification of primary Raynaud's phenomenon, highlighting its role in differentiating functional from disease-associated RP [1]. This concept was subsequently reinforced by the international expert consensus published in 2014 by Maverakis et al., which formalized the presence of a normal capillaroscopic pattern as a key criterion in the diagnosis of primary RP [18].

However, some uncertainty remained, as evidence emerged that nonspecific capillary alterations may also be present in individuals without any underlying disease. In a large population study, Andrade et al. found that about one-third of healthy subjects displayed at least one minor capillaroscopic anomaly. More specifically, 25% of participants showed a single alteration, 8% had two, and only 1% exhibited three distinct abnormalities [7]. These data suggest that isolated findings may occur sporadically in healthy individuals and should not be considered pathognomonic [7, 19, 20].

Similar findings were reported by Ingegnoli et al., who also observed capillary abnormalities in healthy subjects, though with a lower frequency compared to previous studies. This reinforces the need for cautious interpretation of nonspecific changes, particularly when they appear in isolation and without associated clinical features [15].

Several studies have investigated the potential correlation between capillaroscopic patterns and connective tissue diseases other than systemic sclerosis that are also frequently associated with Raynaud's phenomenon, particularly systemic lupus erythematosus (SLE), primary Sjögren's syndrome (pSS), and antiphospholipid syndrome (APS). However, these investigations have generally not demonstrated strong associations with specific or disease-defining capillaroscopic patterns. Most patients with these conditions exhibit either normal capillary morphology or nonspecific abnormalities, limiting the diagnostic value of capillaroscopy in these settings [20–25].

An exception may be emerging in the context of APS, where recent studies have suggested a possible association with a distinctive pattern characterized by multiple microhemorrhages and a "comb-like" appearance, although further validation is needed before it can be considered diagnostically reliable [23–25].

In contrast, capillaroscopy plays a well-established role in the evaluation of systemic sclerosis, where the identification of a scleroderma pattern is not only diagnostically informative but has also been included as a classification criterion since 2013 [26–29]. Consequently, mixed connective tissue disease (MCTD), which frequently exhibits overlapping features with systemic sclerosis, is similarly associated with scleroderma-type patterns [30].

More recently, the role of capillaroscopy has expanded to include idiopathic inflammatory myopathies (IIMs). The EULAR Study Group on Microcirculation in Rheumatic Diseases has provided recent guidance on the standardized interpretation of capillaroscopy in this context, recognizing its potential utility in IIM diagnosis.

In the following sections, we will focus on these three disease groups—systemic sclerosis, MCTD, and inflammatory myopathies—illustrating their characteristic capillaroscopic findings. The clinical correlation between nailfold capillaroscopy (NVC) findings and the underlying etiology of Raynaud's phenomenon is summarized in Fig. 13.4, which outlines how capillaroscopic patterns vary across primary RP, non-rheumatologic secondary forms, and rheumatologic conditions, including those within the scleroderma spectrum.

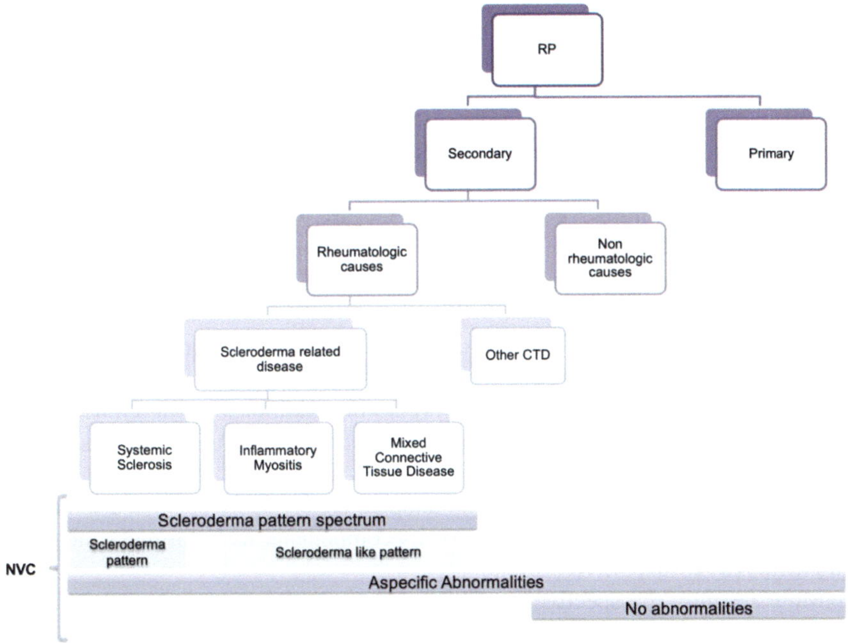

Fig. 13.4 Association between capillaroscopic characteristics and primary and secondary Raynaud Phenomenon

The Diagnostic Role of the *Scleroderma Pattern* for Very Early and Definite Systemic Sclerosis Diagnosis

The standardization of the scleroderma pattern definition by the EULAR Study Group on Microcirculation in Rheumatic Diseases and the Scleroderma Clinical Trials Consortium Group on Capillaroscopy, along with the development of a Fast Track algorithm (as detailed at the beginning of this chapter), became necessary following the inclusion of the scleroderma pattern among the items of the 2013 ACR/EULAR classification criteria for systemic sclerosis (SSc) [26]. This marked a turning point in the recognition of the disease at earlier stages. By assigning a weighted score to the presence of a scleroderma pattern on nailfold videocapillaroscopy (NVC), alongside other clinical and serological features, the criteria acknowledged the diagnostic relevance of microvascular damage in the disease trajectory. This was the result of a progressive evolution in the understanding of how capillaroscopic abnormalities, especially the scleroderma pattern, can anticipate overt clinical manifestations [28].

Well before the introduction of the 2013 criteria, efforts were already underway to identify predictors of disease evolution in patients presenting with Raynaud's phenomenon (RP). A pivotal contribution came from LeRoy and Medsger, who in 2001 proposed that the combination of RP, SSc-specific autoantibodies, and capillaroscopic changes suggestive of SSc could define a subset of patients in a preclinical phase of the disease [1].

This hypothesis was later substantiated by a longitudinal cohort study involving patients with isolated RP, which followed them over a 20-year period. The findings revealed that individuals who had both SSc-specific antibodies and capillaroscopic features consistent with a scleroderma pattern at baseline developed definite SSc in approximately two-thirds of cases within 5 years, with the proportion rising to nearly 80% after two decades. In stark contrast, patients lacking both immunological and microvascular markers rarely transitioned to SSc, with a progression rate of just 1.3% at 5 years [29].

To enhance early recognition even further, the concept of Very Early Diagnosis of Systemic Sclerosis (VEDOSS) was introduced in 2011. This initiative expanded the LeRoy–Medsger framework by incorporating additional subtle clinical signs, most notably the presence of puffy fingers, which is often one of the first visible clues in evolving disease [30].

The VEDOSS concept was not only adopted conceptually but was also embedded in clinical classification. Several of its components were formally integrated into the 2013 ACR/EULAR criteria.

More recently, prospective data have validated the prognostic value of this approach. In 2021, Bellando Randone and colleagues published a prospective multicenter study from the VEDOSS cohort specifically designed to assess the predictive performance of the VEDOSS criteria in patients with Raynaud's phenomenon. Over a 5-year follow-up period, up to 94% of individuals presenting both puffy fingers and SSc-specific autoantibodies fulfilled the 2013 ACR/EULAR criteria [27].

Importantly, the same study further clarified the prognostic value of nailfold capillaroscopy. Among those with abnormal capillaroscopic findings at baseline, 70.1% progressed to definite SSc within 5 years, compared to only 41.5% of those without abnormalities. Although its predictive strength was slightly lower than that of puffy fingers or SSc-specific autoantibodies in multivariable models, capillaroscopic abnormalities remained an independent and statistically significant predictor of progression (RR 1.70; 95% CI 1.18–2.46; $p = 0.004$). Moreover, when combined with SSc-specific autoantibodies, the progression rate increased to 82.2%, underscoring the additive prognostic impact of microvascular changes. These findings confirm that nailfold capillaroscopy, beyond its diagnostic utility, plays a central role in stratifying risk and guiding early management in individuals at the preclinical stage of systemic sclerosis [27].

The Supportive Role of *Scleroderma-Like Pattern* for Idiopathic Inflammatory Myopathies (IIMs) and Mixed Connective Tissue Disease (MCTD) Diagnosis

IIMs

Although nailfold videocapillaroscopy (NVC) findings are not included in the current classification criteria for idiopathic inflammatory myopathies (IIMs), they should be considered in clinical practice given the growing body of evidence supporting their diagnostic relevance [32–38].

A recent systematic evaluation of NVC in IIMs aimed to critically review the available literature and reclassify published findings using the standardized framework proposed by the EULAR Study Group on Microcirculation in Rheumatic Diseases and the Scleroderma Clinical Trials Consortium (SCTC) Group on Capillaroscopy. The analysis revealed that a subset of IIM patients exhibited microvascular abnormalities resembling those typically seen in systemic sclerosis (SSc). However, in most cases, the findings did not fit neatly into the classical "early," "active," or "late" scleroderma stages and were therefore described as "scleroderma-like patterns" [32].

Prevalence estimates varied across studies but consistently showed that dermatomyositis (DM) patients exhibited a higher frequency of scleroderma-like patterns than polymyositis (PM) patients. For instance, Manfredi et al. reported a scleroderma pattern in 69% of DM patients and 0% of PM patients and healthy controls [33, 34]. Similarly, Kubo et al. found both scleroderma and scleroderma-like patterns in 32.6% and 32.7% of DM patients, compared to 5.6% and 22.2% in PM, respectively [35].

These findings highlight the potential of NVC as a supportive tool in the diagnostic assessment of IIMs, particularly in patients with clinical or serological overlap with the scleroderma spectrum.

MCTD

Although not included in current classification criteria, NVC should be considered in the clinical assessment of MCTD, a condition frequently associated with Raynaud's phenomenon. Capillaroscopic findings in MCTD are heterogeneous, ranging from normal or nonspecific changes to scleroderma and scleroderma-like patterns, but, as observed in idiopathic inflammatory myopathies (IIMs), consistently show an increased prevalence of scleroderma-like features. In a comparative study, Granier et al. identified a scleroderma-like pattern in 64% of MCTD patients, suggesting its potential to differentiate MCTD from other autoimmune rheumatic diseases [39–42].

Additionally, a large prospective study by Pavlov et al. found a significant association between the presence of a scleroderma-like pattern and the future development of MCTD in patients with Raynaud's phenomenon [28].

While MCTD patients typically show less capillary loss and higher capillary density than those with systemic sclerosis (SSc), the presence of scleroderma-like features may provide diagnostic and prognostic value, particularly when integrated with clinical and serological data.

The Role of NVC in a Longitudinal, Multidimensional Approach

Although nailfold videocapillaroscopy (NVC) is widely recognized as a valuable tool in the assessment of Raynaud's phenomenon (RP) and in identifying patients at risk for systemic sclerosis (SSc), recent prospective evidence has questioned its use as an isolated predictor. A randomized controlled study re-evaluating the utility of NVC in ANA-positive patients with RP showed that capillaroscopic abnormalities alone were insufficient to reliably predict progression to definite SSc, with only a minority of patients fulfilling classification criteria over time. These findings underscore the risk of diagnostic overestimation when NVC is interpreted without adequate clinical and serological context [31].

This concept is consistent with the approach promoted by the VEDOSS (Very Early Diagnosis of Systemic Sclerosis) initiative and incorporated in the 2013 ACR/EULAR classification criteria, which emphasize the need for a multidimensional evaluation, integrating clinical features, autoantibody status, and NVC findings.

Notably, the prospective study supports the idea that NVC may be more useful when employed as a monitoring tool within a structured follow-up protocol [31]. Serial NVC assessments can offer valuable insight into the evolution of microvascular damage, particularly when interpreted in conjunction with dynamic changes in clinical and immunological parameters. As such, the strength of NVC may lie not in its isolated diagnostic value but in its integration into a longitudinal, multiparametric strategy for the early identification and stratification of patients within the SSc spectrum.

Clinical Cases

The following clinical cases illustrate the practical utility of nailfold videocapillaroscopy in the assessment of Raynaud's phenomenon, highlighting its role in distinguishing between primary and secondary forms, supporting early diagnosis, and guiding follow-up.

Case 1: Primar Raynaud Phenomenon

A 25-year-old patient with a 5-year history of Raynaud's phenomenon, negative ANA, no systemic symptoms, and a family history of Raynaud's. Nailfold videocapillaroscopy shows a normal capillary density and morphology, with single capillary loops characterized by a convex tip, the presence of crossing capillaries as a normal variant, and normal dimensions (Fig. 13.5). Applying the Fast Track algorithm, capillary density is within normal limits, and no giant capillaries are detected. The overall pattern supports a diagnosis of primary Raynaud's phenomenon, with no features suggestive of a secondary form.

Case 2: Progression to Very Early Diagnosis of Systemic Sclerosis (VEDOSS)

A patient developed Raynaud's phenomenon at the age of 17 but did not undergo further evaluation. Two years later, a first nailfold videocapillaroscopy (Fig. 13.6) revealed nonspecific abnormalities, including a few microhemorrhages, some microaneurysms, and a few dilated capillaries, with preserved capillary density and no giant capillaries. Autoantibody testing was requested, revealing ANA positivity at 1:640 with an anti-centromere pattern; puffiness of the fingers was absent at that time.

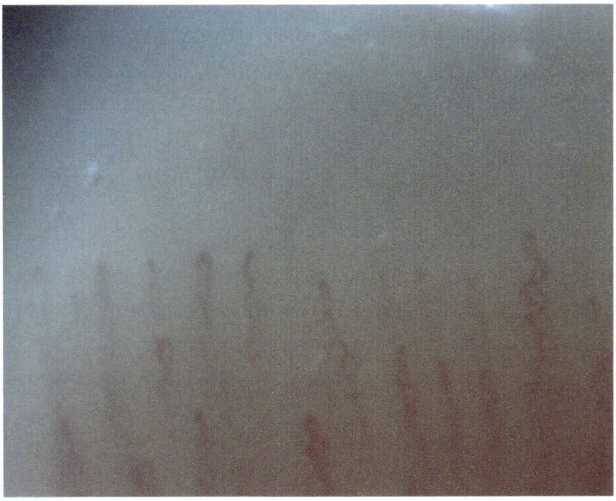

Fig. 13.5 NVC of clinical case 1

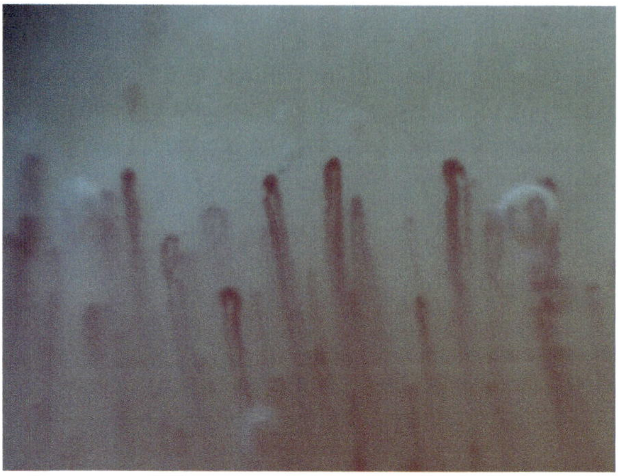

Fig. 13.6 First NVC performed

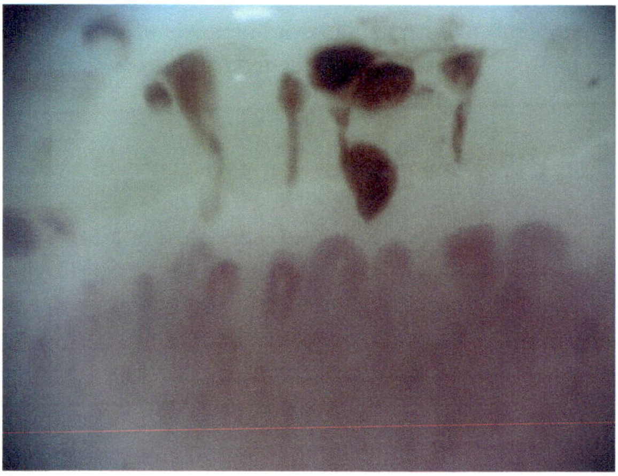

Fig. 13.7 NVC after 2 years

The patient was placed under clinical follow-up, and 2 years later, a second capillaroscopy (Fig. 13.7) was performed. This showed preserved capillary density but the appearance of overt giant capillaries and recurrent microhemorrhages, consistent with an "early" scleroderma pattern. Clinically, the patient had also developed puffy fingers. Based on these findings, the diagnosis of Very Early Diagnosis of Systemic Sclerosis (VEDOSS) was made.

Case 3: Mixed Connective Tissue Disease and Scleroderma-Like Pattern

A young woman presented at 18 years of age with photosensitive cutaneous plaques, puffy fingers, and classic biphasic Raynaud's phenomenon. Laboratory work-up showed a high-titer ANA (> 1:320, speckled) with strong anti-RNP positivity; creatine-kinase was normal, and mild leucopenia (WBC < 1.7×10^9/L) was noted.

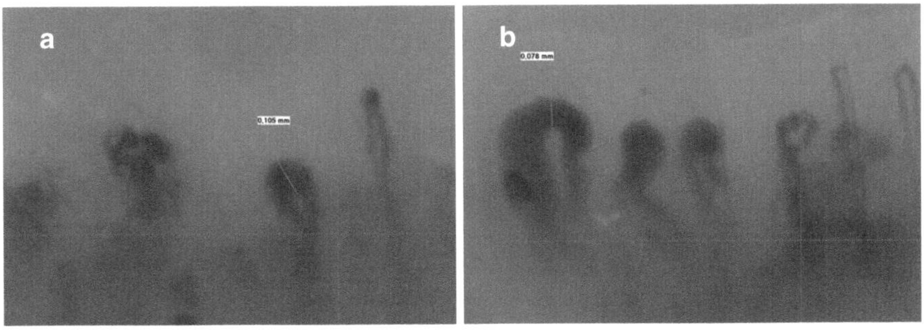

Fig. 13.8 Scleroderma-like pattern with giant megacapillaries and markedly reduced capillary density

Nailfold videocapillaroscopy revealed a frankly scleroderma-like pattern, characterized by megacapillaries coexisting with markedly reduced capillary density. This microvascular picture, together with anti-RNP antibodies and the clinical triad of cutaneous lupus features, Raynaud's, and digital edema, firmly supported the diagnosis of mixed connective tissue disease (MCTD) (Fig. 13.8).

Case 4: Early Reynolds Syndrome Uncovered Through Serial Capillaroscopy

A 68-year-old woman came to medical attention after routine blood work revealed persistently elevated γ-glutamyl-transferase. Serology showed strong anti-mitochondrial antibodies (AMA-M2) together with anti-centromere positivity, yet abdominal ultrasound and elastography were entirely normal, and there was no imaging evidence of biliary cirrhosis.

Two years later (age 70), she developed biphasic Raynaud's phenomenon but remained free of skin thickening, digital edema, arthralgia, myalgia, or sicca complaints. Nailfold videocapillaroscopy performed at that time (Fig. 13.9a) was normal with only rare microhemorrhages. Because of the combined AMA and centromere positivity, she was enrolled in a tight clinical follow-up program.

At age 74, her fingers became puffy, and repeat capillaroscopy now demonstrated an early scleroderma pattern characterized by a few giant capillary loops (Fig. 13.9b and c). Although detailed organ staging is still underway, the constellation fulfills the criteria for VEDOSS (Very Early Diagnosis of Systemic Sclerosis). The clinical picture is highly suggestive of a very early Reynolds syndrome—the association of primary biliary cholangitis and limited cutaneous systemic sclerosis—at a stage in which no overt organ damage is yet detectable by imaging.

From this case, we see that serial nailfold capillaroscopy can serve as the first objective marker of ongoing disease activity and progression in patients who harbor systemic-sclerosis-specific autoantibodies but lack definite clinical manifestations. When a patient with AMA-positive cholestasis develops Raynaud's phenomenon and evolves from a normal to an early scleroderma pattern, clinicians should

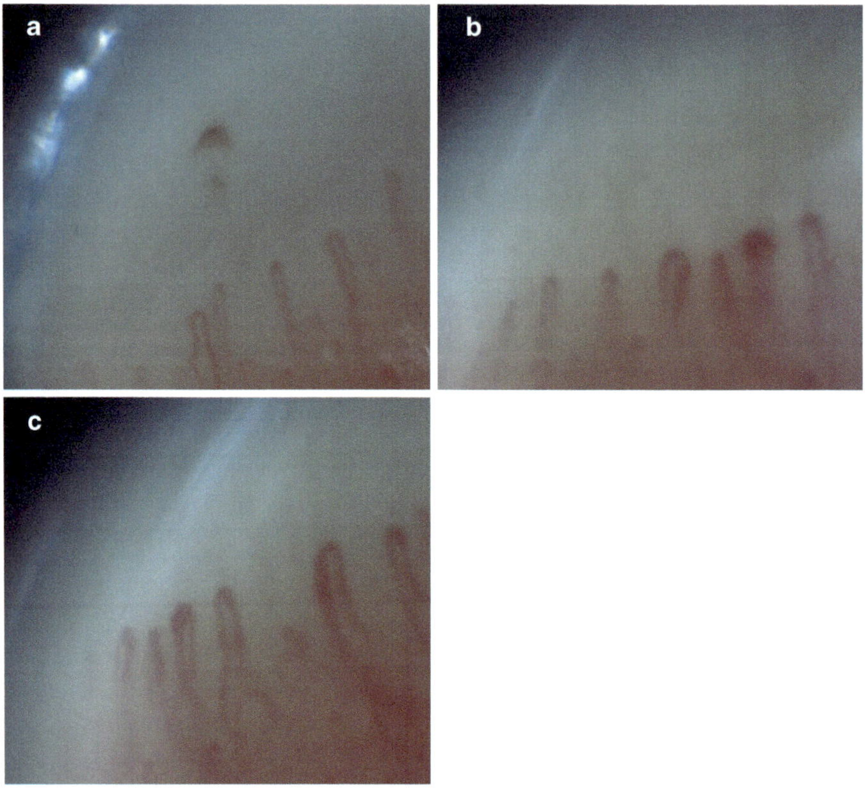

Fig. 13.9 (**a**) Baseline study (age 70): normal capillary density and morphology, one apical micro-hemorrhage. (**b**, **c**) Follow-up study (age 74): early scleroderma pattern with isolated giant capillaries

consider Reynolds syndrome and initiate comprehensive organ screening even before imaging evidence of biliary or systemic-sclerosis damage emerges.

Case 5: Anti-Pm/Scl Scleromyositis Revealed by Scleroderma-Like Capillaroscopy

A 65-year-old man presented after 12 months of dermatologic and joint complaints: progressive palmar desquamation, erythema over the metacarpophalangeal joints, distal fissures, intermittent digital swelling, and arthralgias. Although he denied long-standing color changes, he recalled brief episodes of finger pallor in the cold, consistent with a mild Raynaud's phenomenon that had never been investigated. Routine serology—including ANA, an extended ENA panel, rheumatoid factor, and anti-CCP—was completely negative, and inflammatory markers (ESR, CRP) remained within the normal range.

On first evaluation, physical examination revealed classic "mechanic's hands," without sclerodactyly, finger puffiness, or telangiectasias. Nailfold videocapillaroscopy proved decisive: it showed a clear scleroderma-like pattern characterized by the copresence of megacapillaries, markedly reduced capillary density, neo-angiogenesis, and abnormally shaped loops. This constellation differed from a late scleroderma pattern, which by definition displays neo-angiogenesis and capillary loss but no megacapillaries.

Because such microvascular changes strongly suggest a systemic sclerosis spectrum disorder, we extended the immunological work-up beyond routine ANA testing. A specialized panel was positive for anti-Pm/Scl-75 and anti-Pm/Scl-100 antibodies, clinching the diagnosis of scleromyositis—the overlap between systemic sclerosis and inflammatory myopathy. High-resolution chest CT further demonstrated approximately 15% subpleural reticulation and ground-glass opacities in the lower lobes, indicating early interstitial lung involvement despite the absence of respiratory symptoms.

This case underscores the pivotal role of capillaroscopy in the diagnostic work-up of patients with nonspecific skin or musculoskeletal manifestations. Even when ANA screening is negative, a scleroderma-like microvascular pattern—especially one combining megacapillaries with density loss and neo-angiogenesis—should prompt targeted testing for rare systemic sclerosis and myositis-associated antibodies. Early recognition through this microvascular "window" not only clarifies the clinical picture—here, a classic anti-Pm/Scl scleromyositis—but also guides timely assessment of internal organ involvement and appropriate management (Fig. 13.10).

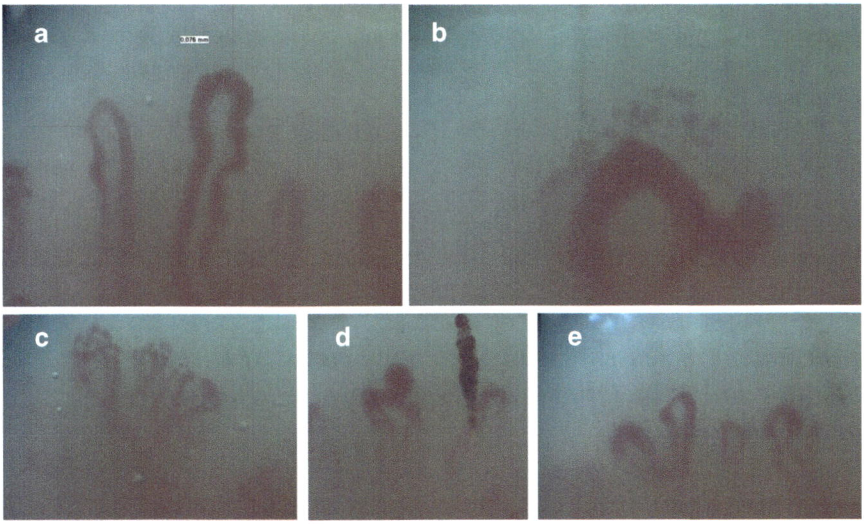

Fig. 13.10 (**a**) Megacapillary (diameter ≈ 76 μm) with only two capillaries visible in a 1-mm field. (**b**) Single megacapillary occupying the entire field. (**c**) Neo-angiogenesis with branching capillary loops. (**d**) Megacapillary showing a microaneurysm and microhemorrhage. (**e**) Dilated, abnormally shaped capillaries with a characteristic "double-tip" morphology

Case 6: Raynaud's Phenomenon with a Scleroderma-Like Capillaroscopic Pattern Unmasking Smoldering Myeloma

A 40-year-old man with a known diagnosis of smoldering multiple myeloma was referred for evaluation of new-onset color changes in his fingers. For the previous 6 months, he had experienced classic biphasic Raynaud's phenomenon triggered by minimal cold exposure, without digital pitting, ulcers, skin thickening, arthralgias, or muscle weakness. He denied dysphagia, dyspnea, sicca symptoms, or constitutional complaints.

Routine autoimmune screening was entirely negative: ANA by indirect immunofluorescence, a full ENA panel, and an extended myositis/SSc antibody profile all returned negative; creatine-phosphokinase and inflammatory markers were normal.

Physical examination showed intact skin texture and normal joint range of motion, but nailfolds exhibited alternating pale areas and subtle erythema. Nailfold videocapillaroscopy revealed a scleroderma-like pattern—megacapillaries, markedly reduced capillary density, scattered microhemorrhages, and focal neoangiogenesis—yet the clinical picture lacked sufficient criteria for either systemic sclerosis or idiopathic inflammatory myopathy.

Given the incongruity between the capillaroscopic findings and the absence of connective tissue disease features or autoantibodies, attention turned to his underlying hematologic condition. In plasma-cell dyscrasias, hyperviscosity, cryoglobulinaemia, and paraneoplastic endothelial injury can all precipitate Raynaud's phenomenon and capillary architectural distortion. Further hematology review confirmed stable smoldering myeloma with mild hyperviscosity but no progression to symptomatic disease. Cryoglobulins and cold agglutinins were negative, and organ function remained preserved, so conservative management was continued.

This case remarks that a scleroderma-like capillaroscopic pattern is not pathognomonic for systemic sclerosis. When the clinical context and serology do not support a connective tissue diagnosis, clinicians should broaden the differential to include hematologic malignancies and dyscrasias, particularly plasma-cell disorders. Recognizing this possibility prompts appropriate hematologic follow-up (Fig. 13.11).

Assessment of Patients with Systemic Sclerosis: Disease Staging and Association with Organ Involvement and Complications

Among the parameters assessable through nailfold videocapillaroscopy (NVC), capillary density, which reflects capillary loss, has emerged as the most reproducible between observers and the most reliable predictor of clinical complications in systemic sclerosis (SSc). Numerous studies have consistently linked reduced capillary density to the development of digital ulcers and pulmonary arterial

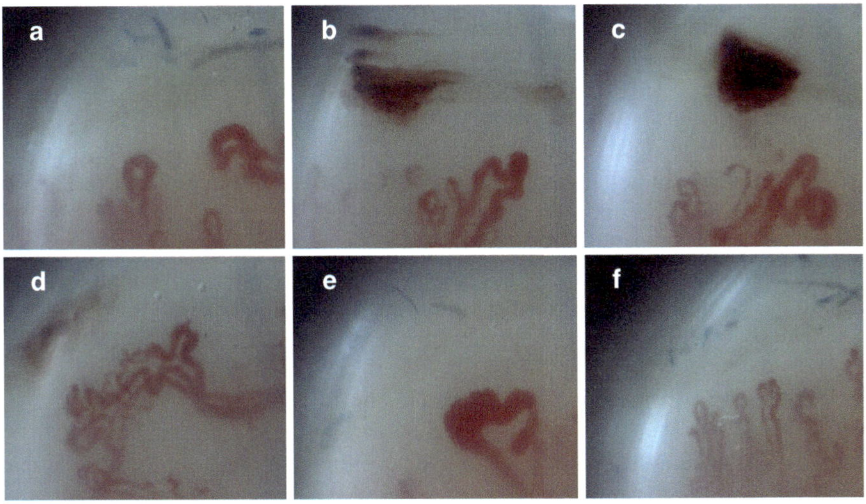

Fig. 13.11 (**a**) Markedly reduced capillary density with loop dilatation. (**b**, **c**) Decreased density with microhemorrhage and capillary aneurysm. (**d**) Disorganization of the capillary bed with overall density loss. (**e**) Megacapillary accompanied by reduced density and a microaneurysm. (**f**) Reduced density with tortuous, abnormally shaped loops displaying a "double-tip" configuration

hypertension (PAH). Some evidence is also for an association with interstitial lung disease (ILD), skin fibrosis progression, and overall worsening of disease severity. In contrast, other NVC parameters, such as capillary enlargement, morphological abnormalities, and microhemorrhages, have a less clearly defined prognostic value, and in the case of microhemorrhages, their limited interrater reliability further hampers their utility as consistent biomarkers [43–57].

The clinical significance of reduced capillary density on nailfold videocapillaroscopy (NVC) in systemic sclerosis largely depends on the type of study design, with different insights emerging from cross-sectional, prospective, and longitudinal studies.

Cross-Sectional Associations of Capillary Density with Organ Involvement

Reduced capillary density has been consistently associated with vascular complications in systemic sclerosis. Several cross-sectional studies have shown that lower capillary density correlates with the presence of digital ulcers (DUs) and pulmonary arterial hypertension (PAH) and has also been linked to interstitial lung disease (ILD) [45, 46].

Prognostic Value of Baseline Capillary Density

The predictive role of capillary loss at baseline has been explored in prospective studies, where reduced density, often reflected by the presence of "active" or "late" scleroderma patterns, has shown strong associations with subsequent disease progression. The multicenter CAP study, with a 6-month follow-up, found that a "late" capillaroscopic pattern at baseline was linked to a higher risk of developing digital ulcers [47]. These results were later confirmed by smaller studies with longer follow-up durations of up to 3 years.

More recently, a large prospective study by the EULAR Study Group on Microcirculation, in collaboration with EUSTAR, demonstrated that severe NVC patterns ("active" or "late") at baseline were significantly associated with an increased risk of both cutaneous progression and new organ involvement (including SSc-ILD and PAH, confirmed either by right heart catheterization or echocardiography) during a follow-up period ranging from 12 to 24 months [48].

Capillaroscopic Progression and Future Complications

Longitudinal studies have also underscored the clinical relevance of capillaroscopic changes over time. Two independent prospective cohorts showed that progression to more severe NVC patterns ("active" or "late") is predictive of new organ involvement and worsening disease [49, 50]. In both studies, progressive capillary loss was associated with the development of PAH, confirmed by right heart catheterization. One of these studies further demonstrated an association with incident ILD over a 7-year period. The other, involving 140 patients followed with serial NVC over 3 years, reported that progression to a "late" pattern was linked to new digital ulcers, PAH, progression of skin fibrosis, and an overall increase in disease activity.

Figure 13.12 summarizes the evidence discussed, illustrating the association between reduced capillary density and major systemic complications in systemic sclerosis.

Clinical Cases

The following clinical cases highlight how specific capillaroscopic findings—particularly reduced capillary density—correlate with internal organ involvement, supporting the role of nailfold videocapillaroscopy not only in disease staging but also in prognostic assessment of systemic sclerosis.

Case 7: Reduced Capillary Density Associated with Severe Skin and Lung Involvement

A 43-year-old woman presented with new-onset Raynaud's phenomenon, marked digital puffiness, early sclerodactyly, and arthralgias. Autoantibody testing revealed ANA positivity with a nuclear pattern (1:1280) and anti-topoisomerase I antibodies (anti-Scl70). Rheumatologic evaluation included nailfold videocapillaroscopy, which demonstrated reduced capillary density with the presence of megacapillaries, consistent with an "active" scleroderma pattern.

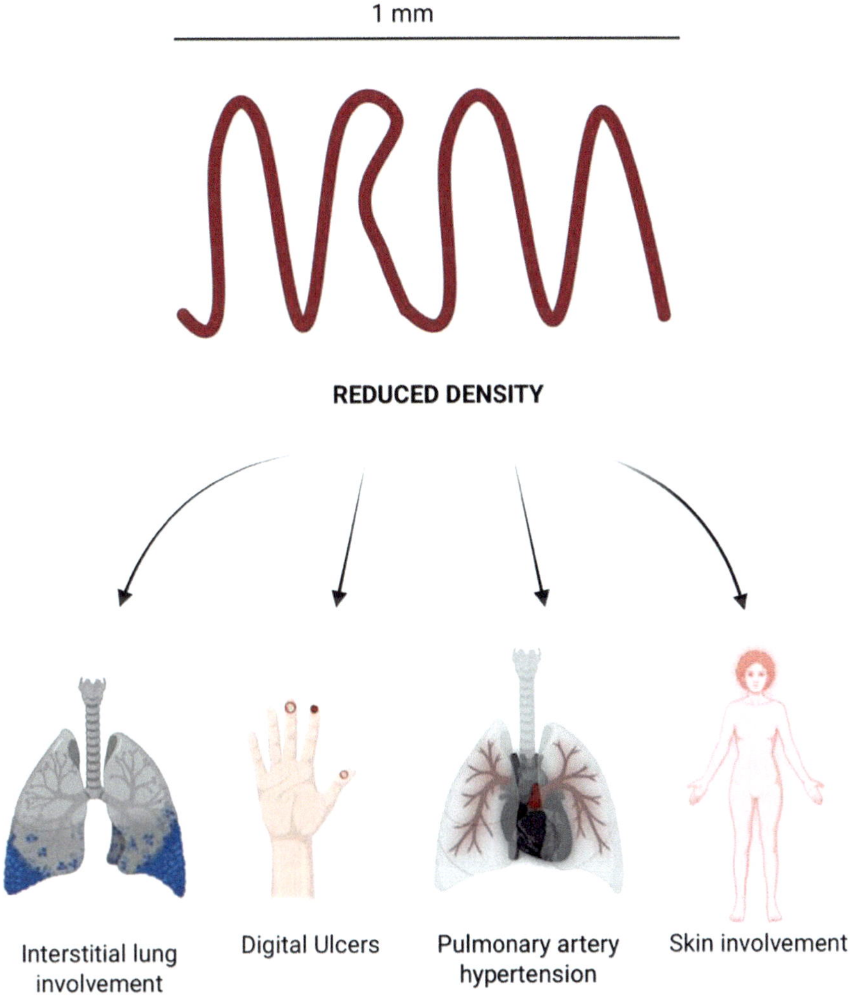

Fig. 13.12 Clinical association of reduced density and major organ involvement in systemic sclerosis

A diagnosis of systemic sclerosis was made, and further investigations revealed interstitial lung disease. Over the following months, the patient developed a rapid progression of skin thickening. This case illustrates the association between reduced capillary density, the presence of a scleroderma pattern on capillaroscopy, and more severe internal organ involvement, particularly pulmonary and cutaneous (Fig. 13.13).

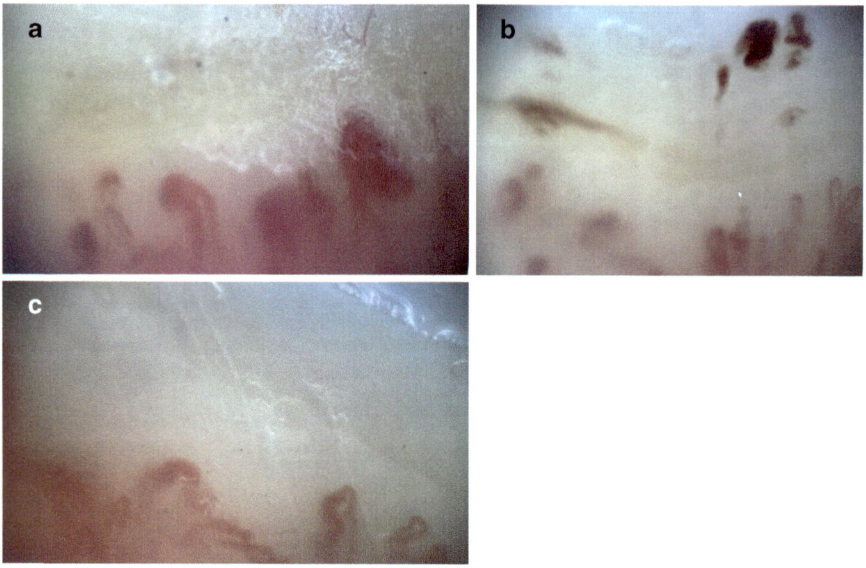

Fig. 13.13 NVC of clinical case 3 with giant capillaries (**a**), microhemorrhages (**b**), reduced density (**c**)

Case 8: Reduced Capillary Density Associated with Digital Ulcers

A 57-year-old woman presented with Raynaud's phenomenon, digital puffiness, arthralgias, and the recent development of painful digital ulcers. Autoantibody testing showed ANA positivity at 1:1280 with anti-PM/Scl-75 antibodies. Nailfold videocapillaroscopy revealed reduced capillary density, the presence of megacapillaries, and frequent microhemorrhages, consistent with a scleroderma pattern.

Further work-up identified interstitial lung disease. This case highlights the link between severe microangiopathy, as indicated by reduced capillary density, and the occurrence of digital ulcers, as well as the presence of internal organ involvement (Fig. 13.14).

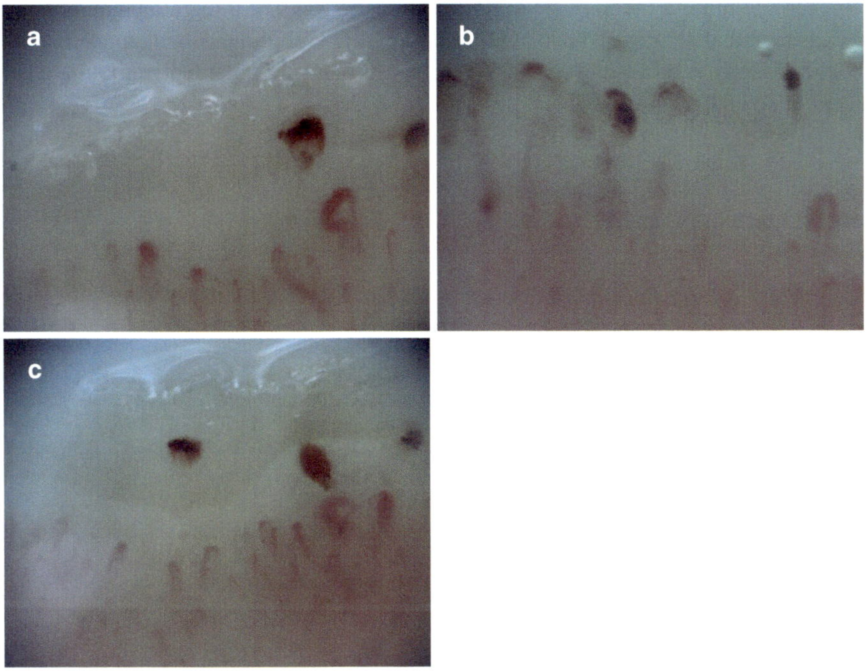

Fig. 13.14 NVC clinical case 4 at first evaluation showing reduced density, giant capillaries and microhemorrhages (**a**, **b**, **c**)

Conclusion

Nailfold videocapillaroscopy (NVC) is a valuable and accessible tool for the in vivo assessment of microvascular abnormalities. Its clinical application is twofold: first, in the evaluation of Raynaud's phenomenon to support early identification of patients at risk for scleroderma-spectrum connective tissue diseases; second, in patients with an established diagnosis of systemic sclerosis, to assess disease severity and predict internal organ involvement.

Over the years, increasing efforts have led to a more precise definition of normal and pathological capillaroscopic patterns, thanks to international consensus initiatives and the development of standardized approaches such as the Fast Track algorithm. These advancements have significantly enhanced the clinical utility of NVC, providing a practical and reproducible framework to support clinicians in the evaluation and follow-up of patients with Raynaud's phenomenon and in the early diagnosis of systemic sclerosis.

Among all NVC parameters, reduced capillary density has shown the strongest correlation with clinical complications, including digital ulcers, interstitial lung disease, and cutaneous progression. Nevertheless, capillaroscopy alone should never be used in isolation. As illustrated through the clinical cases presented in this chapter, the interpretation of NVC findings must always be integrated with clinical assessment and serological data. Only through this multidimensional approach can capillaroscopy achieve its full diagnostic and prognostic potential in the management of scleroderma-related conditions.

References

1. LeRoy EC, Medsger JTA. Raynaud's phenomenon: a proposal for classification. Clin Exp Rheumatol. 1992;10(5):485–8.
2. Cutolo M, Smith V. Detection of microvascular changes in systemic sclerosis and other rheumatic diseases. Nat Rev Rheumatol. 2021;17(11):665–77.
3. Dinsdale G, Peytrignet S, Moore T, et al. The assessment of nailfold capillaries: comparison of dermoscopy and nailfoldvideocapillaroscopy. Rheumatology. 2018;57(6):1115–6.
4. Smith V, Beeckman S, Herrick AL, et al. An EULAR study group pilot study on reliability of simple capillaroscopic definitionsto describe capillary morphology in rheumatic diseases. Rheumatology. 2016;55(5):883–90.
5. Cutolo M, Melsens K, Herrick AL, et al. Reliability of simple capillaroscopic definitions in describing capillary morphology in rheumatic diseases. Rheumatology. 2018;57(4):757–9.
6. Smith V, Herrick AL, Ingegnoli F, et al. Standardisation of nailfold capillaroscopy for the assessment of patients with Raynaud's phenomenon and systemic sclerosis. Autoimmun Rev. 2020;19(3):102458.
7. Andrade LE, Gabriel Júnior A, Assad RL, Ferrari AJ, Atra E. Panoramic nailfold capillaroscopy: a new reading method and normal range. Semin Arthritis Rheum. 1990;20(1):21–31. https://doi.org/10.1016/0049-0172(90)90091-s.
8. Smith V, Vanhaecke A, Herrick AL, et al. Fast track algorithm: how to differentiate a "scleroderma pattern" from a "nonsclerodermapattern". Autoimmun Rev. 2019;18(11):102394.
9. Maricq HR, LeRoy EC. Patterns of finger capillary abnormalities in connective tissue disease by "wide-field" microscopy. Arthritis Rheum. 1973;16(5):619–28.
10. Dernie F, Prats-Uribe A, Man WY, et al. POS1412 incidence, prevalence, and baseline characteristics of primary and secondary Raynaud's phenomenon in the United Kingdom, 2000–2022: a population-based cohort Study. Ann Rheum Dis. 2024;83:674–5.
11. Meier FM, Frommer KW, Dinser R, et al. Update on the profile of the EUSTAR cohort: an analysis of the EULAR scleroderma trials and research group database. Ann Rheum Dis. 2012;71(8):1355–60.
12. Herrick AL, Wigley FM. Raynaud's phenomenon. Best Pract Res Clin Rheumatol. 2020;34(1):101474.
13. Garner R, Kumari R, Lanyon P, Doherty M, Zhang W. Prevalence, risk factors and associations of primary Raynaud's phenomenon: systematic review and meta-analysis of observational studies. BMJ Open. 2015;5(3):e006389. Published 2015 Mar 16. https://doi.org/10.1136/bmjopen-2014-00638.
14. Ingegnoli F, Ughi N, Dinsdale G, Orenti A, Boracchi P, Allanore Y, et al. An international SUrvey on non-iNvaSive tecHniques to assess the mIcrocirculation in patients with RayNaud's phEnomenon (SUNSHINE survey). Rheumatol Int. 2017;37(11):1879–90.
15. Ingegnoli F, Gualtierotti R, Lubatti C, Bertolazzi C, Gutierrez M, Boracchi P, Fornili M, De Angelis R. Nailfold capillary patterns in healthy subjects: a real issue in capillaroscopy. Microvasc Res. 2013;90:90–5. https://doi.org/10.1016/j.mvr.2013.07.001. Epub 2013 Jul 21. PMID: 23880032.
16. Maricq HR. Wide-field capillary microscopy. Technique and rating scale for ab- normalities seen in scleroderma and related disorders. Arthritis Rheum. 1981;24(9):1159–65.

17. Maricq HR. Comparison of quantitative and semiquantitative estimates of nailfold capillary abnormalities in scleroderma spectrum disorders. Microvasc Res. 1986;32(2):271–6.
18. Maverakis E, Patel F, Kronenberg DG, et al. InternationalconsensuscriteriaforthediagnosisofR aynaud'sphenomenon. J Autoimmun. 2014;48-49:60–5.
19. Kabasakal Y, Elvins DM, Ring EF, McHugh NJ. Quantitative nailfold capillaroscopy findings in a population with connective tissue disease and in normal healthy controls. Ann Rheum Dis. 1996;55:507–12.
20. Jouanny P, Schmidt C, Feldmann L, Schmitt J. Peri-ungual capillaroscopy. Value in the diagnosis of systemic diseases. Presse Med. 1993;22:1256–60.
21. Cutolo M, Melsens K, Wijnant S, et al. Nailfold capillaroscopy in systemic lupus erythematosus: a systematic review and critical appraisal. Autoimmun Rev. 2018;17(4):344–52.
22. Melsens K, Leone MC, Paolino S, et al. Nailfold capillaroscopy in Sjogren's syndrome: a systematic literature review and standardised interpretation. Clin Exp Rheumatol. 2020;38(4):150–7.
23. Sulli A, Pizzorni C, Cutolo M. Nailfold videocapillaroscopy abnormalities in patients with antiphospholipid antibodies. J Rheumatol. 2000;27(6):1574–6.
24. Schreiber K, Sciascia S, de Groot PG, et al. Antiphospholipid syndrome. Nat Rev Dis Prim. 2018;4(1):17103.
25. Vaz JL, Dancour MA, Bottino DA, Bouskela E. Nailfold videocapillaroscopy in primary antiphospholipid syndrome (PAPS). Rheumatology. 2004;43(8):1025–7.
26. van den Hoogen F, Khanna D, Fransen J, et al. 2013 classification criteria for systemic sclerosis: an American college of rheumatology/European league against rheumatism collaborative initiative. Ann Rheum Dis. 2013;72(11):1747–55. https://doi.org/10.1136/annrheumdis-2013-204424. PMID: 24092682.
27. Bellando-Randone S, Del Galdo F, Lepri G, Minier T, Huscher D, Furst DE, Allanore Y, Distler O, Czirják L, Bruni C, Guiducci S, Avouac J, Cutolo M, Smith V, Matucci-Cerinic M, Very Early Diagnosis of Systemic Sclerosis collaborators. Progression of patients with Raynaud's phenomenon to systemic sclerosis: a five-year analysis of the European scleroderma trial and research group multicentre, longitudinal registry study for Very Early Diagnosis of Systemic Sclerosis (VEDOSS). Lancet Rheumatol. 2021;3(12):e834–43. https://doi.org/10.1016/S2665-9913(21)00244-7. PMID: 38287630.
28. Pavlov-Dolijanovic S, Damjanov NS, Stojanovic RM, Vujasinovic Stupar NZ, Stanisavljevic DM. Scleroderma pattern of nailfold capillary changes as predictive value for the development of a connective tissue disease: a follow-up study of 3,029 patients with primary Raynaud's phenomenon. Rheumatol Int. 2012;32(10):3039–45.
29. Koenig M, Joyal F, Fritzler MJ, et al. Autoantibodies and microvascular damage are independent predictive factors for the progression of Raynaud's phenomenon to systemic sclerosis: a twenty-year prospective study of 586 patients, with validation of proposed criteria for early systemic sclerosis. Arthritis Rheum. 2008;58(12):3902–12.
30. Avouac J, Fransen J, Walker UA, Riccieri V, Smith V, Muller C, Miniati I, Tarner IH, Randone SB, Cutolo M, Allanore Y, Distler O, Valentini G, Czirjak L, Müller-Ladner U, Furst DE, Tyndall A, Matucci-Cerinic M, EUSTAR Group. Preliminary criteria for the very early diagnosis of systemic sclerosis: results of a Delphi consensus study from EULAR scleroderma trials and research group. Ann Rheum Dis. 2011;70(3):476–81. https://doi.org/10.1136/ard.2010.136929. Epub 2010 Nov 15. PMID: 21081523.
31. Amaral MC, Paula FS, Caetano J, Ames PR, Alves JD. Re-evaluation of nailfold capillaroscopy in discriminating primary from secondary Raynaud's phenomenon and in predicting systemic sclerosis: a randomised observational prospective cohort study. Expert Rev Clin Immunol. 2024;20(6):665–72. https://doi.org/10.1080/1744666X.2024.2313642.
32. Bogojevic M, Markovic Vlaisavljevic M, Medjedovic R, Strujic E, Pravilovic Lutovac D, Pavlov-Dolijanovic S. Nailfold Capillaroscopy changes in patients with idiopathic inflammatory myopathies. J Clin Med. 2024;13(18):5550. Published 2024 Sep 19. https://doi.org/10.3390/jcm13185550.

33. Manfredi A, Sebastiani M, Cassone G, Pipitone N, Giuggioli D, Colaci M, et al. Nailfold capillaroscopic changes in dermatomyositis and polymyositis. Clin Rheumatol. 2015;34(2):279–84.
34. Manfredi A, Sebastiani M, Campomori F, Pipitone N, Giuggioli D, Colaci M, et al. Nailfold Videocapillaroscopy alterations in dermatomyositis and systemic sclerosis: toward identification of a specific pattern. J Rheumatol. 2016;43(8):1575–80.
35. Kubo S, Todoroki Y, Nakayamada S, Nakano K, Satoh M, Nawata A, et al. Significance of nailfold videocapillaroscopy in patients with idiopathic inflammatory myopathies. Rheumatology (Oxford). 2019;58(1):120–30.
36. Piette Y, Reynaert V, Vanhaecke A, et al. Standardised interpretation of capillaroscopy in autoimmune idiopathic inflammatory myopathies: a structured review on behalf of the EULAR study group on microcirculation in rheumatic diseases. Autoimmun Rev. 2022;21(6):10308.
37. Pizzorni C, Cutolo M, Sulli A, et al. Long-term follow-up of nailfold videocapillaroscopic changes in dermatomyositis versus systemic sclerosis patients. Clin Rheumatol. 2018;37(10):2723–9.
38. Sebastiani M, Triantafyllias K, Manfredi A, et al. Nailfold capillaroscopy characteristics of antisynthetase syndrome andpossible clinical associations: results of a multicenter international study. J Rheumatol. 2019;46(3):279–84.
39. Granier F, Vayssairat M, Priollet P, Housset E. Nailfold capillary microscopy in mixed connective tissue disease. Com- parison with systemic sclerosis and systemic lupus erythematosus. Arthritis Rheum. 1986;29(2):189–95.
40. John KJ, Sadiq M, George T, et al. Clinical and immunological profile of mixed connective tissue disease and a comparisonof four diagnostic criteria. Internet J Rheumatol. 2020;2020:9692030.
41. Granier F, Vayssairat M, Priollet P, Housset E. Nailfold capillary microscopy in mixed connective tissue disease. Comparison with systemic sclerosis and systemic lupus erythematosus. Arthritis Rheum. 1986;29(2):189–95.
42. Celinska-Lowenhoff M, Pastuszczak M, Pełka K, Stec-Polak M, Wojas-Pelc A, Musiał J. Associations between nailfold capillaroscopy findings and interstitial lung disease in patients with mixed connective tissue disease. Arch Med Sci. 2020;16(2):297–301.
43. Sebastiani M, Manfredi A, Colaci M, D'Amico R, Malagoli V, Giuggioli D, et al. Capillaroscopic skin ulcer risk index: a new prognostic tool for digital skin ulcer development in systemic sclerosis patients. Arthritis Rheum. 2009;61(5):688–94.
44. Riccieri V, Vasile M, Iannace N, et al. Systemic sclerosis patients with and without pulmonary arterial hypertension: a nailfold capillaroscopy study. Rheumatology. 2013;52(8):1525–8.
45. Hofstee HM, Vonk Noordegraaf A, Voskuyl AE, et al. Nailfold capillary density is associated with the presence and severity of pulmonary arterial hypertension in systemic sclerosis. Ann Rheum Dis. 2009;68(2):191–5.
46. Guillen-Del-Castillo A, Simeon-Aznar CP, Callejas-Moraga EL, et al. Quantitative videocapillaroscopy correlates with functional respiratory parameters: a clue for vasculopathy as a pathogenic mechanism for lung injury in systemic sclerosis. Arthritis Res Ther. 2018;20(1):281.
47. Cutolo M, Herrick AL, Distler O, et al. Nailfold videocapillaroscopic features and other clinical risk factors for digital ulcers in systemic sclerosis: a multicenter, prospective cohort study. Arthritis Rheumatol. 2016;68(10):2527–39.
48. Vanhaecke A, Cutolo M, Distler O, Riccieri V, Allanore Y, Denton CP, Hachulla E, Ingegnoli F, Deschepper E, Avouac J, Jordan S, Launay D, Melsens K, Pizzorni C, Sulli A, Vasile M, Herrick AL, Smith V. Nailfold capillaroscopy in SSc: innocent bystander or promising biomarker for novel severe organ involvement/progression? Rheumatology (Oxford). 2022;61(11):4384–96. https://doi.org/10.1093/rheumatology/keac079. PMID: 35176132; PMCID: PMC9629390.
49. Sulli A, Pizzorni C, Smith V, Zampogna G, Ravera F, Cutolo M. Timing of transition between capillaroscopic patterns in systemic sclerosis. Arthritis Rheum. 2012;64(3):821–5.
50. Avouac J, Lepri G, Smith V, et al. Sequential nailfold videocapillaroscopy examinations have responsiveness to detect organ progression in systemic sclerosis. Semin Arthritis Rheum. 2017;47(1):86–94.

51. Smith V, De Keyser F, Pizzorni C, et al. Nailfold capillaroscopy for day-to-day clinical use: construction of a simple scoring modality as a clinical prognostic index for digital trophic lesions. Ann Rheum Dis. 2011;70(1):180–3.
52. Smith V, Ickinger C, Mihai C, et al. 2nd Online Course on Capillaroscopy & Microcirculation, Module 4, Main Review. Capillaroscopic patterns in systemic sclerosis: predictive indices, links with functional methods analysing the microcirculation and with clinical complications. https://doi.org/10.1016/j.berh.2023.101849.
53. Ingegnoli F, Ardoino I, Boracchi P, et al. Nailfold capillaroscopy in systemic sclerosis: data from the EULAR sclerodermatrials and research (EUSTAR) database. Microvasc Res. 2013;89:122e8.
54. Smith V, Riccieri V, Pizzorni C, et al. Nailfold capillaroscopy for prediction of novel future severe organ involvement in systemic sclerosis. J Rheumatol. 2013;40(12):2023–8.
55. Ennis H, Moore T, Murray A, Vail A, Herrick AL. Further confirmation that digital ulcers are associated with the severity of abnormality on nailfold capillaroscopy in patients with systemic sclerosis. Rheumatology. 2014;53(2):376–7.
56. Smith V, Vanhaecke A, Vandecasteele E, et al. Nailfold videocapillaroscopy in systemic sclerosis-related pulmonary arterial hypertension: a systematic literature review. J Rheumatol. 2020;47(6):888–95.
57. Silva I, Teixeira A, Oliveira J, et al. Endothelial dysfunction and nailfold videocapillaroscopy pattern as predictors of digital ulcers in systemic sclerosis: a cohort study and review of the literature. Clin Rev Allergy Immunol. 2015;49(2):240–52.

Chapter 14
Capillaroscopy: Advanced Techniques

Antonia Valenzuela and Yazmin Espinosa

Introduction

Capillaroscopy is a noninvasive diagnostic tool used to evaluate the microcirculation in the nailfold region. It plays a fundamental role in the early detection of Raynaud phenomenon (RP) and systemic autoimmune diseases, especially connective tissue diseases (CTDs) such as systemic sclerosis (SSc) [1] Over the past few decades, technological advances have led to the development of new methodologies that facilitate its application and enhance both the diagnostic accuracy and analytical capacity of the technique.

This chapter explores the evolution of capillaroscopy from conventional optical systems to sophisticated digital platforms supported by quantitative analysis and artificial intelligence (AI). These innovations not only improve image quality and objectivity but also lead to more personalized and real-time medical approaches.

The purpose of this chapter is to provide an in-depth overview of these advanced techniques, discuss their current clinical applications, evaluate their limitations, and propose future directions in research and practice.

A. Valenzuela (✉)
Clinical Immunology and Rheumatology Department, Pontificia Universidad Catolica de Chile, Santiago, Chile
e-mail: antonia.valenzuela@uc.cl

Y. Espinosa
Rheumatology and Immunology Department, Hospital Roberto Del Río, Santiago, Chile

Y. El Miedany, R. A. Elziaty (eds.), *Capillaroscopy*, Contemporary Rheumatology,
https://doi.org/10.1007/978-3-032-22966-3_14

Advanced Techniques in Capillaroscopy

The evaluation of microcirculation plays a crucial role in the early diagnosis and monitoring of various systemic and autoimmune diseases. Among the available techniques, nailfold videocapillaroscopy (NVC) has long been considered a fundamental tool for assessing microvascular abnormalities [2]. Recent technological advances, however, have broadened the diagnostic possibilities by incorporating novel imaging modalities that provide more detailed and dynamic insights into capillary morphology and blood flow.

Digital Capillaroscopy

Digital capillaroscopy is the enhanced form of traditional capillaroscopy. While conventional capillaroscopy uses an optical microscope (often with a manual camera or none at all) to directly observe the capillaries, digital capillaroscopy uses a digital video camera connected to a computer (or other electronic devices) to capture and display high-resolution images on a screen [3]. This technique allows clinicians to observe capillary architecture in greater detail, supporting more precise and reliable assessments of capillary morphology. Traditional capillaroscopy relies on handheld microscopes and real-time observation through ocular lenses. Although effective, it does not allow for long-term tracking. In contrast, digital systems enable longitudinal follow-up and comparisons, which are essential for monitoring disease progression.

Digital capillaroscopy offers several advantages. Its high-resolution imaging provides superior clarity compared to conventional optical devices, allowing for more detailed visualization of capillary structures. The ability to store digital images facilitates longitudinal follow-up, easy access to past records, and seamless sharing among specialists for collaborative evaluation. Additionally, the digital format supports more precise measurements and enables the use of automated software tools, improving the accuracy and efficiency of capillary analysis [4]. The main differences between conventional and digital capillaroscopy are summarized in Table 14.1.

Table 14.1 Main differences between conventional capillaroscopy and digital capillaroscopy

Feature	Conventional capillaroscopy	Digital capillaroscopy
Imaging method	Optical microscope	Digital video camera with computer interface
Magnification	5–200×	Up to 500×
Image capture	Manual sketches or photos	Digital storage and sharing
Analysis	Visual assessment	Automated software-based evaluations
Resolution	Lower	High-resolution
Documentation	Limited	Comprehensive and longitudinal

More recently, low-cost USB microscopes have expanded access to digital imaging techniques, with the following studies demonstrating good performance results comparable to those obtained using traditional NVC.

A pilot study compared nailfold capillaroscopy images obtained from 20 patients with SSc and 20 healthy controls using both videocapillaroscopy (a high-frame-rate camera and lens system mounted on a software-controlled stage, enabling fast and precise video capture across the nailfold) and a low-cost USB microscope. USB microscopy produced high-quality images comparable to those from videocapillaroscopy. Both methods effectively differentiated SSc from controls based on capillary width, although videocapillaroscopy performed better in assessing capillary density. The authors concluded that USB capillaroscopy is an accessible alternative for identifying SSc-related capillary changes [5].

Another study involving 22 patients with diffuse cutaneous SSc (dcSSc), 20 with limited cutaneous SSc (lcSSc), and 42 controls evaluated nailfold capillaries using a digital microscope at 30× and 100× magnification. The results demonstrated that this technique effectively visualized all the changes previously described in studies using videocapillaroscopy, providing comparable image quality and successfully distinguishing between SSc skin subtypes and healthy controls [6].

Finally, a study on a relatively higher number of patients compared nailfold capillary abnormalities among the three most common CTDs and the normal population with USB digital microscopy. The study included 245 participants—54 with systemic lupus erythematosus (SLE), 32 with dermatomyositis (DM), 51 with SSc, and 108 healthy controls—and demonstrated that this method effectively identified capillary alterations associated with CTDs. Moreover, distinct morphological patterns and their severity proved useful in differentiating between these conditions [7].

These studies demonstrate that USB digital capillaroscopy is a reliable procedure compared to videocapillaroscopy, which is much more expensive, and that it allows for similar conclusions to be drawn at a reduced cost.

Other Novel Techniques

Additional alternative approaches have been investigated to assess the microcirculation and enhance the image quality provided by capillaroscopy. Novel and sensitive methods for visualizing longitudinal and even functional changes—such as capillary perfusion and oxygenation—are generating growing interest and are discussed in the following section.

Optical Coherence Tomography

Optical coherence tomography (OCT) is a noninvasive imaging technique that uses an infrared laser to produce detailed images of blood flow. Dynamic OCT (D-OCT) allows visualization of microvasculature and detection of blood flow by using repeated scans and algorithms that filter out non-blood flow movements [8]. A small case series of two patients with SSc, one patient with DM, and one healthy volunteer showed that D-OCT capillaroscopy detected flow status, giant capillaries, and vascular dropouts, as well as characteristic changes in the surrounding skin of the capillaries in the nailfold (such as loss of a well-defined distinct dermo-epidermal junction and more compact dermis with loss of adnexal structures) in patients with SSc, providing more information than traditional capillaroscopy in a single scan [9]. Similarly, a pilot case-controlled study of 40 patients with SSc, classified by NVC pattern in four age- and sex-matched groups (normal/nonspecific, early, active, and late) and ten age- and sex-matched healthy controls, found reduced microvascular flow density with D-OCT in SSc patients, negatively correlating with NVC analysis and demonstrating excellent interobserver reliability [10]. This technique is represented in Fig. 14.1.

Raster-Scan Optoacoustic Mesoscopy (RSOM)

This advanced imaging technique combines optical and ultrasound technologies to provide high-resolution, three-dimensional images of capillaries and deeper microvascular structures. It enables visualization of both superficial and deeper microvasculature, which is helpful in SSc, where deeper vascular involvement and skin thickening are common. Ultra-wideband RSOM (UWB-RSOM) (Fig. 14.2) can reach a penetration depth of 5 mm while keeping high resolution [11]. A study of six healthy volunteers investigated the use of UWB-RSOM to visualize nailfold microvascular structures, including small capillaries and deeper structures like venules and arterioles. The study demonstrated that UWB-RSOM quantified capillary density and diameter, providing results comparable to those of traditional capillaroscopy [11]. Another study explored the use of RSOM to visualize the nailfold capillaries of 23 SSc patients and 19 healthy controls and compared them with dermoscopy and high-magnification capillaroscopy. The vascular volume in the nailfold capillaries was calculated from the RSOM images, showing a significant difference between the SSc patients and controls [12]. RSOM shows potential as an advanced imaging technique for exploring the microcirculation.

Laser Speckle Contrast Analysis (LASCA)

Laser speckle contrast analysis (LASCA) is a noninvasive, high-resolution technique that measures peripheral blood perfusion (PBP) by analyzing changes in laser-induced speckle patterns. (Fig. 14.3) A study involving 61 SSc patients and 61 healthy controls demonstrated that LASCA detected significantly lower PBP in SSc patients compared to healthy subjects and that LASCA perfusion values were found to correlate with the progression of microangiopathy as assessed by NVC patterns [13]. A single-center pilot study of 15 SSc patients and 30 healthy controls showed that LACSA had good to excellent inter-rater agreement and intra-rater reliability

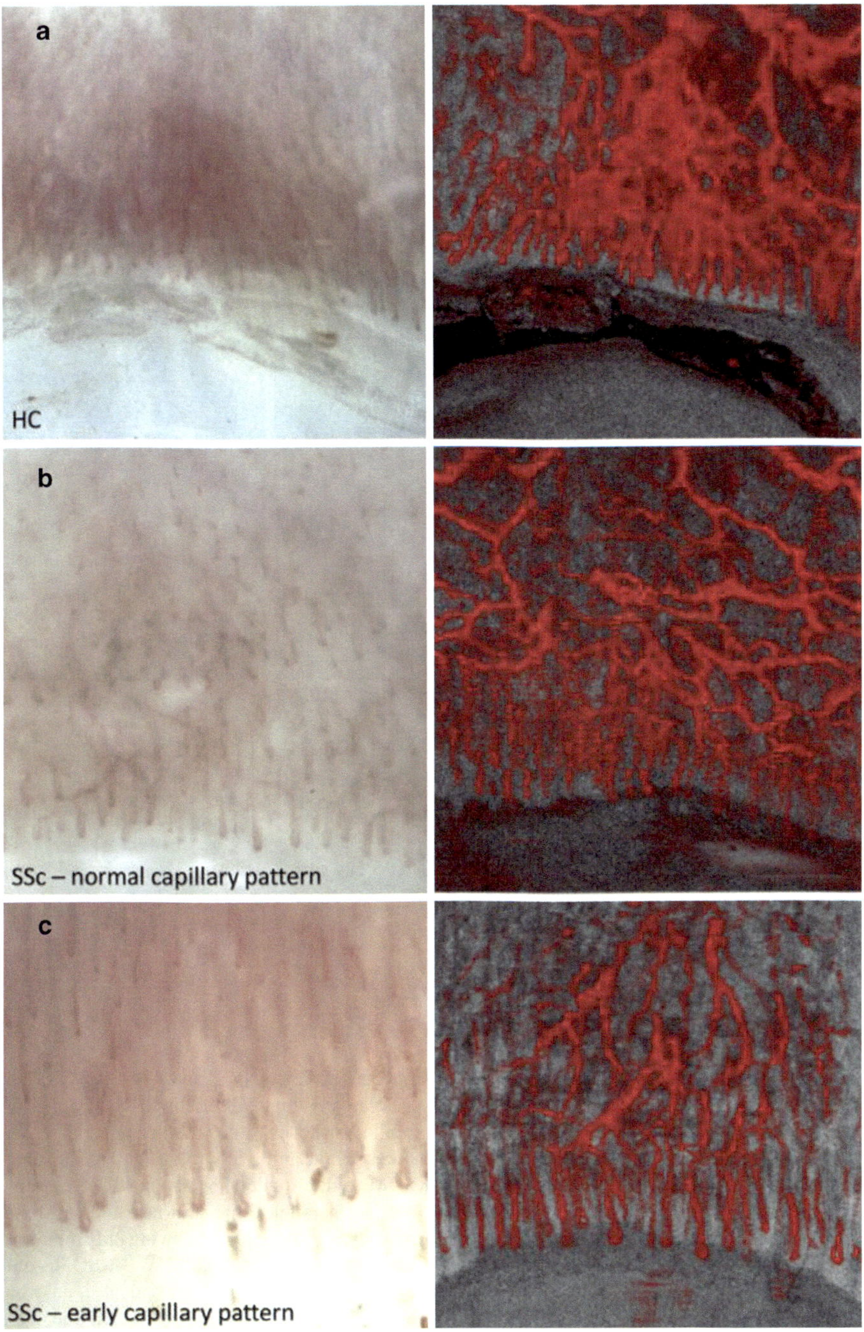

Fig. 14.1 Representative images illustrate capillary loops, their distribution, morphology, presence of hemorrhages, and the overall capillary pattern in NVC and nailfold D-OCT in (**a**) healthy controls, (**b**) SSc patients with a normal pattern, and (**c**) SSc patients with an early capillary pattern. (Reproduced with permission from Abignano et al., J Invest Dermatol. 2022)

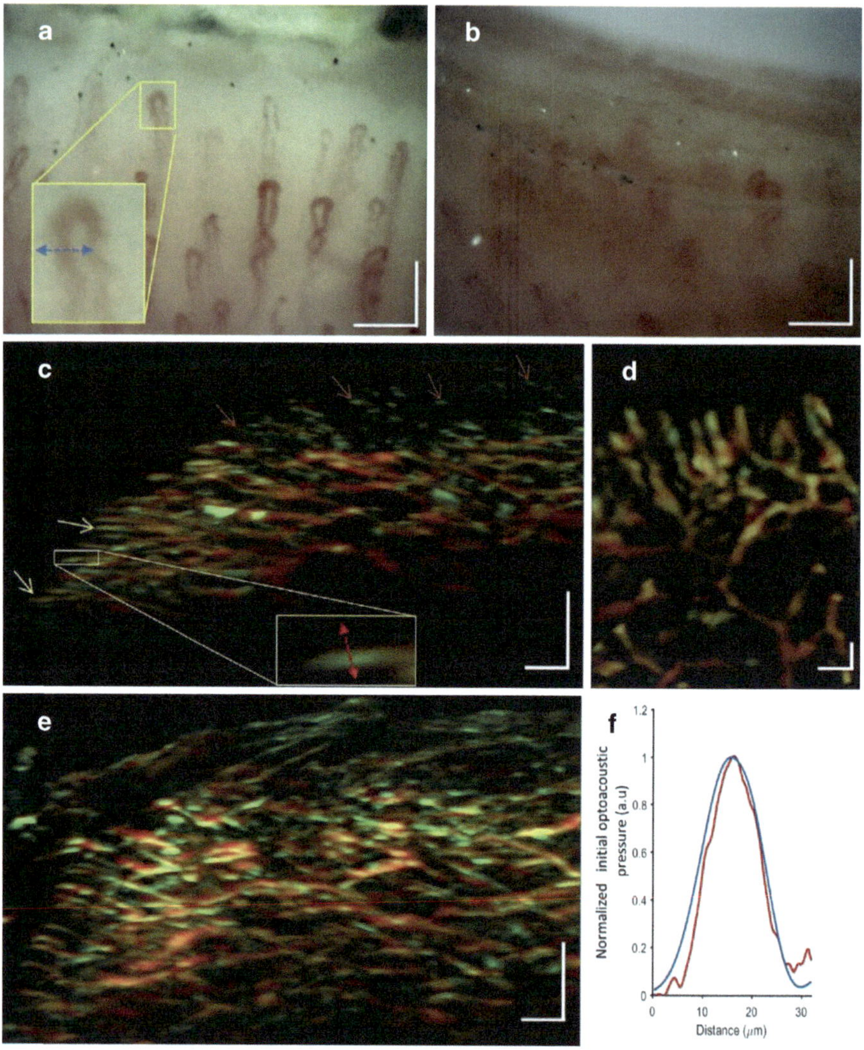

Fig. 14.2 Comparison of capillary imaging using conventional NVC and UWB-RSOM. (**a**) Nailfold capillaroscopy image of Subject 1, who has relatively thin, light-colored skin. Capillaries are clearly visible. The yellow box highlights one capillary, whose profile is shown in panel (f). (**b**) Capillaroscopy image of Subject 2, with thicker, darker skin. Capillaries are difficult to see, making vascular assessment challenging. (**c**) UWB-RSOM sagittal (side view) image near the same area as in (a). Yellow arrows point to capillaries running parallel to the skin near the nail base; brown arrows point to deeper capillaries running perpendicular to the skin, showing only their tips. (**d**) UWB-RSOM coronal (frontal view) image near the same area as in (a). (**e**) UWB-RSOM sagittal image of the region near that shown in (b). (**f**) Capillary profile comparison: optical signal from capillaroscopy (blue line, from panel a) vs. optoacoustic signal from UWB-RSOM (red line, from panel c). (Reproduced with permission from Aguirre et al., Photoacoustics. 2018 Feb 21;10:31–37)

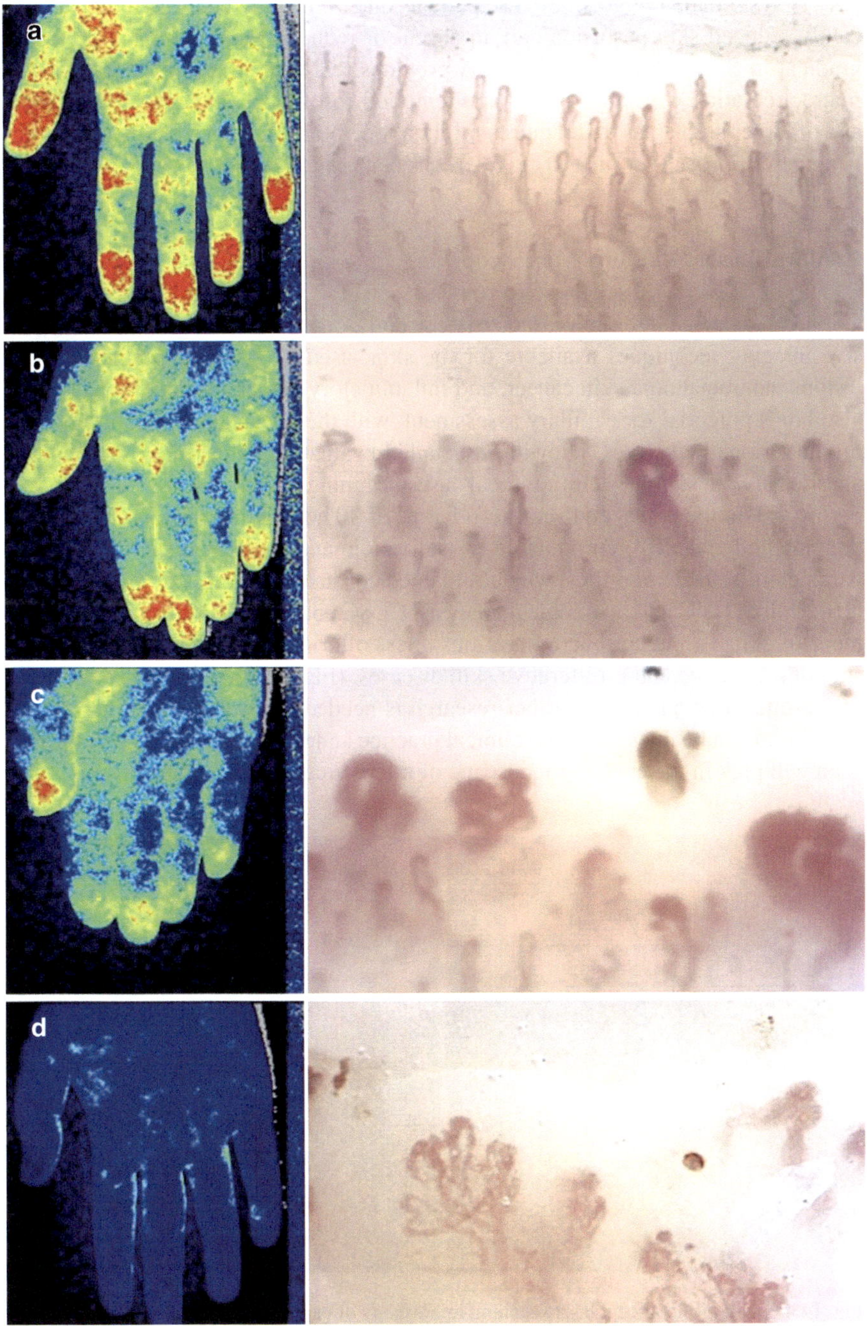

Fig. 14.3 Laser speckle contrast analysis image of right hands and related NVC pictures in a healthy subject (**a**) and in SSc patients with an 'Early' (**b**), 'Active' (**c**), or 'Late' (**d**) pattern of microangiopathy (NVC picture magnification 200×). (Reproduced with permission from Ruaro B et al. Ann Rheum Dis. 2014;73(6):1181–5)

[14]. A systematic review of 30 SSc patients and 30 healthy controls found significantly reduced skin perfusion and an absent or reduced proximal-distal perfusion gradient in SSc patients [15]. LASCA provides real-time, dynamic assessment of microcirculation with high spatial and temporal resolution. It enables rapid coverage of larger skin areas and requires minimal operator effort, presenting as a promising new approach for measuring microcirculation.

Confocal Laser Scanning Microscopy

Confocal laser scanning microscopy is currently one of the most precise noninvasive imaging techniques available for the skin, used to visualize pigmented skin lesions, nonmelanoma skin cancer, and inflammatory cutaneous conditions [16]. It also holds potential for capillary assessment, with the advantage of enabling imaging at various body sites, allowing a detailed evaluation of capillary morphology and density. A study where confocal laser scanning capillaroscopy (CLSC) was performed on the dorsal and ventral forearms of 30 healthy individuals showed that this method enabled reproducible visualization and measurement of capillary parameters at the extremities, which remained constant regardless of the skin depth [16]. Unlike NVC and histological analysis, CLSC enabled accurate, in vivo assessment of skin vasculature across various sites, offering a significant advantage in studying systemic and proliferative skin diseases. (Fig. 14.4).

Despite these advances, further research is needed to evaluate how these novel techniques can be integrated into clinical practice and research and to define the role each will play in the evolving landscape of microcirculation assessment.

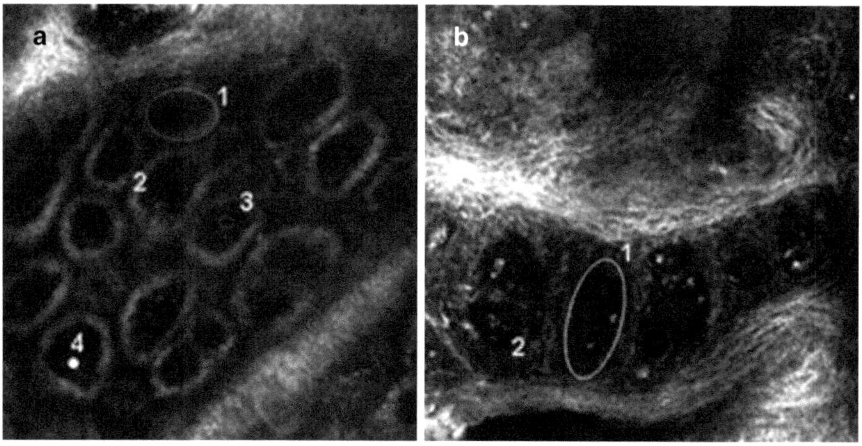

Fig. 14.4 Images of confocal laser scanning microscopy of capillaries in the skin in vivo of (**a**) a healthy volunteer and (**b**) a lesion of a psoriasis patient (500 × 500 μm, 1, papilla; 2, Feret's diameter; 3, perimeter; 4, area). (Reproduced with permission from Hegyi et al., Skin Res Technol. 2009 Nov;15(4):476–81)

Quantitative Analysis

Most analyses of nailfold capillaroscopy images have been qualitative or semi-quantitative, depending largely on subjective interpretation. Manual measurements have been traditionally used to assess various characteristics of individual capillaries, including their dimensions and density, which helps in identifying abnormalities and classifying different patterns. Despite international efforts to standardize image interpretation, significant subjectivity remains in the assessment of nailfold capillary images [17].

The semi-quantitative evaluation of capillary density, capillary dimensions, microhemorrhages, and ramified capillaries has more recently been replaced by a fully quantitative approach. This method involves counting all microhemorrhages and all capillaries, as well as identifying irregularly enlarged and giant capillaries and abnormal shapes in the distal row. Quantitative capillaroscopy introduces computational methods to objectively analyze these capillary parameters. Automated measurement seeks to eliminate subjectivity and enables near-instant image analysis, though image acquisition still requires time [18].

A quantitative approach to capillaroscopy is important for several reasons. First, the broad range of normal nailfold capillary appearances makes it difficult to reliably distinguish normal from abnormal using qualitative or semi-quantitative methods. Second, tracking microvascular changes over time—crucial for understanding disease progression and evaluating treatment response—requires precise, sensitive measurements that only quantitative tools can offer. Third, establishing robust associations between capillary abnormalities and clinical outcomes depends on fast, consistent, and objective assessments. Together, these factors highlight the need for a standardized, quantitative framework in both clinical practice and research [18].

Artificial Intelligence (AI)

AI has emerged as a transformative element in medical diagnostics, and capillaroscopy is no exception. Several automated assistive tools, both open-source and commercial, are now available to facilitate quantitative capillaroscopic analysis. These programs include machine learning and deep learning components that assist in pattern recognition and classification. Algorithms can be programmed to detect and measure various capillaroscopic parameters, including capillary dimensions (such as width and length), intercapillary distance, capillary density, and capillary loop shape patterns. These algorithms serve multiple purposes, from promoting standardization in research and clinical settings to offering an objective approach for evaluating therapeutic response. Additionally, they are instrumental in detecting early microvascular changes [19].

However, successful deployment requires access to extensive, diverse datasets and rigorous, multicenter validation to ensure robustness across different patient populations and imaging systems. Additionally, there is a significant learning curve: operators must acquire consistently high-quality images to enable accurate, quantitative assessment. Despite these challenges, early studies—especially in the context of SSc—have yielded encouraging results, underscoring the potential of advanced capillaroscopic algorithms in improving early detection and monitoring of microvascular disease [18].

In the context of advancing automation in the quantitative assessment of NVC images, the few clinical systems that have been developed and systematically evaluated will be reviewed below.

Capillary.io

Capillary.io is an interactive, web-based tool designed to recognize capillaries in images obtained with any microscope and automatically generate measurements for each capillary, which can measure most nailfold vessel parameters. This enables an exhaustive analysis and the production of detailed, patient-specific reports. The tool was developed using a deep learning and data-driven approach to nailfold capillaroscopy, trained on a dataset of 2713 images and 18,000 measurements. The software demonstrated strong performance in detecting most capillaries in NVC images, with high precision in identifying and classifying capillaries and hemorrhages by shape and size. It achieved a standard metric precision of 83.84% and a recall of 92.44% in capillary identification obtained with machine learning algorithms [20].

This was externally validated in a study of 1164 NVC images obtained during routine examinations of patients with RP at five Spanish hospitals and evaluated by five experienced capillaroscopists and the software-based algorithm. When ≥3 observers agreed (86.9% of images), the algorithm matched 75.8% of the time, and when ≥4 agreed (52% of cases), the match rate rose to 87.1%. The algorithm demonstrated strong performance, with a positive predictive value over 80% for key abnormalities and specificity and negative predictive value exceeding 89% across all categories (normal capillaries, dilations, giant capillaries, abnormal shapes, tortuosity, and microhemorrhages) [21].

Furthermore, these automated quantitative metrics were combined with the consensus expertise of trained capillaroscopists to develop the CAPI-Score algorithm, designed to objectively classify disease patterns, drawing inspiration from the Fast Track model. A total of 851 NVC images, each classified according to consensus-based disease patterns, were examined by nine capillaroscopists, and key variables—such as capillary density, the presence of abnormal and giant capillaries, tortuosity, and hemorrhages—were used. The algorithm was able to reliably distinguish between SSc and non-SSc NVC patterns and accurately identify specific stages of SSc. Accuracy improved with higher interobserver consensus [22].

Finally, a more advanced machine learning model, the CAPI-Detect, was developed to enhance capillaroscopic pattern identification by incorporating a broader range of statistical variables than those used in the CAPI-Score. Among 1490 capillaroscopy images with consensus classifications analyzed by three to four trained observers, images with at least partial consensus (agreement by all but one observer) were used to train machine learning classification models. The model achieved high accuracy for distinguishing SSc from non-SSc patterns, differentiating among SSc patterns, and distinguishing between normal and nonspecific patterns. Accuracy improved when evaluated on the subset of full consensus data (unanimous agreement), outperforming the CAPI-Score algorithm and identifying novel capillary features relevant to machine learning–based classification. These findings highlight CAPI-Detect as an unbiased, quantitative tool that significantly advances capillaroscopic pattern recognition [23] (Fig. 14.5).

AUTOCAPI

The AUTOCAPI system provides vessel density results that are in good agreement with expert assessments for a single field of view (preselected by the operator) [24]. This automated software, designed to assess absolute nailfold capillary number and density from NVC images in SSc, was developed and trained using exploratory and training image sets. Its reliability was tested by comparing automated and manual counts across four independent observers, showing high intraclass correlation coefficients, particularly in SSc patients [24]. The software was optimized to evaluate capillary number in the shortest possible time and with the lowest possible error, in patients with SSc, as well as in healthy subjects. This was further investigated in 183 SSc patients classified by NVC into one of the following patterns: 28 "not specific," 37 "Early," 89 "Active," and 29 "Late." Good reliability of the AUTOCAPI software in nailfold capillary number counting in SSc patients with different patterns of microangiopathy [25].

ViT: Vision Transformer

ViT is a widely adopted deep learning architecture that represents the current state-of-the-art in computer vision, outperforming convolutional neural networks and other previously developed AI models. ViT was applied to identify disease-associated microangiopathic changes—such as enlarged capillaries, giant capillaries, capillary loss, and microhemorrhages—as well as SSc capillaroscopic patterns, using a dataset of 17,126 images from patients enrolled in the EUSTAR and VEDOSS registries. Its performance was also compared to that of rheumatologists using a reliability set of 464 nailfold capillaroscopy images. The ViT showed good performance, with area under the curve (AUC) values ranging from 81.8% to 84.5%.

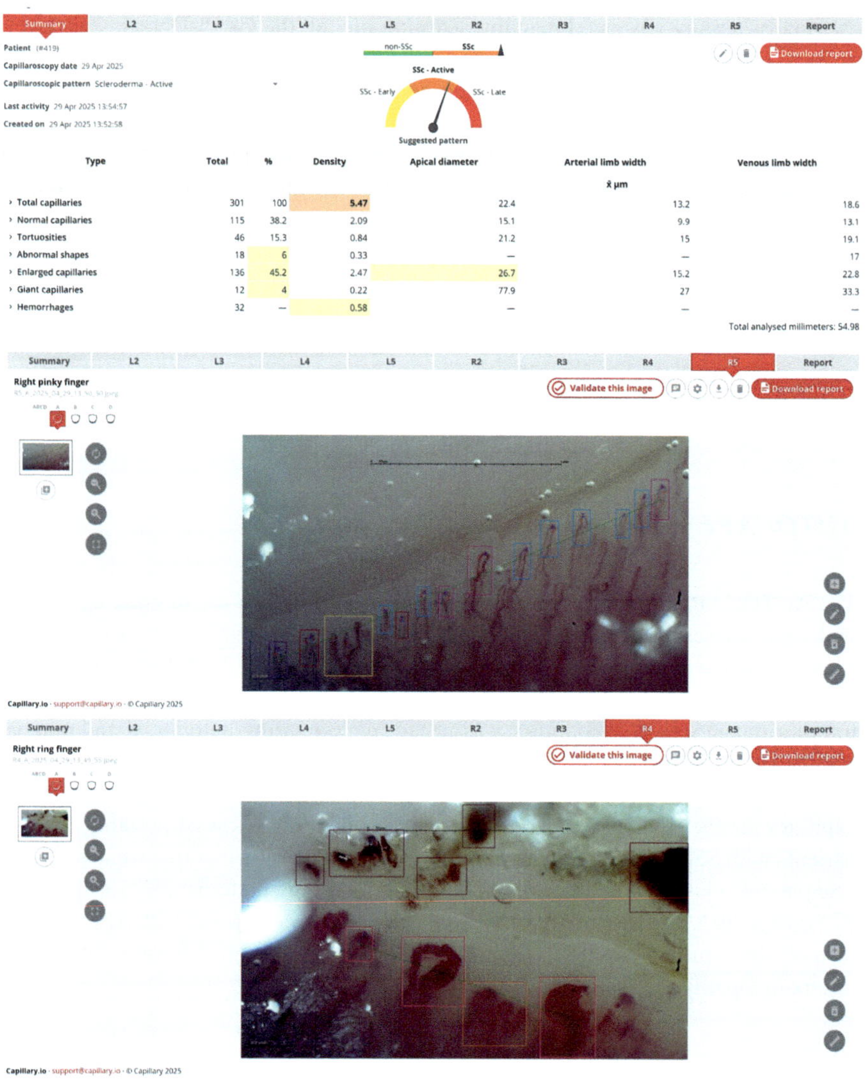

Fig. 14.5 Representative images from Capillary.io software showing the features analyzed for reporting

However, rheumatologists outperformed the ViT in terms of accuracy and sensitivity/specificity balance, though one rheumatologist had performance equal to or worse than the ViT [26]. Authors concluded that the ViT is a modern, reliable tool for analyzing NVC images and may support rheumatologists in producing consistent, high-quality reports, though final diagnosis of an SSc pattern should involve experienced clinical judgment [27].

Manchester University Automated Capillaroscopy Analysis System

Berks et al. developed an automated system to detect individual capillaries using a set of 455 images. This system proved to perform as well as human experts and was able to differentiate between patients with primary RP based on measurements of vessel morphology [28]. A subsequent study tested whether adding blood flow measurements to automated capillary morphology from high-quality nailfold capillaroscopy images could distinguish between SSc patients and those with primary RP and healthy controls. They imaged 50 SSc patients, 12 with primary RP, and 50 healthy individuals, and measured different metrics, which differed significantly between SSc and the other groups. A combined structural score outperformed the best single feature, and adding flow data further increased accuracy [29]. However, this system requires the images to be manually compounded into a single mosaic showing the whole nailfold bed, which could be time-consuming. Bharatti et al. developed and validated a fully automatic image analysis system combining data from each capillary in the distal row of capillaries from multiple fingers to produce a subject-level probability of SSc. Their proposed method was based on a deep learning–based, fully automated system trained on high-resolution images from 111 SSc subjects (group A), which was tested on additional high-resolution (group B) and low-cost digital microscope images (group C). The automated analysis showed strong diagnostic performance, with an area under the ROC curve (AUC) of 97% for group B and 95% for group C, achieving equal sensitivity and specificity of 91% and 89%, respectively. In comparison, SSc expert consensus achieved a sensitivity of 82% and specificity of 73% [19].

Other Automated Systems and AI Applications in NVC Analysis

One of the earliest efforts in this area was the development of CapiAna (capillary analysis), a semi-automated image analysis tool designed to evaluate skin capillary density. Conducted in 20 individuals, the study demonstrated good agreement between CapiAna and the traditional manual method, while offering significant time savings and improved reproducibility compared to manual capillary counting [30].

In a study focused on juvenile DM (JDM), researchers analyzed 1120 NVC images from 111 children with active JDM and 321 images from 31 healthy controls using NFC-Net, a lightweight and explainable deep neural network (downscaled using interpolation techniques to reduce computational cost). The model effectively distinguished JDM patients from healthy controls (ROC AUC: 0.93; accuracy: 0.91; sensitivity: 0.85; specificity: 0.90) and showed moderate success in predicting clinical disease activity (AUC: 0.75; accuracy: 0.74) [31].

Korendovych et al. utilized a digital capillaroscope in combination with deep learning algorithms to differentiate between SSc and non-SSc capillary patterns. They analyzed 1076 NVC images from 70 patients, divided into training (780), validation (196), and test (100) datasets, with balanced representation of both pattern types. The model achieved 87.8% accuracy on the validation set (sensitivity: 94.9%, specificity: 80.6%, AUC: 0.9326) and improved performance on the test set (accuracy: 92%, sensitivity: 96%, specificity: 88%, AUC: 0.9742) [32].

Significant progress has also been made using YOLO (You Only Look Once), a convolutional neural network-based, deep learning algorithm for object detection. In two studies focused on advancing automated nailfold capillaroscopy for microvascular research, researchers utilized different versions of the YOLO algorithm to enhance capillary detection and measurement. In one study, researchers enhanced YOLO to detect distal nailfold capillaries and measure density. The YOLOv5 model, applied to images from 20 healthy volunteers, showed high agreement with expert manual counts, providing a fast and reliable method for capillary density assessment [33].

A second study introduced a low-cost, portable system based on YOLOv8, capable of detecting microvascular changes in conditions like SSc and RP. Running on a single-board computer, the system automatically quantified capillary number, thickness, and density with a mean average precision of 0.882. It proved effective for early diagnosis and monitoring of microvascular disorders, combining speed, objectivity, and affordability [34]. Together, these studies highlight the promising application of YOLO-based systems in microcirculation research, providing efficient, cost-effective, and accurate automated tools for capillary analysis.

Ozturk et al. evaluated machine learning and deep learning techniques using capillaroscopy images from the French prospective multicenter observational study SCLEROCAP, previously annotated by experts. Among various machine learning models, Random Forest (RF), LightGBM (LGB), and XGBoost (XGB) were fairly accurate in analyzing nailfold capillaroscopy images—correctly identifying most of the important patterns about 75–79% of the time (F1 scores between 0.75 and 0.79). Deep learning approaches outperformed them, with F1 scores ranging from 0.87 to 0.94. DenseNet-121 delivered the best results [35].

These studies underscore the potential of automated systems to transform capillaroscopy by improving objectivity, reproducibility, and growth potential. They demonstrate strong performance in detecting and classifying key capillary features, including abnormalities like hemorrhages and tortuosities. Moreover, the ability of AI-driven tools to match expert consensus highlights their promise for widespread clinical implementation in the diagnosis and monitoring of diseases such as SSc, RP, and JDM.

Challenges and Limitations of Advanced Techniques

Comparisons between conventional and advanced techniques have consistently favored digital approaches in terms of diagnostic accuracy, reproducibility, and time efficiency. AI-supported systems also provide a second opinion, reducing operator bias and supporting less experienced clinicians in training environments. Even so, an expert observer's assessment is essential for the final evaluation [27].

Despite their clear benefits, adopting advanced capillaroscopic technologies presents significant challenges. The high cost of specialized analysis software limits access, particularly in low-resource settings. Effective use also requires specialized training in software operation, image acquisition protocols, and AI-driven interpretation, along with an understanding of each tool's limitations to prevent overreliance. Many of these techniques remain in clinical validation, necessitating multicenter trials and standardized protocols for acquisition, analysis, and interpretation. Finally, integrating AI into diagnostics raises ethical and regulatory concerns—such as data privacy, algorithmic transparency, and clinical responsibility—that must be addressed to ensure safe and responsible implementation.

Future Directions

AI is positioned to transform NVC by enabling individualized care through the analysis of large datasets, identifying disease-specific microvascular patterns, and supporting predictive, personalized treatment strategies. Advances in imaging technology—such as 3D visualization, multispectral analysis, and integration with modalities like ultrasound or OCT—will enhance diagnostic precision. Real-time automated systems promise faster, more accessible assessments, potentially bringing capillaroscopy to point-of-care settings, including primary care and telemedicine. Furthermore, integrating capillaroscopic data with laboratory, imaging, and patient-reported outcomes will promote a more comprehensive understanding of disease, with interoperability between digital platforms becoming increasingly essential.

Moving forward, promoting the use of low-cost, handheld devices—such as USB-based microscopes—could significantly expand access to capillaroscopy, enabling broader implementation in clinical settings and facilitating large-scale, multicenter randomized controlled trials that include capillaroscopic parameters as outcome measures. However, challenges remain. Interpretation of findings can still be complex, and current AI tools, while promising, are not without limitations. Additionally, the accessibility of advanced automated systems may be hindered by costs, often tied to licensing, memberships, or proprietary platforms, potentially restricting widespread adoption. Balancing the integration of AI into routine medical practice—ensuring it supports innovation and enhances care—while addressing these ongoing barriers is essential to fully realize the potential of automated capillaroscopy in both research and clinical care.

Conclusions

Advanced techniques in capillaroscopy represent a significant leap forward in the evaluation of microvascular health. Digital capillaroscopy, quantitative image analysis, and AI-assisted interpretation collectively enhance diagnostic accuracy, objectivity, and reproducibility.

These innovations are particularly valuable in the early diagnosis and monitoring of systemic autoimmune diseases such as systemic sclerosis and lupus. Case studies and preliminary research have demonstrated the practical benefits of advanced capillaroscopy, especially when integrated into multidisciplinary care.

Despite their promise, these technologies face challenges related to cost, training, validation, and ethical use. Addressing these barriers will require coordinated efforts among researchers, clinicians, engineers, and policymakers.

The future of capillaroscopy is likely to be increasingly automated, integrated, and patient-centered. Further studies are needed to validate these tools in diverse clinical settings and to explore their full potential in personalized medicine. Continued technological development, along with educational initiatives and infrastructure support, will be essential to fully implement advanced capillaroscopy in routine clinical practice.

The advances in quantitative capillaroscopy described above, including automation, have the potential to improve patient care and to facilitate research into the pathophysiology, measurement, and treatment of SSc-spectrum disorders and hold promise as objective clinical-trial outcome measures. Finally, if the goal is to broaden the clinical use of nailfold capillaroscopy—from early diagnosis to monitoring disease progression and treatment response—then the ability to accurately track changes over time is essential. Automated analysis could be instrumental in meeting this need, offering rheumatologists objective, point-of-care assessments to support clinical decision-making.

Clinical Case 1

A 47-year-old female patient with no relevant medical history presents with RP, evolving over the past 2 years. Initially episodic, it has now become more frequent and painful. She reports progressive skin thickening and swelling of the hands that have prevented her from wearing rings for the past 8 months. Additionally, she experiences episodes of mild dysphagia. She also reports arthralgias in both hands, without dyspnea or fever. Laboratory tests reveal positive ANA antibodies at titers of 1:1280 and a centromere pattern. She is referred for capillaroscopy.

Images were obtained using a digital microscope with 200X optical magnification (Dino-Lite®) and processed manually and with Capillary.io® software. Based on the analysis, an active SSc pattern (Cutolo classification) is identified, highlighting the presence of giant capillaries and decreased capillary density.

In the image of the fourth left finger, the manual analysis using Dino-Capture (A) software is compared to the AI-based analysis (B), which automatically detects capillaries.

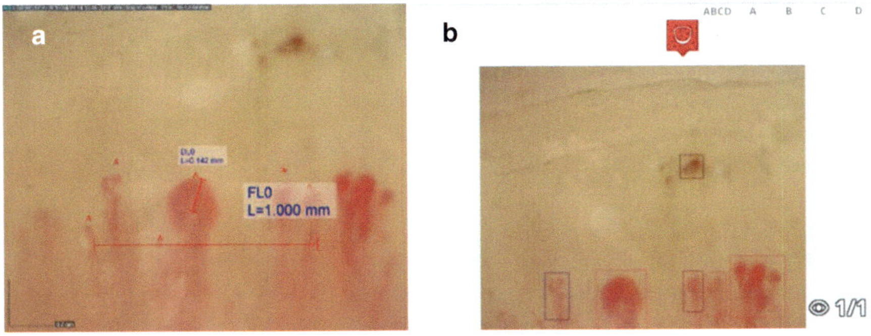

The capillary.io report was as follows:

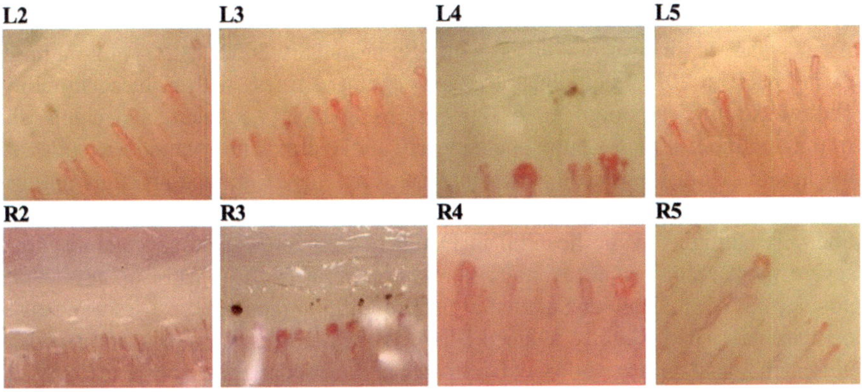

Capillary density: Slightly lowered, with an average density of 6.5 capillaries/mm.

Capillary enlargement: Frequent, affecting 42.9% of capillaries (2/3 on a semi-quantitative scale). The average apical diameter was 32.1 µm, venous 24.9 µm, and arterial 19.7 µm. Giant capillaries were found with a percentage of 20.2% and an average surface area of 45357.7 µm^2.

Capillary deformities:

- *Tortuosities:* Infrequent, affecting 8.3% of capillaries (1/3 on a semi-quantitative scale).
- *Abnormal shapes*: None.

Hemorrhages: Hemorrhages were found, with an average density of 0.5 hemorrhages/mm and an average surface area of 10956.8 µm^2.

Capillary density						
	Total	%	Quant. / mm	Apical diameter	Arterial limb width	Venous limb width
				x̄ µm		
Total capillaries	84	100.0	6.5	32.1	19.7	24.9
Normal capillaries	29	34.5	2.3	13.0	7.9	10.5
Tortuosities	7	8.3	0.5	28.4	17.8	25.9
Abnormal shapes	0	0.0	0.0	–	–	–
Enlarged capillaries	36	42.9	2.8	32.1	21.5	27.8
Giant capillaries	17	20.2	1.3	69.7	38.4	48.0
Hemorrhages	7	–	0.5	–	–	–

Total analyzed millimeters: 12.86

Clinical Case 2

An 11-year-old girl was diagnosed with SSc in January 2022, with symptom onset dating back to 2020, including progressive joint stiffness with reduced mobility, photosensitivity, hypopigmented skin lesions, muscle weakness, and calcinosis. Initial treatment with mycophenolate mofetil and hydroxychloroquine was followed by rituximab infusions due to persistent disease activity, resulting in partial improvement in mobility, though calcinosis persisted, particularly in the knees and back. She was admitted to the hospital in October 2023 for worsening calcinosis and severe pain, receiving intravenous immunoglobulin (IVIG). Work-up revealed a positive ANA >1:320 with a nucleolar pattern, mild to moderate restrictive changes on spirometry with slightly reduced DLCO, subcutaneous calcinosis confirmed by ultrasound, and gastroesophageal reflux. Capillaroscopy was consistent with an active scleroderma pattern (Cutolo classification).

The capillary.io report was as follows:

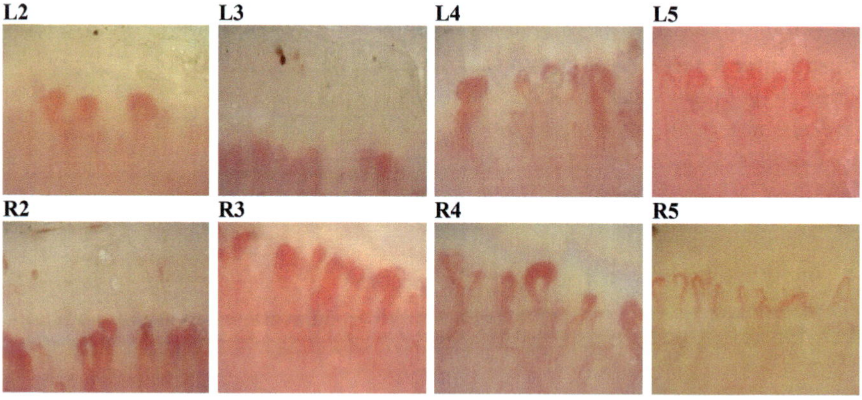

Capillary density: Very low, with an average density of 3.9 capillaries/mm.

Capillary enlargement: Frequent, affecting 35.4% of capillaries (2/3 on a semi-quantitative scale). The average apical diameter was 68.6 μm, venous 60.2 μm, and arterial 42.4 μm. Giant capillaries were found with a percentage of 62.5% and an average surface area of 103047.6 μm².

Capillary deformities:

- *Tortuosities:* Infrequent, affecting 2.1% of capillaries (1/3 on a semi-quantitative scale).
- *Abnormal shapes*: None.

Hemorrhages: Hemorrhages were found, with an average density of 0.4 hemorrhages/mm and an average surface area of 13857.4 μm².

Capillary density						
	Total	%	Quant. / mm	Apical diameter x̄ μm	Arterial limb width	Venous limb width
Total capillaries	48	100.0	3.9	68.6	42.4	60.2
Normal capillaries	1	2.1	0.1	8.7	–	–
Tortuosities	1	2.1	0.1	31.5	24.4	28.3
Abnormal shapes	0	0.0	0.0	–	–	–
Enlarged capillaries	17	35.4	1.4	36.2	24.7	34.3
Giant capillaries	30	62.5	2.5	95.6	52.4	74.7
Hemorrhages	5	–	0.4	–	–	–

Total analyzed millimeters: 12.20

Clinical Case 3

A 47-year-old female with a 10-year history of Raynaud's phenomenon was referred by her primary care physician for nailfold capillaroscopy. She was not taking any vasodilator medications at the time of evaluation, only fluoxetine, clotiazepam, and hormone replacement therapy. Her capillaroscopy was normal, with preserved capillary density, morphology, and architecture. The absence of a scleroderma pattern or microangiopathic changes suggests that her Raynaud's phenomenon is likely primary rather than secondary to a connective tissue disease.

The capillary.io report was as follows:

Capillary density: Conserved with an average density of 8.0 capillaries/mm.

Capillary enlargement: Infrequent, affecting 21.1% of capillaries (1/3 on a semi-quantitative scale). The average apical diameter was 24.5 μm, venous 19.1 μm, and arterial 15.0 μm. No giant capillaries were found.

Capillary deformities:

- *Tortuosities:* Infrequent, affecting 2.1% of capillaries (1/3 on a semi-quantitative scale).
- *Abnormal shapes*: None.

Hemorrhages: Hemorrhages were found, with an average density of 0.1 hemorrhages/mm and an average surface area of 9622.7 μm^2.

Capillary density						
	Total	%	Quant. / mm	Apical diameter	Arterial limb width	Venous limb width
				x̄ μm		
Total capillaries	237	100.0	8.0	24.5	15.0	19.1
Normal capillaries	182	76.8	6.1	22.4	14.0	17.9
Tortuosities	5	2.1	0.2	21.9	15.7	18.8
Abnormal shapes	0	0.0	0.0	–	–	–
Enlarged capillaries	50	21.1	1.7	31.8	19.0	23.5
Giant capillaries	0	0.0	0.0	–	–	–
Hemorrhages	2	–	0.1	–	–	–

Total analyzed millimeters: 29.68

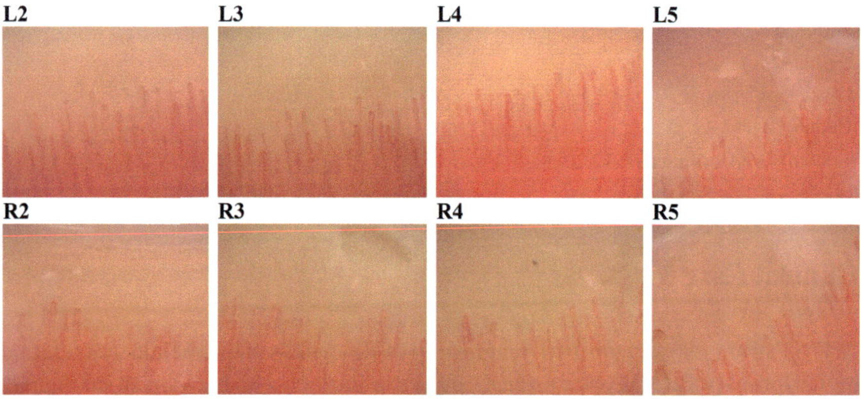

Clinical Case 4

A teenage girl developed progressive muscle weakness and a skin rash and was diagnosed with juvenile dermatomyositis in January 2022. She presented with malar erythema, Gottron's papules, periorbital edema, and markedly elevated CK (19,043 U/L), with positive ANA (1:2560, fine speckled) and Mi-2 alpha/beta antibodies. MRI showed bilateral muscle inflammation, and skin biopsy confirmed inflammatory infiltrates. Nailfold capillaroscopy revealed decreased capillary density, giant capillaries, abnormal morphology, and sparse hemorrhages, consistent with a late SSc pattern (Cutolo classification). She was initially treated with corticosteroids, hydroxychloroquine, and IVIG, followed by mycophenolate, resulting in improved strength and normalization of CK levels.

The capillary.io report was as follows:

Capillary density: Very low, with an average density of 3.7 capillaries/mm.

Capillary enlargement: Very frequent, affecting 67.4% of capillaries (3/3 on a semi-quantitative scale). The average apical diameter was 41.3 μm, venous 35.5 μm, and arterial 25.6 μm. Giant capillaries were found with a percentage of 18.6% and an average surface area of 55249.5 μm^2.

Capillary deformities:

- *Tortuosities:* Infrequent, affecting 7.0% of capillaries (1/3 on a semi-quantitative scale).
- *Abnormal shapes*: Infrequent, affecting 18.6% of capillaries (1/3 on a semi-quantitative scale).

Hemorrhages: Hemorrhages were found, with an average density of 0.1 hemorrhages/mm and an average surface area of 202553.9 μm^2.

Capillary density

	Total	%	Quant. / mm	Apical diameter	Arterial limb width	Venous limb width
				x̄ μm		
Total capillaries	43	100.0	3.7	41.3	25.6	35.5
Normal capillaries	3	7.0	0.3	–	–	–
Tortuosities	3	7.0	0.3	37.7	18.1	32.8
Abnormal shapes	8	18.6	0.7	–	–	–
Enlarged capillaries	29	67.4	2.5	33.6	20.7	29.1
Giant capillaries	8	18.6	0.7	62.4	36.2	49.5
Hemorrhages	1	–	0.1	–	–	–

Total analyzed millimeters: 11.58

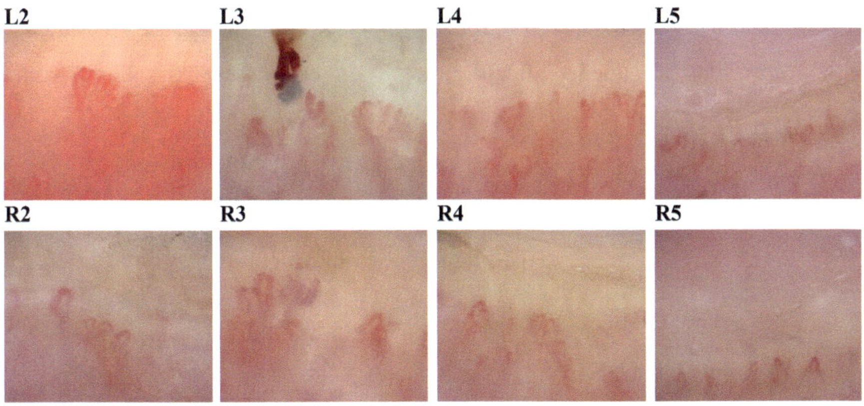

Clinical Case 5

A 49-year-old female patient was referred for nailfold capillaroscopy by her rheumatologist. She has a 3-year history of Raynaud's phenomenon and a diagnosis of undifferentiated connective tissue disease. Her current medications include hydroxychloroquine, omeprazole, and ursodeoxycholic acid for comorbid primary biliary cholangitis. She works as a cook and has never experienced digital ulcers. Capillaroscopy revealed an early SSc pattern based on the Cutolo classification, characterized by the presence of a few giant capillaries, microhemorrhages, and generally preserved capillary architecture, with normal density and no extensive avascular areas. Due to decreased image transparency, the software generated the report using only ten images instead of the usual 12, as shown below:

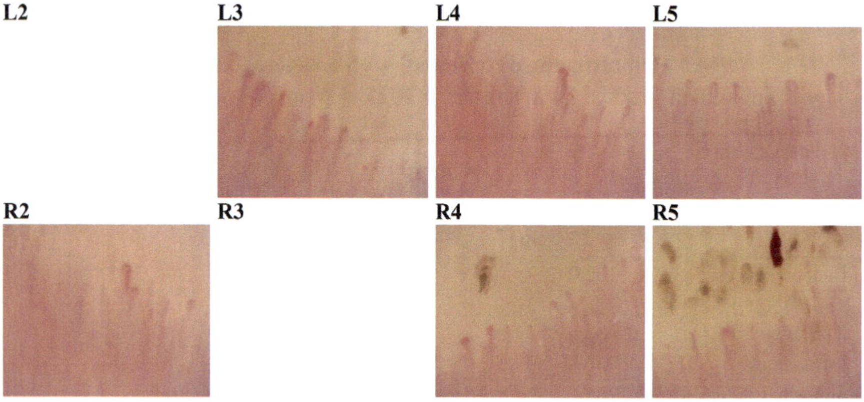

Capillary density: Very low, with an average density of 5.6 capillaries/mm.

Capillary enlargement: Very frequent, affecting 70.0% of capillaries (3/3 on a semi-quantitative scale). The average apical diameter was 33.4 µm, venous 25.6 µm, and arterial 18.3 µm. Giant capillaries were found with a percentage of 12.2% and an average surface area of 34707.6 μm^2.

Capillary deformities:

- *Tortuosities:* Infrequent, affecting 1.1% of capillaries (1/3 on a semi-quantitative scale).
- *Abnormal shapes:* None.

Hemorrhages: Hemorrhages were found, with an average density of 1.2 hemorrhages/mm and an average surface area of 35752.1 μm^2.

Capillary density						
	Total	%	Quant. / mm	Apical diameter x̄ μm	Arterial limb width	Venous limb width
Total capillaries	90	100.0	5.6	33.4	18.3	25.6
Normal capillaries	16	17.8	1.0	17.6	8.4	14.8
Tortuosities	1	1.1	0.1	41.0	20.3	23.9
Abnormal shapes	0	0.0	0.0	–	–	–
Enlarged capillaries	63	70.0	3.9	31.8	18.3	24.9
Giant capillaries	11	12.2	0.7	60.9	28.1	40.8
Hemorrhages	19	–	1.2	–	–	–

Total analyzed millimeters: 16.06
Total analyzed images: 10

References

1. Smith V, Ickinger C, Hysa E, Snow M, Frech T, Sulli A, et al. Nailfold capillaroscopy. Best Pract Res Clin Rheumatol. 2023;37(1):101849.
2. Smith V, Herrick AL, Ingegnoli F, Damjanov N, De Angelis R, Denton CP, et al. Standardisation of nailfold capillaroscopy for the assessment of patients with Raynaud's phenomenon and systemic sclerosis. Autoimmun Rev. 2020;19(3):102458.
3. Cutolo M, Smith V. State of the art on nailfold capillaroscopy: a reliable diagnostic tool and putative biomarker in rheumatology? Rheumatology (Oxford). 2013;52(11):1933–40.
4. Ma Z, Mulder DJ, Gniadecki R, Cohen Tervaert JW, Osman M. Methods of assessing nailfold capillaroscopy compared to video capillaroscopy in patients with systemic sclerosis-a critical review of the literature. Diagnostics (Basel). 2023;13(13):2204.
5. Berks M, Dinsdale G, Marjanovic E, Murray A, Taylor C, Herrick AL. Comparison between low cost USB nailfold capillaroscopy and videocapillaroscopy: a pilot study. Rheumatology (Oxford). 2021;60(8):3862–7.
6. Bhakuni DS, Vasdev V, Garg MK, Narayanan K, Jain R, Mullick G. Nailfold capillaroscopy by digital microscope in an Indian population with systemic sclerosis. Int J Rheum Dis. 2012;15(1):95–101.
7. Chanprapaph K, Fakprapai W, Limtong P, Suchonwanit P. Nailfold capillaroscopy with USB digital microscopy in connective tissue diseases: a comparative study of 245 patients and healthy controls. Front Med (Lausanne). 2021;8:683900.
8. González JM, Valenzuela A. Vascular, soft tissue, and musculoskeletal imaging in systemic sclerosis. Rheum Dis Clin N Am. 2024;50(4):661–81.
9. Ring HC, Themstrup L, Banzhaf CA, Jemec GB, Mogensen M. Dynamic optical coherence tomography capillaroscopy: a new imaging tool in autoimmune connective tissue disease. JAMA Dermatol. 2016;152(10):1142–6.
10. Abignano G, Green L, Eng S, Emery P, Del Galdo F. Nailfold microvascular imaging by dynamic optical coherence tomography in systemic sclerosis: a case-controlled pilot study. J Invest Dermatol. 2022;142(4):1050–7.
11. Aguirre J, Hindelang B, Berezhnoi A, Darsow U, Lauffer F, Eyerich K, et al. Assessing nailfold microvascular structure with ultra-wideband raster-scan optoacoustic mesoscopy. Photoacoustics. 2018;10:31–7.

12. Nitkunanantharajah S, Haedicke K, Moore TB, Manning JB, Dinsdale G, Berks M, et al. Three-dimensional optoacoustic imaging of nailfold capillaries in systemic sclerosis and its potential for disease differentiation using deep learning. Sci Rep. 2020;10(1):16444.
13. Ruaro B, Sulli A, Alessandri E, Pizzorni C, Ferrari G, Cutolo M. Laser speckle contrast analysis: a new method to evaluate peripheral blood perfusion in systemic sclerosis patients. Ann Rheum Dis. 2014;73(6):1181–5.
14. Cutolo M, Vanhaecke A, Ruaro B, Deschepper E, Ickinger C, Melsens K, et al. Is laser speckle contrast analysis (LASCA) the new kid on the block in systemic sclerosis? A systematic literature review and pilot study to evaluate reliability of LASCA to measure peripheral blood perfusion in scleroderma patients. Autoimmun Rev. 2018;17(8):775–80.
15. Ruaro B, Bruni C, Wade B, Baratella E, Confalonieri P, Antonaglia C, et al. Laser speckle contrast analysis: functional evaluation of microvascular damage in connective tissue diseases. Is there evidence of correlations with organ involvement, such as pulmonary damage? Front Physiol. 2021;12:710298.
16. Hegyi J, Hegyi V, Messer G, Arenberger P, Ruzicka T, Berking C. Confocal laser-scanning capillaroscopy: a novel approach to the analysis of skin capillaries in vivo. Skin Res Technol. 2009;15(4):476–81.
17. Valenzuela A, Concha S, Kayser C. The power of quantitative algorithms in nailfold videocapillaroscopy. Rheumatology (Oxford). 2024;63(12):3203–4.
18. Herrick AL, Berks M, Taylor CJ. Quantitative nailfold capillaroscopy-update and possible next steps. Rheumatology (Oxford). 2021;60(5):2054–65.
19. Bharathi PG, Berks M, Dinsdale G, Murray A, Manning J, Wilkinson S, et al. A deep learning system for quantitative assessment of microvascular abnormalities in nailfold capillary images. Rheumatology (Oxford). 2023;62(6):2325–9.
20. Gracia Tello B, Ramos Ibañez E, Fanlo Mateo P, Sáez Cómet L, Martínez Robles E, Ríos Blanco JJ, et al. The challenge of comprehensive nailfold videocapillaroscopy practice: a further contribution. Clin Exp Rheumatol. 2022;40(10):1926–32.
21. Gracia Tello BC, Ramos Ibañez E, Saez Comet L, Guillén Del Castillo A, Simeón Aznar CP, Selva-O'Callaghan A, et al. External clinical validation of automated software to identify structural abnormalities and microhaemorrhages in nailfold videocapillaroscopy images. Clin Exp Rheumatol. 2023;41(8):1605–11.
22. Gracia Tello BC, Sáez Comet L, Lledó G, Freire Dapena M, Mesa MA, Martín-Cascón M, et al. Capi-score: a quantitative algorithm for identifying disease patterns in nailfold videocapillaroscopy. Rheumatology (Oxford). 2024;63(12):3315–21.
23. Lledó-Ibáñez GM, Sáez Comet L, Freire Dapena M, Mesa Navas M, Martín Cascón M, Guillén Del Castillo A, et al. CAPI-detect: machine learning in capillaroscopy reveals new variables influencing diagnosis. Rheumatology (Oxford). 2025;64:3667.
24. Cutolo M, Trombetta AC, Melsens K, Pizzorni C, Sulli A, Ruaro B, et al. Automated assessment of absolute nailfold capillary number on videocapillaroscopic images: proof of principle and validation in systemic sclerosis. Microcirculation. 2018;25(4):e12447.
25. Sulli A VA, Pizzorni C, Ferrari G, Tomatis V, Pendolino M, Smith V, Cutolo M. Automated Nailfold Capillary Counting System (AUTOCAPI) in systemic sclerosis patients with different capillaroscopic patterns [abstract]. Arthritis Rheumatol. 2019;71 (suppl 10).
26. Garaiman A, Nooralahzadeh F, Mihai C, Gonzalez NP, Gkikopoulos N, Becker MO, et al. Vision transformer assisting rheumatologists in screening for capillaroscopy changes in systemic sclerosis: an artificial intelligence model. Rheumatology (Oxford). 2023;62(7):2492–500.
27. Cutolo M, Gotelli E, Smith V. Reading nailfold capillaroscopic images in systemic sclerosis: manual and/or automated detection? Rheumatology (Oxford). 2023;62(7):2335–7.
28. Berks M, Tresadern P, Dinsdale G, Murray A, Moore T, Herrick A, et al. An automated system for detecting and measuring nailfold capillaries. Med Image Comput Comput Assist Interv. 2014;17(Pt 1):658–65.

29. Berks M, Dinsdale G, Murray A, Moore T, Manning J, Taylor C, et al. Automated structure and flow measurement - a promising tool in nailfold capillaroscopy. Microvasc Res. 2018;118:173–7.
30. Gronenschild EH, Muris DM, Schram MT, Karaca U, Stehouwer CD, Houben AJ. Semi-automatic assessment of skin capillary density: proof of principle and validation. Microvasc Res. 2013;90:192–8.
31. Kassani PH, Ehwerhemuepha L, Martin-King C, Kassab R, Gibbs E, Morgan G, et al. Artificial intelligence for nailfold capillaroscopy analyses - a proof of concept application in juvenile dermatomyositis. Pediatr Res. 2024;95(4):981–7.
32. Korendovych V, Korsten P. POS1328 differentiating "scleroderma" with non-scleroderma patterns in nailfold capillary microscopy using a deep learning model. Ann Rheum Dis. 2023;82:1014.
33. Yin H, Wu Z, Huang A, Luo J, Liang J, Lin J, et al. Automated nailfold capillary density measurement method based on improved YOLOv5. Microvasc Res. 2023;150:104593.
34. Tuncer SA, Yildirim M, Tuncer T, Mülayim MK. YOLOv8-based system for nail capillary detection on a single-board computer. Diagnostics (Basel). 2024;14(17):1843.
35. Ozturk L, Laclau C, Boulon C, Mangin M, Braz-Ma E, Constans J, et al. Analysis of nailfold capillaroscopy images with artificial intelligence: data from literature and performance of machine learning and deep learning from images acquired in the SCLEROCAP study. Microvasc Res. 2025;157:104753.

Chapter 15
Clinical Cases

Rahma A. Elziaty and Yasser El Miedany

Introduction

Nailfold capillaroscopy (NFC) is a noninvasive, reliable, and reproducible tool. Its ability to visualize the microcirculation in vivo makes it indispensable for early detection of scleroderma-spectrum disorders and for monitoring disease progression and therapeutic response. Beyond systemic sclerosis, NFC has been increasingly applied to other autoimmune diseases, vasculitides, and even non-rheumatological conditions, broadening its diagnostic scope [1].

The present chapter showcases a diverse selection of clinical cases that emphasize the spectrum of NFC findings across different pathologies. Each case includes a concise patient history, high-resolution NFC images, and a focused discussion linking the observed microvascular changes to the clinical presentation and diagnosis. The diversity of cases—ranging from typical scleroderma patterns to unusual and overlapping features—provides the reader with practical insights into recognizing, interpreting, and differentiating various NFC findings.

By integrating real-world scenarios from multiple expert contributors, the chapter aims to serve as a practical reference for clinicians, highlighting how capillaroscopic interpretation can impact diagnostic reasoning and patient management. The detailed visual documentation and correlation with systemic features make this compilation an essential learning resource for both beginners and experienced practitioners in the field.

R. A. Elziaty (✉)
Internal Medicine Department, Rheumatology Division, Faculty of Medicine, Ain Shams University, Cairo, Egypt

Y. El Miedany (✉)
Canterbury Christ Church University, Canterbury, UK

Rheumatology and Rehabilitation, Ain Shams University, Cairo, Egypt

King's College, London, UK

Y. El Miedany, R. A. Elziaty (eds.), *Capillaroscopy*, Contemporary Rheumatology, https://doi.org/10.1007/978-3-032-22966-3_15

Systemic Sclerosis Cases

Case 1: A Case of Very Early Diagnosis of Systemic Sclerosis (VEDOSS)

Minrui Liang
Department of Rheumatology, Huashan Hospital, Fudan University, Shanghai, China

Patient: 48-year-old Female

History

- Raynaud's phenomenon (RP): 2 years
- Swollen fingers: 6 months

Clinical Examination

- Puffy fingers with RP (Fig. 15.1); no obvious signs of skin sclerosis, fingertip lesions, or telangiectasia
- Chest, cardiac, abdominal exams: unremarkable

Current Medications

- Not started yet

Outcome of Investigations

- Antinuclear antibody (ANA) positive (centromere pattern) (Fig. 15.2) and anti-Centromere antibody (ACA) positive

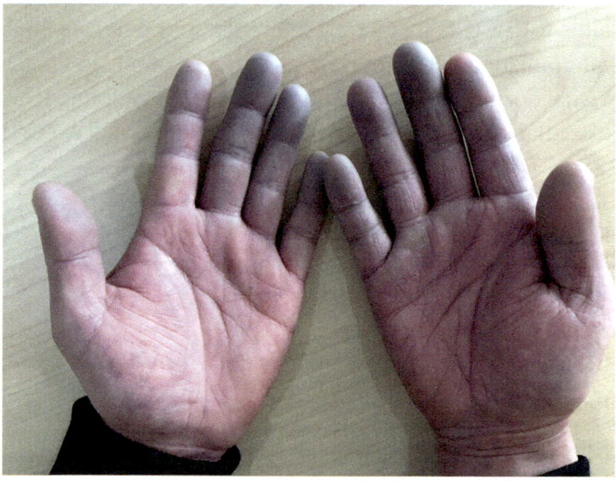

Fig. 15.1 Puffy fingers with RP

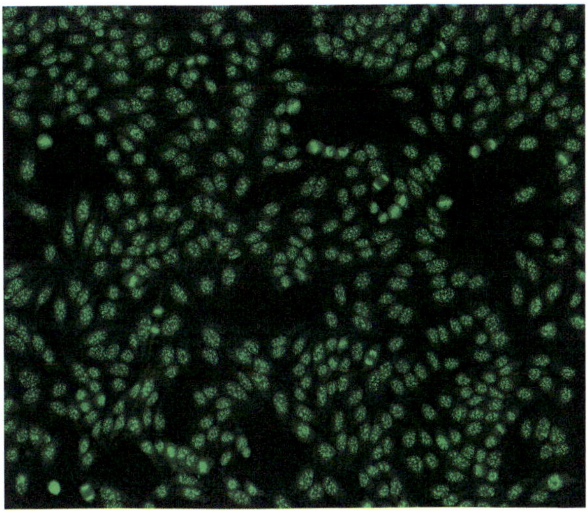

Fig. 15.2 ANA positivity in immunofluorescence (centromere pattern)

- Chest high-resolution computed tomography (HRCT) and echocardiography: no evidence of interstitial lung disease (ILD) or pulmonary hypertension (PH).
- Nailfold capillaroscopy (NFC) showing the reduced capillary density, enlarged/giant loops, and microhemorrhage, indicative of an active scleroderma pattern (Fig. 15.3).

Questions to Challenge the Reader Regarding Possible Findings and Outcomes

- Does the combination of puffy fingers, active scleroderma pattern on NFC, and ACA positivity render this RP patient a definite systemic sclerosis (SSc) according to the 2013 ACR/EULAR criteria?
- Alternatively, should this patient be labeled as "Very Early Diagnosis of Systemic Sclerosis" (VEDOSS), and what are the implications for follow-up and treatment?

Discussion

This 48-year-old female patient presents with three classic red flags: Raynaud's phenomenon, puffy fingers, and ANA positivity, together with the typical active scleroderma pattern on NFC and the SSc-specific antibody ACA. Consequently, this patient fulfills the criteria of the Very Early Diagnosis of Systemic Sclerosis (VEDOSS) proposed by the EULAR Scleroderma Trials and Research Group in 2011 [2] but remains below the threshold of the 2013 ACR/EULAR criteria for a definite SSc due to the lack of evident cutaneous or visceral fibrosis (the total score = 7) [3]. A longitudinal cohort study indicated that 52.4% of patients with VEDOSS would progress and meet the criteria of definite SSc within 5 years, while the combination of puffy fingers and SSc-specific antibody profile confers the highest risk of 94.1% for the progression to a definite SSc [4]. Even at this pre-diagnostic stage, subclinical gastrointestinal and heart involvement can be detected [5, 6], and the skin biopsies from VEDOSS patients have already exhibited SSc-linked tissue remolding, highlighting VEDOSS as a "window of opportunity" for early detection and early intervention [7, 8].

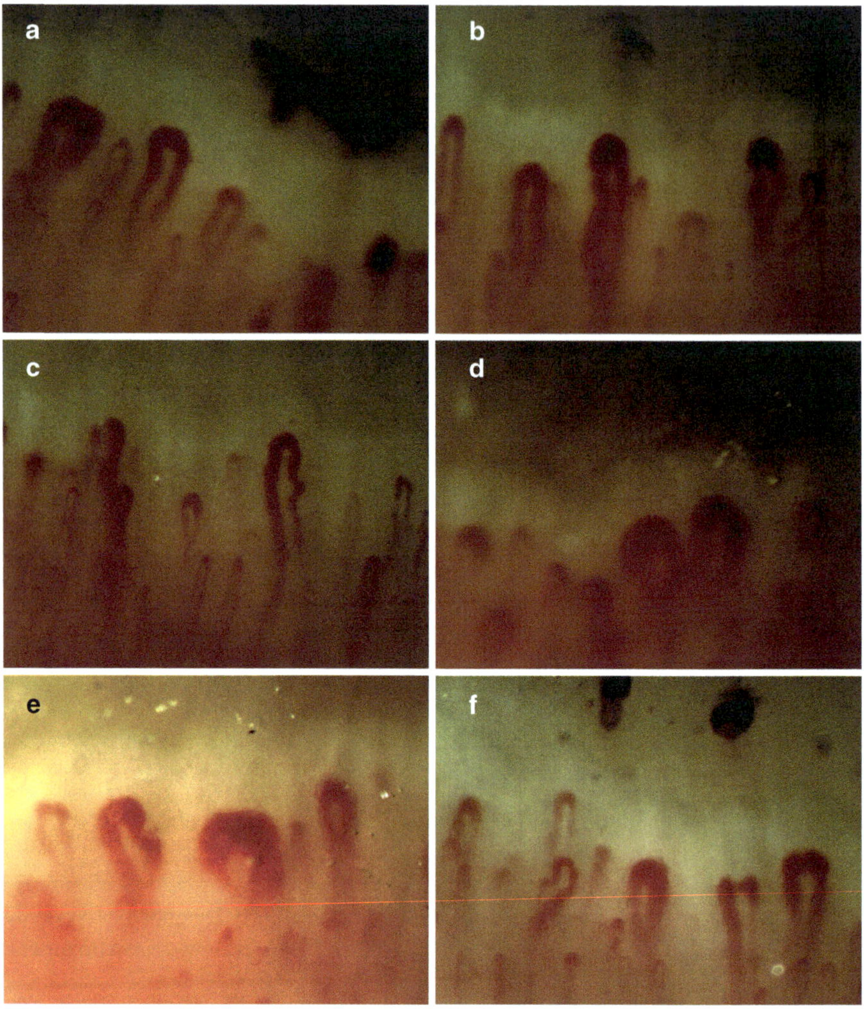

Fig. 15.3 NFC images of active scleroderma pattern from six different fields of nailfolds (250-fold magnification)

Key Learning Points

- VEDOSS is defined as Raynaud phenomenon, puffy fingers, and positive ANA, corroborated by characteristic nailfold capillaroscopy changes and SSc-specific autoantibody profile [2]; however, it does not yet fulfill the 2013 ACR/EULAR criteria for definite SSc [3].
- Identification of VEDOSS is of crucial importance: it not only indicates the entrance to the SSc spectrum disease continuum but also provides a unique "opportunity of window" for patient stratification and precise intervention.

Case 2: Late-Presenting Raynaud's Phenomenon and Its Capillaroscopic Signature

Sara Alves Costa, Maria João Cadório, Maria João Salvador, and Tânia Santiago
Rheumathology Department, Coimbra's Local Health Unit, Coimbra, Portugal

A 51-year-old woman presented with a 5-year history of late-onset Raynaud's phenomenon affecting the fingers, with episodes lasting longer than one hour and showing progressively increasing frequency. The episodes were exacerbated during cold exposure but were not invariably triggered by it. She also reported diffuse swelling of the fingers over the same time period. There was no history of digital ulcers. The patient denied any additional symptoms suggestive of connective tissue disease, namely cutaneous thickening, respiratory complaints, dysphagia, other gastrointestinal disturbances, or muscle weakness. She also denied inflammatory arthralgia in any location.

Her past medical history included bilateral carpal tunnel syndrome, surgically treated on the right side. There were no other relevant comorbidities. She was not taking any regular medication and reported no smoking or alcohol use.

Question 1 *Which clinical features in this presentation should raise suspicion for secondary Raynaud's phenomenon rather than a primary form?*

On physical examination, she exhibited facial skin thickening and microstomia but no cutaneous thickening of the extremities or anterior chest wall and no telangiectasias. Examination of the hands revealed puffy fingers without digital ulcers. There was no joint tenderness or swelling. Additionally, she presented with mild lower limb edema up to the knees, with signs of associated chronic venous insufficiency (Fig. 15.4).

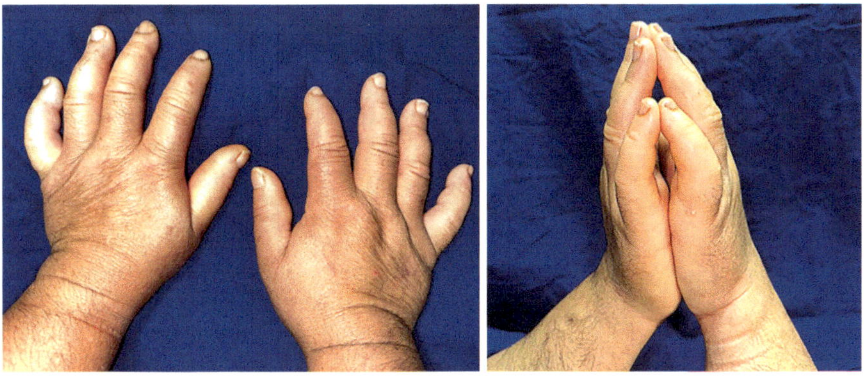

Fig. 15.4 Diffuse edema of the fingers compatible with puffy fingers, causing limited finger mobility

Question 2 *Given this clinical presentation, what are the most likely diagnoses? What investigations would you perform?*

Laboratory studies showed positive antinuclear antibodies (ANA) at a titer >1:1280, with an AC-3 nuclear centromere pattern. Anti-CENP-A and anti-CENP-B antibodies were strongly positive. The remaining laboratory evaluation was unremarkable, including complete blood count, complement levels, serum protein electrophoresis, and assessment of renal function, with both rheumatoid factor and anti-CCP antibodies testing negative (Fig. 15.5).

Question 3 *What abnormalities are visible in the capillaroscopic image? What pattern is represented in the image?*

Nailfold videocapillaroscopy revealed decreased density (<7 capillaries per mm) in most examined fields. Enlarged capillaries (apical diameter ≥20 μm), two giant capillaries (apical diameter ≥50 μm), and microhemorrhages were observed, without avascular areas. These findings were consistent with an active scleroderma pattern [9].

A high-resolution computed tomography (HRCT) showed no signs of interstitial lung disease.

Based on clinical, serological, and capillaroscopic findings, the diagnosis of systemic sclerosis, limited cutaneous form, was established. The patient received education regarding the disease and counseling on cold protection measures. Nifedipine 30 mg daily was initiated to reduce the frequency and severity of Raynaud's phenomenon [10, 11].

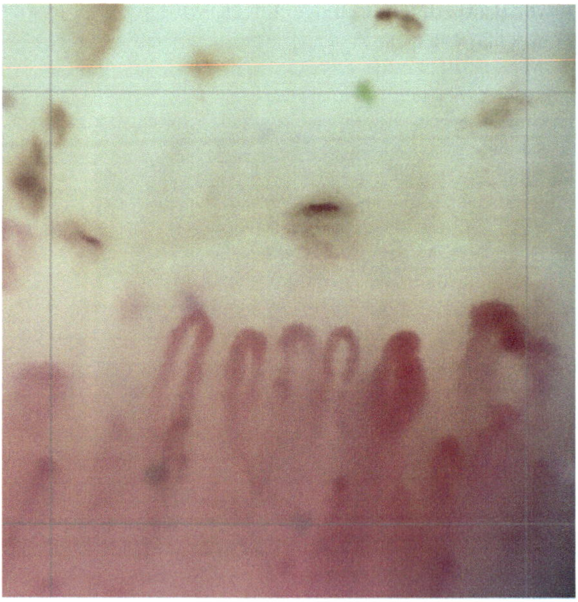

Fig. 15.5 Capillaroscopic image of the patient obtained with a nailfold videocapillaroscope with a 200× magnification in a 1 linear millimeter. (VideoCap 3.0; DS Medica, Italy)

Question 4 *Considering the early-stage presentation, what baseline assessments for organ involvement should be performed, and why are they important for prognosis and management?*

Discussion

Raynaud's phenomenon is generally the most common and earliest clinical manifestation of systemic sclerosis. Late-onset Raynaud's phenomenon, particularly when presenting after the age of 45, is always a red flag and warrants investigation for an underlying connective tissue disease. The other clinical features that should raise suspicion for a secondary Raynaud's phenomenon, in this case, rather than a primary form, include the female sex, the presence of puffy fingers, facial skin thickening, and microstomia.

Nailfold videocapillaroscopy plays a pivotal role in differentiating between primary and secondary Raynaud's phenomenon and in the subsequent monitoring of disease progression. In this patient, the diagnosis of systemic sclerosis was made at an early stage, characterized by longstanding puffy fingers, Raynaud's phenomenon, capillaroscopic findings compatible with an early scleroderma pattern, and strongly positive antinuclear and anticentromere antibodies.

Despite the absence of cardiopulmonary symptoms, baseline assessment of target organ involvement is mandatory. Transthoracic echocardiography, pulmonary function tests, and HRCT of the chest were requested, since the presence of pulmonary arterial hypertension or interstitial lung disease has a significant impact on prognosis and therapeutic strategy.

In the long term, patient follow-up should include regular monitoring of skin thickening and Raynaud's phenomenon to prevent the development of digital ulcers. Serial capillaroscopic examinations may be useful in assessing microvascular damage, and the evaluation of possible involvement of other organ systems, particularly the gastrointestinal tract, is also essential [9, 12].

Optimal management of systemic sclerosis requires a multidisciplinary approach, involving not only rheumatology but also cardiology, pulmonology, and physical and rehabilitation medicine, to ensure comprehensive assessment and control of systemic involvement. This strategy aims to improve patients' quality of life and long-term prognosis [11].

Key Learning Points

- Systemic sclerosis is a rare and complex disorder affecting multiple systems. Clinical features such as late-onset Raynaud's phenomenon and puffy fingers can serve as early indicators of disease, even when cutaneous involvement appears minimal.
- Assessment of the microcirculation is recommended in patients with suspected or confirmed systemic sclerosis, with nailfold videocapillaroscopy serving as a crucial diagnostic and prognostic tool. Capillaroscopic findings, including megacapillaries, microhemorrhages, and tortuous capillaries, allow differentiation between primary and secondary Raynaud's phenomenon and enable early identification of microvascular damage.

- Baseline evaluation of target organs, including the heart, lungs, and gastrointestinal tract, is essential for prognostic stratification and to guide therapeutic decisions, even in asymptomatic patients.
- Regular, multidisciplinary follow-up is essential to optimize management, facilitate timely intervention, and mitigate the risk of complications, including digital ulcers and progressive organ involvement, thereby enhancing long-term outcomes.

Case 3: Diagnostic Redefinition in a Patient with Undifferentiated Connective Tissue Disease

Sherif Ismail
Rheumatology and Rehabilitation, Internal Medicine Department, Medical Research and Clinical Studies Institute, National Research Center, Cairo, Egypt

Clinical Presentation

A 32-year-old woman presented at the Rheumatology outpatient clinic for follow-up with complaints of persistent fatigue, mild arthralgias, myalgias, and a recurrent malar-like facial rash. She also reported progressive dyspnea and alopecia. Her past medical history was significant for well-controlled hypothyroidism and moderate obesity (BMI 31.2).

The patient was tentatively managed for Systemic Lupus Erythematosus (SLE) and coexistent knee osteoarthritis (OA), the latter diagnosed five months prior.

- *Musculoskeletal Symptoms*: Pain was primarily centered in the knee joints, described as effort-associated and consistent with her OA diagnosis. She also reported involvement of the small joints of the hands and wrists. No objective joint swelling or sclerodactyly was noted on physical examination.
- *Medications*: Hydroxychloroquine (400 mg/day), prednisolone (5 mg/day), occasional NSAIDs, and topical analgesics.

Initial Investigations and Diagnostic Uncertainty

Recent laboratory workup suggested low-grade systemic activity but did not confirm a clear SLE diagnosis:

- *Serology*: ANA positive (1:80, low titer), anti-dsDNA negative, rheumatoid factor (RF) negative, anti-CCP negative.
- *Inflammatory/Hematologic Markers*: erythrocyte sedimentation rate (ESR) 33 mm/h, mild anemia (hemoglobin 10.9 g/dL).
- *Renal Function*: No proteinuria detected.

Given the nonspecific symptoms, low ANA titer, and negative SLE-specific antibodies (anti-dsDNA), the provisional diagnosis of SLE remained uncertain and required further classification.

The Vascular Clue: Nailfold Capillaroscopy (NFC)

The patient reported mild Raynaud's Phenomenon (RP), prompting referral for NFC to search for microvascular abnormalities that could strengthen the suspected diagnosis of SLE or suggest an alternative diagnosis.

NFC was performed on eight fingers (excluding the thumbs) at 200X magnification by a single operator.

- *Key Findings*: The examination revealed significant microvascular anomalies, including marked tortuousity, branching, and irregular capillary crossings. See Figs. 15.6, 15.7, 15.8, and 15.9.
  Capillary enlargements were prominent, and the most critical finding was the unequivocal presence of a few giant capillaries in two digits. See Figs. 15.10 and 15.11.
- *Absent Features*: Importantly, no microhemorrhages or neoangiogenesis were observed. The average capillary density was mildly affected.

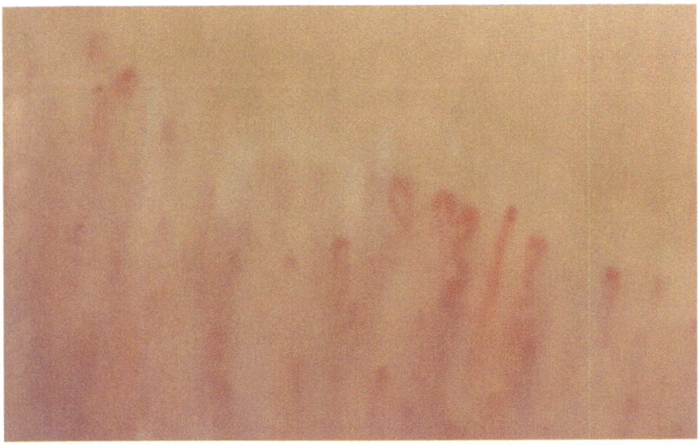

Fig. 15.6 Tourtiosities, meandering capillaries, and crossings

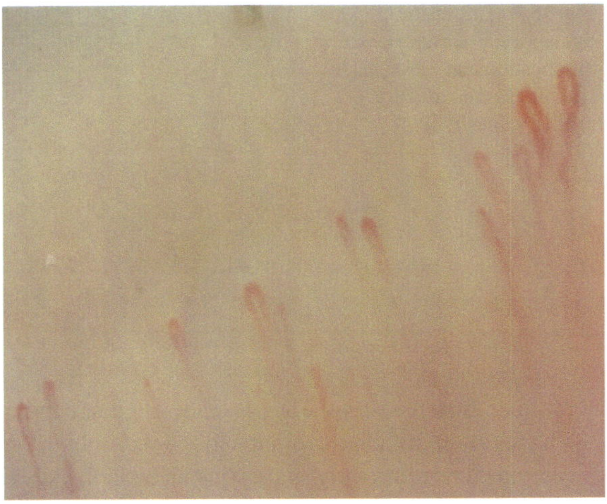

Fig. 15.7 Crossed capillary, branching, and apical dilatations with moderately low capillary density

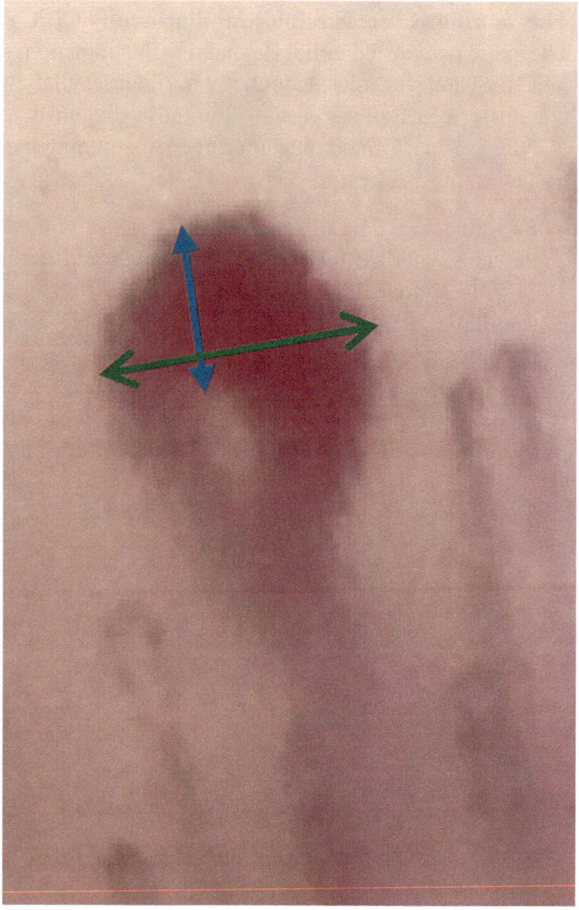

Fig. 15.8 Tortuosities, meandering capillaries, fusions, and crossings with moderate reduction of capillary density

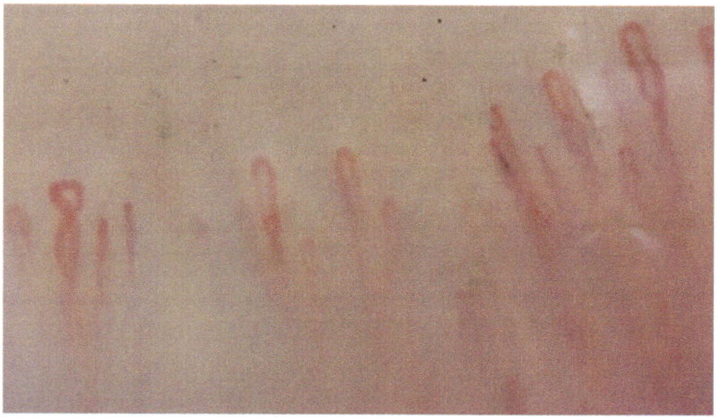

Fig. 15.9 Tortuosities, dilatations, extravasations, ramification and crossings with moderate reduction of capillary density

- *Pattern Interpretation*: The presence of giant capillaries in the absence of hemorrhages or significant capillary loss was highly consistent with an early scleroderma pattern, strongly suggesting an evolving systemic sclerosis (SSc) spectrum disease rather than active SLE vasculopathy.

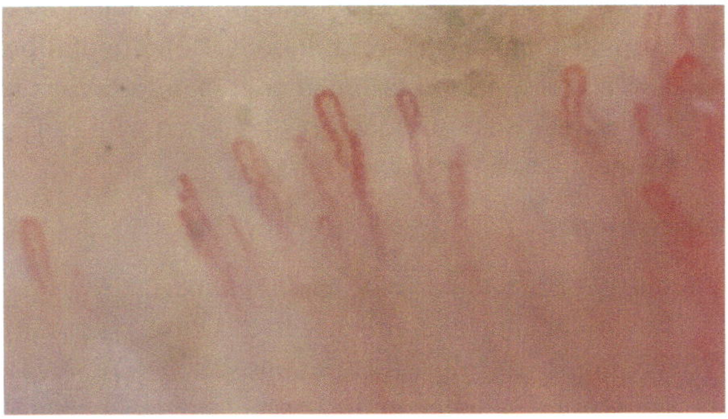

Fig. 15.10 A giant capillary, measured by both apical diameter and total width

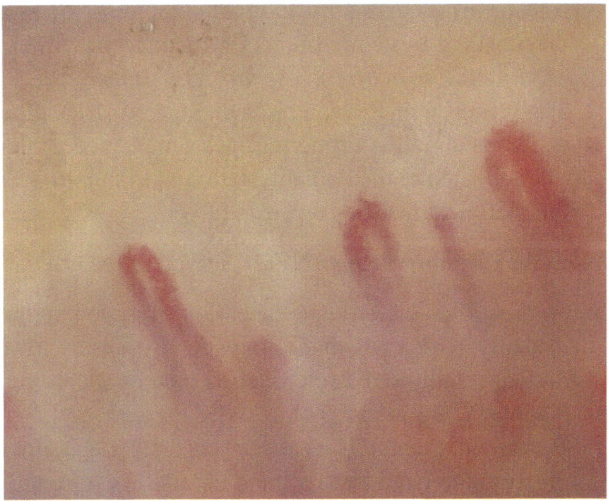

Fig. 15.11 Mega-capillaries, apical thrombosis with significantly lowered capillary density

Diagnostic Redefinition and Final Confirmation

The NFC findings mandated a clinical reassessment and follow-up inquiry.

- *Reevaluation*: On follow-up phone contact, the patient reported a recent increase in the frequency of RP attacks accompanied by digital "puffiness" (swelling of fingers and toes) during these episodes.
- *Algorithm and Serology*: The combination of Raynaud's Phenomenon, digital puffiness (suggestive of edematous phase scleroderma/sclerodactyly), and the positive ANA fulfilled the three entry criteria for Very Early Diagnosis of Systemic Sclerosis (VEDOSS). It was further fortified by the NFC changes that completed the algorithm and also prompted immediate testing for SSc-specific antibodies:
  - Anti-centromere and anti-RNA polymerase III were negative.
  - Anti-topoisomerase I (Scl-70) was positive.
  - Anti-U1RNP was negative (ruling out mixed connective tissue disease, MCTD).
- *Conclusion*

  The NFC findings served as the critical pivot point, shifting the diagnosis from an uncertain SLE/undifferentiated connective tissue diseases (CTD) to systemic sclerosis (SSc), specifically the diffuse cutaneous form (suggested by the positive anti-topoisomerase I antibody). The digital puffiness, initially subtle, was correctly recognized as a cutaneous manifestation of SSc upon closer questioning. The patient was subsequently diagnosed with early systemic sclerosis, and management was adjusted accordingly.

Discussion

Diagnostic Pivot to early systemic sclerosis

The initial clinical ambiguity in this case, characterized by nonspecific systemic symptoms and low-titer seropositivity (ANA 1:80), highlights a common diagnostic challenge in the nascent stages of connective tissue diseases (CTDs). The coexistence of effort-associated knee pain (attributable to obesity and likely osteoarthritis) and constitutional symptoms led to a preliminary, but uncertain, diagnosis of Systemic Lupus Erythematosus (SLE).

The Critical Role of Microvascular Assessment

The presence of Raynaud's Phenomenon (RP), alongside the patient's report of insidious digital swelling/puffiness, mandated a microvascular assessment. RP is often the first clinical manifestation of systemic sclerosis (SSc) and may precede other clinical features by years [13].

Nailfold Capillaroscopy (NFC) served as the critical diagnostic tool.

- *Pattern Recognition*: The detection of giant capillaries, even if few in number, instantly redirected the diagnostic hypothesis toward the SSc spectrum. This finding established a scleroderma pattern according to the established fast track diagnostic algorithm [14].
- *Pattern Subtyping*: The pattern was further classified as early SSc microangiopathy, characterized by few giant capillaries, minimal hemorrhages, and relatively preserved capillary distribution, consistent with the initial stages of microvascular damage that precedes widespread capillary loss [15]. This observation strongly supports the utility of NFC in differentiating secondary RP (associated with CTD) from primary RP, especially at the very beginning of disease onset, as documented in similar cases by Cutolo et al. [16].

Differentiating SSc from SLE

The capillaroscopic pattern provided a powerful exclusionary clue against typical SLE microangiopathy:

- *SLE Pattern*: While approximately 50% of SLE patients exhibit nonspecific NFC abnormalities (e.g., tortuous loops, meandering capillaries, prominent subcapillary plexus), the specific presence of giant capillaries is highly uncharacteristic. Studies, including a systematic review by the EULAR microcirculation study group [17], confirm that the key capillaroscopic findings prevalent in active SLE are tortuous capillaries, abnormal morphology, and hemorrhages, but not the hallmark SSc triad components (giant capillaries, avascular areas, and bushy capillaries).

- *Diagnostic Weight*: The NFC findings, therefore, diminished the likelihood of primary SLE and strongly amplified the suspicion of SSc.

Validation by VEDOSS Criteria
The diagnostic shift was formalized by applying the *Very Early Diagnosis of Systemic Sclerosis (VEDOSS)* criteria. This scheme bypasses the limitations of the older ACR/EULAR classification criteria (which require definitive skin or organ involvement) by identifying patients at a stage where intervention may be most effective.

- *Criteria Fulfillment*: This patient fulfilled the three necessary VEDOSS entry criteria: Raynaud's phenomenon, digital swelling/puffiness (representing the insidious edema/sclerodactyly), and a positive ANA.
- *Scl-70 Confirmation*: The subsequent positive finding of Anti-Topoisomerase I (Scl-70) antibodies definitively cemented the diagnosis of early systemic sclerosis. This confirms the hypothesis proposed by LeRoy [18] and Medsger years ago and subsequently validated in large cohorts by Koenig et al. [19], demonstrating that patients who evolve into SSc almost universally meet these early criteria at baseline.

Conclusion and Future Management
The patient's initial diagnosis was likely misdirected toward more common rheumatologic disorders (SLE, RA, etc.). The microvascular findings provided an essential, objective biomarker that prevented this diagnostic oversight.

Based on the VEDOSS criteria, the characteristic NFC pattern, and the confirmatory Scl-70 positivity, the patient is now definitively managed as having early systemic sclerosis. Aggressive screening for potential visceral involvement—including pulmonary function tests (PFTs), High-resolution CT (HRCT) of the chest, and echocardiography—is now urgently required to establish a comprehensive baseline and initiate proactive, organ-specific management.

Key Learning Points
The most important learning points from this case—the diagnostic shift from uncertain SLE to confirmed early systemic sclerosis (SSc) based on microvascular findings—are centered on the critical role of nailfold capillaroscopy (NFC) in the early diagnosis of connective tissue diseases.

1. *NFC as a Pivotal Diagnostic Filter in Undifferentiated CTD*

    - *Microvascular Diagnosis Trump's Serology*: In patients with nonspecific symptoms, low-titer positive ANA, and ambiguous clinical features (like the overlap of SLE and osteoarthritis symptoms), NFC serves as an essential, objective biomarker. The presence of a pathognomonic microvascular pattern can overrule weak serological evidence and guide the differential diagnosis.
    - *Exclusion of SLE*: The finding of giant capillaries strongly steered the diagnosis away from typical SLE microangiopathy, where such features are rare. The characteristic NFC patterns of the SSc spectrum are highly specific and aid in excluding other CTDs when clinical presentations overlap [20].

2. *Validation of the Very Early Diagnosis of SSc (VEDOSS)*
   - *Early Detection is Possible*: This case reinforces the value of the VEDOSS criteria. The combination of Raynaud's Phenomenon, digital swelling/puffiness (representing the insidious edema phase of sclerodactyly), and the scleroderma capillaroscopy pattern identifies patients at risk for SSc years before they meet the traditional ACR/EULAR classification criteria.
   - *The Power of the Triad*: The prompt and correct recognition of digital puffiness (swelling) combined with the NFC findings provided the necessary clinical weight to pursue SSc-specific serology, leading directly to the confirmation via the Anti-Topoisomerase I (Scl-70) antibody.
3. *The Prognostic Importance of Early Pattern Recognition*
   - *Pattern Subtyping Is Key*: The detection of an early scleroderma pattern (even with only a few giant capillaries and absent avascularity/hemorrhages) mandates aggressive follow-up. This pattern signals an underlying systemic vasculopathy that requires immediate screening for potentially life-threatening visceral complications (e.g., ILD, pulmonary hypertension).
   - *Scl-70 Implications*: The positive Anti-Topoisomerase I (Scl-70) antibody is associated with a higher risk for diffuse cutaneous involvement, interstitial lung disease, and scleroderma renal crisis. This dictates the urgency of commencing comprehensive visceral screening (PFTs, HRCT, echocardiography) immediately upon re-diagnosis.

Case 4: Refractory Vasculopathy and Severe Disease Progression

Caroline Evers and Carina Mihai
Department of Rheumatology, University Hospital Zurich, Zurich, Switzerland

We present the case of a 50-year-old patient who was referred to our rheumatology department after consulting the emergency service of another hospital for arthralgia, Raynaud's phenomenon, and positive antinuclear antibodies, with suspected systemic sclerosis (SSc).

On clinical examination, we found an active polyarthritis as well as tendon friction rubs, puffy fingers, and minimal skin fibrosis in the fingers, with a modified Rodnan skin score of 2/51 points. Blood tests showed highly elevated inflammatory parameters (C-reactive protein up to 150 mg/l and blood sedimentation rate of 90 mm/h) and positive antinuclear antibodies (1:5120, AC-29 pattern) correlating with markedly elevated anti-Scl70 antibodies. Regarding vasculopathy, the patient reported frequent Raynaud's phenomenon attacks without the occurrence of ulcers or pitting scars, and the first capillaroscopy already showed a severe microangiopathy of the scleroderma active pattern, with frequent giant capillaries, extensive dysangiogenesis with ramified capillaries, frequent microhemorrhages, and slight

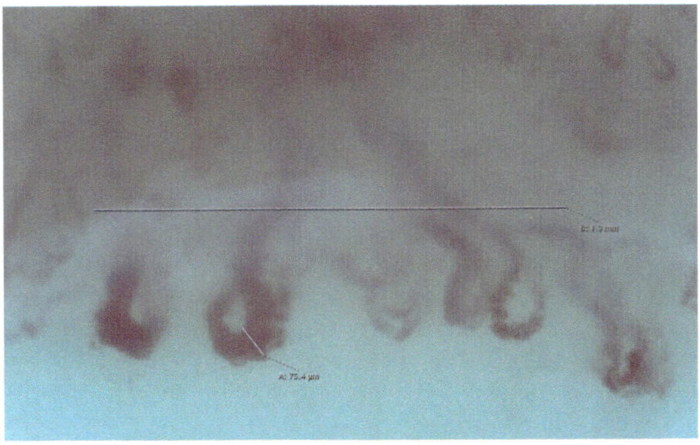

Fig. 15.12 Giant capillaries and slight rarefaction of capillaries, defining a scleroderma active pattern

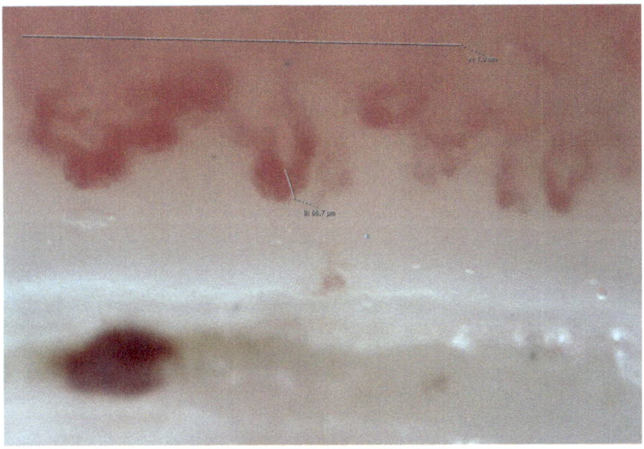

Fig. 15.13 Distorted architecture of the capillary network as a sign of dysangiogenesis. Capillary loss and giant capillaries define the presence of an active scleroderma active pattern

capillary loss, as shown in Figs. 15.12 and 15.13. Internal organ assessment, including high-resolution thorax computer tomography, showed an interstitial lung disease of a nonspecific interstitial pneumopathy pattern. Based on all these findings, the diagnosis of limited cutaneous SSc was made, and therapy with calcium channel blockers and with tocilizumab was started.

Initially, the disease course was favorable, without further organ progression and even with remission of the skin fibrosis and of arthritis. However, two years later, the patient presented with critical digital ischemia and digital ulcers (Fig. 15.14). Follow-up nailfold capillaroscopies consistently showed a scleroderma late pattern, with severe rarefaction, as seen in Fig. 15.15. After initiating antiplatelet therapy, the patient received several cycles of intravenous prostacyclin analog (Iloprost) treatment. Furthermore, we diagnosed a cryoglobulinemia, which could be attributed to Waldenström's disease, but which however showed no further signs of activity. The patient responded very well to prostacyclin treatment, with complete healing of his digital ulcers. To prevent further ulcerations, an endothelin receptor blocker, bosentan, was added to aspirin and calcium channel blockers.

While arthritis was well controlled with tocilizumab and there was barely any more skin fibrosis observable, yearly organ assessments showed a progression of

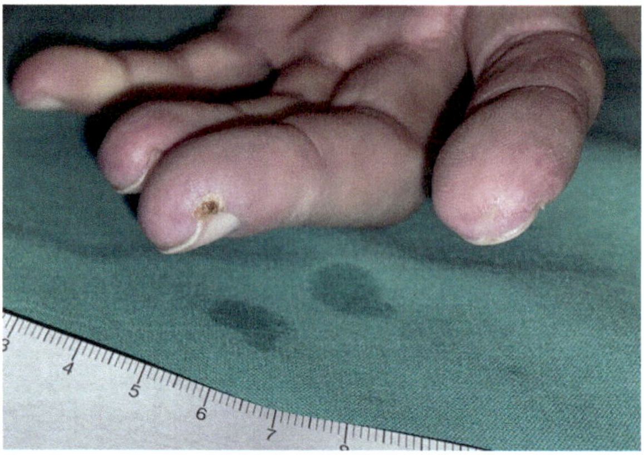

Fig. 15.14 Periungual digital ulceration

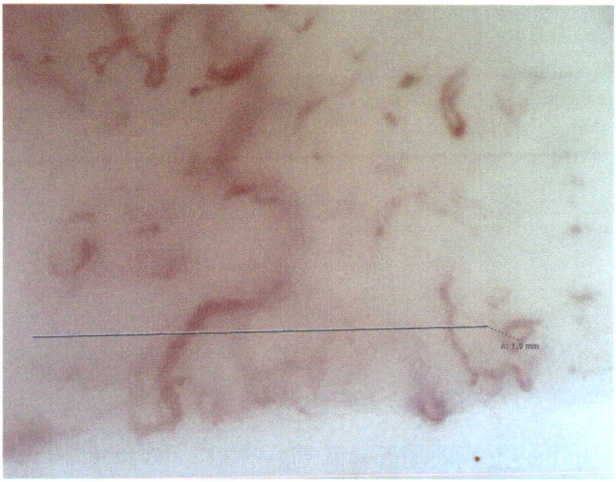

Fig. 15.15 Markedly distorted architecture of the capillary network and capillary loss, defining a scleroderma late pattern

the interstitial lung disease, for which antifibrotic treatment with nintedanib was initiated, in addition to tocilizumab.

Approximately four years after the first presentation, the disease course turned aggressive, and the patients needed an emergency hospitalization for scleroderma renal crisis with accompanying critical digital ischemia. Furthermore, there was also severe progression of his skin fibrosis, with—for the first time in the course of his disease—diffuse cutaneous fibrosis with a modified Rodnan skin score of 20/51 points. High-resolution computer tomography showed progression of the interstitial lung disease, and heart magnetic resonance imaging, performed due to elevated troponin, showed myocardial inflammation in a pattern suggestive of SSc-associated heart involvement. Under treatment with ACE inhibitors, severe renal failure could be avoided. Immunosuppressive therapy was intensified by adding mycophenolate to the already established treatment with tocilizumab. Digital ischemia was successfully treated with intravenous iloprost.

However, vasculopathy deteriorated further, with recurrent digital ulcerations on hands and feet. Occlusive disease of large arteries was ruled out by duplex sonography, and phosphodiesterase-5-inhibitor treatment with sildenafil was added to bosentan and aspirin. Under this combination therapy, the ulcers finally healed; however, there was no improvement in the recurring Raynaud's phenomenon episodes.

While skin and lung fibrosis could be stabilized under intensified immunosuppressive therapy, the patient experienced another episode of renal failure, this time due to nephrotic syndrome caused by cryoglobulinemic glomerulonephritis due to his Waldenström gammopathy. Therefore, tocilizumab was switched to rituximab, which needed to be discontinued after the first dose due to decompensated heart failure. Unfortunately, there was no improvement in the kidney function (eGFR <10 ml/min), and due to the uncertain prognosis as well as the patient's wish, no dialysis was initiated. He was also suffering from new painful acral ischemia and ulcers, the latter complicated by digital infections. Finally, he was transferred to the palliative care station, where he died 20 days later, 6 years after being diagnosed with SSc.

Discussion

This case illustrates how severe peripheral vasculopathy is associated with progressive organ involvement, leading to a fatal outcome in this case [21]. Cohort studies showed that progression from an early or active to a late scleroderma pattern [22] in nailfold capillaroscopy is associated with an elevated risk of new digital ulcers and also progression of lung fibrosis [23]. Also, capillaroscopy patterns have been shown to be directly associated with disease severity and prognosis [24, 25].

Even though this patient was under combined vasoactive medication, including an endothelin-1 receptor blocker, a phosphodiesterase-5 inhibitor, and a calcium antagonist, as well as repetitive iloprost infusions, his vasculopathy stayed active with persistent severe Raynaud's phenomenon and recurrent digital ulcers and ischemia. This shows how vasculopathy can be refractory to maximal therapy, with no further conventional therapeutic options [26].

Small studies show a possible effect of palmar botulinum toxin injections on digital ulcers and Raynaud's phenomenon [27]; also, digital sympathectomy could have a positive effect on abnormal digital vasoreactivity [28]. However, those invasive therapy options are not evidence-based so far, and it remains unclear whether our patient would have been able to benefit from such a treatment.

Learning Points

Vasculopathy in SSc can be difficult to treat, even under maximal drug therapy. Calcium channel antagonists are most often used to treat Raynaud's phenomenon; phosphodiesterase-5 inhibitors and intravenous iloprost can be used for digital ulcers aiming at healing, while bosentan can be used for secondary prevention. Other therapeutic options, like botulinum toxin injections, are supported only by a low level of evidence. This case illustrates how the progression of a scleroderma pattern from active to late on nailfold capillaroscopy is a marker of overall disease progression and severe outcome.

Acknowledgment The patient provided written informed consent for the use of his clinical data and images for teaching and research purposes. We express our sincere gratitude and regret his premature passing.

Case 5: Refractory Digital Ulcers in Systemic Sclerosis—The Role of NVC and Capillaroscopic Skin Ulcer Risk Index (CSURI) in Guiding Management

Rahma A. Elziaty
Internal Medicine Department, Rheumatology Division, Faculty of Medicine, Ain Shams University, Cairo, Egypt

A 42-year-old female began, in *2018*, to experience severe Raynaud's phenomenon, puffy fingers, telangiectasia, and polyarthritis. The autoimmune profile showed ANA 1:320 (speckled), anti-centromere antibody (ACA): positive, and anti-Scl-70: negative. Baseline HRCT chest, PFT, and echocardiography were normal. Nailfold capillaroscopy was not available at that time. According to the EULAR/ACR 2013 Classification Criteria for systemic sclerosis, the patient scored ten points, confirming the diagnosis. Initial management included calcium channel blockers, methotrexate, and low-dose corticosteroids.

Progression in *2022*: the patient developed bilateral sclerodactyly, new digital ulcers, and finger pitting scars. Nailfold videocapillaroscopy (NVC) demonstrated an active scleroderma pattern. CSURI calculation: D = 65, M = 2, N = 5; *CSURI = 5.2* > cutoff value "2.94." Figures 15.16 and 15.17. Accordingly, the patient received IV prostaglandin (PGE1) for 5 days, resulting in marked improvement, and then she was maintained on CCB, sildenafil, and methotrexate 25 mg/week. The digital ulcers almost healed after 6 months, as demonstrated in Fig. 15.18.

Progression in *2023*: the patient developed a new digital ulcer, pitting scars, features of interstitial lung disease (ILD), and NVC: active scleroderma pattern. *CSURI = 4.8*, again >2.94. Investigations revealed PFT: moderate restrictive pattern, HRCT: ground-glass opacities, and Echo: normal PAP (18 mmHg) (Fig. 15.19).

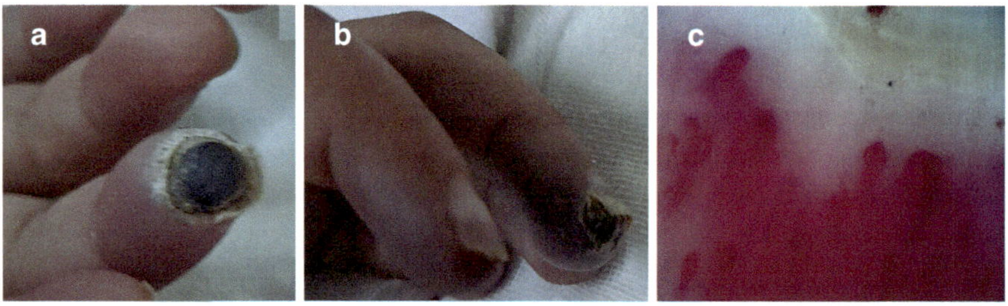

Fig. 15.16 Demonstrates puffy fingers, digital ulcer (**a**, **b**), and sclerodactyly (**b**). Also, active scleroderma pattern (**c**). "Decreased capillary density, giant capillaries and microhemorrhages"

Capillaroscopic Skin Ulcer Risk Index: CSURI ($D \times M / N^2$)	
D	The *maximum loop diameter* (the diameter of the largest giant capillary present in the capillaroscopic image
M	*Number of giant capillaries* (image with highest M among examined fingers)
N	The lowest number of capillaries in the distal (image with the lowest n among examined fingers)
CSURI > 2.94 : high risk of digital ulcer **CSURI < 2.94 : low risk of digital ulcer**	

Fig. 15.17 How to use and calculate Capillaroscopic Skin Risk Index "CSURI" **(2)**

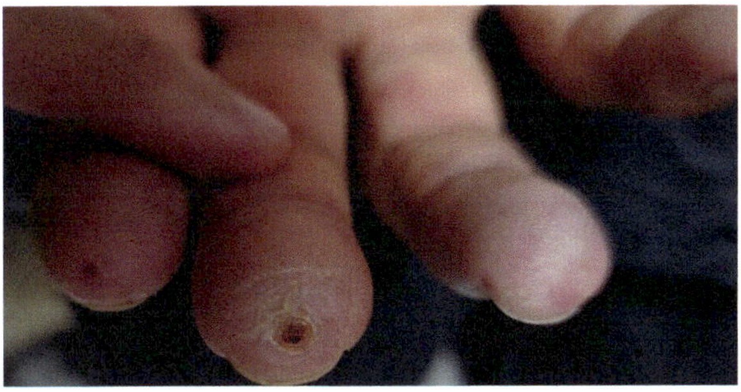

Fig. 15.18 Demonstrates healed digital ulcers of the ring and little fingers

The patient received IV prostaglandin (PGE1) and cyclophosphamide IV 800 mg monthly × 6 months and then was maintained on long-term therapy: mycophenolate mofetil, endothelin receptor blocker, CCB, sildenafil, and atorvastatin, with marked improvement of the digital ulcer as demonstrated in Fig. 15.20. Since then, the patient did not experience any new digital ulcers. Currently, she is continuing follow-up at the outpatient clinic of rheumatology, pulmonology, and dermatology as MTD

Discussion

Digital ulcers (DU) are a major vascular complication of systemic sclerosis and are linked to early microangiopathy and progressive ischemia. The patient initially

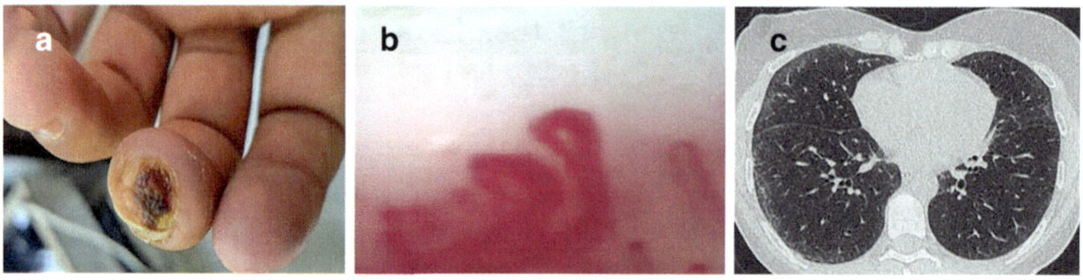

Fig. 15.19 New digital ulcers of the left middle finger (**a**). Active scleroderma pattern (**b**). HRCT chest demonstrates interstitial lung disease with the presence of GGO (**c**)

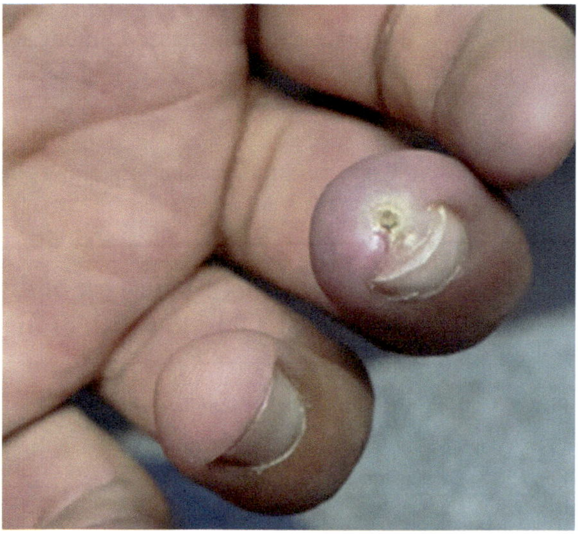

Fig. 15.20 Healed digital ulcers of the middle finger

presented with early vasculopathic manifestations (Raynaud's, puffy fingers, and telangiectasia) and an autoantibody profile (positive ACA), meeting the 2013 EULAR/ACR criteria for limited cutaneous systemic sclerosis [29].

Nailfold videocapillaroscopy (NVC) is essential for assessing SSc microvascular damage. The presence of giant capillaries, microhemorrhages, capillary loss, and abnormal architecture is strongly associated with DU risk.

The Capillaroscopic Skin Ulcer Risk Index (CSURI) is validated as a predictor of DU formation within 3 months, with CSURI >2.94 indicating high risk [30]. In this case, both assessments (2022 and 2023) showed high CSURI scores (5.2 and 4.8), correlating with the occurrence of recurrent DU.

The refractory nature of digital ulcers in systemic sclerosis is attributed to the combined microvascular vasculopathy (endothelial dysfunction, capillary rarefaction). Macrovascular dysfunction (fixed arterial stenosis and impaired blood flow) [31]. Early intervention with vasodilators such as calcium channel blockers, phosphodiesterase-5 inhibitors (sildenafil), and IV prostaglandins is recommended [31, 32].

For patients with progressive disease and ILD, cyclophosphamide or mycophenolate mofetil is advised. In this patient, the development of ILD (ground-glass opacities and restrictive PFT pattern) represented systemic disease progression, requiring escalation to cyclophosphamide followed by mycophenolate [32].

Learning Outcome Points

- Use Nailfold videocapillaroscopy to assess microangiopathy and monitor disease progression.
- Interpret CSURI to identify patients at high risk of digital ulcer development.
- Appreciate that digital ulcers in SSc may be refractory due to combined micro- and macrovascular vasculopathy.
- Recognize when to escalate treatment to include IV prostaglandins, cyclophosphamide, or mycophenolate.

Case 6: From Nailfold to Kidney: Correlation Between Capillaroscopic and Renal Doppler Findings During Scleroderma Renal Crisis and Recovery

Rahma A. Elziaty and Nada Mahmoud
Internal Medicine Department, Rheumatology Division, Faculty of Medicine, Ain Shams University, Cairo, Egypt

A 48-year-old woman with a 3-year history of diffuse cutaneous systemic sclerosis (dcSSc) presented with new-onset severe hypertension (BP 200/120 mmHg), headache, and oliguria. She had progressive skin thickening, digital ulcers, and Raynaud's phenomenon (Fig. 15.21).

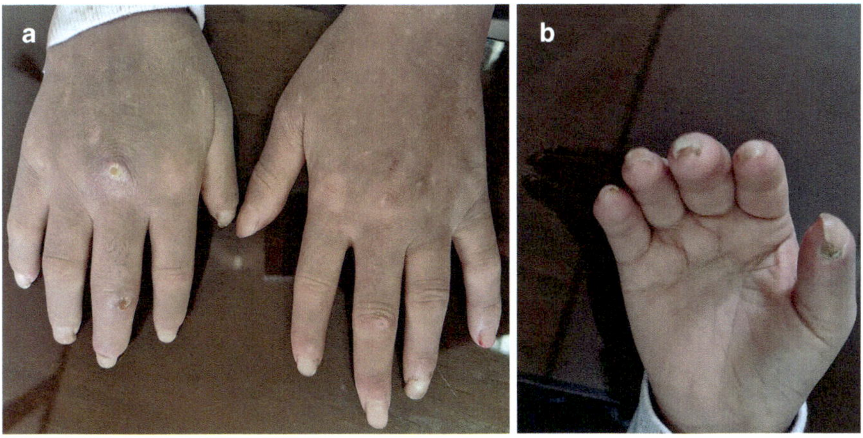

Fig. 15.21 (**a**) Puffy fingers of both hands, digital ulcers, and pitting scars on the dorsal surface. (**b**) Fingertip ulcers and pseudo clubbing

Baseline laboratory results revealed serum creatinine: 3.2 mg/dL (baseline 0.9 mg/dL), urea: 85 mg/dL, mild proteinuria (1+) without hematuria, hemoglobin: 9.8 g/dL with fragmented red cells on peripheral smear, platelets: 110 × 10^9/L, ANA: 1:640 (speckled pattern), anti-Scl-70 positive, and anti-RNA polymerase III strongly positive. These findings were consistent with *scleroderma renal crisis (SRC) complicated by microangiopathic hemolytic anemia.*

Capillaroscopy Findings at Admission Nailfold video capillaroscopy showed an active scleroderma pattern with giant capillaries, frequent microhemorrhages, severe architectural disorganization, capillary density of 3–4/mm, and extensive avascular areas. These features reflected severe ongoing microangiopathy (Fig. 15.22).

Renal Artery Duplex at Admission renal artery resistive index (RI): left renal RI: 0.78 and right renal RI: 0.85. Increased vascular resistance and reduced cortical perfusion, consistent with microvascular ischemia secondary to SRC. No evidence of large-vessel stenosis (Fig. 15.23).

Management and Clinical Course: The patient was treated aggressively with *plasma exchange* (5 sessions) to control microangiopathic hemolysis, and this *ACE inhibitor* (captopril) was titrated to the maximal tolerated dose with other antihypertensive medications (CCB and nitroprusside). Endothelin receptor antagonist (*Bosentan*) for endothelial protection and digital ischemia. Rituximab (1 g IV, two doses 2 weeks apart) for systemic disease control.

After 4 weeks, blood pressure stabilized at 130/80 mmHg, serum creatinine decreased to 1.5 mg/dL, and digital ischemia improved.

Follow-Up Findings (3 Months Postcrisis)
Capillaroscopy: remaining active scleroderma pattern with partial revascularization. Reduction in giant capillaries and microhemorrhages. Capillary density improved to 5–6/mm. Better organization of capillary loops, indicating vascular recovery (Fig. 15.24).

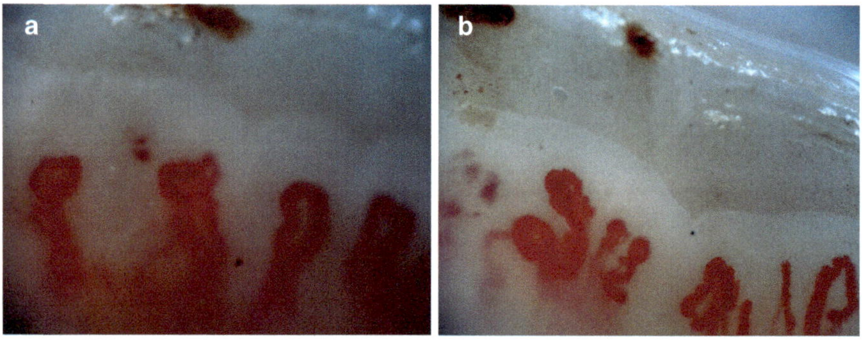

Fig. 15.22 NFC demonstrates an active scleroderma pattern: decreased capillary density, giant capillaries, and microhemorrhages with the presence of some neoangiogenic vessels, indicating disease progression (**a**, **b**)

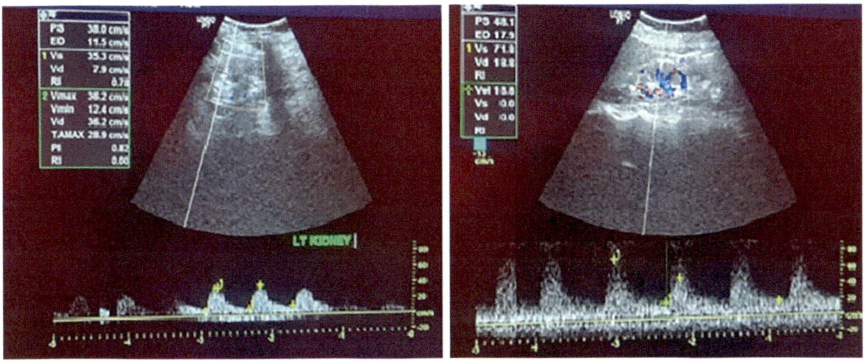

Fig. 15.23 Renal artery resistive index (RI) on admission; left renal RI: 0.78 and right renal RI: 0.85

Fig. 15.24 NFC demonstrates an active scleroderma pattern, improved capillary density, and giant capillaries

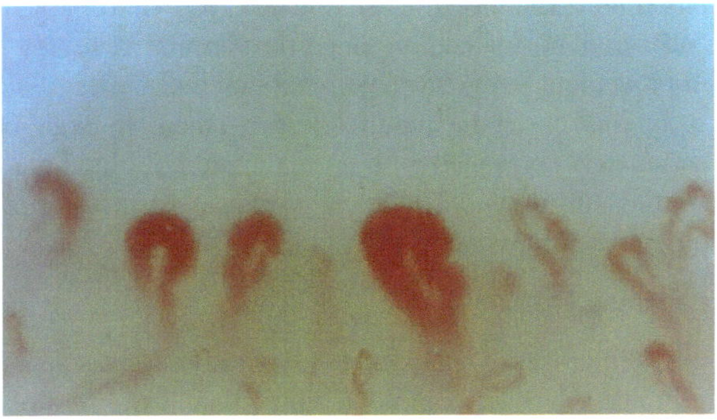

Renal Artery Duplex: Resistive index (RI): normalized to *left renal RI: 0.65*, and *right renal RI: 0.54*. Improved cortical perfusion and renal size were preserved (Fig. 15.25).

6-Month Follow-up: Renal function remained stable (creatinine 1.3 mg/dL), and blood pressure was controlled without recurrence of SRC.

Discussion

Scleroderma renal crisis is a severe manifestation of systemic sclerosis that occurs in approximately 5–10% of patients, more frequently in those with diffuse cutaneous involvement and anti-RNA polymerase III antibodies. The hallmark features include abrupt hypertension, rapidly progressive renal impairment, and microangiopathic hemolysis [33, 34].

Early diagnosis and monitoring are essential for prognosis. Traditionally, evaluation relies on clinical and laboratory parameters, but microvascular imaging tools offer additional insights into disease activity and response to therapy.

Nailfold capillaroscopy provides a noninvasive "window" into systemic microangiopathy. The active pattern observed during SRC reflects severe endothelial injury and microvascular dropout, paralleling renal microvascular pathology. Following treatment, improvements in capillary density and organization may mirror systemic endothelial repair [35–37].

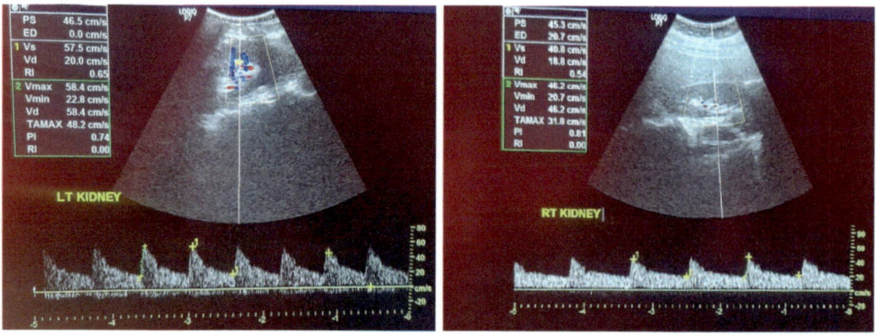

Fig. 15.25 Renal artery resistive index (RI) on admission; left renal RI: 0.65 and right renal RI: 0.54

Similarly, renal Doppler ultrasonography offers dynamic evaluation of renal blood flow. Increased resistive index (RI > 0.8) indicates impaired renal perfusion, and serial normalization suggests vascular recovery. Studies have correlated RI improvement with favorable renal outcomes after ACE inhibitor therapy [38].

In this case, the parallel improvement in both capillaroscopic and Doppler parameters correlated with normalization of blood pressure and creatinine, demonstrating the potential of these noninvasive modalities in disease monitoring and prognostic assessment.

Learning Outcomes

- Capillaroscopy can detect systemic microvascular injury and recovery in systemic sclerosis, complementing clinical and serological data.
- Renal Doppler ultrasonography provides a valuable, radiation-free method for monitoring renal perfusion in scleroderma renal crisis.
- Early and aggressive therapy with ACE inhibitors, endothelin blockers, and B-cell–targeted therapy can reverse microangiopathic changes.
- Integration of microvascular imaging improves patient follow-up, allowing noninvasive tracking of systemic vascular health.

Case 7: Nailfold Capillaroscopy as a Risk Predictor in Systemic Sclerosis: Beyond a Mere Diagnostic Tool

Carlos Valera-Ribera
Department of Rheumatology, Hospital Universitario Dr. Peset, Valencia, Spain

1. *Patient's History and Clinical Examination*

A 55-year-old Hispanic male construction worker was referred to the rheumatology department for evaluation of suspected systemic sclerosis (SSc). He reported a

7-month history of Raynaud's in both hands and progressive dyspnea on moderate exertion over the past year. He denied orthopnea, peripheral edema, dysphagia, or gastroesophageal reflux. There was no history of previous or active smoking or alcohol intake.

His medical history included vitiligo affecting the hands and face, arterial hypertension treated with amlodipine 5 mg daily, and dyslipidemia managed with atorvastatin 20 mg per day.

On physical examination, he presented with mild sclerodactyly and periungual telangiectasias (Fig. 15.26). Skin thickening involved the forearms, face, thorax, abdomen, and feet, with a modified Rodnan skin score of 9. Blood pressure was 127/91 mmHg, oxygen saturation was 97%, and cardiopulmonary auscultation was unremarkable. No digital ulcers or pitting scars were observed. Complete laboratory testing, nailfold capillaroscopy (NFC), pulmonary function tests (PFTs), lung high-resolution computed tomography (HRCT), and echocardiography were performed.

2. *Outcome of Investigations*

Laboratory results showed a positive antinuclear antibody (ANA) with a speckled and nucleolar pattern at a titer of 1:320 and markedly elevated anti-topoisomerase I (Scl-70) antibodies (238 U/mL), confirming the diagnosis of diffuse cutaneous systemic sclerosis (dcSSc). Complete blood count, inflammatory markers, hepatic and renal function tests, and NT-proBNP were all within normal limits.

HRCT of the chest revealed bibasilar ground-glass opacities and reticular changes with traction bronchiectasis, consistent with a nonspecific interstitial pneumonia (NSIP) pattern (Fig. 15.27). PFTs demonstrated a moderate restrictive defect with preserved diffusing capacity for carbon monoxide (DLCO). Echocardiography showed normal biventricular function and no indirect signs of pulmonary hypertension.

NFC displayed architectural disorganization with reduced capillary density, frequent megacapillaries, and microhemorrhages (Fig. 15.28). In several nailfolds, extensive avascular areas (further lowered capillary density) were evident, indicating the coexistence of active and late scleroderma patterns (Fig. 15.29).

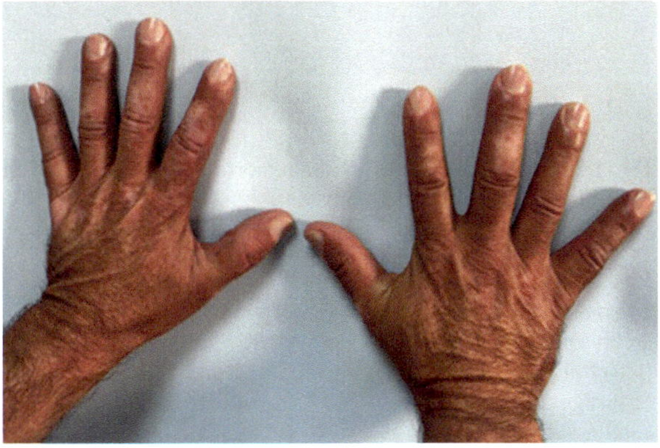

Fig. 15.26 Hands showing mild sclerodactyly, periungual telangiectasias, and vitiligo-associated hypopigmentation

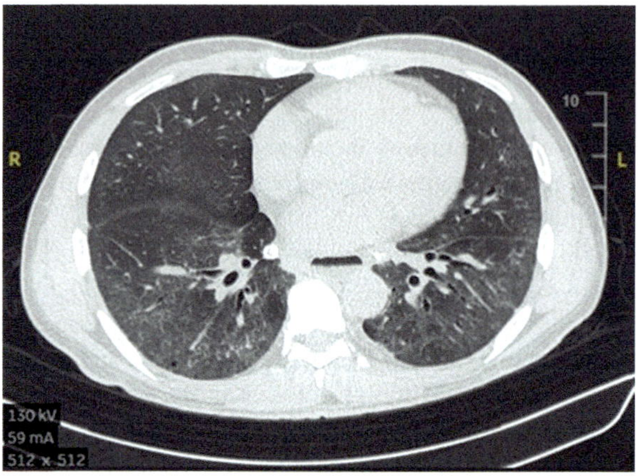

Fig. 15.27 Lung HCT demonstrating basal ground-glass opacities and reticulation consistent with an NSIP pattern

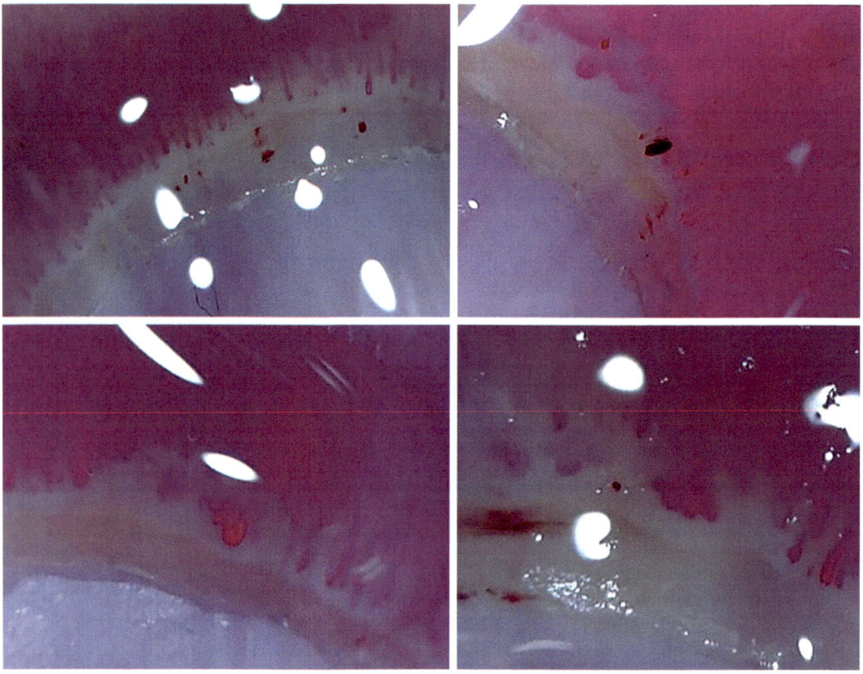

Fig. 15.28 Megacapillaries, microhemorrhages, and reduced capillary density, findings compatible with an active scleroderma pattern

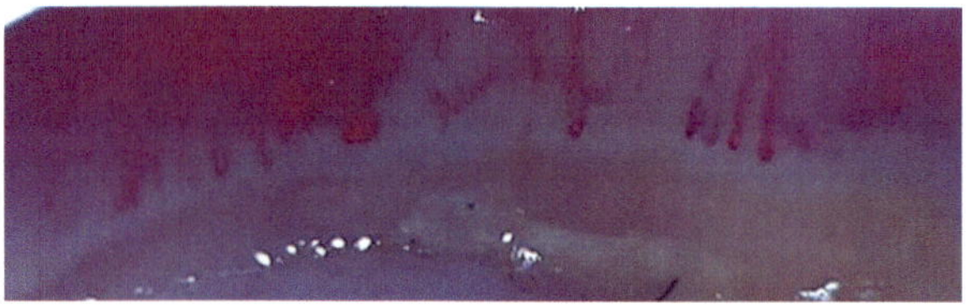

Fig. 15.29 Mecapillaries and mild capillary architectural disruption (left) followed by an area of further decreased capillary density (right)

3. *Figures*
4. *Questions for the Reader*

   - What is the current definition of further lowered capillary density in NFC according to EULAR/STCT recommendations?
   - How can NFC contribute to systemic risk assessment in systemic sclerosis?
   - What is the relationship between microangiopathic changes in NFC and cardiovascular risk in systemic sclerosis?

5. *Discussion*

This case illustrates a classic presentation of diffuse cutaneous systemic sclerosis (dcSSc) with Anti-Topoisomerase I (Scl-70) positivity and early interstitial lung disease (ILD). NFC findings demonstrated an active scleroderma pattern with focal transition to late pattern morphology. Therefore, beyond the categorical classification of NFC patterns, detailed reporting of specific morphological findings remains essential for accurate disease characterization [39]. Notably, the presence of late pattern NFC at baseline has been associated with a higher risk of ILD development [40].

The extent of avascular areas (further lowered capillary density) has been associated with increased mortality and cardiovascular risk, as demonstrated in recent cohort studies, where the presence of further lowered capillary density independently predicted major adverse cardiovascular events and all-cause mortality [41, 42].

These observations reinforce the concept that nailfold microangiopathy mirrors systemic vasculopathy, providing clinically relevant prognostic insight into both cardiovascular and overall risk assessment. Accordingly, in this patient, meticulous control of cardiovascular risk factors and longitudinal monitoring are strongly warranted.

6. *Key Learning Points*

   - Nailfold capillaroscopy is a noninvasive technique that provides insight into both disease activity and systemic vasculopathy in systemic sclerosis.
   - The presence of avascular areas (further lowered capillary density) correlates with more severe disease and higher cardiovascular event risk.
   - Integrating NFC findings with cardiopulmonary evaluation (HRCT, echocardiography, PFTs) enhances early detection of organ involvement.
   - Patients with diffuse cutaneous SSc and Scl-70 positivity should undergo multisystemic evaluation, even in the absence of overt symptoms.

Case 8: Post-COVID-19 New-Onset Systemic Sclerosis in a Young Female: A Rare Case Highlighting Possible Viral Trigger and Rapid Disease Evolution

Rahma A. Elziaty and Rasha M. Hammoda
Internal Medicine Department, Rheumatology Division, Faculty of Medicine, Ain Shams University, Cairo, Egypt

A 26-year-old female with no previous autoimmune or chronic medical illnesses contracted symptomatic *COVID-19 infection in 2021*. The condition was mild and just required isolation and home treatment. She fully recovered with no immediate complications.

Approximately one year later *(2022), she developed severe Raynaud's phenomenon* with frequent digital color changes and cold intolerance. She sought medical advice and received vasodilator therapy, including calcium channel blockers, but experienced minimal symptomatic improvement.

Over the following six months, she developed *puffy fingers*, *progressive hand swelling*, *arthralgia*, and *dysphagia for solids*, associated with *reflux symptoms*. Capillaroscopy; early scleroderma pattern. Laboratory evaluation at that time revealed: ANA positive (titer not stated), anti-centromere antibody strongly positive, normal creatine kinase (CK), and ESR mildly elevated. She was diagnosed with limited cutaneous systemic sclerosis (Fig. 15.30).

Regarding the treatment strategy at that time, she received methotrexate 25 mg/week, folic acid 5 mg, calcium channel blockers, hydroxychloroquine 400 mg daily, a proton pump inhibitor (PPI), and prokinetic therapy.

By 2023, the patient developed *progressive exertional dyspnea and a dry cough.* Capillaroscopy: Active scleroderma pattern. Investigations showed: Pulmonary function tests → moderate restrictive pattern, High-resolution CT chest → findings consistent with systemic-sclerosis-associated ILD. Echocardiography did not suggest pulmonary hypertension (Fig. 15.31).

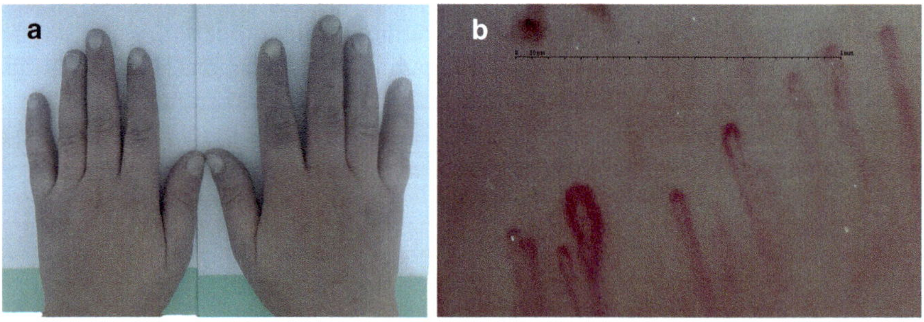

Fig. 15.30 (**a**) Demonstrates puffy fingers and Raynaud's of both hands (**b**) NFC demonstrates an early scleroderma pattern, normal capillary density, giant capillaries, and the presence of microhemorrhages

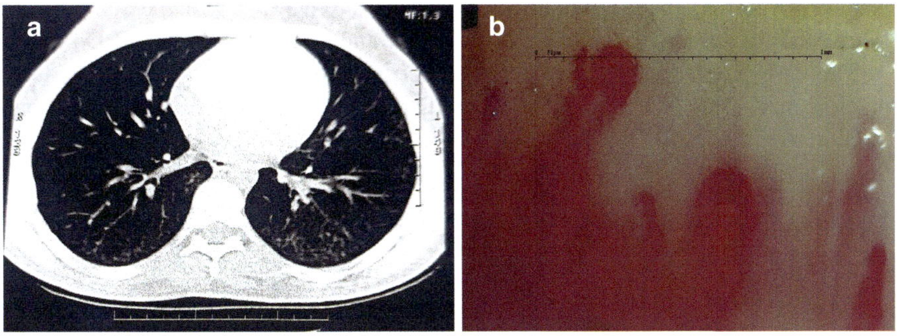

Fig. 15.31 (**a**) Early ILD demonstrated in HRCT chest with the presence of Ground-Glass Opacities (GGOs), (**b**) NFC demonstrates an active scleroderma pattern, decreased capillary density, giant capillaries, presence of microhemorrhages, and pericapillary edema

Accordingly, she received rituximab 1 g with the regimen (0–2 weeks every 6 months) for 2 years till *June 2025* and was then maintained on mycophenolate mofetil (MMF) 2 g daily, calcium channel blockers, hydroxychloroquine 400 mg daily, proton pump inhibitor (PPI), and prokinetic therapy. The patient showed marked improvement of the symptoms, and she is under regular follow-up with rheumatology, pulmonology, and gastroenterology.

Discussion

Systemic sclerosis is a complex autoimmune disease characterized by microvascular injury, immune dysregulation, and progressive fibrosis. COVID-19 has emerged as a potential environmental trigger for autoimmune conditions, including SSc. Proposed mechanisms include molecular mimicry, bystander T-cell activation, hyperactive type I interferon pathways, and endothelial injury, which may accelerate microvascular dysfunction characteristic of SSc [43].

In this patient, Raynaud's phenomenon developed one year post-COVID-19, followed by rapid evolution to puffy fingers, dysphagia, arthralgia, and SSc-specific capillaroscopic changes. While anti-centromere antibody positivity is generally associated with a slower disease course and lower risk of ILD, post-COVID immune dysregulation may modify classical phenotypes, leading to earlier internal organ involvement [44–46].

Nailfold capillaroscopy showed progression from an early to active scleroderma pattern, reflecting ongoing microvascular injury. Capillaroscopic monitoring is critical for early detection of SSc progression and correlates with internal organ involvement.

The development of SSc-associated ILD within two years of Raynaud's onset emphasizes the aggressive nature of post-COVID SSc. SARS-CoV-2–related pulmonary inflammation and fibrosis may amplify autoimmunity, contributing to early ILD development [47].

The therapeutic strategy included rituximab, which has evidence for stabilizing skin and lung involvement in SSc, particularly in early or rapidly progressive disease [48]. Maintenance with mycophenolate mofetil aligns with the Scleroderma Lung Study II, which demonstrated its efficacy and tolerability in SSc-ILD [49].

This case underscores the need for vigilance in patients with new-onset Raynaud's phenomenon after COVID-19, early capillaroscopy, autoantibody screening, and pulmonary evaluation. Prompt immunomodulatory therapy can prevent irreversible organ damage.

Learning Outcome Points

- COVID-19 may trigger systemic autoimmune diseases, including systemic sclerosis.
- Rapid progression from Raynaud's to systemic sclerosis warrants early evaluation.
- Nailfold capillaroscopy is crucial for detecting early SSc microangiopathy and monitoring disease activity.
- Anti-centromere antibodies do not preclude early ILD, particularly in post-COVID SSc.
- Rituximab and mycophenolate mofetil are effective therapies for skin and lung involvement.
- Early recognition and multidisciplinary care optimize patient outcomes.

Case 9: Severe Vascular Involvement in Patient with Systemic Sclerosis and a Long History of Smoking

Maria Lungu
Rheumatology and Nephrology Discipline, Nicolae Testemiţanu University, Chişinău, Republic of Moldova

Timofei Moşneaga Republican Clinical Hospital, Chişinău, Republic of Moldova

Svetlana Agachi
Rheumatology and Nephrology Discipline, Nicolae Testemiţanu University, Chişinău, Republic of Moldova

Patient's History
Female aged 65, active smoker (for approximately 20 years), known to have puffy fingers and Raynaud's phenomenon for approximately 2 years, with exacerbation of episodes during the last year, especially upon exposure to cold, with the appearance of digital ulcers in January 2025. Then dysphagia with solid foods and heartburn were associated. She suffers from peripheral arteriopathy of the lower limbs, hypertension, C.I., ventricular extrasystole, and atrial fibrillation for 5 years. No family history of autoimmune diseases.

On Clinical Examination indurated skin on the fingers (sclerodactyly), radial folds around the mouth, microstomia, fine telangiectasias on the face and hands, and active ischemic ulcers on the II and III fingers bilaterally. Cold extremities. Obesity gr.II. Auscultation of the lungs—diminished basal vesicular murmur, single crepitant rales. Muffled heart sounds, arrhythmic. Hemodynamic parameters: BP-145/80 mmHg, FCC-72 b/min, SpO_2-98%, FR-17/min.

Current Medication Tab. Lercanidipine 10 mg/day, Tab. Omeprazole 20 mg/day, Tab. Sildenafil 20 mg/day, Tab. Mycophenolate mofetil 500 mg, 2 tabs × 2 times a day.

Outcome of Investigations ANA: positive, 9.4 AU/ml; anti-CENP A antibodies, IgG: positive (990.8 U/mL); anti-CENP B antibodies, IgG: positive (990.8 U/mL); anti-Ro52 antibodies, IgG: positive (569.6 U/mL); ESR: 5 mm/h; C-reactive protein (CRP): 3 mg/L; RF: 18.3 IU/mL.

Chest X-Ray: Venous congestion and basal pneumofibrotic changes. *Thoracic HRCT*: basal nonspecific interstitial pneumonia pattern changes. *Echocardiography*: EF 52%, TAPSE N, estimated pulmonary pressure 46 mmHg, considerable dilatation of the LA, moderate RA and RV, and thin pericardial leaflets. Thickening of the aortic, mitral, tricuspid, and pulmonary valves. *Pulmonary Function Tests*—FVC 70.6%, FEV1/FVC—90.85. Pulmonary diffusion test (DLCO): 37.8% of the theoretical value.

Nailfold Capillaroscopy (NFC) Pictures Digital videocapillaroscopy (200x) performed on fingers II–V bilaterally: Numerous giant capillaries, diameter >50 μm; moderate pericapillary hemorrhages; moderate reduction in capillary density (3–5 capillaries/mm); absence of marked neoangiogenesis.

Right Hand

Finger II: density 5 capillaries/mm, size >50 μm (megacapillaries), normal morphology, absent hemorrhage.

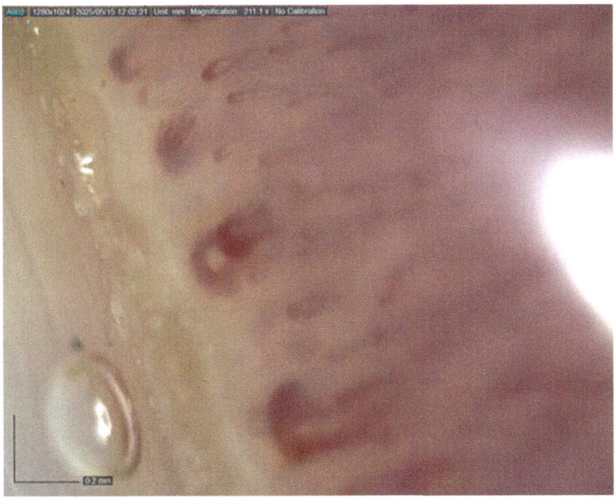

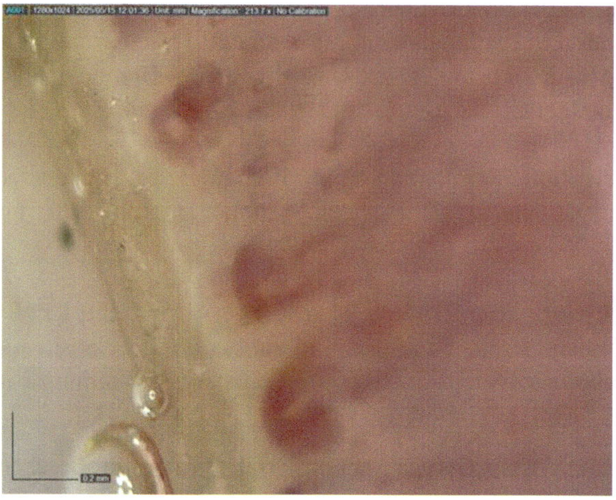

Finger III: density 7 capillaries/mm, size 20–50 μm, normal morphology, absent hemorrhage.

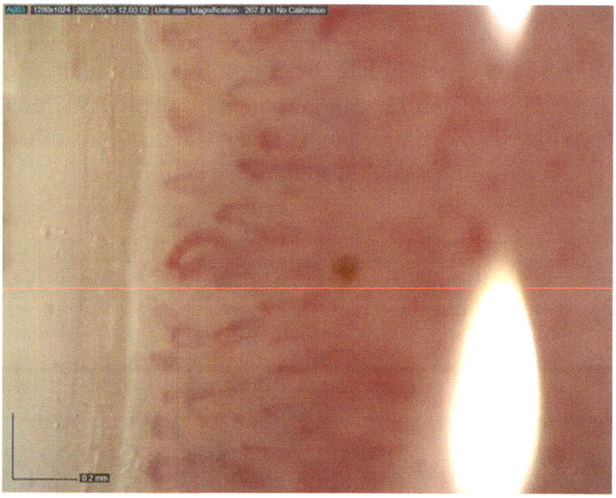

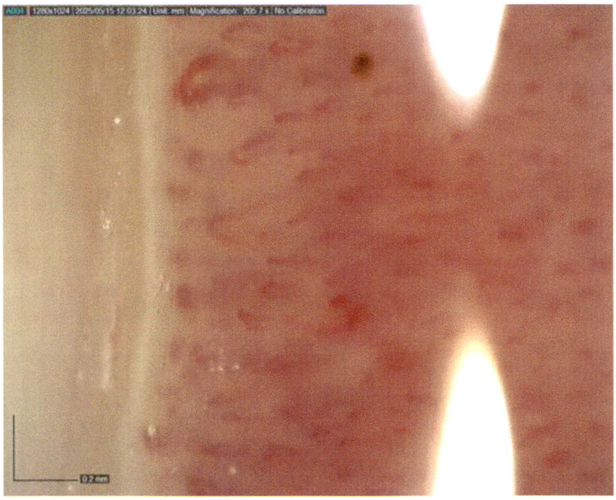

Finger IV: density 5 capillaries/mm, size >50 μm (megacapillaries), normal morphology, absent hemorrhage.

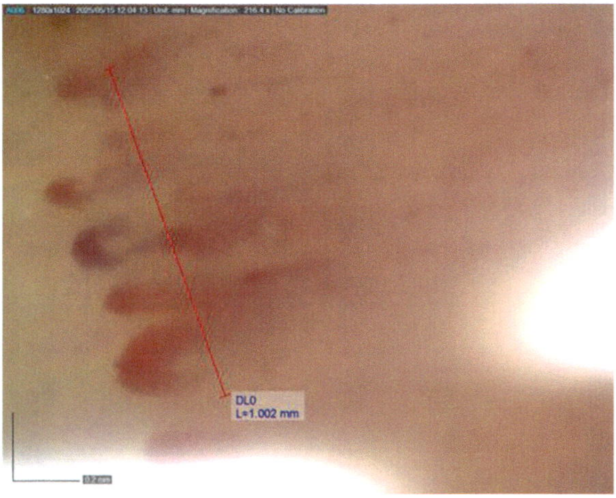

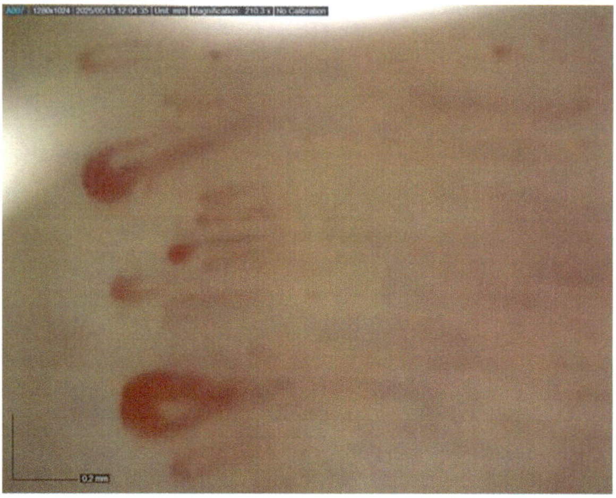

Finger V: density >7 capillaries/mm, size 20–50, normal morphology, absent hemorrhage.

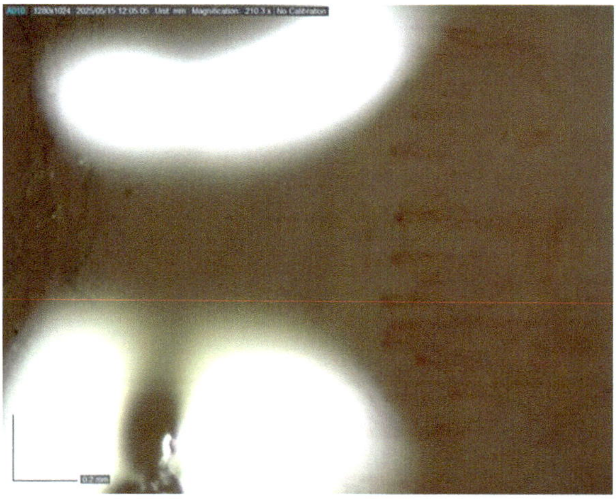

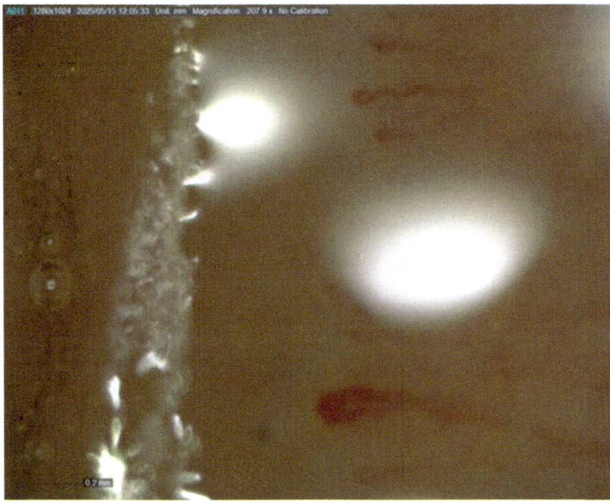

Left Hand

Finger II: density 4 capillaries/mm, size >50 μm (megacapillaries), normal morphology, present hemorrhage.

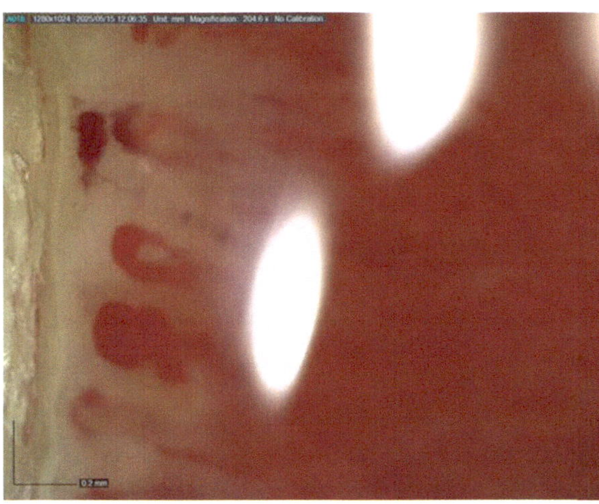

Finger III: density 3 capillaries/mm, size >50 μm (megacapillaries), regular morphology, hemorrhages present.

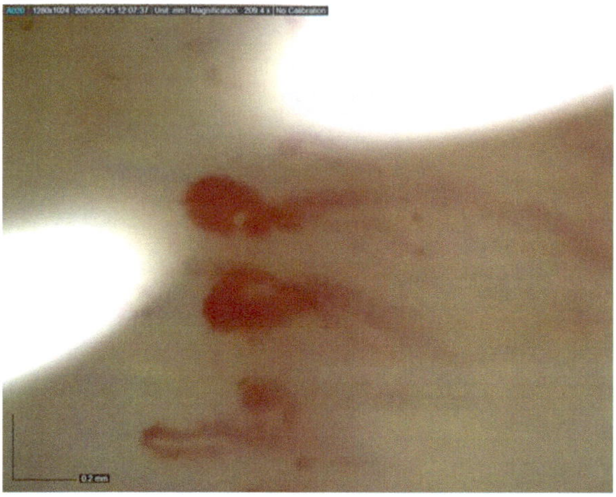

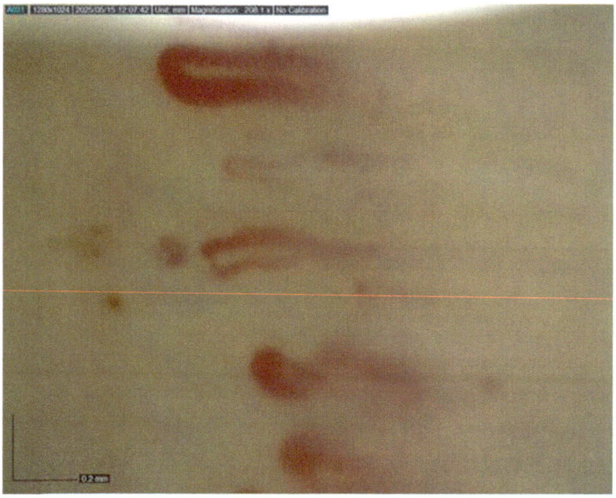

Finger IV: density 3 capillaries/mm, size >50 μm (megacapillaries), regular morphology, hemorrhages absent.

Finger V: density >7 capillaries/mm, size <20 μm, crossed capillary morphology, hemorrhages absent.

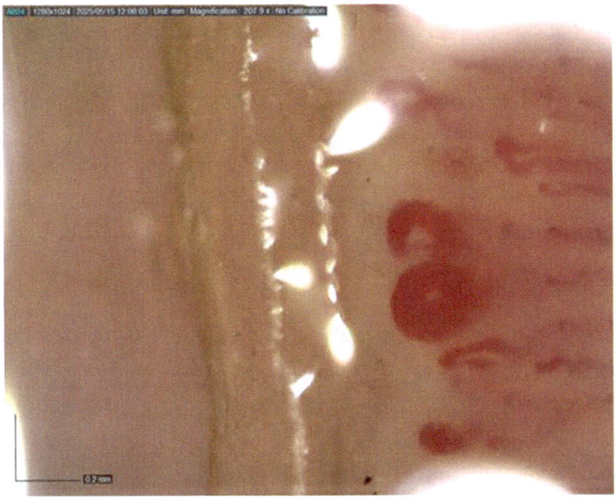

Conclusion Capillaroscopic picture with scleroderma pattern-like changes in the active phase (moderate-low capillary density, presence of megacapillaries and hemorrhages), lack of signs of neoangiogenesis.

Questions to Challenge the Reader Regarding Possible Findings and Outcomes

- What is the significance of the presence of megacapillaries in the context of a reduced capillary density?
- What does the presence of pericapillary hemorrhages imply in the active stage of scleroderma microangiopathy?
- How does the active capillaroscopic pattern correlate with the risk of visceral involvement?
- What monitoring strategies are recommended at this stage?

Discussion

The observed capillaroscopic pattern corresponds to the "active" phase of scleroderma microangiopathy, characterized by the alternation of megacapillaries with areas of capillary rarefaction and the appearance of pericapillary hemorrhages. This phase reflects a dynamic process of endothelial injury and incomplete regeneration, often preceding the development of visceral manifestations.

The recent onset of the disease, but with a rapid evolution of vascular changes with progression to digital ulcers, can be explained by the association of atherosclerotic cardiovascular pathology and long-term smoking [50–52].

Periodic capillaroscopic monitoring, associated with the assessment of pulmonary and cardiac function, has prognostic value and allows early adjustment of vascular therapy (calcium channel blockers, possibly PDE5 inhibitors).

Key Learning Points

- Capillaroscopy is an essential noninvasive tool in the early diagnosis and assessment of the progression of systemic scleroderma.
- The active pattern indicates an evolutionary phase of microangiopathy, with a risk of progression to late forms.
- The presence of megacapillaries and hemorrhages is a marker of microvascular activity.
- Correlation with autoantibodies and evaluation of target organs is mandatory in establishing the prognosis.

Case 10: Capillaroscopy as an Important Clue to Diagnosis

Caroline Evers and Carina Mihai
Department of Rheumatology, University Hospital Zurich, Zurich, Switzerland

A 48-year-old male patient was referred to our rheumatology department due to recurring occlusions of digital arteries, leading to osteomyelitis of the distal phalanx of the second digit of his right hand, with subsequent amputation. The patient had been diagnosed with Gitelman's disease at age 28. This is an autosomal recessive tubular disorder caused by mutations of genes encoding the sodium, chloride, and magnesium carriers in the apical membrane of the distal convoluted tubule, mainly of SLC12A3 or TRP6M [53]. Most patients are heterozygous for SLC12A3 mutations. The patient had a family history of Gitelman's disease and two heterozygous pathogenic variants of the SLC12A3 gene. As a complication, he developed chronic kidney disease (KDIGO grade 4a) and calcium pyrophosphate dihydrate (CPPD) arthropathy involving both knees before the age of 40.

Case History Before Presentation to the Rheumatology Department

Peripheral vasculopathy onset, with persistent painful discoloration of the fingers of the left hand (distal pallor and proximal bluish-purple discoloration), had occurred 5 years before the first presentation in the rheumatology department. During the previous winter, short self-limiting episodes of finger discoloration had started to occur on cold exposure, leading to a diagnosis of Raynaud's phenomenon. Painful discoloration of several other fingers, including some of the right hand, led to referral to the angiology clinic of our hospital, where duplex sonography showed no relevant stenosis of the brachial arteries, no significant atherosclerosis, and no signs of vascular thoracic outlet syndrome. However, oscillography demonstrated pathological perfusion in two fingers, suggestive of digital artery occlusions. Video nailfold capillaroscopy performed by the department of angiology was unremarkable. Low-titer antinuclear antibodies with an AC-4 pattern were detected by indirect immunofluorescence, with negative results in ELISA for anti-dsDNA, anti-SSA, anti-SSB, and rheumatic factor, and negative immunoblot for systemic sclerosis-associated antibodies. Antiphospholipid antibodies and lupus anticoagulants were negative.

Transthoracic and subsequently transesophageal echocardiography, as well as 48-hour Holter electrocardiographic monitoring, did not reveal cardiac sources of emboli such as atrial fibrillation, endocarditis, or intracardiac thrombi. The underlying cause of the digital occlusions remained unclear. Given the patient's history of persistent smoking (approximately 30 pack-years, with current consumption of around ten cigarettes/day at that time), thrombangiitis obliterans (Buerger's disease) was considered the most likely diagnosis, and complete smoking cessation was recommended. The patient was subsequently able to reduce smoking to two cigarettes per day.

Initial treatment included anticoagulation with low molecular weight heparin and initiation of antiplatelet therapy with low-dose aspirin. However, the symptoms progressed to permanent discoloration of further fingers, which led to the initiation of a 10-day course of intravenous iloprost and a switch of the anticoagulant treatment from heparin to rivaroxaban, a direct factor Xa inhibitor. Lack of response prompted emergency hospitalization followed by direct angiography (Fig. 15.32). This showed total occlusion of the distal right radial artery, which prompted intra-arterial thrombolysis with urokinase, leading to a significant improvement. One month later, the patient presented with a new painful digital lesion (Fig. 15.33), which persisted despite topical wound therapy and led to osteomyelitis, requiring amputation of the distal phalanx. After anticoagulation was discontinued, the patient experienced recurrent episodes of critical digital ischemia, requiring repeated intravenous iloprost infusions, at times for up to 14 consecutive days.

In the continued search for an underlying cause of the digital artery stenoses and occlusions, the patient was referred to the hematology department, where no hereditary or acquired thrombophilia could be identified. Subsequent direct angiography of the left brachial arterial system showed patent radial and ulnar arteries without stenosis but confirmed distal digital artery occlusions. Anticoagulation with rivaroxaban was reinitiated with 2.5 mg daily and switched to apixaban due to recurrent ulcers in the later course.

Additional workup in the department of cardiology showed no signs of intracardiac thrombi again. Due to multiple ventricular extrasystoles and several short self-limiting ventricular tachycardias on 48-hour electrocardiography, a heart MRI was conducted, which was normal except for midmyocardial fibrosis of the left ventricle of uncertain cause. Genetic testing for storage diseases, including Fabry disease and hemochromatosis, was negative.

Case Management in the Rheumatology Department

Due to recurring acral ischemia, the patient was referred to the department of rheumatology, more than 5 years after initial symptoms of peripheral vasculopathy, as already mentioned before. Digital capillaroscopy was repeated (Fig. 15.34) and showed only nonspecific abnormalities, consisting of frequent dilated capillaries, with normal capillary density and no hemorrhages or giant capillaries. Antinuclear antibody (ANA) testing in immunofluorescence was positive, with a titer of 1:320, negative ELISA for anti-SSA, anti-SSB, and anti-dsDNA, and negative immunoblot testing for antibodies associated with systemic sclerosis (SSc). X-rays of the hands showed acro-osteolysis of several digits (Fig. 15.35), in which fingertip pitting scars were visible on physical examination. Therapeutically, bosentan, an endothelin-1

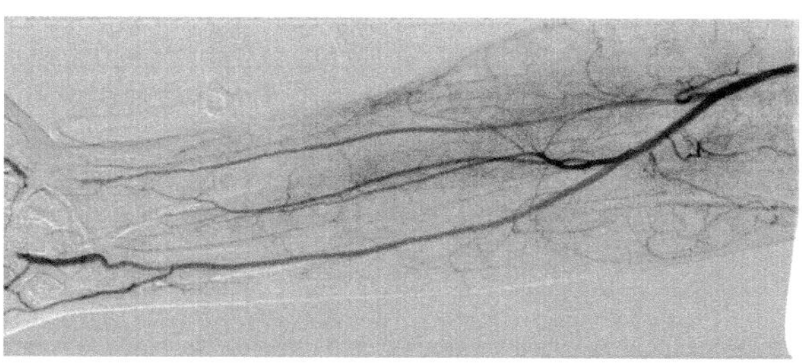

Fig. 15.32 Arteriography of the right forearm demonstrating complete occlusion of the distal radial artery, performed five years before the patient first presented to the rheumatology department

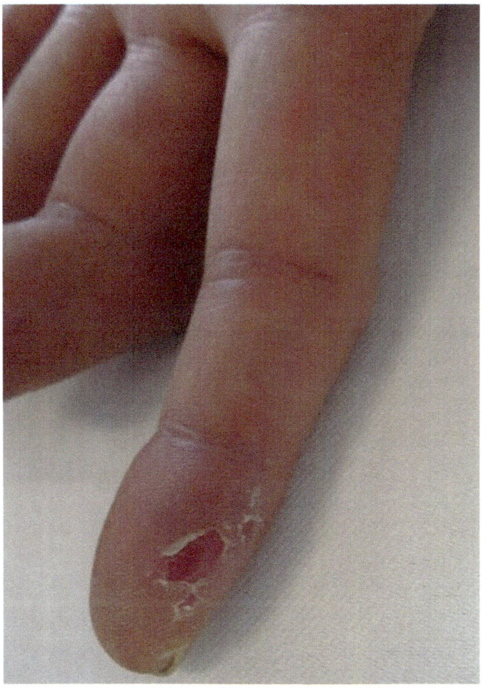

Fig. 15.33 Bluish discoloration of the fingertip of the second right digit, with painful ulceration

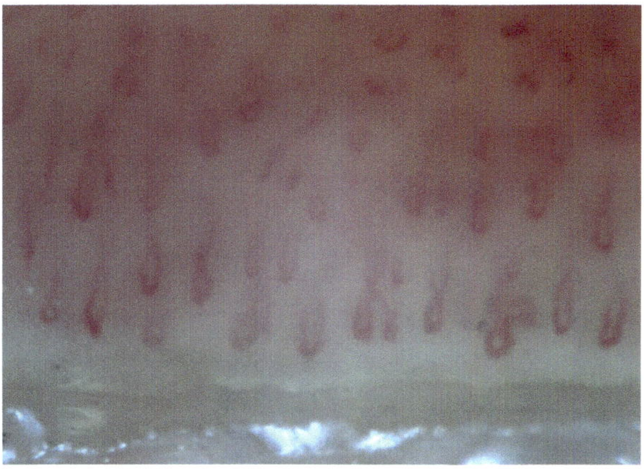

Fig. 15.34 Unremarkable nailfold capillaroscopy image at the first presentation in the rheumatology department

receptor blocker, as well as amlodipine, a calcium channel blocker, were added to the existing regimen with apixaban and aspirin. Furthermore, occupational hand therapy was initiated, and digital botulinum toxin injections were conducted by hand surgeons, with subsequent healing of the digital ulcers.

Follow-up capillaroscopy one year later showed again unspecific changes with moderately frequent dilated capillaries, otherwise still unremarkable. Due to these

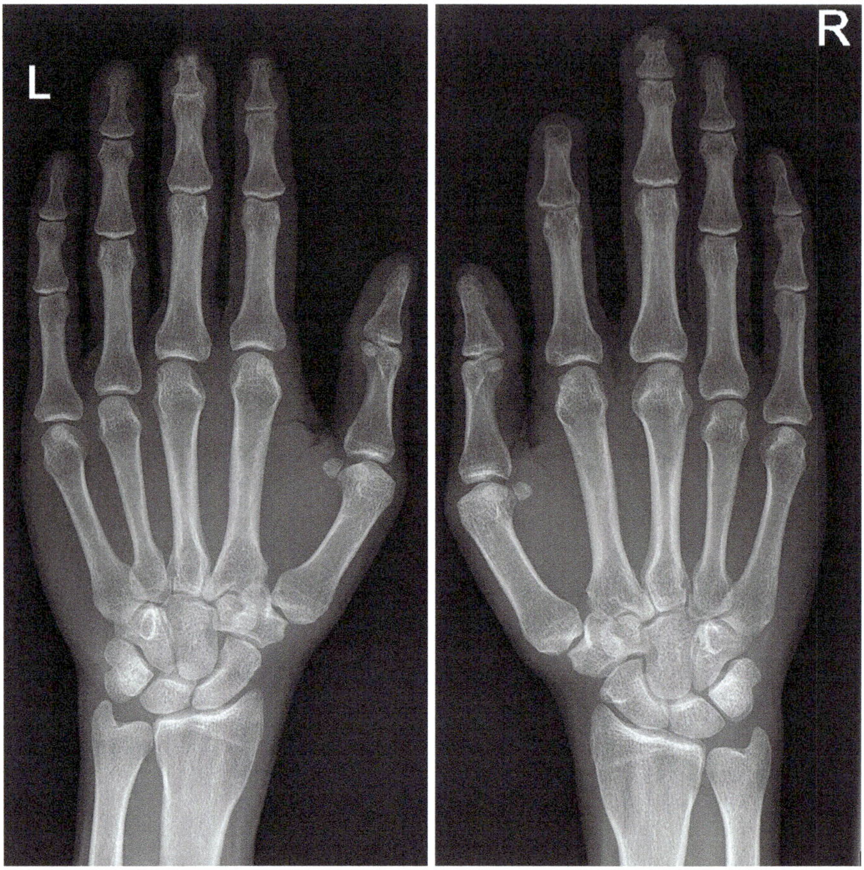

Fig. 15.35 Hand X-ray examination at the first presentation in the rheumatology department, showing apical resorption of the distal phalanx of both middle fingers. The distal phalanx of the right index finger is missing due to surgical amputation

Fig. 15.36 Most recent nailfold capillaroscopy, showing frequent apical dilatation of capillaries, with some reaching the dimension of giant dilatation (>50 μm)

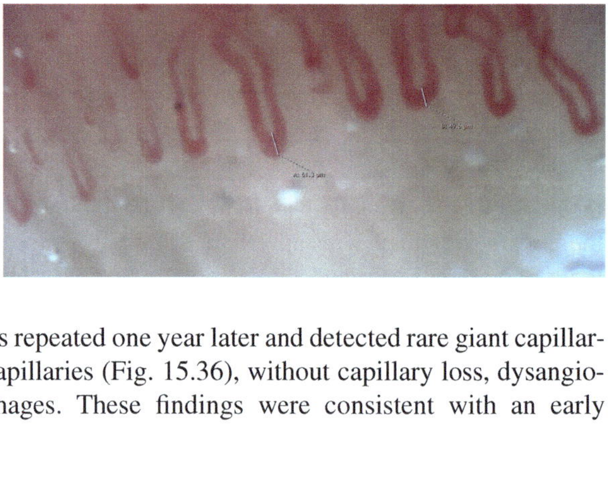

changes, capillaroscopy was repeated one year later and detected rare giant capillaries, in addition to dilated capillaries (Fig. 15.36), without capillary loss, dysangiogenesis, or microhaemorrhages. These findings were consistent with an early scleroderma pattern, which, together with the clinical picture of severe Raynaud's phenomenon, recurrent digital ischemia with fingertip ulcers and pitting scars, acro-osteolysis on hand X-ray examination, and positive ANA with AC-4 pattern, led to the diagnosis of systemic sclerosis *sine scleroderma*. In retrospect, the changes in the heart MRI with diffuse mild myocardial fibrosis might be associated with this condition.

Discussion

This case report highlights the importance of nailfold capillaroscopy in the diagnosis of SSc. As shown, it can be the last piece of the puzzle necessary for making a diagnosis, which also has strong implications for further treatment and prognosis. Since SSc is a disease with frequent and possibly life-limiting internal organ involvement, regular organ screening has a positive effect on survival and prognosis, especially in patients with the diffuse cutaneous subset [54]. However, also in limited cutaneous subtypes (such as this patient), one should think of pulmonary hypertension, developing in about 10% of all patients with SSc [55], and consider regularly screening for it using the help of the DETECT algorithm [56].

Highly particular in this case is the preexisting Gitelman's disease, complicated by chronic kidney disease and CPPD arthropathy. To our best knowledge, there are no similar cases published so far. The only associations of Gitelman's disease (GD) with systemic autoimmune rheumatic disease (SARD) were a few cases in whom Gitelman's syndrome occurred years later after the onset of SSc [57, 58]; the patients had no family history of GD and were negative on genetic testing, suggesting the possibility of "acquired GD." In our case, GD preceded the severe vasculopathy by almost two decades, and we could not find any risk factor attributable to GD or to its complications for developing SSc. Moreover, arterial calcifications were not detectable upon X-ray, so the long-standing, occlusive peripheral vasculopathy of these patients can hardly be attributed to medial arterial calcification (see Fig. 15.35). On the other hand, occlusion of the distal radial or ulnar artery in SSc is not infrequent, the latter being detectable by duplex arterial sonography in up to 37% of consecutive patients enrolled in a French cohort study [59].

Learning Points

This case powerfully demonstrates how capillaroscopy findings can make a difference in the recognition of SSc by representing an important piece of the diagnostic puzzle of this rare condition. Furthermore, this case shows how follow-up nailfold capillaroscopy examinations can be important, since capillaroscopy patterns can change and get more severe over time.

Acknowledgment The patient provided written informed consent for the use of his clinical data and images for teaching and research purposes. We express our sincere gratitude.

Case 11: A Vascular Clue to a Silent Disease: Capillaroscopy in Sine Scleroderma

Rahma A. Elziaty and Hanan Ewais
Internal Medicine Department, Rheumatology Division, Faculty of Medicine, Ain Shams University, Cairo, Egypt

Yasser El Miedany
Canterbury Christ Church University, Canterbury, UK

Rheumatology and Rehabilitation, Ain Shams University, Cairo, Egypt

King's College, London, UK

A 45-year-old female with no significant past medical history presented with *a 4-month history of Raynaud's phenomenon*, characterized by triphasic color changes in her fingers upon cold exposure. She denied any skin thickening, joint pain, or photosensitivity.

Over the subsequent months, she developed mild exertional dyspnea without cough or chest pain. On examination, skin texture was normal, with no evidence of digital ulcers or telangiectasia (Fig. 15.37).

Given the new-onset Raynaud's and respiratory symptoms, nailfold capillaroscopy was performed and demonstrated an *early scleroderma pattern* characterized by giant capillaries, mild architectural disorganization, and occasional microhemorrhages. No avascular areas were observed (Fig. 15.38).

Autoimmune serology revealed: ANA: Positive (1:320, speckled pattern), *Anti-centromere antibodies*: *Positive*, Anti-Scl-70 and anti-RNP: Negative, and Complement (C3, C4): Normal

Pulmonary function tests showed a reduced diffusing capacity for carbon monoxide (DLCO). High-resolution CT (HRCT) of the chest demonstrated *early interstitial lung disease (ILD)* with ground-glass opacities. Echocardiography revealed normal cardiac structure and function with normal pulmonary arterial pressure (PAP: 15 mmHg).

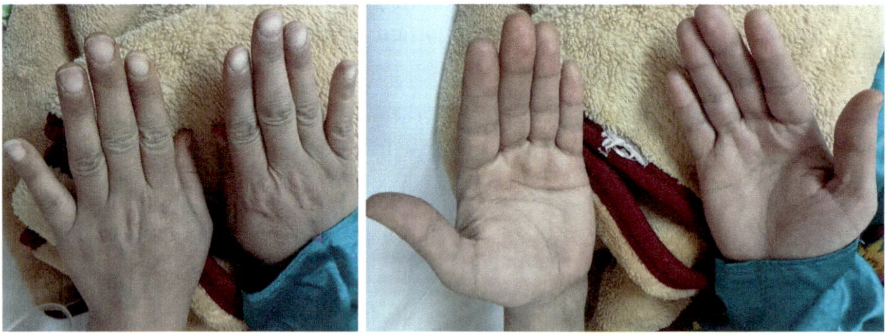

Fig. 15.37 The hands of the patient reveal Raynaud's phenomenon but no skin tightness or puffy fingers

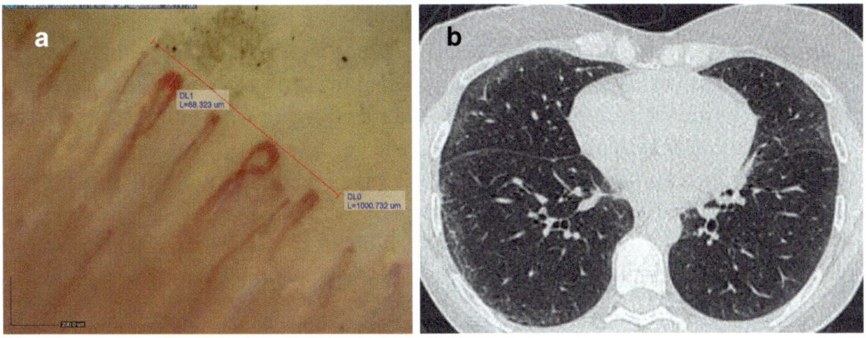

Fig. 15.38 (**a**) NFC reveals an early scleroderma pattern "normal capillary density, presence of giant capillary and microhemorrhages." (**b**) Ground-glass opacities in the HRCT chest

Apart from Raynaud's phenomenon, *no cutaneous involvement* was detected on serial follow-up examinations. A diagnosis of *systemic sclerosis sine scleroderma* was established.

The patient was started on *mycophenolate mofetil (2 g/day)* and *oral prednisolone (10 mg/day)* for ILD, along with *calcium channel blockers* for Raynaud's phenomenon. She also received *proton pump inhibitors, calcium, and vitamin D supplementation.*

After 3 months, *prednisolone was tapered to 7.5 mg/day, with improvement in respiratory symptoms and DLCO results* and a *stationary course on high-resolution chest CT (HRCT).*

During follow-up, she demonstrated *marked improvement in both respiratory symptoms and Raynaud's attacks* under *close clinical and functional monitoring*, with *plans to gradually withdraw corticosteroids as soon as clinical stabilization is maintained.*

Discussion

Systemic sclerosis sine scleroderma accounts for up to 10% of all SSc cases and is characterized by the absence of cutaneous manifestations, despite the presence of Raynaud's phenomenon, positive SSc-specific autoantibodies, and visceral organ involvement such as interstitial lung disease or pulmonary hypertension [60, 61].

This case illustrates the central role of capillaroscopy in detecting early microvascular abnormalities in the absence of skin fibrosis. The early scleroderma pattern on capillaroscopy—particularly the presence of giant capillaries—supported the hypothesis of a systemic autoimmune process [62].

In systemic sclerosis sine scleroderma, early identification is vital because internal organ involvement may progress silently. ILD is a major cause of morbidity and mortality in SSc, and its early detection—using HRCT and PFTs—is crucial [61]. This patient's subtle pulmonary findings, confirmed by imaging and physiology, were consistent with early ILD, justifying early immunosuppression with mycophenolate, a treatment supported by randomized clinical trials [63].

Early recognition and treatment may improve long-term outcomes, delay disease progression, and reduce morbidity in sine scleroderma patients.

Learning Points

- In patients with positive serology and ILD but no skin changes, capillaroscopy findings may be the first clue toward diagnosis of early systemic sclerosis, including sine scleroderma; guiding further investigations, confirming diagnosis, and initiating timely treatment is invaluable
- Early immunosuppressive therapy (e.g., mycophenolate mofetil) can prevent progression of ILD and improve prognosis.
- Rheumatologists should maintain a high index of suspicion for sine scleroderma in Raynaud's patients with abnormal capillaroscopy and systemic symptoms.

Case 12: Capillaroscopic Evidence of Vascular Repair Following Autologous HSCT in Diffuse Systemic Sclerosis

Cristiana Sieiro Santos
Center for Musculoskeletal Research, School of Biological Sciences, Faculty of Biology, Medicine and Health, University of Manchester, Manchester, UK

A 42-year-old man was diagnosed with diffuse cutaneous systemic sclerosis (dcSSc) after a history of Raynaud's phenomenon of less than one year and inflammatory arthralgia. Over the next 6 months, his disease evolved aggressively. He developed progressive skin tightening involving the hands, forearms, and chest, together with active polyarthritis predominantly affecting the wrists and knees. He reported worsening exertional dyspnea to the extent that climbing a single flight of stairs became difficult and intermittent palpitations. Subcutaneous calcinosis emerged over the elbows and fingertips, at times discharging chalky material. During this period, he experienced an unintentional weight loss of 8 kg, associated with anorexia and profound fatigue. He also developed proximal muscle weakness, struggling to rise from a chair or lift objects overhead [64–69].

Clinical Examination

On examination, the patient exhibited diffuse cutaneous sclerosis with a modified Rodnan skin score (mRSS) of 28/51, indicating extensive skin involvement. The skin was taut and adherent over the arms and trunk. Subcutaneous calcinosis nodules were palpable over the olecranon and extensor surfaces of the fingers. The hands demonstrated sclerodactyly with fixed flexion contractures. The small joints of the wrists and knees were swollen and tender, accompanied by tendon friction rubs. Neuromuscular assessment revealed mild-to-moderate proximal weakness. Cardiac auscultation was regular but notable for a pericardial rub, while pulmonary examination disclosed bibasilar crackles.

Investigations

Serology showed a strongly positive antinuclear antibody (ANA, 1:1280 speckled) and positivity for PM-Scl100 and PM-Scl75 antibodies. Muscle enzymes were elevated (creatine kinase 950 U/L). Pulmonary function tests (PFTs) showed a restrictive pattern with a moderate decrease in DLCO of 45%. High-resolution CT (HRCT) revealed fibrosing interstitial lung disease with a basal nonspecific interstitial (NSIP) pattern, involving >20% of the parenchyma. Echocardiography demonstrated a mild pericardial effusion with preserved left ventricular function and no evidence of pulmonary hypertension.

Crucially, nailfold capillaroscopy (NFC) revealed a late scleroderma pattern. There were large avascular areas with severe capillary dropout (<3 capillaries per mm). The remaining loops were often ramified ("bushy") and irregular, reflecting disorganized angiogenesis. Giant capillaries and hemorrhages were scarce.

Diagnosis and Initial Management

The constellation of findings confirmed rapidly progressive dcSSc with multiorgan involvement. Over two years, he received multiple immunosuppressive therapies, including methotrexate (MTX), mycophenolate mofetil (MMF), rituximab (RTX), tocilizumab (TCZ), tofacitinib, and intravenous immunoglobulins (IVIg). Despite this extensive treatment history, his disease remained refractory: skin thickening progressed (mRSS from 20 to 28), lung function declined (DLCO from 50% to 40%), and both muscle weakness and arthritis persisted.

Given the rapid progression, organ-threatening disease, and lack of response to conventional immunosuppression, autologous hematopoietic stem cell transplantation (AHSCT) was considered. In line with international recommendations, he met the criteria for AHSCT in systemic sclerosis. Following comprehensive counseling regarding risks and benefits, the patient underwent transplantation (Table 15.1).

Treatment and Follow-Up After AHSCT

At follow-up between 6 and 12 months posttransplant, the patient showed striking multisystem improvement. He regained 6 kg in weight (from 69 to 75 kg), with restoration of appetite and energy. Dyspnea improved substantially, with PFTs

Table 15.1 Clinical, functional, and capillaroscopic findings before and after autologous HSCT

Domain	Before HSCT	After HSCT (6–12 months)
mRSS	22	18
Weight/Nutrition	69 kg (−10 kg vs. baseline, anorexia, asthenia)	75 kg (+6 kg, improved appetite and energy)
Pulmonary function tests	FVC 61%, DLCO 45%	FVC 68%, DLCO 54% (functional improvement)
HRCT	Fibrotic NSIP with ≥20% involvement	Fibrotic NSIP with <20% involvement
Cardiac	Symptomatic ventricular extrasystoles	Symptoms improved, no new dysfunction
Muscle involvement	Proximal weakness, MMT-8 = 76/150	Muscle enzymes normalized (CK, aldolase), MMT-8 110/150
Articular involvement	Active polyarthritis	Persistent activity (no major change)
Nailfold capillaroscopy (NFC)	Late SSc pattern: giant capillaries, frequent hemorrhages, reduced density, early avascular areas	Early SSc pattern: Normal capillary density, no avascular areas, few hemorrhages

showing FVC 68% and DLCO 54%, and HRCT demonstrated regression of fibrotic NSIP (<20% involvement). Skin thickening softened with the mRSS decreasing to 18. Muscle strength stabilized, with normalization of CK and aldolase and an improvement in the MMT-8 score. Arthritis and calcinosis persisted, remaining the only domains with limited response.

Most remarkable was the evolution of NFC. Repeated examination demonstrated a clear transition from a late pattern to an active pattern, characterized by restoration of capillary density, disappearance of avascular areas, and scattered hemorrhages. This transformation reflected vascular repair and neovascularization following immune reconstitution, providing a direct visual correlate of his systemic improvement.

Discussion

This case involves a patient with rapidly progressive, treatment-refractory diffuse cutaneous systemic sclerosis (dcSSc). The patient had severe multisystem involvement, including interstitial lung disease, cardiac manifestations, inflammatory myopathy, arthritis, and advanced microangiopathy evident on nailfold capillaroscopy (NFC). Despite multiple immunosuppressive treatments, the disease continued to worsen, underscoring the poor prognosis associated with aggressive dcSSc and high-risk features.

Autologous hematopoietic stem cell transplantation (AHSCT) was pursued as a rescue therapy for this high-risk SSc. In recent years, AHSCT has emerged as the most effective disease-modifying treatment for selected patients with severe SSc. Randomized trials (ASSIST, ASTIS, and SCOT) have consistently demonstrated that AHSCT leads to better outcomes than cyclophosphamide, including improvement in skin fibrosis, stabilization of pulmonary function, and superior event-free survivalfrontiersin.org. The therapeutic mechanism of AHSCT is thought to involve an immune "reset," wherein intensive immunoablation eliminates autoreactive immune clones and allows reconstitution of a new, self-tolerant immune systemfrontiersin.org. In essence, AHSCT can halt the autoimmune-driven fibrotic process and alter the natural history of aggressive SSc.

A striking feature of this case was the evolution of the nailfold capillaroscopy findings after AHSCT. At baseline, the patient's NFC showed a late scleroderma pattern, characterized by severe capillary loss and avascular areas (a finding associated with worse outcomes, including higher mortality). Following AHSCT and immune reconstitution, the capillaroscopic pattern transitioned markedly to an active scleroderma pattern. On follow-up NFC, there was restoration of capillary density, disappearance of avascular fields, and the reappearance of giant capillaries with microhemorrhages. This dramatic "reverse remodeling" provides visual evidence of vascular repair and new microangiogenesis after transplant. Notably, such capillaroscopic improvements have been reported in previous studies as well. For example, Miniati et al. observed that patients undergoing AHSCT showed a shift from a late to an active capillaroscopy pattern within months, whereas those on conventional cyclophosphamide therapy had no change. These observations support the concept that intensive immune ablation can foster microvascular regeneration in SSc (Fig. 15.39).

Importantly, the patient's systemic improvements after transplant paralleled the capillaroscopic changes. Pulmonary function stabilized (and even improved), skin

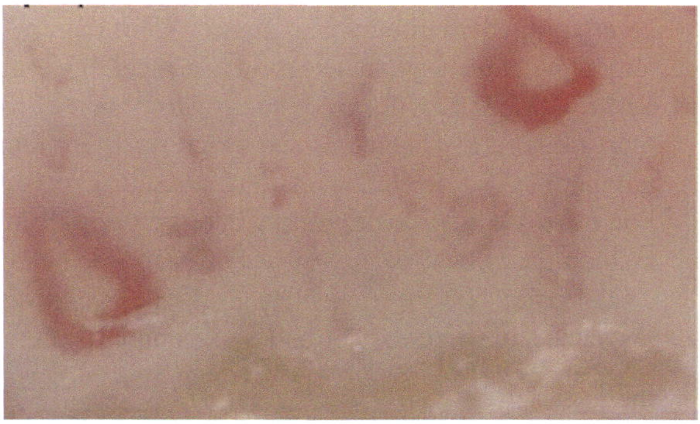

Fig. 15.39 Nailfold capillaroscopy before autologous HSCT in systemic sclerosis
Late scleroderma pattern with marked capillary dropout, avascular areas, and a few giant/ramified capillaries, consistent with advanced microangiopathy

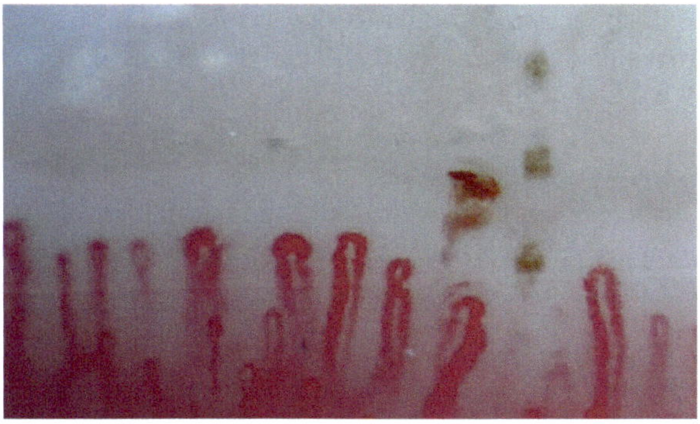

Fig. 15.40 Nailfold capillaroscopy after autologous HSCT in systemic sclerosis
Capillaroscopic image of the periungual area demonstrating an *active pattern* following HSCT. Compared with baseline, *giant capillaries* and *microhemorrhages*, together with a *reduction in avascular areas and partial restoration of capillary density* compared with baseline

thickening regressed, and the patient's overall nutritional status and performance improved in concert with the microvascular repair observed on NFC. This suggests that nailfold capillaroscopy may serve not only as a diagnostic and prognostic tool, but also as a dynamic biomarker of treatment response. Serial NFC examinations provided a noninvasive window into the ongoing vascular recovery in this patient, complementing clinical and imaging assessments. In fact, capillaroscopic analysis has been noted to correlate with disease activity and can help evaluate response to therapy in SSc. Nevertheless, it is worth noting that not all disease manifestations responded equally in this case—for instance, the patient's arthritis (articular involvement) persisted despite transplant. This highlights that organ-specific responses to AHSCT can vary, and some disease domains (e.g., chronic joint damage or inflammation) may be less reversible than skin or vascular changes (Fig. 15.40).

Key Messages

- *AHSCT can profoundly alter the course of severe dcSSc*: Even in rapidly progressive, refractory cases, autologous stem cell transplant can stabilize or improve major organ involvement and skin fibrosis, improving long-term outcomes compared to standard immunosuppression. This therapy offers hope in high-risk SSc, although careful patient selection is critical due to the procedure's risks.

- *Serial nailfold capillaroscopy is a valuable tool for monitoring SSc*: NFC not only aids in early diagnosis and prognosis of systemic sclerosis, but in this case, it dynamically reflected the patient's vascular recovery after AHSCT. The transition from a late (poor prognosis) capillaroscopic pattern to an active pattern with increased capillary density provided real-time evidence of microvascular repair. Thus, serial NFC exams offer a unique, noninvasive window into treatment response and vascular health in SSc, complementing functional and radiographic assessments.

Questions

- After AHSCT, the nailfold capillaroscopy evolved to an active pattern. What does this transition suggest about the potential for *vascular repair* in systemic sclerosis?
- How can *serial NFC examinations* complement pulmonary function tests and imaging in monitoring treatment response in SSc?
- Could *NFC changes* serve as a surrogate endpoint in clinical trials for systemic sclerosis therapies, particularly those targeting vascular and immune repair?

Case 13: Rapidly Progressive Paraneoplastic Systemic Sclerosis in a Patient with Breast Cancer: A Capillaroscopy-Guided Diagnosis

Rahma A. Elziaty and Merna M. Sidky
Internal Medicine Department, Rheumatology Division, Faculty of Medicine, Ain Shams University, Cairo, Egypt

A 38-year-old woman with a history of left-sided breast cancer, treated with mastectomy and hormonal therapy three years prior, presented to dermatology with a progressively enlarging, firm mass in the scalp (Fig. 15.41). Initially presumed to be a dermatologic lesion, empirical treatments failed to yield improvement. A skin biopsy revealed *calcinosis cutis*, raising suspicion for an underlying connective tissue disorder.

To exclude metastatic recurrence, a PET scan was performed, which was negative for malignancy. Six months later, she developed Raynaud's phenomenon, characterized by digital pallor and cyanosis upon cold exposure. She was referred to rheumatology for further evaluation.

Nailfold capillaroscopy at the initial rheumatologic visit showed an *early scleroderma pattern*: the presence of a few giant capillaries, mild hemorrhages, and slightly disorganized architecture (Fig. 15.42). Autoimmune serologies were positive for ANA 1/160 "speckled pattern" anti-centromere antibodies, with negative

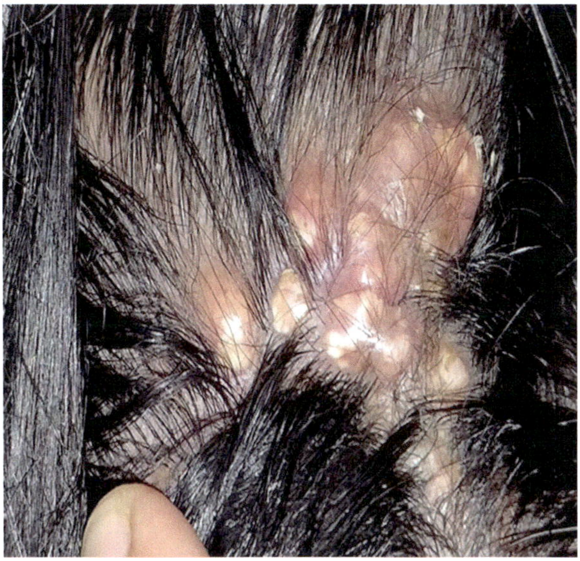

Fig. 15.41 Calcinosis cutis of the scalp

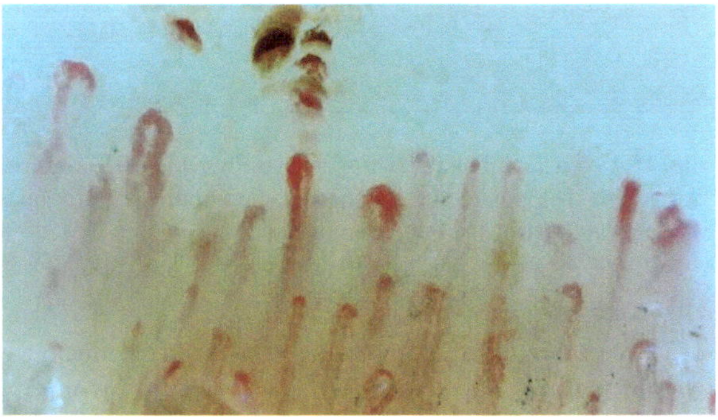

Fig. 15.42 NFC reveals an early scleroderma pattern: normal capillary density, presence of giant capillaries, and microhemorrhages

anti-Scl-70. She was started on methotrexate 15 mg/week for early systemic sclerosis.

Six months later, she returned with progressive exertional dyspnea and a dry cough. Chest high-resolution computed tomography (HRCT) findings are consistent with *severe ILD*. Repeat nailfold capillaroscopy demonstrated an *active scleroderma pattern*, including increased frequency of capillary hemorrhages, architectural disarray, and emerging avascular areas—indicative of capillary destruction and systemic progression (Fig. 15.43).

Given the rapid clinical progression, internal organ involvement, and her oncologic history, she was diagnosed with *paraneoplastic systemic sclerosis*. Methotrexate was discontinued and replaced with mycophenolate mofetil 2 g/day to manage ILD and vasculopathy. The patient was closely followed by both oncology and rheumatology teams.

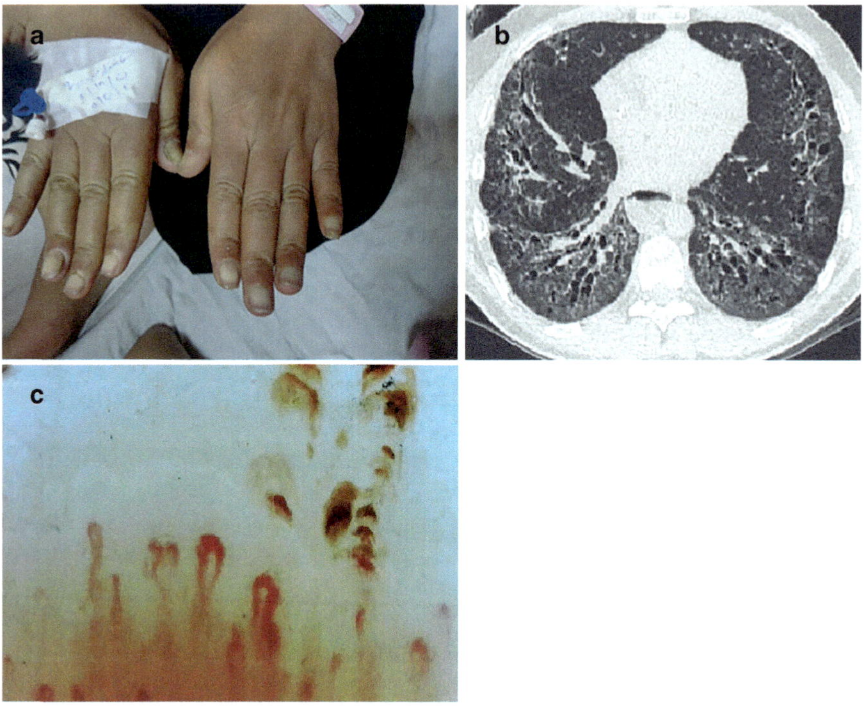

Fig. 15.43 (**a**) Swollen puffy fingers and Raynaud's. (**b**) Severe interstitial lung disease with honeycombing. (**c**) NFC reveals an active scleroderma pattern: decreased capillary density, presence of giant capillaries, and microhemorrhages

Discussion

This case exemplifies a paraneoplastic presentation of systemic sclerosis, where classic features developed in close temporal proximity to a history of malignancy. Paraneoplastic SSc is believed to be driven by tumor-induced immune dysregulation, potentially through cross-reactive antigen expression or cytokine overproduction [70, 71].

Calcinosis cutis was the initial clue, preceding the more classic features of SSc, such as Raynaud's phenomenon and interstitial lung disease. While calcinosis is more common in limited cutaneous SSc, its early presentation in this patient without initial skin thickening raises suspicion of an atypical or aggressive disease variant.

Nailfold capillaroscopy was central to the diagnostic process. It not only identified the scleroderma-spectrum vascular changes but also allowed monitoring of disease progression. Transitioning from an early to an active capillaroscopic pattern paralleled the evolution of internal organ involvement, notably ILD—a known determinant of morbidity and mortality in SSc [72].

The paraneoplastic form of SSc is often associated with a more rapid disease course than idiopathic forms and may present with atypical features. It was noted that patients with paraneoplastic SSc tend to be older, have fewer autoantibodies, and show more aggressive organ involvement [73].

Immunosuppressive therapy is often needed, though careful coordination with oncologic management is essential to balance cancer recurrence risks. Mycophenolate mofetil is now a preferred agent for SSc-related ILD due to its efficacy and tolerability, as shown in trials such as SLS II [74].

Learning Points

- *Paraneoplastic systemic sclerosis* should be considered in patients with recent or remote breast or gynecologic malignancies who present with rapidly evolving SSc features.
- Rapid transition from Raynaud's phenomenon to interstitial lung disease suggests a more aggressive disease course, as seen in paraneoplastic variants.
- *Calcinosis cutis* can be an early feature and should prompt investigation for autoimmune connective tissue diseases.
- Nailfold capillaroscopy is valuable not only for diagnosing early systemic sclerosis but also for monitoring vascular progression.
- Mycophenolate mofetil is an effective and well-tolerated treatment for SSc-ILD, particularly suitable for patients with prior hormonal therapy.

Scleroderma Mimickers Cases

Case 14: A Case of Hydroxyurea-Induced Sclerodermiform Dermatitis with Scleroderma-Like Vasculopathy on nailfold capillaroscopy

Houssem Abida and Nadia ben Abdelhafidh
Faculty of Medicine of Tunis, Tunis El Manar University, Tunis, Tunisia

Internal Medicine and Clinical Immunology Department, Principal Military Hospital of Tunis, Tunis, Tunisia

Hela Ghedira, Amine Ben Moussa, and Fathi Msadak
Faculty of Medicine of Tunis, Tunis El Manar University, Tunis, Tunisia

Clinical Hematology Department, Principal Military Hospital of Tunis, Tunis, Tunisia

Nour El Houda Gueddiche and Faida Ajili
Faculty of Medicine of Tunis, Tunis El Manar University, Tunis, Tunisia

Internal Medicine and Clinical Immunology Department, Principal Military Hospital of Tunis, Tunis, Tunisia

Research Unit for Autoimmune Diseases UR17DNO2, Principal Military Hospital of Tunis, Tunis, Tunisia

A 52-year-old woman with a medical history of uterine fibroma and arterial hypertension was referred to the hematology department for a two-year history of thrombocytosis with chronic headaches and diffuse paresthesia.

Physical examination was unremarkable. Cardiovascular auscultation was normal. No hepatomegaly or splenomegaly was found. Skin, articular, and neurological examinations were normal.

Laboratory investigations revealed a high platelet count of 1237×10^9/L. The remaining hematologic parameters and peripheral blood smear were normal. Inflammatory markers, including ferritin, C-reactive protein (CRP), serum protein electrophoresis, and erythrocyte sedimentation rate (ESR), were within normal ranges. Renal and hepatic function tests were normal. Molecular testing ruled out BCR-ABL transcript and JAK2-V617F mutation. Bone marrow biopsy demonstrated a hypercellular and hyperplastic marrow with multiple clusters of morphologically normal or slightly dysplastic megakaryocytes.

According to the 2016 WHO criteria, essential thrombocythemia without myelofibrosis was retained as a diagnosis. Treatment was initiated with aspirin (100 mg/day) and hydroxyurea (1000 mg/day), later increased to 1500 mg/day because of persistent thrombocytosis. After three years of follow-up, platelet counts remained high at 600×10^9/L. The hydroxyurea dose was therefore increased to 1500–2000 mg/day on alternate days, leading to significant improvement, with a reduction in platelet count to below 400×10^9/L.

One year after the last dose increase, the patient started noticing erythromelalgia and progressive thickening of the skin on her hands. She denied shortness of breath, dry cough, arthralgia, dysphagia, or acid reflux symptoms. She also denied any finger color changes suggestive of Raynaud Phenomenon (RP).

On examination, she had puffy fingers on both hands without digital ulcers or sclerodactyly, along with hyperpigmented, finely squamous plaques approximately 2 cm in diameter around the fingers. Besides, she had black longitudinal nail striae, palmoplantar keratoderma, and diffuse xerosis (Fig. 15.44a). She also had some telangiectasia on her face. The rest of the cutaneous examination was normal. Cardiopulmonary auscultation and muscle strength were normal. There was no evidence of active peripheral joint synovitis.

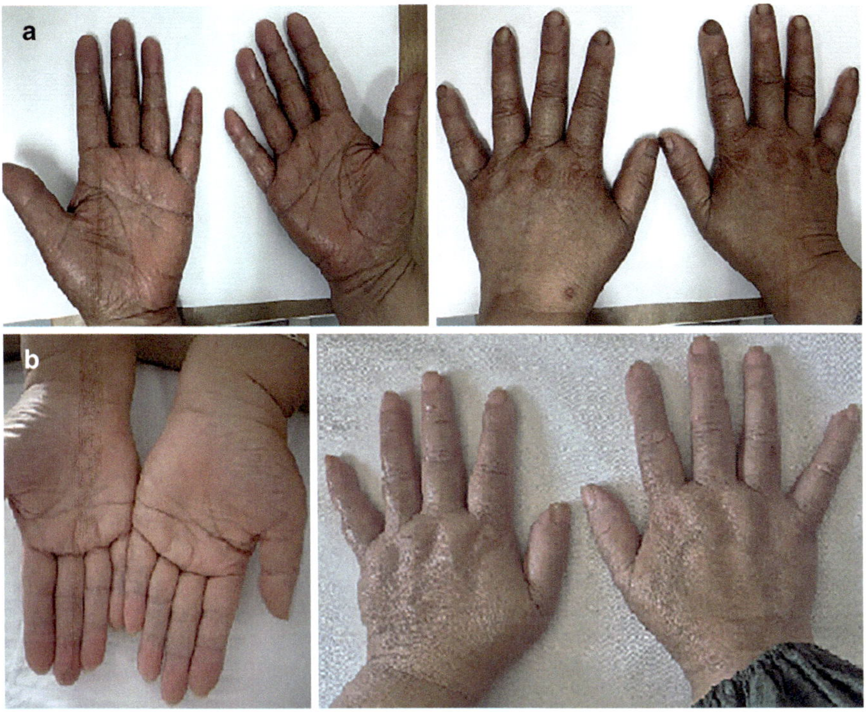

Fig. 15.44 (**a**) Patient's hands after a year with a high-dose hydroxyurea regimen: Puffy fingers with pigmentation abnormalities. (**b**) Patient's hand after 2 years of hydroxyurea withdrawal: resolution of puffy fingers and pigmentation abnormalities

Hematologic markers were normal on repeated blood counts. Inflammatory markers were negative, and the rest of the biological tests were normal (Fig. 15.44).

Q1: What would you expect the nailfold capillaroscopy to show?
Nailfold capillaroscopy (NFC) revealed a scleroderma-like pattern with decreased capillary density, giant and widened capillaries, multiple microhemorrhages, and diffuse edema (Fig. 15.45a).

Skin biopsy showed focal epidermal atrophy with hyperkeratosis, dermal fibrosis with thick collagen bundles, reduced capillary lumina, and absence of inflammatory infiltrates, consistent with scleroderma-like changes.

Chest computed tomography excluded interstitial lung disease, and cardiac ultrasound showed no evidence of pulmonary arterial hypertension. Gastrointestinal endoscopy revealed antral gastritis with a prepyloric ulcer, likely related to aspirin use. Antinuclear antibodies (ANA) by indirect immunofluorescence on HEp-2 cells were negative. A second bone marrow biopsy excluded fibrotic transformation.

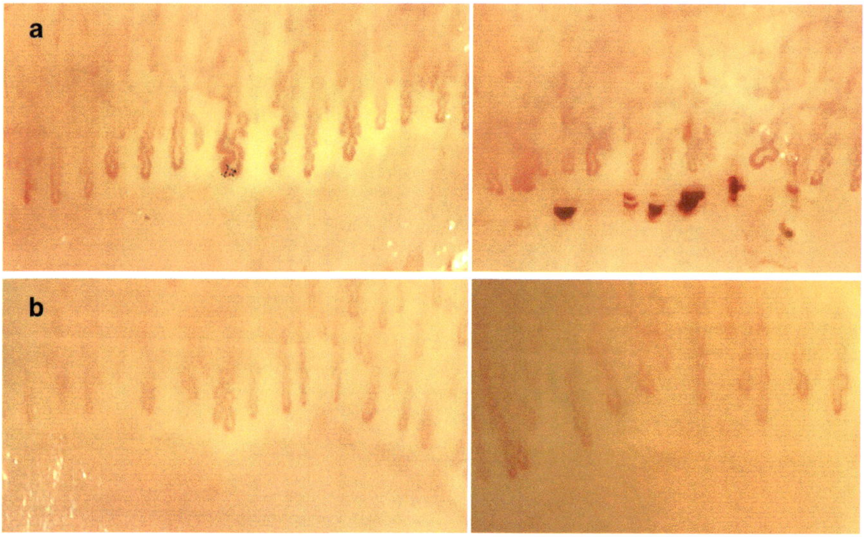

Fig. 15.45 (**a**) Baseline nailfold capillaroscopy with a hydroxyurea high-dose regimen: Giant capillary with multiple widened loops and microhemorrhages. (**b**) Follow-up nailfold capillaroscopy after 2 years of hydroxyurea withdrawal: Resolution of vascular changes apart from a few widened loops

Q2: Would you consider the presentation consistent with a Very Early Diagnosis of Systemic Sclerosis (VEDOSS)?

A diagnosis of drug-induced sclerodermiform dermatitis (SD) was suspected. Hydroxyurea was therefore discontinued.

Q3: What clinical changes would you anticipate after hydroxyurea discontinuation?

Remarkable improvement of erythromelalgia and cutaneous lesions was noted within six weeks of drug withdrawal. Skin thickening and pigmentation abnormalities resolved, and telangiectasia disappeared. Repeated NFC showed improvement of the peripheral vasculopathy. No giant capillaries were found, and only a few widened capillaries remained. She was subsequently started on anagrelide (2 tablets/day) as second-line therapy, achieving a complete hematologic response within three months. After two years of follow-up, the patient remains in sustained clinical and biological remission, with no recurrence of cutaneous (Fig. 15.44b) or vascular (Fig. 15.45b) features.

Discussion

This case illustrates a rare instance of hydroxyurea-induced SD, presenting with both cutaneous and vasculopathic features mimicking systemic sclerosis (SSc). The patient exhibited puffy fingers, fibrotic changes confirmed by histopathology, pigmentation abnormalities, telangiectasia, and scleroderma-related microangiopathy on NFC. Notably, the symptoms appeared following an increase in hydroxyurea dose and resolved within 6 months after drug discontinuation, strongly suggesting causality.

SD is a recognized cutaneous side effect of various chemotherapeutic agents. Skin sclerosis typically occurs on the lower extremities and can occasionally mimic conditions such as Shulman fasciitis [75, 76]. Skin sclerosis severity varies and has been reported to lead to functional impairment in some cases [75]. Additional features such as telangiectasia, calcinosis, and even positivity of ANAs have also been reported [75]. Drugs implicated in inducing such reactions include bleomycin, taxanes, gemcitabine, and, more recently, immune checkpoint inhibitors [75, 76]. Yet, RP, digital ulcers, organ involvement, and vascular changes on NFC are uncommon in this set and are barely reported [75].

Concerning hydroxyurea, and similar to our patient, erythromelalgia has been documented in approximately 6% of patients receiving the drug [76]. Isolated RP is also reported but less frequently than erythromelalgia in this context [77, 78].

Thus said, hydroxyurea-induced SD is barely reported in the literature. To our knowledge, only two cases resembling ours have been documented. The first reported case involved a patient with progressive, pruritic, woody induration symmetrically affecting both legs, which resolved six months after hydroxyurea withdrawal [79]. The second case described sclerodactyly, facial skin fibrosis, microstomia, and buccal fissures. All skin symptoms significantly improved after hydroxyurea withdrawal as well [80]. Apart from SSc-like disease, cases of dermatomyositis-like dermatitis induced by hydroxyurea have also been reported with significant improvement after disease withdrawal [81]. None of the patients reported RP or had organ involvement. No NFC data is available for these patients [81].

Key Learning Points

- Drug-induced scleroderma-like disease should always be considered before concluding a diagnosis of VEDOSS or definite SSc, particularly in the presence of atypical features such as the absence of RP or organ involvement.
- The onset of dose increase and the resolution within 6 months of hydroxyurea discontinuation strongly support a drug-induced mechanism of SC.
- Even though treatment's main goal was met, drug-induced SD onset led to treatment change with switching to second-line therapy with anagrelide.

Case 15: When a Normal Capillaroscopy Completes the Diagnostic Puzzle

Sara Alves Costa, Maria João Cadório, Tânia Santiago, and Maria João Salvador
Rheumathology Department, Coimbra's Local Health Unit, Coimbra, Portugal

A 21-year-old woman presented with a progressive onset of proximal muscle weakness, associated diffuse myalgias, and inflammatory arthralgias affecting the wrists, small joints of the hands, knees, and ankles. She reported prolonged morning stiffness, with progressive difficulty performing activities of daily living. The symptoms had evolved over 8 months and were initially attributed by the patient to the initiation of topical isotretinoin for acne; however, the complaints persisted for more than 6 months following cessation of the medication. She additionally reported recent-onset skin thickening of the forearms, thighs, and legs, with a duration of one month. Systemic review just revealed longstanding fatigue. She denied Raynaud's phenomenon. Her medical history was notable for hypothyroidism, treated with levothyroxine, and acne.

On physical examination, vital signs and cardiopulmonary auscultation were unremarkable, and there were no palpable lymphadenopathies. Diffuse skin thickening was noted, with reduced skin foldability, involving the arms, forearms, legs, and thighs (Fig. 15.46). Hand joints demonstrated limited extension and flexion, without evident sclerodactyly or tendon friction rubs. There was no apparent involvement of the face, trunk, or abdomen. Musculoskeletal examination revealed difficulty performing a full squat, attributed to restricted tendon mobility in the lower limbs. Both elbows had 20° flexion, without overt swelling, and only one knee demonstrated active arthritis, with no other significant musculoskeletal findings.

Question 1 *Given this clinical presentation, which differential diagnoses should be considered?*

The case was characterized by an insidious onset of limb skin thickening, accompanied by myalgias, subjective proximal muscle weakness, and inflammatory arthralgias. The differential diagnosis included connective tissue diseases such as systemic sclerosis, where skin thickening represents a hallmark feature; however, in this patient, Raynaud's phenomenon and sclerodactyly were absent. Mixed connective tissue disease, which can present with arthritis, myopathy, and skin thickening, as well as overlap syndromes, were also considered. Inflammatory myopathies were contemplated due to the presence of proximal weakness and myalgias, although skin thickening is not typically observed in these conditions. Eosinophilic fasciitis was likewise considered, given its characteristic involvement of the subcutaneous tissue and fascia predominantly in the limbs, in the absence of Raynaud's phenomenon or sclerodactyly, often resulting in stiffness and functional limitation. Less common causes, such as drug exposure or radiation, were also taken into account as potential contributors to skin thickening [82].

Question 2 *Which additional diagnostic tests are most useful and would allow us to reach a definitive diagnosis?*

Laboratory investigations revealed peripheral eosinophilia (0.75×10^9/L), microcytic hypochromic anemia (Hb 11.5 g/dL), and thrombocytosis (407×10^9/L). C-reactive protein was elevated (3.26 mg/dL) along with erythrocyte sedimentation rate (49 mm/h). Serum protein electrophoresis demonstrated polyclonal hypergammaglobulinemia. Creatine phosphokinase and aldolase were normal, as was renal function. Autoimmune serology revealed ANA 1:320, homogeneous pattern, and strongly positive anti-cN-1A antibodies, with the remainder of the study negative.

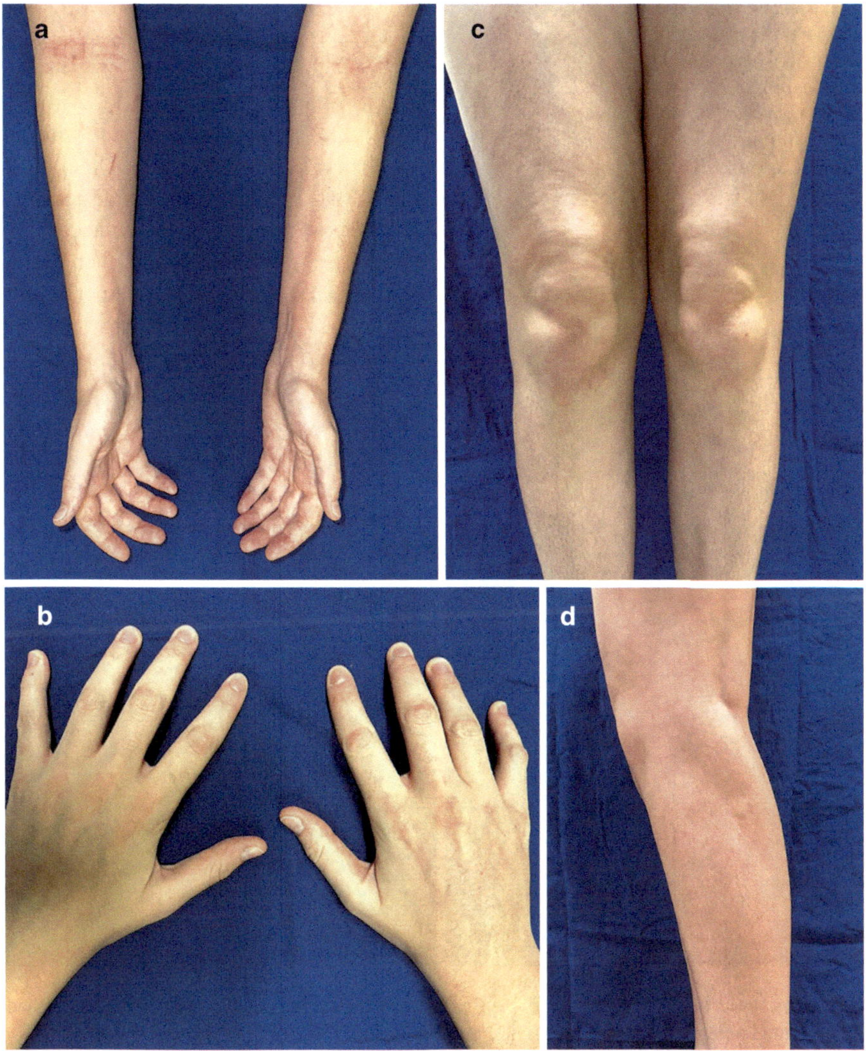

Fig. 15.46 (**a**) Patient's forearms with a shiny appearance due to the skin thickening. (**b**) Patient's hands demonstrating a semi-flexed posture of the fingers. (**c**) Peau d'orange sign and tumefaction of the right knee. (**d**) Skin thickening of the leg

Question 3 *Would capillaroscopy be useful in this case?*

Nailfold videocapillaroscopy demonstrated normal capillary density (≥7 capillaries/mm), dimension (apical diameter <20/tm), and morphology, without microhemorrhages. The screening for systemic sclerosis target organ involvement with pulmonary function tests, high-resolution thoracic computed tomography, and transthoracic echocardiography revealed no abnormalities. Electromyography of the limbs showed no evidence of muscle fiber injury (Fig. 15.47).

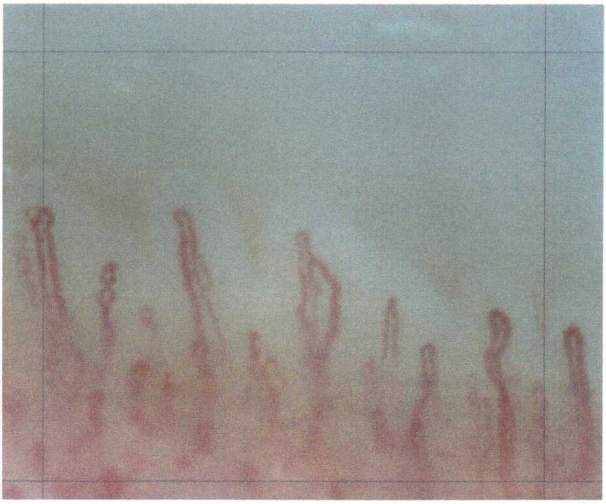

Fig. 15.47 Capillaroscopic image of the patient obtained with a nailfold videocapillaroscope with a 200× magnification in a 1 linear millimeter. (VideoCap 3.0; DS Medica, Italy)

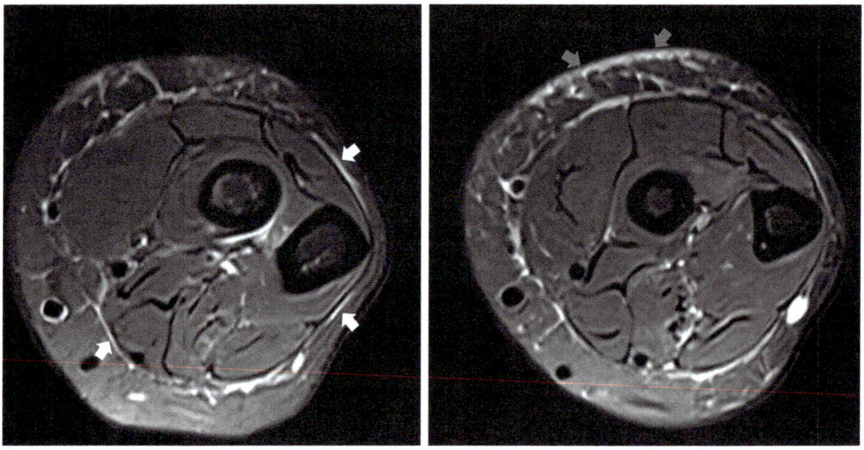

Fig. 15.48 MRI of the forearm demonstrating thickened muscular fascia on axial fat-suppressed T2-weighted images, with increased signal intensity within muscular fascial layers (white arrows) and hyperintensity in the subcutaneous fat and skin (grey arrows)

Question 4 *Given these findings, what is the most likely diagnosis?*

The most likely diagnosis was deemed to be eosinophilic fasciitis, based on diffuse cutaneous and subcutaneous thickening in a young woman with peripheral eosinophilia, elevated acute-phase reactants, and hypergammaglobulinemia, alongside otherwise normal investigations.

Magnetic resonance imaging (MRI) of the left forearm demonstrated moderate diffuse thickening of the muscular fascia across multiple muscle groups, with hyperintensity on contrast-sensitive sequences and relatively homogeneous gadolinium enhancement. Diffuse skin thickening of the proximal forearm and edematous infiltration of subcutaneous fat were also noted (Fig. 15.48).

With the diagnosis of eosinophilic fasciitis established, the patient commenced oral prednisolone (1 mg/kg/day, tapered) and oral methotrexate (10 mg/week). A biopsy of skin, subcutaneous tissue, and fascia from the proximal third of the left forearm was subsequently performed, which later confirmed the clinical diagnosis [83].

After three months of follow-up, the patient demonstrated a favorable response to treatment, with normalization of laboratory parameters and improvement in myalgia and fatigue. Currently she is on prednisolone 20 mg/day and methotrexate 15 mg/week. Physiotherapy was included to aid recovery of mobility.

Discussion

This case highlights the complexity of differential diagnosis in patients presenting with skin thickening and musculoskeletal symptoms. Systemic sclerosis and overlap syndromes with myositis were considered; however, the absence of capillaroscopic abnormalities, negative disease-specific autoantibodies, and lack of visceral involvement made these diagnoses unlikely. Normal muscle enzymes, electromyography, and absence of muscular oedema on MRI further excluded inflammatory myopathy.

Functional limitation was attributable not only to skin thickening but also to involvement of subcutaneous tissue and muscular fascia, impairing joint mobility. The isolated positivity of anti-cN-1A antibodies, typically associated with inclusion body myositis but occasionally found in other systemic autoimmune rheumatic diseases, was interpreted as clinically non-specific in this context [84].

Nailfold videocapillaroscopy was essential to exclude microvascular pathology and reinforce the exclusion of connective tissue disease.

In conclusion, this case demonstrates that eosinophilic fasciitis should be considered in patients with extremities skin thickening and muscular complaints in the absence of Raynaud's phenomenon, with normal capillaroscopy and peripheral eosinophilia. Integration of clinical, laboratory, imaging, and histopathological findings is essential for accurate diagnosis.

Key Learning Points

- Eosinophilic fasciitis should be considered in the differential diagnosis of scleroderma-like diseases.
- A normal nailfold videocapillaroscopy can be a pivotal clue, supporting the exclusion of scleroderma-like diseases.
- MRI plays a crucial role in confirming fascial involvement and in guiding biopsy site selection.

Case 16: Morphea Profunda Mimicking Systemic Sclerosis

Rahma A. Elziaty and Merna M. Sidky
Internal Medicine Department, Rheumatology Division, Faculty of Medicine, Ain Shams University, Cairo, Egypt

Ahmed Nassar
Department of Dermatology, Venereology and Andrology, Faculty of Medicine, Ain Shams University, Cairo, Egypt

A 40-year-old Egyptian man presented to the rheumatology clinic with a 10-month history of Raynaud's phenomenon and slowly progressive skin erythema and swelling of both hands. Over months, the swelling progressed to extensive, symmetrical thickening of the hands, ending in bilateral sclerodactyly. The patient reported an unintended weight loss of 20 kg over 6 months. He denied other systemic features, a family history of similar disease, or preceding cutaneous trauma.

On examination, the hands showed erythematous, indurated plaques with deep-seated thickening and fixed sclerodactyly. No obvious telangiectasia, digital ulcers, or signs of severe internal organ involvement were found (Fig. 15.49).

Laboratory tests: ESR 15 mm/h, CRP 5 mg/L, ANA 1:80 speckled. Tumor markers were negative. CT neck/chest/abdomen–pelvis with contrast, transthoracic echocardiography, and pulmonary function testing were all within normal limits.

Nailfold videocapillaroscopy (NFC) showed a non-scleroderma (normal) pattern: capillary density $\approx$ 8 capillaries/mm, apical loop width <20 μm, no giant capillaries, no abnormal shapes, and no microhemorrhages (Fig. 15.50).

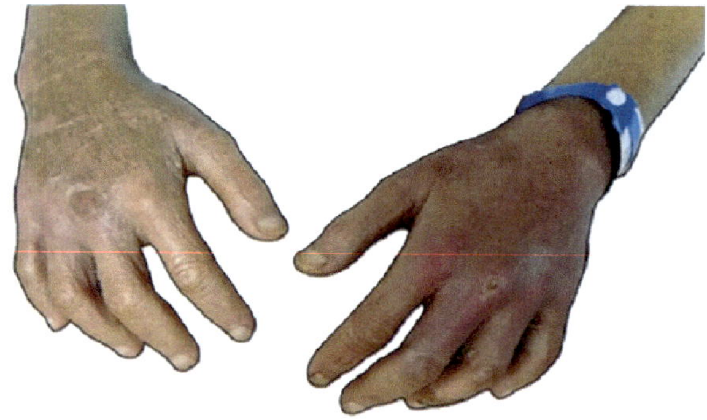

Fig. 15.49 Deep-seated thickening and fixed bilateral sclerodactyly

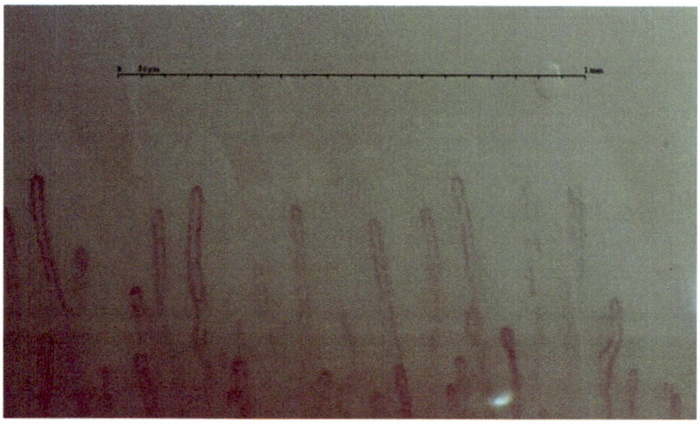

Fig. 15.50 Nailfold capillaroscopy of the case reveals a normal pattern: normal capillary density, no microhemorrhages, or abnormal-shaped capillaries

A full-thickness skin biopsy demonstrated the absence of dermal sclerotic bundles in the superficial and mid-dermis with prominent sclerosis in the deep reticular dermis and subcutaneous tissue, findings interpreted as consistent with morphea profunda (deep morphea).

In collaboration with dermatology, the patient was started on UVA-1 phototherapy combined with mycophenolate mofetil (MMF). The clinical course was stable with no further progression of skin tightness on short-term follow-up.

Discussion

Morphea profunda is an uncommon variant of localized scleroderma characterized by fibrosis extending into the deep reticular dermis, subcutaneous tissue, and occasionally the fascia. Because it may present with progressive skin thickening of the extremities and even sclerodactyly-like changes, it can closely mimic early diffuse cutaneous systemic sclerosis (dcSSc). This overlap creates significant diagnostic challenges, especially when Raynaud's phenomenon is present, as in our patient. Distinguishing deep morphea from SSc is of major importance because their prognoses and therapeutic requirements differ substantially. While systemic sclerosis carries a risk of multiorgan involvement and potential mortality, morphea—regardless of depth—remains confined to the skin and subcutis in nearly all cases [85].

In this case, several key features argued against systemic sclerosis. First, the absence of internal organ involvement on pulmonary function testing, echocardiography, and thoracic imaging strongly suggested a localized rather than systemic fibrosing process. Organ involvement is a defining feature of SSc and typically appears early in dcSSc [86]. Second, nailfold videocapillaroscopy (NFC) revealed a normal (non-scleroderma) pattern with preserved capillary density and no giant capillaries or microhemorrhages. NFC is a validated tool for differentiating SSc from other causes of Raynaud's phenomenon; over 90% of SSc patients demonstrate a characteristic "scleroderma pattern," while morphea patients generally show normal findings [87, 88]. Thus, the microvascular assessment in our case provided strong evidence against SSc despite the presence of Raynaud's.

Histopathological analysis ultimately confirmed the diagnosis. The biopsy demonstrated sclerosis predominantly in the deep dermis and subcutaneous tissue with sparing of the papillary and mid-dermis, a classic pattern for morphea profunda. In contrast, systemic sclerosis is characterized by diffuse dermal sclerosis, loss of adnexal structures, and homogenization of collagen bundles throughout the entire dermis. Deep morphea often requires full-thickness or deep incisional biopsy, as superficial sampling may miss diagnostic changes, leading to misclassification. Prior studies highlight that the depth of sclerosis is a critical discriminator between morphea profunda and SSc, particularly when clinical findings overlap [89, 90].

Management of morphea profunda typically includes phototherapy and/or systemic immunomodulatory therapy, depending on the extent and depth of disease. In this case, the patient improved with a combination of UVA-1 phototherapy and mycophenolate mofetil (MMF). UVA-1 phototherapy has demonstrated benefit in morphea by inducing matrix metalloproteinases and reducing collagen deposition and is considered a first-line therapy for active or inflammatory lesions. MMF has gained increasing support as an effective therapeutic option for extensive or refractory morphea, with observational studies reporting improvement in skin induration and disease activity, particularly in deep variants and in patients who do not respond adequately to methotrexate. The combination used in this case aligns with current expert recommendations favoring individualized therapy guided by disease severity, depth, and functional impairment [91].

This case underscores the importance of a structured diagnostic approach when evaluating patients with sclerotic skin changes affecting the hands. Although sclerodactyly and Raynaud's phenomenon are hallmark features of SSc, their presence does not exclude morphea profunda, which can present with similar features but carries a vastly different prognosis. Integrating NFC, targeted evaluation for systemic involvement, and deep histopathologic examination provides a reliable framework for distinguishing systemic from localized sclerotic disorders. Early recognition prevents unnecessary anxiety, avoids excessive immunosuppression, and ensures timely initiation of appropriate therapy.

Learning Outcome Points

- Morphea profunda (deep morphea) can clinically mimic systemic sclerosis (sclerodactyly, Raynaud's, and progressive skin thickening) but is a localized fibrosing disease confined to skin, subcutis, and sometimes fascia. Histology from a deep biopsy is often required to confirm the diagnosis.
- Nailfold videocapillaroscopy is an important differentiating tool: a scleroderma pattern strongly suggests systemic sclerosis, whereas a normal/non-scleroderma pattern supports localized morphea in the right clinical context. NFC should be used together with organ screening and histopathology.
- Absence of internal organ involvement (normal PFTs, echocardiography, and CT imaging) further supports a localized process and significantly changes prognosis and management compared with SSc.
- Treatment is tailored to depth and extent: phototherapy (UVA-1/PUVA) is useful for many morphea cases; for extensive or deep disease, systemic agents such as mycophenolate mofetil are effective alternatives to methotrexate in refractory cases. Combination dermatology–rheumatology care optimizes outcomes.

Inflammatory Myositis Cases

Case 17: New-Onset Raynaud in a Patient with Refractory Rash: Could Nailfold Capillaroscopy Be the Missing Piece?

Maria João Cadório, Sara Alves Costa, and Tânia Santiago
Rheumathology Department, Coimbra's Local Health Unit, Coimbra, Portugal

João Teixeira
Dermatology Department, Coimbra's Local Health Unit, Coimbra, Portugal

A 38-year-old woman presented to the emergency department with pruriginous erythematous–violaceous cutaneous lesions evolving over 4 months. The eruption began on the face and scalp line and progressively extended to the chest, shoulders, thighs, and dorsal aspects of the hands. She had received multiple topical and systemic treatments without improvement. On systematic questioning, the patient recalled new-onset Raynaud's phenomenon beginning one year earlier, to which she had not considered significant and had not been previously investigated. She also reported asthenia and mild proximal myalgias but denied arthralgia; photosensitivity beyond the rash; dysphagia; dyspnea; fever or weight loss; as well as new medications, statin use, recent infections, or toxic exposures. She had no past medical history, chronic medication, or family history of autoimmune disease.

On physical examination, she presented with erythematous–violaceous plaques with fine scaling, superficial erosions, and poikilodermatous changes involving the face, anterior chest, shoulders, and upper back (photoexposed and seborrheic areas). The periocular region showed a violaceous discoloration with mild edema, consistent with a heliotrope rash. Poikiloderma was evident in "V-sign" and "shawl sign" distributions, and similar lesions were noted on the lateral thighs, consistent with "holster sign," and dorsal hands, consistent with Gottron's papules, accompanied by periungual erythema and cuticular hypertrophy (Fig. 15.51). No skin thickening, sclerodactyly, telangiectasias, digital ulcers, or pitting scars were noted. Muscle examination revealed mild symmetric proximal weakness of the shoulder and hip girdles (Manual Muscle Testing-8 score: 139/150), with preserved distal strength and tendon reflexes.

Given the refractory rash and late-onset Raynaud's phenomenon, the patient was referred for urgent evaluation by rheumatology and dermatology. Nailfold videocapillaroscopy (NVC) revealed a scleroderma-like pattern, with marked capillary rarefaction, giant capillaries, architectural disorganization, and pericapillary microhemorrhages (Fig. 15.52), consistent with a microangiopathic process strongly suggestive of an underlying connective tissue disease, particularly dermatomyositis. Laboratory tests showed elevated muscle enzymes, including creatine kinase (464 U/L; N: <145), lactate dehydrogenase (328 U/L; N <247), aspartate aminotransferase (60 U/L; N: <31), alanine aminotransferase (97 U/L; N: <34), and myoglobin (166 ng/mL; N: 9-82). Complete blood count, serum electrolytes, renal, thyroid, and hepatic function tests (apart from transaminases), and aldolase levels were normal, as were inflammatory markers and complement fractions. Urinalysis showed no evidence of proteinuria or hematuria. Autoimmune serology was negative for antinuclear antibodies (ANA), extractable nuclear antigens (ENA), and anti-double-stranded DNA antibodies. However, given the clinical suspicion of an inflammatory myopathy, a myositis-specific antibody panel was performed, which revealed a moderately positive anti-p155/140 (transcription intermediary factor 1-gamma; TIF1γ) antibody. Electromyography demonstrated a myopathic pattern with acute denervation, most prominent in the iliopsoas muscle, consistent with active muscle fiber injury. Skin biopsy revealed interface dermatitis with vacuolar basal layer changes, scattered keratinocyte apoptosis, and superficial perivascular lymphomononuclear infiltrate with prominent dermal mucin deposition, findings compatible with dermatomyositis.

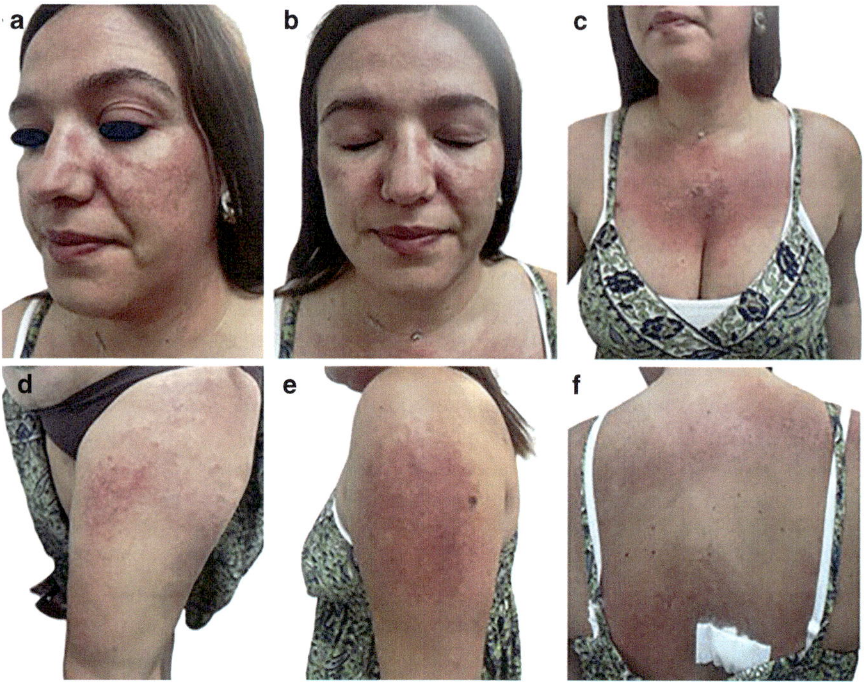

Fig. 15.51 Cutaneous manifestations at presentation. (**a**, **b**) Facial erythematous–violaceous rash involving the malar region and nasolabial fold, forehead, scalp line, and periocular area with subtle edema, consistent with a heliotrope rash. (**c**, **f**) Poikiloderma and erythema of the anterior chest ("V-sign") and upper back ("shawl sign") involving photoexposed areas. (**d**, **e**) Violaceous erythematous plaques on the lateral thighs ("holster sign") and deltoid regions, with fine scaling and early poikilodermatous changes

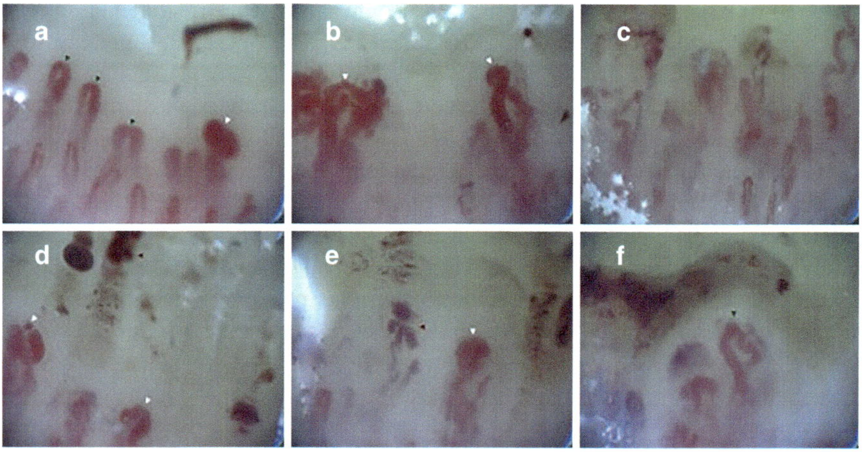

Fig. 15.52 Nailfold videocapillaroscopy obtained with a videocapillaroscopy at ×200 magnification (Videocap, DS Medica, Milan, Italy). Images **a**–**f** show giant capillaries >50 microns (white arrowheads), enlarged capillaries >20 microns (green arrowheads), ramifications, marked reduction in capillary density, and numerous pericapillary microhemorrhages (red arrowheads)

Considering clinical, serological, and skin histopathological findings, the patient was diagnosed with dermatomyositis (DM) and started on prednisolone 1 mg/kg/day plus methotrexate 15 mg weekly, hydroxychloroquine 400 mg/day, and strict photoprotection. She showed progressive improvement in skin lesions and muscle strength, with normalization of muscle enzymes and resolution of pruritus.

Comprehensive systemic assessment, including pulmonary function tests with diffusing capacity for carbon monoxide, high-resolution computed tomography of the lungs, electrocardiogram, and transthoracic echocardiography, revealed no cardiopulmonary involvement. Given anti–TIF1γ antibody positivity, malignancy screening was performed with age-appropriate oncologic surveillance (mammography, pelvic and gynecologic ultrasound, and cytology and HPV testing), and 18-fluorodeoxyglucose positron emission tomography scan, with no evidence of occult malignancy or inflammatory organ involvement.

At 26 months of follow-up, the patient remains clinically stable and asymptomatic under gradual corticosteroid tapering and methotrexate 25 mg weekly.

Questions to Challenge the Reader

1. How can NVC aid in differentiating connective tissue diseases presenting with Raynaud's phenomenon?
2. What specific NVC features help distinguish DM from systemic sclerosis (SSc)?
3. In a patient presenting with a refractory rash and newly developed Raynaud's phenomenon, how can early NVC alter the diagnostic pathway?
4. Can NVC findings correlate with disease activity or internal organ involvement in DM?
5. Can NVC findings correlate with autoantibody profiles in DM?
6. What is the prognostic significance of a scleroderma-like capillaroscopic pattern outside systemic sclerosis?
7. How can a DM patient have a positive anti–TIF1γ antibody while testing negative for ANA?

Discussion

NVC is an invaluable, non-invasive tool for the assessment of microvascular architecture in rheumatic diseases [92]. While it has long been considered a hallmark diagnostic instrument for SS), its application in other connective tissue diseases is increasingly recognized [92–94]. This case highlights the diagnostic value of NVC in DM, where early detection of microangiopathy can be crucial to raise diagnostic suspicion and initiate prompt immunosuppression.

Microangiopathy represents a central pathophysiological mechanism in DM, contributing to both cutaneous ischemia and myofiber necrosis. The capillaroscopic findings in this case, namely marked capillary rarefaction, giant capillaries, and pericapillary microhemorrhages, reflect the same vascular injury observed histologically in DM muscle and skin. These features closely resemble the "scleroderma pattern" described in SSc, characterized by enlarged loops, capillary dropout, and hemorrhages [95–99]. However, subtle distinctions exist: in DM, capillary loss and microhemorrhages are often more pronounced, whereas the neoangiogenic, bushy, or ramified loops typically seen in late SSc stages are less frequent [100]. This underscores a shared vascular pathology but differing patterns of vascular remodeling between the two conditions.

In this patient, NVC provided the first objective clue to systemic disease. The presence of a scleroderma-like pattern in a patient with refractory dermatitis and new-onset Raynaud's phenomenon prompted targeted myositis testing, leading to the identification of anti-TIF1γ-positive DM. Importantly, this serologic subtype is associated with a higher risk of malignancy, justifying comprehensive oncologic screening despite a negative ANA test [101].

The coexistence of a positive anti-TIF1γ antibody with a negative ANA test is not uncommon in DM. Anti-TIF1γ is a myositis-specific antibody directed against a cytoplasmic transcription intermediary factor rather than a nuclear antigen. Standard ANA testing by indirect immunofluorescence (HEp-2 cells) detects antibodies targeting nuclear or nucleolar components and therefore may miss antibodies against cytoplasmic or non-nuclear antigens such as TIF1γ, MDA5, or Jo-1. In addition, low antibody titers or epitope masking can result in false-negative ANA results despite disease-specific autoimmunity, highlighting the importance of extended myositis antibody panels in patients with compatible clinical features, regardless of ANA status [102].

Beyond diagnosis, NVC also has prognostic and monitoring value in DM. Capillary density correlates with disease activity, and serial NVC can track therapeutic response [103, 104]. On the other hand, improvement in capillary density and reduction in microhemorrhages may parallel decreases in muscle enzyme levels and cutaneous inflammation, reflecting microvascular recovery under immunosuppressive therapy [103, 104]. In adult DM, NVC abnormalities have been associated with myositis-specific antibodies including anti-TIF1γ, and more frequent and severe microvascular alterations have been observed in those antibody subgroups [105].

This case therefore reinforces that NVC serves as a window to systemic microangiopathy across connective tissue diseases. When integrated early in clinical evaluation, it can reveal subtle yet decisive evidence of disease activity, guiding both diagnosis and management.

Key Learning Points

- NVC is a powerful diagnostic and monitoring tool that extends beyond systemic sclerosis, offering insights into microvascular injury in diseases such as DM.
- The scleroderma-like capillaroscopic pattern (giant capillaries, microhemorrhages, and avascular areas) can occur in both DM and systemic sclerosis, but DM usually shows more capillary dropout and less neoangiogenesis.
- Capillaroscopic abnormalities in DM reflect disease activity and may improve following immunosuppressive treatment.
- ANA negativity does not exclude autoimmune myopathy; antibodies against cytoplasmic targets such as TIF1γ may be present even with a negative ANA test.
- In patients presenting with refractory rash and Raynaud's phenomenon, early NVC can redirect diagnostic reasoning toward an inflammatory myopathy, leading to earlier diagnosis and improved outcomes.

Case 18: Anti-MDA5-Positive Dermatomyositis with a Scleroderma-Like Capillaroscopic Pattern

Claudia Cobilinschi and Laura-Maria Groşeanu
Department of Rheumatology, "Sf. Maria" Clinical Hospital, Carol Davila University of Medicine and Pharmacy, Bucharest, Romania

This case illustrates the evolving understanding of vasculopathic changes in anti-MDA5-positive dermatomyositis, a subset of idiopathic inflammatory myopathies (IIMs) frequently associated with severe cutaneous and pulmonary involvement. It emphasizes the diagnostic and prognostic value of nailfold capillaroscopy (NFC) in recognizing and following microvascular injury in this challenging disease.

A 54-year-old man with a history of permanent atrial fibrillation, hypercholesterolemia, and benign prostatic hypertrophy was confirmed with dermatomyositis. The onset of the disease was four years earlier, while he was living in Germany, with symmetric ankle swelling and inflammatory-type arthralgias affecting the metacarpophalangeal and shoulder joints. Sarcoidosis was initially suspected because of arthritis, mediastinal lymphadenopathy, and a high CD4/CD8 ratio in broncho-alveolar lavage, and he was started on corticosteroids (30 mg equivalent of prednisone).

Over the following months, the patient developed new cutaneous manifestations—heliotrope rash, Gottron's papules on the hands, and erythematous rash on the V-area of the chest—followed by secondary Raynaud phenomenon with painful digital ischemia and ulcerations (Fig. 15.53). Laboratory tests revealed a marked inflammatory response and positivity for anti-MDA5 antibodies, establishing the diagnosis of dermatomyositis with severe vasculopathic features. Muscle enzyme levels were only mildly elevated, and muscle weakness was minimal, indicating a hypomyopathic form.

Despite sustained corticosteroid therapy, the disease course was complicated by interstitial lung disease (ILD) and recurrent digital ischemic events. Over time, the patient received multiple immunosuppressive regimens, including intravenous cyclophosphamide pulses (cumulative 5 g), methotrexate and azathioprine (both discontinued because of leukopenia), and later mycophenolate mofetil (up to 2 g/day). Vasodilator therapy with iloprost and alprostadil was added to manage severe Raynaud's phenomenon and digital ulcers. Because of incomplete control and persistent pulmonary involvement, he was enrolled in a clinical trial (brepocitinib vs placebo) and maintained on low-dose prednisone and hydroxychloroquine.

At the most recent follow-up, the patient was clinically stable but still had heliotrope rash, mild erythema of the face and neck, Gottron's papules on hands and feet, and residual scars from previous digital ischemia (Fig. 15.54). Fingertip ulcerations were minimal, and there was no sign of active myositis or joint synovitis. Fine bibasal crackles were audible on pulmonary examination, consistent with known ILD.

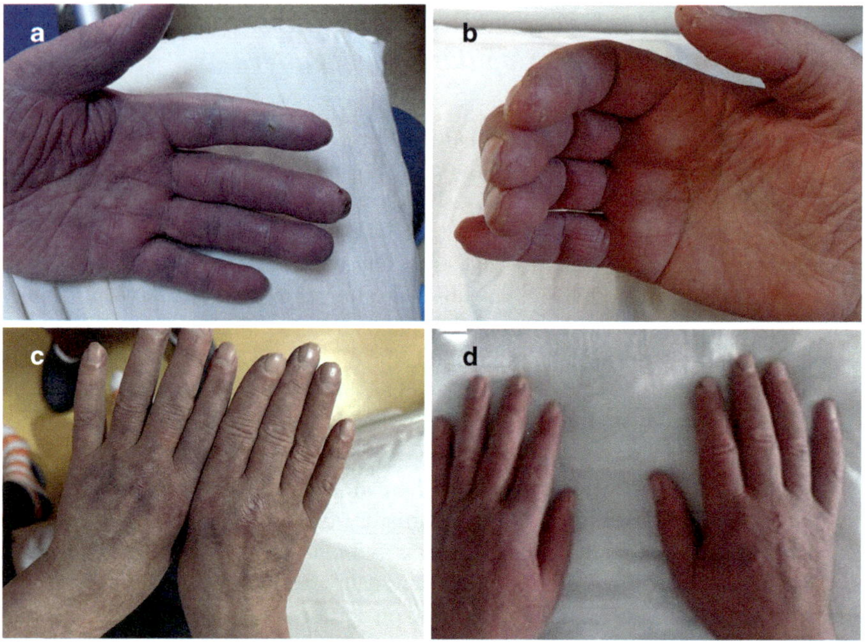

Fig. 15.53 (**a**) Severe acrocyanosis and digital ulcerations on the right hand before treatment. (**b**) Improvement of color and healing of lesions after vasodilator and immunomodulatory therapy

Fig. 15.54 (**a***) Erythematous poikilodermatous rash over the anterior chest forming a characteristic *V-sign*, associated with gynecomastia

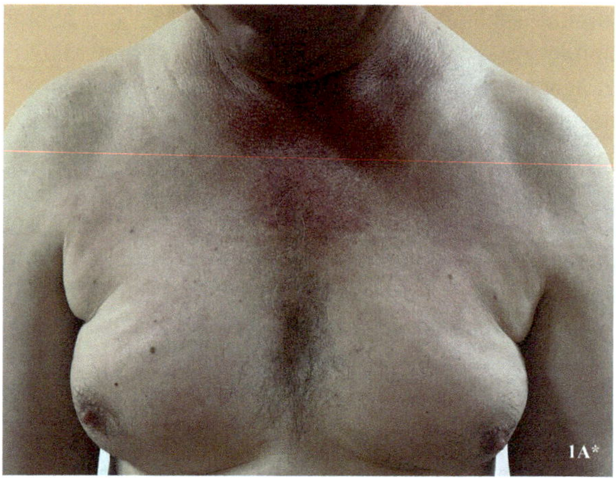

High-resolution CT of the chest demonstrated bilateral, predominantly basal and peripheral reticular infiltrates with traction bronchiectasis, stable compared with prior imaging (Fig. 15.55), while pulmonary function tests showed a mild restrictive pattern and a moderately reduced diffusing capacity (DLCO 56–57% of predicted). Cardiac ultrasound excluded pulmonary hypertension.

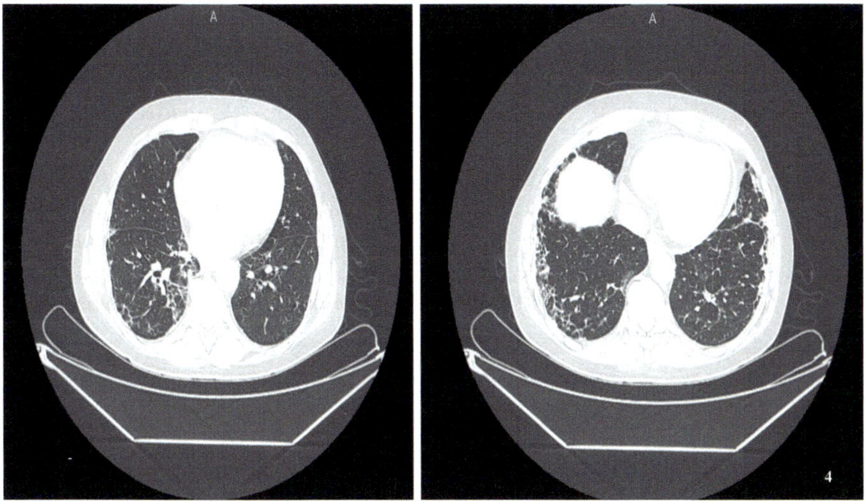

Fig. 15.55 High-resolution computed tomography showing bilateral, predominantly basal and peripheral reticular infiltrates with traction bronchiectasis

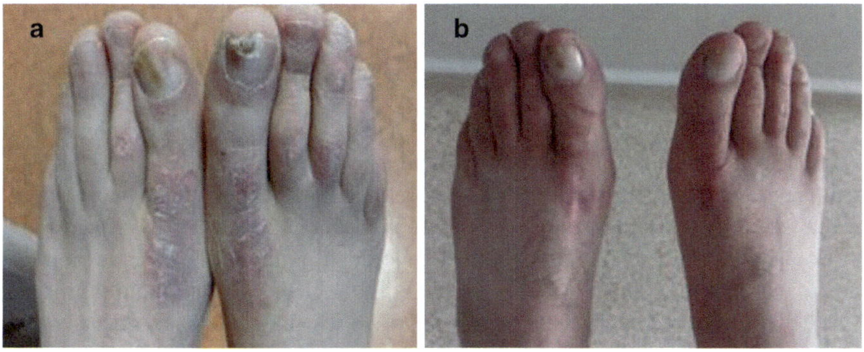

Fig. 15.56 (a) Erythematous and scaly lesions on the dorsal feet with nail involvement at baseline. (b) Resolution of skin changes following treatment

Nailfold capillaroscopy, performed during disease activity, revealed a markedly reduced capillary density, numerous dilated and giant capillaries, scattered recent microhemorrhages, and mild architectural disorganization, corresponding to an active "scleroderma-like" pattern (Fig. 15.56). After treatment intensification with vasodilators and JAK-inhibitor therapy from a clinical trial, a follow-up examination showed partial restoration of normal architecture and fewer hemorrhages (Fig. 15.56). Clinically, the cutaneous lesions improved, and new digital ulcers no longer occurred (Fig. 15.57).

The presence of an active scleroderma-like pattern in anti-MDA5 dermatomyositis is clinically relevant, as it correlates with severe microangiopathy, ischemic complications, and ILD progression. In this case, capillaroscopy findings mirrored

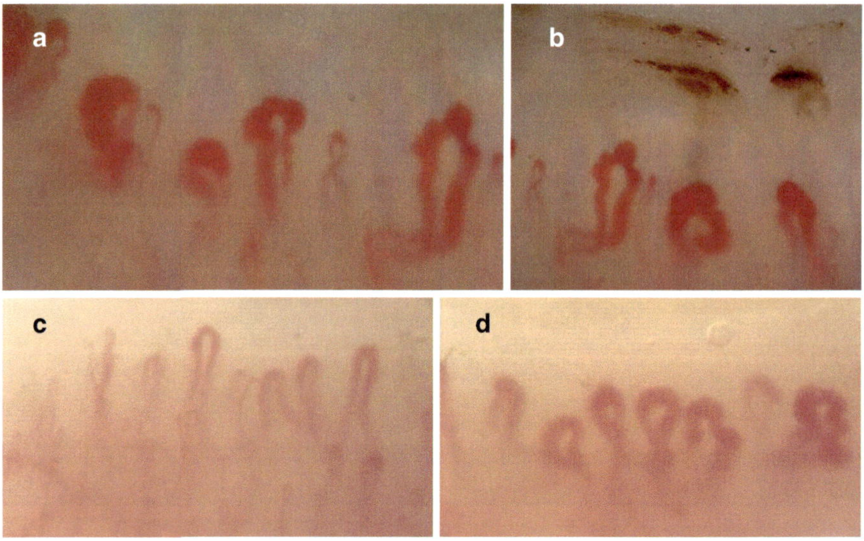

Fig. 15.57 (**a**, **b**) Baseline nailfold capillaroscopy showing markedly dilated and giant capillaries, microhemorrhages, and reduced density—an active scleroderma-like pattern. (**c**, **d**) Follow-up capillaroscopy demonstrates decreased hemorrhages and improved capillary organization

disease activity and supported ongoing vasodilator therapy and close multidisciplinary monitoring.

This observation illustrates the overlap between dermatomyositis and scleroderma-spectrum vasculopathy. Although anti-MDA5-positive dermatomyositis is recognized as a distinct myositis subset, capillaroscopic studies increasingly reveal scleroderma-like changes such as capillary enlargement, hemorrhages, and avascular areas. These alterations reflect endothelial injury and can serve as prognostic markers for complications, including digital ulceration and rapidly progressive ILD. Early recognition of these abnormalities may influence management, prompting timely vasodilator therapy, closer pulmonary follow-up, and more aggressive immunomodulation when appropriate.

This case underlines several points, namely that NFC is a simple, noninvasive tool that extends beyond systemic sclerosis to other connective tissue diseases with vascular involvement.

Secondly, detecting a modified NFC pattern in anti-MDA5-positive dermatomyositis captures patients at higher risk for ischemic and lung complications.

Finally, dynamic capillaroscopic assessments can complement serologic and clinical data in monitoring disease course and therapeutic response.

In summary, this patient with anti-MDA5-positive hypomyopathic dermatomyositis exhibited a "scleroderma-like" capillaroscopic pattern that pointed to severe microvascular injury and paralleled his clinical picture of Raynaud phenomenon, digital ulcerations, and ILD. The integration of NFC into routine evaluation proved essential for understanding disease mechanisms and optimizing individualized management.

Case 19 Beyond the Skin: The Diagnostic Value of Capillaroscopy in Amyopathic JDM

Rahma A. Elziaty
Internal Medicine Department, Rheumatology Division, Faculty of Medicine, Ain Shams University, Cairo, Egypt

Yasser El Miedany
Canterbury Christ Church University, Canterbury, UK

Rheumatology and Rehabilitation, Ain Shams University, Cairo, Egypt

King's College, London, UK

Waleed Hassan
Rheumatology and Rehabilitation Department, Faculty of Medicine, Benha University, Benha, Egypt

Mohammed Hassan Abu-Zaid
Rheumatology and Rehabilitation Department, Faculty of Medicine, Tanta University, Tanta, Egypt

A 10-year-old previously healthy girl presented to the dermatology clinic with a 2-month history of a violaceous rash around her eyes (heliotrope rash), erythematous scaly papules over the extensor surfaces of her fingers (Gottron's papules), and periungual erythema. The patient denied any muscle weakness, fatigue, or myalgia. There was no history of fever, photosensitivity, Raynaud's phenomenon, or respiratory symptoms.

On physical examination, periorbital discoloration was noted with mild eyelid edema. Gottron's papules were present over the MCP and IP joints. No objective muscle weakness was found on neurological examination; proximal strength in both upper and lower limbs was preserved (5/5 on the MRC scale). No joint swelling or tenderness.

Laboratory investigations: Creatine kinase (CK): Normal, ANA: Positive at 1:320 (speckled), Anti-Mi-2, Anti-MDA5, Anti-TIF1γ, and Anti-NXP2: Negative, ESR: 37 mm/h, and CRP: 18 mg/L. Electromyography (EMG): Normal. Nailfold capillaroscopy was performed and revealed dilated capillary loops, capillary dropout, ramified (bushy) capillaries, and microhemorrhages in some areas. These capillaroscopic features were consistent with a scleroderma-like pattern commonly seen in dermatomyositis, which reflects Active Dermatomyositis Microangiopathy.

Based on the pathognomonic skin findings, absence of muscle involvement for >6 weeks, normal muscle enzymes, and abnormal capillaroscopy, a diagnosis of clinically amyopathic juvenile dermatomyositis was established. Treatment was initiated with oral prednisolone (1 mg/kg/day) and methotrexate (15 mg/m^2/week).

At the 4-month follow-up, there was marked improvement in cutaneous lesions. Repeat nailfold capillaroscopy showed a decrease in capillary dropout and normalization of most dilated loops. The patient remained free of muscle symptoms and was monitored regularly (Figs. 15.58 and 15.59).

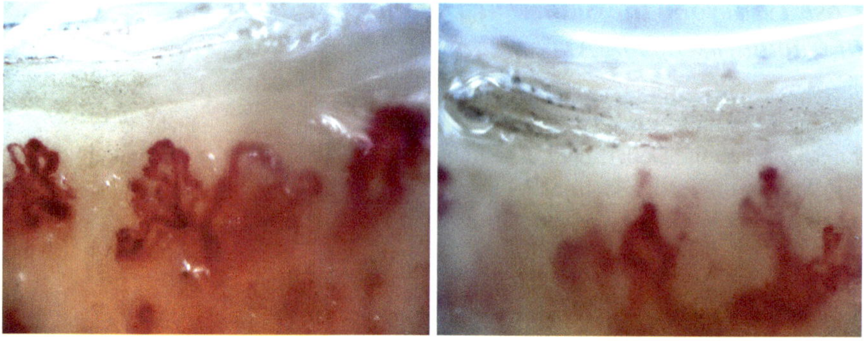

Fig. 15.58 Dilated capillary loops, capillary dropout, ramified (bushy) capillaries, and microhemorrhages in some areas; "scleroderma-like pattern."

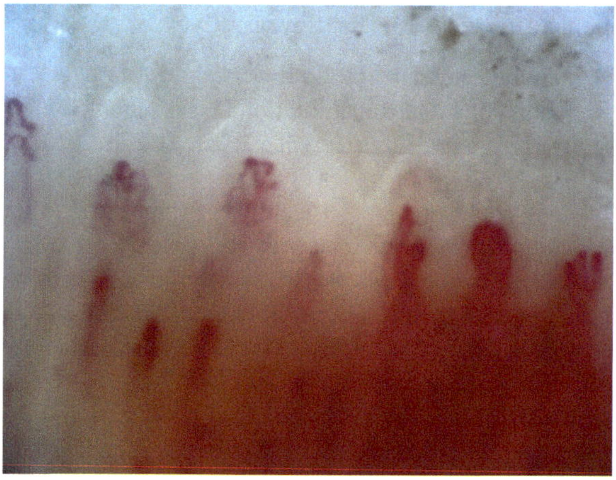

Fig. 15.59 Follow-up capillaroscopy after 4 months revealed a decrease in capillary dropout and no microhemorrhages

Discussion

Clinically amyopathic juvenile dermatomyositis is a subtype of juvenile dermatomyositis (JDM) characterized by hallmark skin manifestations without clinical, laboratory, or radiologic evidence of muscle involvement for at least 6 months. It accounts for approximately 5–20% of JDM cases [106].

Despite the absence of myositis, clinically amyopathic juvenile dermatomyositis can follow a chronic course and may involve complications such as calcinosis cutis, interstitial lung disease, and vasculopathy. Therefore, early diagnosis and treatment are crucial to prevent long-term sequelae.

Nailfold capillaroscopy is a noninvasive, sensitive tool that reveals microvascular abnormalities typical of dermatomyositis. Findings such as dilated loops, bushy capillaries, and capillary loss correlate with disease activity and can assist in diagnosis when muscle involvement is absent. In this case, capillaroscopy helped confirm the diagnosis and served as a baseline for monitoring response to treatment [107, 108].

Management of clinically amyopathic juvenile dermatomyositis generally mirrors that of classic JDM, with corticosteroids and immunosuppressants like methotrexate being first-line therapies. MTX was initiated early to achieve a rapid steroid-sparing effect and manage the cutaneous disease, consistent with current JDM guidelines. Long-term follow-up is needed to monitor for the delayed onset of myositis or other systemic complications.

Learning Points

- Clinically amyopathic juvenile dermatomyositis should be considered in children presenting with classic dermatomyositis skin changes but no muscle weakness.
- Nailfold capillaroscopy is valuable for diagnosis and follow-up, especially in amyopathic forms where muscle biomarkers and myositis-specific antibodies are normal.
- Clinically amyopathic juvenile dermatomyositis is not a benign variant that carries risks including calcinosis, lipodystrophy, and Interstitial Lung Disease (ILD), necessitating aggressive treatment, and requires careful long-term follow-up for emerging muscle or pulmonary involvement.

Case 20: From Raynaud to a Unified Diagnosis: Amyopathic Dermatomyositis and Colonic Carcinoma In Situ

Miriam Retuerto Guerrero, Elvira Díez Álvarez, and Ignacio González Fernández
Department of Rheumatology, Complejo Asistencial Universitario de León, León, Spain

72-year-old woman with a 2-year history of triphasic Raynaud phenomenon of the hands, with winter-*worsening fingertip* fissures. She denies oral ulcers, photosensitivity, alopecia, dyspnea, or reflux. Past history: remote tobacco use (quit ~30 years ago) and hyperlipidemia; on rosuvastatin 10 mg nightly.

Examination. No cutaneous ulcers or inflammatory rash. No sclerodactyly, pitting scars, or other stigmata of systemic sclerosis [109–111].

Initial Raynaud Workup

- *Immunology*. ANA *negative* by indirect immunofluorescence; cryoglobulins, antiphospholipid antibodies, and lupus anticoagulant *negative*.
- *Inflammation and muscle enzymes*. ESR 5 mm/h, CRP 0.7 mg/L; CK 61 U/L, aldolase 1.8 U/L; *CBC normal*.
- *Chest radiograph*. Basal bilateral ground-glass pattern with reticular bands and bronchial dilatations (first consideration viral/infectious); normal cardiothoracic index; calcified aortic-arch atheroma; small para-esophageal bulge compatible with a tiny hiatal hernia; diffuse axial osteopenia with mild anterior wedging of mid-thoracic vertebrae.

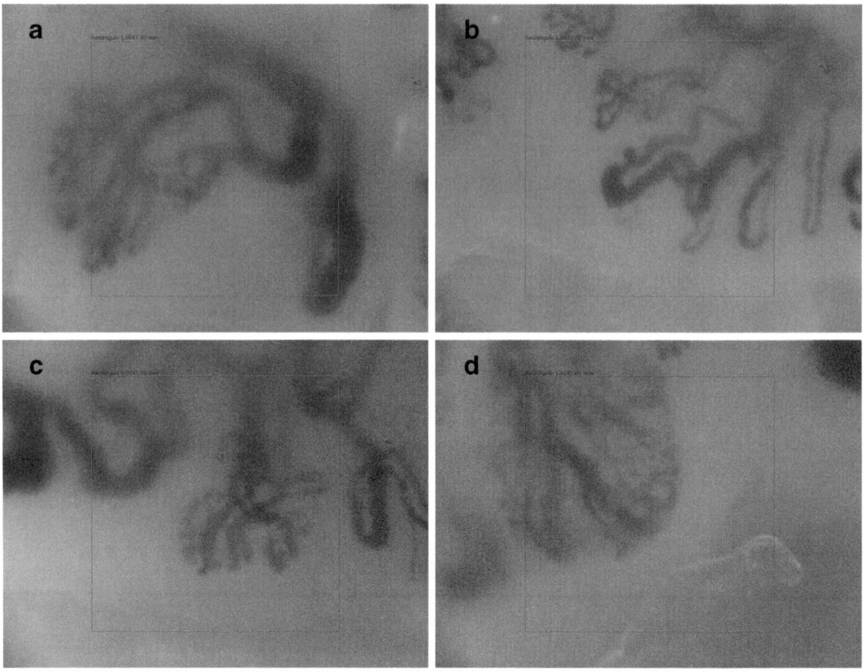

Fig. 15.60 Nailfold capillaroscopy: decreased density with arborizing loops and complex tortuosities (representative images)

- *Nailfold videocapillaroscopy (NVC).* Reduced capillary density with focal avascular areas, irregular alignment, dilated loops without some giants, numerous ramified/arborizing loops, and complex tortuosities, no microhemorrhages. Overall pattern *compatible with inflammatory myopathy* (Fig. 15.60).

Extended Workup (Given IIM Suspicion and CXR Abnormalities)

- *Autoimmunity (repeat).* ANA *1:80* (IIF). Myositis immunoblot: *anti-TIF1γ positive, anti-Ku positive*; remaining MSA/MAA negative.
- *High-resolution CT (HRCT).* Bilateral *ground-glass opacities* in *peripheral–subpleural* and *peribronchovascular* distributions with *confluent consolidations*; dependent atelectatic/scar bands; thin-walled cyst in the anterior LUL; mediastinal/hilar nodes ≤1.1 cm; no pleural or pericardial effusion. *Overall impression: organizing pneumonia (OP)* (Figs. 15.61 and 15.62).

Outcome of Investigations

Because of *anti-TIF1γ positivity*, a structured occult-malignancy screen was completed:

- *Breast imaging.* Mammography and breast ultrasound *BI-RADS 2* (benign).
- *Gynecologic assessment.* Pelvic exam, transvaginal ultrasound and cervical cytology *unremarkable*.

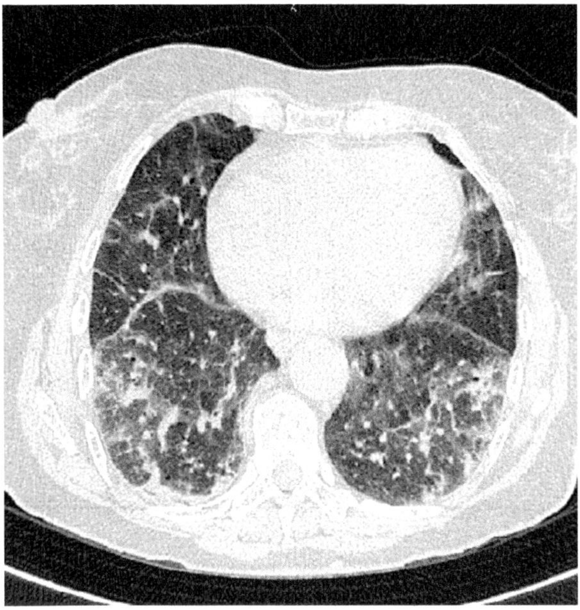

Fig. 15.61 HRCT demonstrating peripheral–subpleural ground-glass and organizing consolidations in the lower lobes

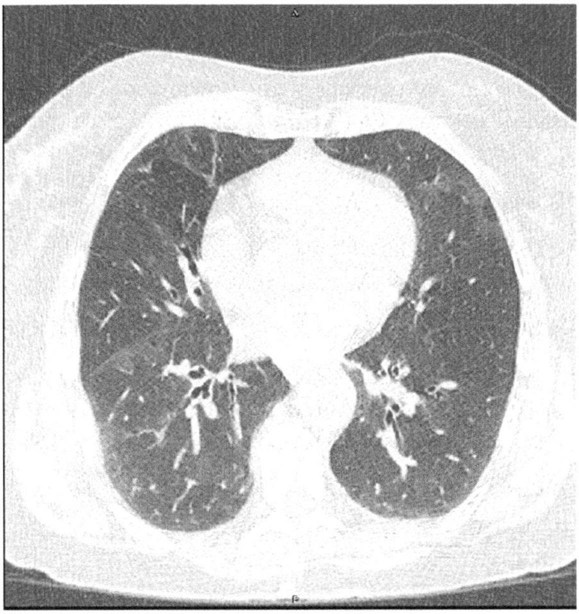

Fig. 15.62 HRCT demonstrating post-corticosteroid imaging showing resolution of consolidations and improvement of ground-glass opacities

- *PET-CT*. Diffuse hypermetabolism in lower lung fields concordant with CT; *focal hypermetabolic lesion (SUVmax 23)* in the transverse colon/hepatic flexure, *suspicious for neoplasia*; no hypermetabolic liver, spleen, adrenal, bone, mesenteric, abdominal, or pelvic nodal disease (Fig. 15.63).

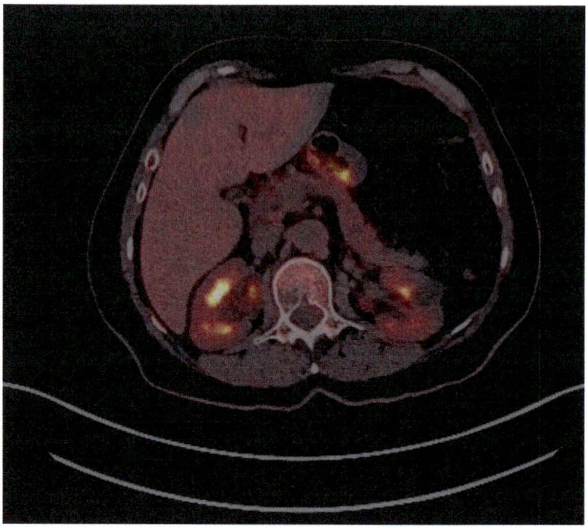

Fig. 15.63 PET-CT: focal hypermetabolism in transverse colon/hepatic flexure

- *Colonoscopy*. At ~60 cm from the anal verge in the transverse colon, *pedunculated polypoid lesion ~10 mm*, endoscopically serrated in appearance; *en-bloc hot-snare resection* and retrieval for histology.
- *Pathology result*. Pedunculated polyp with *carcinoma in situ (Tis)*, *R0* after en-bloc hot-snare resection (*clear margins*).

Concomitant pulmonary assessment showed preserved spirometry with mildly reduced gas transfer: *FVC 3010 mL (133% predicted), FEV_1 2470 mL, FEV_1/FVC 82%, DLCO 79%.*

Management

- *Therapy*. Prednisone *0.5 mg/kg/day* with taper for OP; *hydroxychloroquine 200 mg/day* for fissuring/mechanic's-hands phenotype.

Follow-Up

- *Ongoing endoscopic surveillance* (per Tis-R0 pathway).
- HRCT after corticosteroids showed resolution of OP (Fig. 15.62); prednisone discontinued; patient continues HCQ (Fig. 15.63).

Questions to Challenge the Reader

Which NVC features in this case support an inflammatory myopathy pattern rather than an early/active scleroderma-spectrum pattern?

How does anti-TIF1γ shape the differential diagnosis and the intensity of malignancy screening?

Which HRCT signs favor organizing pneumonia (OP) over other ILD patterns (e.g., NSIP, UIP)?

Would you escalate immunosuppression beyond corticosteroids in an amyopathic phenotype with improving OP?

Discussion

This case illustrates amyopathic dermatomyositis (anti-TIF1γ+, anti-Ku+) presenting with Raynaud phenomenon and mechanic's-hands–like fissuring, supported by a nailfold videocapillaroscopy pattern of reduced density with branching/arborizing loops and complex tortuosity, but without the giant loops and hemorrhagic burden typical of early scleroderma-spectrum microangiopathy. Anti-TIF1γ positivity mandates structured and repeated malignancy screening; in this patient, it unveiled a hypermetabolic colonic lesion subsequently proven to be carcinoma in situ (Tis) and curatively removed by en-bloc hot-snare polypectomy with clear margins (R0), allowing surveillance rather than surgery.

Pulmonary involvement was consistent with organizing pneumonia: peripheral–subpleural and peribronchovascular ground-glass opacities with confluent consolidations and dependent bands, with preserved spirometry and mildly reduced DLCO. A prednisone taper (≈0.5–1 mg/kg/day) led to radiologic resolution, permitting steroid discontinuation while maintaining hydroxychloroquine for cutaneous/mechanic's-hands features. The overall course emphasizes the importance of (i) integrating NVC with serology and imaging to refine phenotype; (ii) early, multidisciplinary malignancy screening in anti-TIF1γ+ dermatomyositis; and (iii) tailoring immunosuppression to response, reserving escalation when OP improves, and physiology remains stable.

Key Learning Points

- NVC showing reduced density with ramified/arborizing loops and complex tortuosity can support an inflammatory myopathy pattern when classic DM rashes are subtle or absent.
- *In this case, nailfold videocapillaroscopy (NVC) was pivotal to flag an inflammatory myopathy, which in turn prompted a targeted malignancy workup and led to the subsequent diagnosis of neoplasia.*
- Anti-TIF1γ positivity requires systematic, repeated cancer screening; anti-Ku may indicate overlapping features.
- Organizing pneumonia can complicate dermatomyositis and often responds to corticosteroids.
- Coordinated rheumatology–pulmonology–gastroenterology care streamlines diagnosis, treatment, and follow-up.

SLE and Antiphospholipid Syndrome (APS) Cases

Case 21: Nailfold Videocapillaroscopy Findings in a Systemic Lupus Erythematosus Patient with a History of Stroke

Marius Cadar, Jacopo Landro, Simona Truglia, and Valeria Riccieri
Rheumatology, Department of Medical and Cardiovascular Sciences, Sapienza University, Rome, Italy

In 2008, a 47-year-old man developed Raynaud phenomenon, malar rash, antinuclear antibody (ANA) positivity, and hypocomplementemia. A diagnosis of undifferentiated connective tissue disease (UCTD) was established. Treatment with cyclosporine A and low-dose glucocorticoids was initiated, resulting in good symptom control.

In 2012, at the age of 51, he experienced an ischemic stroke involving the right cerebral hemisphere, leading to left hemiplegia. During the recovery phase, the patient tested positive for anti-dsDNA and anti-RNP antibodies, and a diagnosis of Systemic Lupus Erythematosus (SLE) was established. Cyclosporine A was discontinued, and therapy with hydroxychloroquine, azathioprine, statins, and antihypertensive agents was introduced.

The patient also underwent physical therapy with gradual improvement in strength and sensitivity of the affected areas, although spastic paralysis of the left hand persisted.

SLE subsequently remained in remission for about 10 years on stable therapy, with no further ischemic events, under regular rheumatological follow-up.

In 2024, at the age of 63, he presented with worsening Raynaud phenomenon affecting only the right hand, while the left spastic hand was spared. He reported a Raynaud Condition Score (RCS) of 8/10, mainly during winter. To investigate the worsening of Raynaud symptoms, nailfold videocapillaroscopy (NVC) was performed for the first time at our tertiary rheumatology center.

What is expected in SLE patients with Raynaud phenomenon? What is the potential role of the nervous system?

NVC findings differed markedly between the two hands. In the right hand, there was a reduced capillary density (~6 capillaries/mm), microhemorrhages, and enlarged but not giant capillaries. In contrast, the left (paralyzed) hand showed a normal capillary density (>8 capillaries/mm) with short, variably shaped capillaries and visible venous plexus, but without hemorrhages (Fig. 15.64).

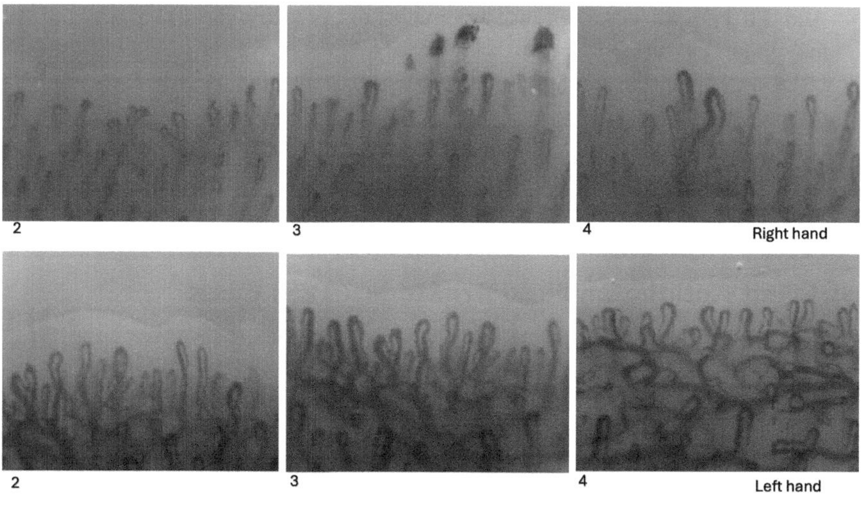

Fig. 15.64 NVC demonstrates different findings in both hands

Discussion
Raynaud phenomenon is a multifactorial vasospastic disorder involving vascular, neural, and intravascular mechanisms [112]. It may occur as a primary (idiopathic) condition or as secondary to connective tissue disease. In SLE, up to 50% of patients may develop Raynaud phenomenon [113, 114].

NVC abnormalities are frequent in SLE. A systematic review and meta-analysis of 40 studies demonstrated that patients with SLE have higher semi-quantitative NVC scores than healthy controls, with more tortuous capillaries, abnormal morphology, and hemorrhages [115]. Moreover, NVC findings and scores have been correlated with disease activity indices such as SLEDAI, ECLAM, and SLAM [116, 117].

In 2025, Ingegnoli et al. identified two clusters of NVC patterns in SLE: cluster 1 (less severe, observed in ~88% of patients) and cluster 2 (more severe, characterized by low capillary density, abnormal morphology, enlarged capillaries, and architectural disorganization) [118].

This case highlights several noteworthy aspects. First, as expected in an SLE patient with Raynaud phenomenon, NVC abnormalities were present. Second, the absence of Raynaud symptoms in the paralyzed hand confirms a key role of neural regulation in Raynaud pathophysiology and, perhaps, in endothelial damage. Interestingly, the paralyzed hand exhibited SLE-related NVC abnormalities without the features of more severe changes demonstrated in the contralateral hand.

Thus, this unique case illustrates the contribution of neural factors to NVC changes in SLE with Raynaud phenomenon. The coexistence of both new NVC clusters in the same patient, probably depending on neural involvement, reinforces the complex interplay between immune-mediated vascular damage and nervous system regulation.

Case 22: Microvascular Insight into Lupus: Capillaroscopic Evolution Following Immunosuppressive Therapy

Rahma A. Elziaty
Internal Medicine Department, Rheumatology Division, Faculty of Medicine, Ain Shams University, Cairo, Egypt

A 32-year-old female with a known history of systemic lupus erythematosus diagnosed two years earlier (positive ANA with high anti-dsDNA titers, low complement during flares, nonerosive arthritis, and mild serositis) presented with a *painful digital ulcer* on the distal aspect of the right index and middle fingers persisting for two weeks. The lesion began as a dusky discoloration progressing despite conservative care (Fig. 15.65). She also reported intermittent Raynaud's-like color changes in cold exposure. There was no history of sclerodactyly, skin tightening, or prior severe vasculitic episodes.

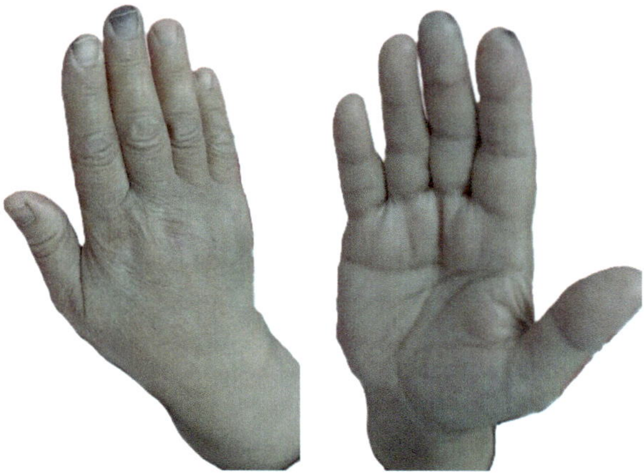

Fig. 15.65 Digital ulcer on the distal aspect of the right index and middle fingers with dusky discoloration

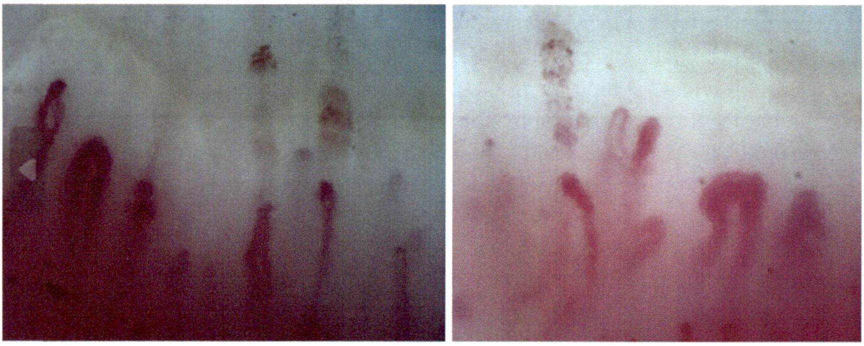

Fig. 15.66 NFC reveals active scleroderma pattern; Decreased capillary density, presence of giant capillaries, and microhemorrhages

On examination, the ulcer had a necrotic center with surrounding erythema. No skin thickening was noted. Laboratory workup showed mild anemia, hemoglobin 10 g/dl, ESR: 43 mm/h, rising anti-dsDNA compared to baseline, and decreased C3/C4, suggesting active lupus. Antiphospholipid antibodies were negative. There was no evidence of large-vessel thrombosis confirmed by arteriovenous duplex.

Given the vascular manifestation, nailfold video capillaroscopy was performed. Findings included giant capillaries, multiple microhemorrhages, and mild architectural disorganization—constituting *a scleroderma pattern* (active pattern) (Fig. 15.66)

The patient received escalation of immunosuppression: oral prednisone (tapering regimen), hydroxychloroquine continuation, and initiation of mycophenolate mofetil 2 gm/day. Local wound care and vasodilator support (calcium channel blocker) were also instituted.

At the 4-month follow-up, the digital ulcer had completely healed (Fig. 15.67). Serologic markers normalized: "anti-dsDNA negative, complements were normal." Repeat nailfold capillaroscopy revealed resolution of microhemorrhages, improved capillary architecture with less disorganization, and persistent dilated capillaries,

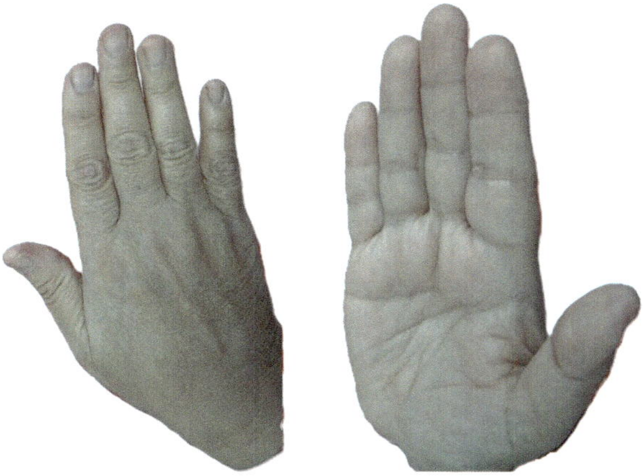

Fig. 15.67 The digital ulcer of the right index and middle fingers had completely healed

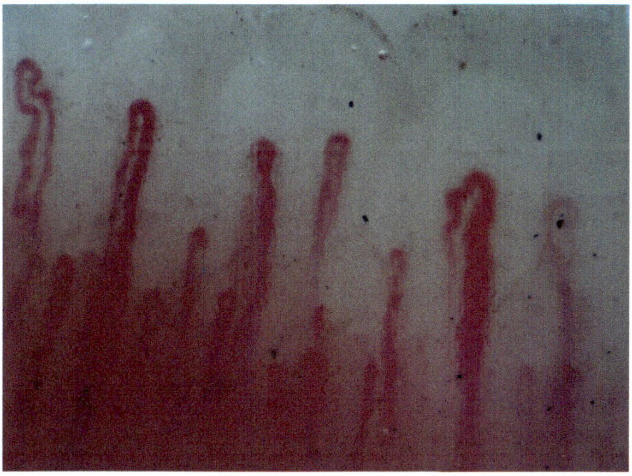

Fig. 15.68 Follow-up NFC after 4 months reveals nonspecific abnormalities: elongated, dilated, tortuous capillaries with an absence of microhemorrhages

but no giant capillaries. This pattern reflected partial microvascular recovery with some residual remodeling (Fig. 15.68).

Discussion

Microvascular dysfunction is a hallmark in systemic autoimmune rheumatic diseases, and nailfold capillaroscopy (NFC) provides a window into these changes. While the classic "scleroderma pattern" (giant capillaries, microhemorrhages, avascular areas, and neoangiogenesis) is prototypically linked to systemic sclerosis, "scleroderma-like" capillaroscopic abnormalities are well described in SLE and other connective tissue diseases, especially during periods of increased disease activity [119, 120].

The presence of giant capillaries and microhemorrhages in this patient raised the index of suspicion for active microvascular lupus involvement beyond simple Raynaud's. Such findings signal endothelial perturbation and capillary leakage, consistent with immune-mediated damage; they have been shown to associate with disease activity and, in some series, with internal organ involvement [121, 122].

Importantly, capillaroscopic abnormalities in SLE are not invariably permanent. Improvement in systemic disease activity—via effective immunosuppression—has been associated with partial reversal of microvascular lesions, particularly resolution of hemorrhages and reduced architectural distortion, while some features like capillary dilation may persist longer due to structural remodeling. This aligns with the concept that some capillary abnormalities reflect active injury (potentially reversible) and others reflect chronic change [119].

In this case, the disappearance of microhemorrhages and improvement in capillary organization after therapy paralleled the clinical remission and serologic improvement, underscoring capillaroscopy's role as a dynamic biomarker of microvascular disease activity. Persistent dilated capillaries likely represent residual morphological alteration from prior injury, a finding seen even in patients who achieve clinical control.

Differential consideration included overlap syndromes (e.g., mixed connective tissue disease or undifferentiated overlap with scleroderma features), but the absence of skin sclerosis, negative specific antibodies for other CTDs, and the temporal relation to lupus serologic flare favored SLE with scleroderma-like microvascular involvement. Regular capillaroscopic monitoring helped avoid premature labeling as systemic sclerosis and guided confidence in adjusting immunosuppression based on microvascular response.

Learning Points

- *Scleroderma pattern can occur in SLE*, especially during active disease, and includes giant capillaries and microhemorrhages.
- *Nail fold capillaroscopy acts as a dynamic biomarker in SLE*, allowing clinicians to monitor microvascular response to immunosuppressive therapy, with the resolution of microhemorrhages and architectural disorganization often paralleling clinical and serologic remission.
- *Serial capillaroscopy allows monitoring* of treatment response and can support clinical decision-making in difficult vascular manifestations.
- *Capillaroscopy acts as a dynamic biomarker in SLE*, allowing clinicians to monitor microvascular response to immunosuppressive therapy, with the resolution of microhemorrhages and architectural disorganization often paralleling clinical and serologic remission.

Case 23: Comb-Like Hemorrhages as a Clue to Antiphospholipid Antibodies in a Patient with Mixed Connective Tissue Disease

Sofia Azevedo
Rheumatology Department, Unidade Local de Saúde da Região de Aveiro, Aveiro, Portugal

CIRA, Centro de Investigação em Reumatologia de Aveiro, Aveiro, Portugal

Carolina Mazeda
Rheumatology Department, Unidade Local de Saúde da Região de Aveiro, Aveiro, Portugal

CIRA, Centro de Investigação em Reumatologia de Aveiro, Aveiro, Portugal

EpiDoC Unit – NOVA Medical School, NOVA University, Lisbon, Portugal

A 60-year-old woman was first evaluated in 2017 with a one year history of severe asthenia, symmetrical inflammatory polyarthralgia, proximal muscle weakness, and progressive functional limitation. She also reported 22 kg weight loss over this period, acrocyanosis, and xerostomia. The patient lived with her husband and had been fully independent in daily activities prior to symptom onset. Her past medical history included arterial hypertension and type 2 diabetes mellitus complicated by diabetic nephropathy. She denied photosensitivity, skin rash, oral ulcers, sicca-related ocular symptoms, ocular redness, respiratory complaints (including dyspnea or cough), chest pain, gastrointestinal symptoms (including dysphagia, dyspepsia, or altered bowel habits), genitourinary symptoms, or neuropsychiatric manifestations. Physical examination revealed puffy hands, Raynaud's phenomenon, and polyarthritis involving the small joints of the hands. No skin thickening, oral or digital ulcers, or alopecia were observed. Muscular strength was globally reduced (MMT8: 42/80), predominantly in proximal limbs [123–129].

Laboratory evaluation revealed elevated creatine phosphokinase (994 U/L; normal range: 34–145 U/L) and myoglobin (438 ng/mL; normal range: <114 ng/mL), with an erythrocyte sedimentation rate of 73 mm/h (normal range: <20 mm/h) and elevated C-reactive protein (2.59 mg/dL, normal range: <0.50 mg/dL). Autoimmune screening showed high-titer antinuclear antibodies (1:1280, speckled pattern), with anti-Ro52, anti-dsDNA, and anti-U1-RNP positivity. Antiphospholipid antibodies were negative at that time.

Transthoracic echocardiography demonstrated an estimated pulmonary artery systolic pressure of 59 mmHg and interventricular septal thickening, with signs of right ventricular pressure overload. Right heart catheterization confirmed combined precapillary and postcapillary pulmonary hypertension (mean pulmonary artery pressure 27 mmHg; pulmonary capillary wedge pressure 9 mmHg; pulmonary vascular resistance 6 WU).

High-resolution computed tomography of the chest revealed no mediastinal or hilar lymphadenopathy. There was pulmonary artery trunk dilatation (diameter 3.9 cm) and a globular cardiac silhouette. Parenchymal window images showed basal reticular opacities and septal thickening, more prominent on the right, suggestive of fibrotic changes.

Electromyography of the upper and lower limbs shows severe muscle fiber abnormalities consistent with a marked proximal myopathic/myositic process. No evidence of peripheral polyneuropathy was observed.

Muscle biopsy confirmed inflammatory myopathy.

Outcome of Investigations

Based on the combination of anti-U1-RNP positivity, myositis, Raynaud's phenomenon, puffy hands, pulmonary hypertension, and arthritis, a diagnosis of mixed connective tissue disease (MCTD) was established. The relation between pulmonary interstitial findings and connective tissue disease was excluded, and a diagnosis of hypersensitivity pneumonitis to birds was made.

She received induction therapy with intravenous (IV) methylprednisolone pulses (1 g × 3 days) followed by oral prednisolone (1 mg/kg/day) and IV cyclophosphamide (500 mg/m^2 monthly for six months), later transitioning to azathioprine maintenance therapy. Pulmonary hypertension was subsequently managed with tadalafil (40 mg/day) and macitentan (10 mg/day).

Over subsequent years, the patient remained stable under azathioprine 100 mg/day, allowing for progressive steroid tapering.

In 2025, she was hospitalized for marantic endocarditis, leading to aortic valve replacement, and later she developed brady-tachycardia syndrome requiring a permanent pacemaker.

After these events, mild left ventricular systolic depression and persistent grade III diastolic dysfunction were observed. Antiphospholipid antibodies (aPL) analysis was repeated, showing high (-titer) positivity for anti-cardiolipin and anti-beta-2-glycoprotein I IgG (358.9 UI/mL and 213.9 UI/mL, respectively).

Nailfold Videocapillaroscopy Findings

Baseline nailfold videocapillaroscopy (NVC) (2015) revealed:

- Preserved global architecture without atypical forms;
- Slight capillary tortuosity and a few ectatic loops without hemorrhages or avascular areas;
- Normal capillary density, irregular coloration, and mild pericapillary edema.

Reevaluation of NVC (2025) showed:

- Preserved global architecture with some arborescent and atypical forms;
- Several ectatic capillaries, no megacapillaries;
- Multiple microhemorrhages, some traumatic but others arranged in parallel rows forming a "comb-like" pattern;
- Normal capillary density, irregular coloration, and mild pericapillary edema.

According to Cutolo's classification, the pattern remained nonspecific, but the combination of numerous findings and the new comb-like hemorrhages suggested progression of microangiopathy and possible secondary aPL-related vascular injury, consistent with her serological conversion (Fig. 15.69).

Questions for the Reader

1. What is the clinical significance of comb-like hemorrhages on NVC?
2. How do capillaroscopic findings guide the reassessment of systemic autoimmunity in MCTD?
3. What mechanisms explain the association between antiphospholipid antibodies and specific microvascular injury patterns?

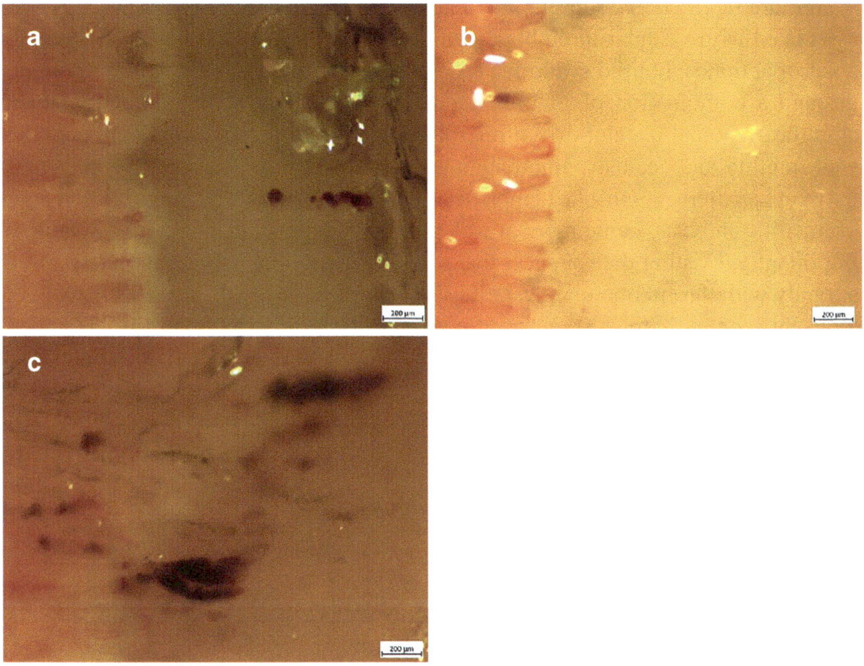

Fig. 15.69 (**a–c**) Nailfold videocapillaroscopy picture; magnification 200x; Density: normal capillary density; Dimension: several ectatic capillaries (<50 µg); Morphology: atypical capillaries, with arborescent forms; microhemorrhages: multiple microhemorrhages, some traumatic but others arranged in parallel rows forming a "comb-like" pattern

Discussion

MCTD is a systemic autoimmune disease characterized by clinical and serological overlap with systemic sclerosis (SSc), systemic lupus erythematosus, and idiopathic inflammatory myopathies. This overlap extends to the microvascular level, where NVC findings range from normal or nonspecific abnormalities to scleroderma-spectrum changes (including scleroderma and scleroderma-like patterns). In cross-sectional and prospective studies, up to two-thirds of patients with MCTD may demonstrate a scleroderma-like capillaroscopic pattern, which has been associated with a more aggressive phenotype and disease progression. However, unlike SSc, MCTD typically demonstrates less severe capillary loss and fewer avascular areas, reflecting a heterogeneous and often less destructive microangiopathy.

In the present case, two NVC evaluations performed ten years apart demonstrated progression of microangiopathy despite formal persistence of a nonspecific pattern according to the Cutolo classification. The most relevant new finding on follow-up NVC was the appearance of comb-like hemorrhages, absent at baseline. This evolution paralleled seroconversion for aPL and the development of nonbacterial thrombotic endocarditis, indicating superimposed thrombotic microvascular involvement.

aPL are reported in a subset of patients with MCTD, and their presence has been associated with vascular thrombotic damage even in the absence of a definite diagnosis of antiphospholipid syndrome (APS). aPL contributes to microvascular injury through a combination of immune-mediated endothelial activation, complement amplification, and platelet-driven microthrombosis, ultimately promoting capillary wall fragility and occlusive microangiopathy. Although APS lacks a specific capillaroscopic pattern, comb-like hemorrhages have emerged as a potential NVC marker of microthrombosis, being more prevalent in APS patients than in healthy controls. Importantly, existing data suggest that this capillaroscopic feature correlates more strongly with thrombotic manifestations than with isolated aPL positivity.

In this context, the appearance of comb-like hemorrhages in an MCTD patient should prompt reevaluation for secondary APS, even if previous aPL testing was negative. Although the prognostic value of this finding is not yet validated, its presence may justify closer vascular surveillance. The association between specific aPL subtypes and distinct NVC abnormalities remains unclear and requires further study.

Key Learning Points

- MCTD exhibits heterogeneous clinical and microvascular phenotypes; NVC can aid in tracking vascular involvement over time.
- The "comb-like hemorrhage" pattern on NVC is highly suggestive of antiphospholipid antibody–associated microangiopathy.
- Although the prognostic value of comb-like hemorrhages in NVC is not yet validated, their presence may justify closer vascular surveillance.
- NVC may represent a noninvasive marker of systemic vascular damage.

Case 24: Dynamic Capillaroscopic Changes in a Patient with SLE and APS

Rahma A. Elziaty
Internal Medicine Department, Rheumatology Division, Faculty of Medicine, Ain Shams University, Cairo, Egypt

Yasser El Miedany
Canterbury Christ Church University, Canterbury, UK

Rheumatology and Rehabilitation, Ain Shams University, Cairo, Egypt

King's College, London, UK

Mary Wadie
Department of Internal Medicine, Faculty of Medicine, Cairo University, Kasr Alainy, Egypt

A 29-year-old woman known with SLE for 2 years (malar rash, arthritis, serositis). Autoantibodies: ANA 1:640 (homogenous), anti-dsDNA positive. Intermittent

Raynaud's phenomenon. No prior digital ulcers. On hydroxychloroquine 400 mg daily and low-dose prednisone 10 mg daily.

New Presentation (March 2025): 3 weeks of worsening triphasic Raynaud's, painful fingertip ischemia (index and middle fingers), and one episode of transient binocular visual blurring. No dyspnea or chest pain. *On examination,* she was vitally stable, with cool fingers and periungual erythema. No synovitis. *Laboratory investigations* revealed: CBC: mild thrombocytopenia (PLT: 120 × 10^9/L), ESR: 48 mm/h, CRP: 8 mg/L, complements low (C3: 58 mg/dL, C4: 9 mg/dL), anti-dsDNA elevated. APS profile on two occasions, 12 weeks apart: LA positive; anticardiolipin IgG positive; anti-β2GPI IgG positive → consistent with APS (laboratory criteria met). Vascular Imaging: Hand duplex: no vessel occlusion. The combination of vascular event "fingertip ischemia" and positive laboratory criteria (LAC, ACL IgG, anti-beta2 glycoprotein I IgG on two occasions) meets the criteria of definite APS.

Nailfold Capillaroscopy (NFC): baseline: normal capillary density, tortuosity common, frequent microhemorrhages (comb-like pattern), sluggish flow with occasional intraluminal dark plugs suggestive of microthrombi. Pattern: non-scleroderma pattern; Findings support active microvascular involvement and micro-thrombotic injury consistent with SLE/APS vasculopathy.

Treat SLE flare: methylprednisolone 500 mg IV × 3 days → tapering oral prednisone 20 mg/day and mycophenolate mofetil 2 g/day, low-dose aspirin 81 mg.

Vascular care: nifedipine ER 30 mg/day; topical wound care; avoidance of cold; smoking status negative.

Follow-Up NFC (16 weeks): capillary density improved; microhemorrhages decreased; no avascular areas; flow normalized. Clinically, Raynaud's is less frequent, and complements and anti-dsDNA are normalized (Figs. 15.70 and 15.71).

Discussion

Nailfold capillaroscopy (NFC) is a noninvasive window to the microcirculation. In SLE, capillaroscopic changes are common but typically nonspecific (tortuosity,

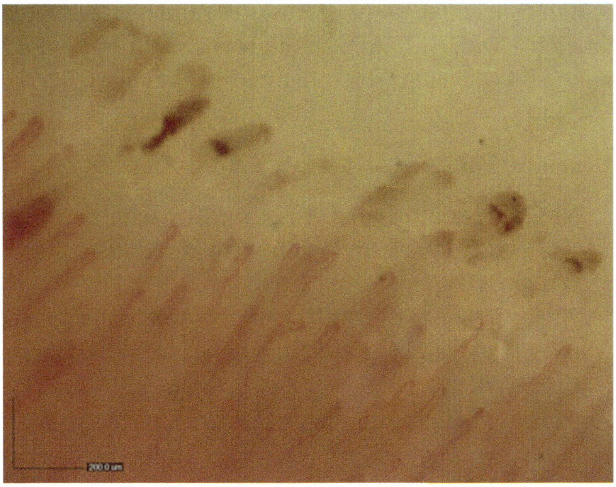

Fig. 15.70 Initial NFC reveals microhemorrhages (comb-like pattern)

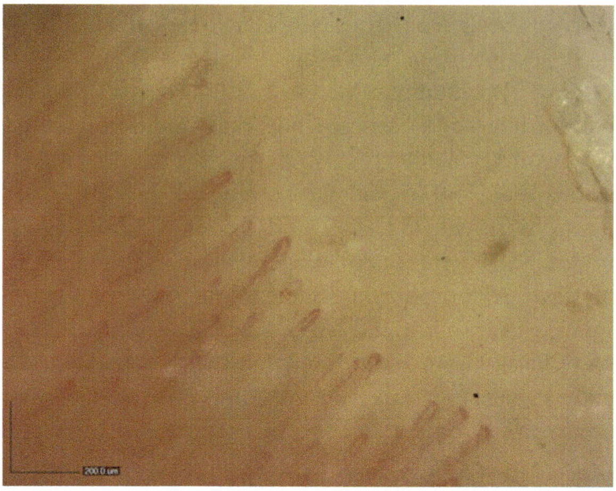

Fig. 15.71 Follow-up NFC reveals dilated capillaries with decreased microhemorrhages

dilated loops, microhemorrhages, and mild density reduction) and do not display the structured "scleroderma pattern." Nevertheless, these changes often correlate with disease activity and endothelial dysfunction [130].

Secondary APS can present with digital ischemia/ulcers driven by micro- and macro-thrombosis. While APS-specific NFC criteria are not established, microhemorrhages, sluggish flow, and capillary loss/avascular areas may reflect microthrombotic injury and ischemia, supporting the clinical suspicion when coupled with a positive aPL profile [131, 132].

Nailfold capillaroscopy (NFC) was valuable in this case by aiding diagnosis, assessing activity, and monitoring response. The abnormal but non-scleroderma pattern helped exclude early systemic sclerosis while supporting SLE/APS-related vasculopathy. The presence of microhemorrhages and reduced capillary density paralleled serologic activity and ischemic symptoms, then improved with immunosuppression and anticoagulation. On follow-up, NFC normalization coincided with ulcer healing and clinical stabilization, underscoring its role as a monitoring tool in connective tissue diseases beyond SSc. Although the absence of giant capillaries fits with SLE/APS, clinicians should stay vigilant since some SLE patients may still develop scleroderma-like changes, indicating overlap or evolving SSc [133].

Learning Points

- NFC is useful beyond SSc: In SLE (with or without APS), NFC often shows nonspecific microangiopathy that correlates with disease activity and ischemic symptoms.
- APS can cause digital ischemia via microthrombosis; NFC may reveal microthrombotic surrogates (sluggish flow, dark intraluminal plugs, microhemorrhages) that complement a positive aPL profile and support the need for anticoagulation/antiplatelet therapy.

- Pattern recognition matters: Non-scleroderma pattern in Raynaud's favors SLE/APS, guiding investigations and management.
- Follow-up value: Serial NFC can document improvement with immunosuppression/anticoagulation and vasodilators, aligning with clinical and serologic recovery.
- Vigilance for APS: Severe digital ischemia in an SLE patient, especially if accompanied by other vascular events (e.g., transient visual blurring) and a non-scleroderma NFC pattern, should prompt immediate and thorough investigation for secondary antiphospholipid syndrome (APS).

Case 25: From Raynaud's to APS: The Diagnostic Value of Nailfold Capillaroscopy in a Patient with Lymphoma

Rahma A. Elziaty
Internal Medicine Department, Rheumatology Division, Faculty of Medicine, Ain Shams University, Cairo, Egypt

A 51-year-old man, previously diagnosed with non-Hodgkin lymphoma and in complete remission for the past three years, presented to the rheumatology clinic with a two-month history of Raynaud's phenomenon involving both hands. He reported episodic discoloration and pain in his fingers upon cold exposure but denied digital ulcers, skin thickening, or systemic symptoms.

There was no family history of autoimmune disorders. On physical examination, peripheral pulses were intact, and the hands showed no signs of trophic changes. Neurological and cardiovascular examinations were normal.

Due to the patient's oncologic history, secondary causes were considered. Nailfold video capillaroscopy was performed, revealing a distinctive "comb-like" capillary pattern characterized by regularly aligned capillaries with pericapillary hemorrhages and irregular spacing, without capillary loss or neo-angiogenesis. These findings have been reported in association with APS (Fig. 15.72).

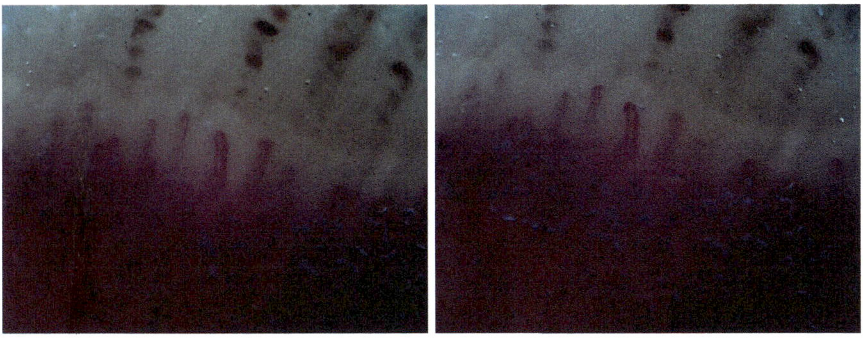

Fig. 15.72 "Comb-like" capillary pattern

Prompted by the capillaroscopic findings, serological testing was conducted: Positive anticardiolipin IgG antibodies, positive anti-β2 glycoprotein I antibodies (IgG and IgM), and positive lupus anticoagulant. Negative ANA and anti-dsDNA. Normal complement (C3, C4).

Repeat testing after 12 weeks confirmed the persistence of antiphospholipid antibodies. Based on the revised Sydney criteria, a diagnosis of APS was made [134]. The patient was maintained on antiplatelet therapy along with prophylactic anticoagulation.

Discussion

This case demonstrates the evolving role of nailfold capillaroscopy beyond classic connective tissue diseases (CTDs), emphasizing its relevance in identifying autoimmune vasculopathies such as APS. The presence of RP in this middle-aged male with no prior autoimmune history but a background of lymphoma raised the index of suspicion for paraneoplastic or autoimmune complications [135, 136].

Capillaroscopy findings in APS are often subtle and variable but may include dilated loops, microhemorrhages, or the "comb-like" pattern—reflecting preserved architecture with parallel orientation and intermittent hemorrhages. Although not specific, this pattern warrants consideration of APS, especially when accompanied by vascular symptoms like RP.

Interestingly, malignancies such as lymphoma may be followed by immune dysregulation and emergence of autoantibodies or autoimmune diseases, either due to immune reconstitution or underlying paraneoplastic processes [135, 136]. This case reinforces the importance of a vigilant approach when new vascular symptoms arise in cancer survivors.

The positive serology confirmed the presence of antiphospholipid antibodies and fulfilled the criteria for APS. Early diagnosis enabled prompt counseling and monitoring for thrombotic risks—critical in preventing serious complications such as stroke, deep vein thrombosis, or pregnancy morbidity in women.

This case supports prior findings that capillaroscopy, while not diagnostic in isolation, can serve as a valuable noninvasive screening tool guiding more specific serologic investigations. Its utility is especially pronounced in atypical presentations, late-onset RP, or patients with a history of malignancy.

Learning Points

- Raynaud's phenomenon in middle-aged individuals, particularly cancer survivors or those with a history of lymphoma, warrants a high index of suspicion for secondary autoimmune causes like APS.
- Nailfold capillaroscopy can provide a crucial initial clue toward non-SSc microangiopathies (like APS) when it reveals signs of microvascular damage (e.g., hemorrhages) but lacks the classic SSc giant loops or avascularity.
- High-risk aPL profiles (e.g., triple positivity) in asymptomatic or low-symptom patients require prompt risk stratification and consideration for antithrombotic therapy (antiplatelet or anticoagulation) to prevent serious thrombotic complications.

– Capillaroscopy's role extends beyond SSc; it is a valuable, noninvasive screening tool for microvascular disease, capable of guiding serologic investigation in patients with atypical vascular symptoms.

Miscellaneous Cases

Case 26: Microcirculatory Insights in Behçet's Disease: Linking Nailfold Capillary Alterations to Ocular Vasculitis

Rahma A. Elziaty
Internal Medicine Department, Rheumatology Division, Faculty of Medicine, Ain Shams University, Cairo, Egypt

Doaa M. Ashour
Department of Ophthalmology, Faculty of Medicine, Ain Shams University, Cairo, Egypt

A 28-year-old man with a 5-year history of Behçet's disease, diagnosed according to the international criteria, presented to the ophthalmology clinic with blurred vision and floaters in both eyes for the past 2 weeks. Fundus examination and fluorescein angiography (FA) revealed bilateral retinal vasculitis involving both arterioles and venules, with diffuse capillary leakage over the posterior pole, including macular and perimacular regions. No areas of retinal neovascularization or major non-perfusion zones were identified. Visual acuity at presentation was moderately reduced (Fig. 15.73).

Given the known systemic vascular involvement in Behçet's disease, the patient was referred for nailfold videocapillaroscopy (NVC) to assess systemic microcirculation status. NVC was performed on eight fingers (excluding thumbs) under standardized conditions.

NVC revealed multiple abnormalities: several tortuous and branched capillaries, occasional enlarged (dilated) loops, and scattered micro-hemorrhages. There was no "scleroderma-type" pattern; capillary density was within lower normal limits but slightly reduced compared to healthy controls (Fig. 15.74).

Based on these findings, the diagnosis of systemic microvascular involvement in Behçet's disease (BD) was affirmed. The ocular findings (retinal vasculitis) were interpreted in the context of underlying systemic microcirculatory changes, suggesting that the retinal vascular inflammation may reflect broader capillary and small-vessel pathology.

The patient was maintained on adalimumab 40 mg subcutaneous injection every 2 weeks and mycophenolate mofetil 2 gm/day with marked improvement of the eye condition. The patient continues follow-up at the uveitis clinic at Ain Shams University hospitals with uveitis MDT, including a rheumatologist and an ophthalmologist.

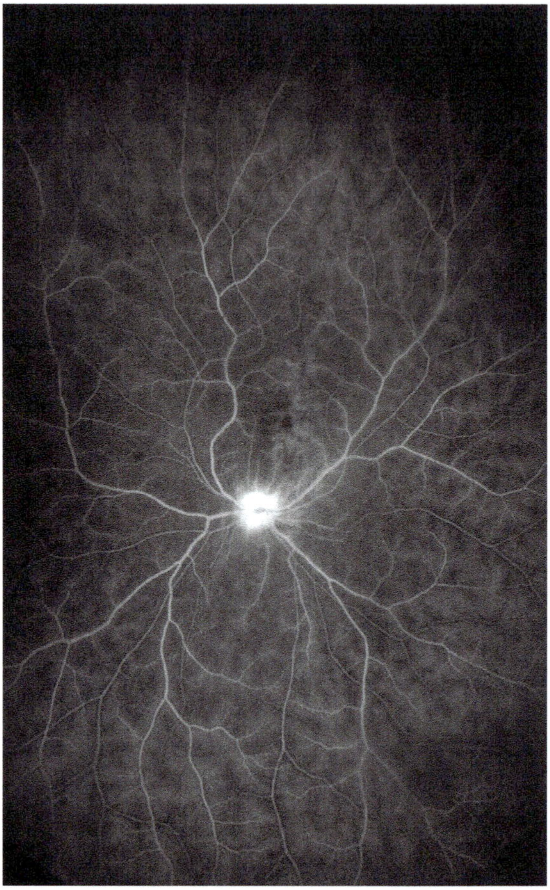

Fig. 15.73 Fundus fluorescein angiography (FFA) revealed retinal vasculitis with diffuse capillary leakage, macular leakage, and hot disk

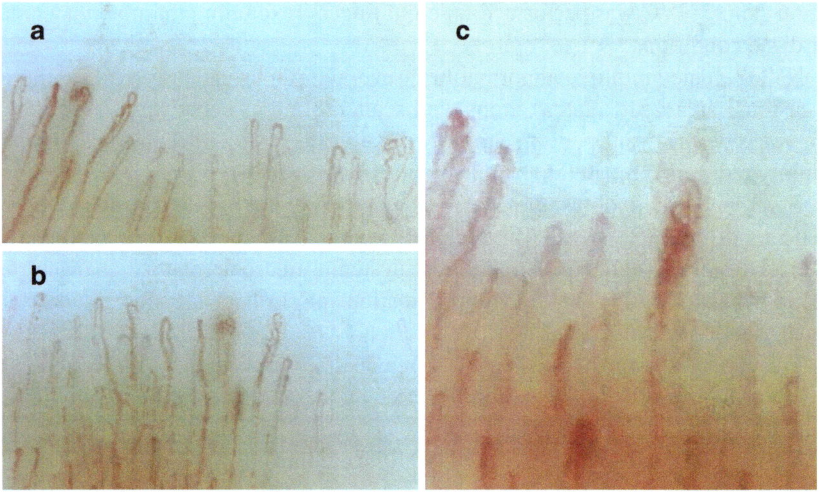

Fig. 15.74 Nailfold capillaroscopy reveals dilated, elongated capillaries with some abnormal-shaped capillaries and microhemorrhages

Discussion

Microvascular involvement is increasingly recognized in Behçet's disease (BD) as an integral component of its vascular phenotype. Nailfold videocapillaroscopy (NVC) offers a noninvasive method for evaluating systemic microcirculation and has been increasingly applied in BD patients both with and without clinically overt vascular manifestations. In a landmark study involving 128 BD patients, approximately 40% demonstrated abnormal nailfold capillaroscopic findings, most frequently enlarged capillaries (26%) and microhemorrhages (16%), while true capillary loss was uncommon [137].

Similarly, subsequent studies comparing BD patients with healthy controls have consistently reported a significantly higher prevalence of capillary dilatation and microhemorrhages in the BD population. In a cohort derived from a national referral center, more than half of BD patients exhibited capillary loop dilatation, increased tortuosity, megacapillaries, and microhemorrhages on periungual capillaroscopy, further supporting the presence of systemic microvascular involvement in this disease [138].

These observations suggest a possible association between systemic microvascular abnormalities detectable by NVC and ocular microvascular inflammation in BD. Capillary dilatation, tortuosity, microhemorrhages, and abnormal capillary morphology likely reflect generalized endothelial dysfunction or microangiopathy, which may predispose to or coexist with retinal vascular involvement.

From an ophthalmologic perspective, retinal vasculitis in BD typically affects both arteries and veins, with diffuse capillary leakage on fluorescein angiography representing a hallmark of active disease. These angiographic changes may precede more advanced manifestations such as vascular occlusion or retinal neovascularization [139, 140]. With the advent of advanced imaging techniques, particularly widefield swept-source optical coherence tomography angiography (OCTA), studies have demonstrated reduced retinal vessel density and enlargement of the foveal avascular zone even during clinically inactive uveitis, indicating persistent microcirculatory damage [141].

Taken together, these findings support the concept that systemic microvascular abnormalities identified by NVC may mirror or even foreshadow ocular microvascular pathology. In the present case, the presence of tortuous, dilated capillaries and microhemorrhages likely reflects generalized capillary fragility and endothelial disruption, which may contribute to the development of retinal vasculitis within the pro-inflammatory environment characteristic of BD.

Nevertheless, it is important to emphasize that capillaroscopic alterations in BD remain nonspecific. Unlike systemic sclerosis, no pathognomonic capillaroscopic pattern has been established for BD. Indeed, in large cohort studies, capillary loss has been rare, and a scleroderma-type pattern has been consistently absent. The variability in reported prevalence and severity of capillaroscopic abnormalities likely reflects heterogeneity in disease duration, activity, and clinical phenotype, including differences between vascular, ocular, and mucocutaneous involvement.

Learning Outcome Points

- Nailfold videocapillaroscopy (NVC) can detect microvascular abnormalities (dilated loops, tortuosity, microhemorrhages, and mega-capillaries) in a substantial subset of patients with Behçet's disease, reflecting systemic microcirculatory involvement.
- In BD patients with ocular involvement (uveitis / retinal vasculitis), NVC seems more likely to show microhemorrhages and abnormal capillary morphology compared to healthy controls—suggesting a potential association between systemic microvascular alterations and ocular microcirculation pathology.
- Systemic microvascular changes (capillary abnormalities) may parallel, or even precede, ocular microvascular involvement; thus, NVC could serve as a noninvasive, supportive tool to identify BD patients at higher risk of ocular vascular complications.
- However, there is no specific capillaroscopic "signature" for BD; findings are nonspecific and cannot substitute for ocular imaging modalities (e.g., FA, OCTA) in diagnosing or monitoring retinal vasculitis.
- Given the heterogeneity of BD and variability of microvascular involvement, combining systemic (NVC) and ocular (OCTA/FA) microcirculation assessments may provide a more comprehensive picture of vascular health and risk stratification in BD patients.

Case 27: Microvascular and Neurological Recovery in RA-Related Vasculitis: Role of Nailfold Capillaroscopy

Rahma A. Elziaty
Internal Medicine Department, Rheumatology Division, Faculty of Medicine, Ain Shams University, Cairo, Egypt

Yasser El Miedany
Canterbury Christ Church University, Canterbury, UK

Rheumatology and Rehabilitation, Ain Shams University, Cairo, Egypt

King's College, London, UK

A 38-year-old woman with a 7-year history of seropositive RA (on methotrexate and low-dose steroids) developed purpuric, tender papules on both lower limbs consistent with cutaneous vasculitis. Simultaneously, she experienced distal limb tingling and sensory disturbance.

Investigations: Elevated ESR/CRP, nerve conduction study revealed *axonal peripheral neuropathy*. Nailfold Capillaroscopy: Showed dilated, tortuous capillaries plus scattered microhemorrhages—indicative of microvascular damage in the context of systemic inflammation.

Other labs: no overlap syndrome identified.

Given the poor response to conventional immunosuppression, rituximab was added (two infusions, anti-CD20 monoclonal antibody) per established protocols.

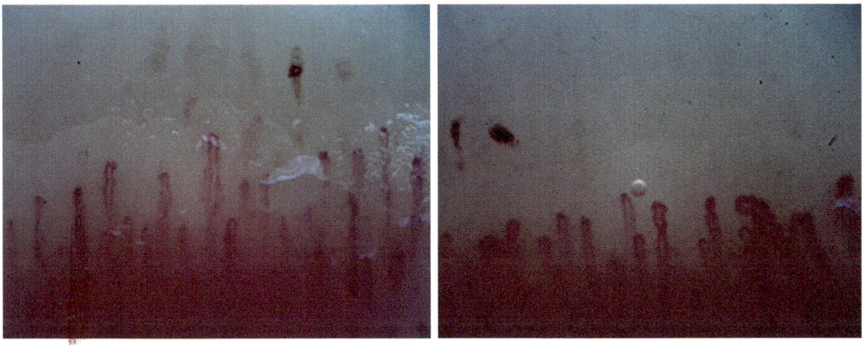

Fig. 15.75 Nailfold capillaroscopy showed normal density, dilated, tortuous capillaries, plus scattered microhemorrhages

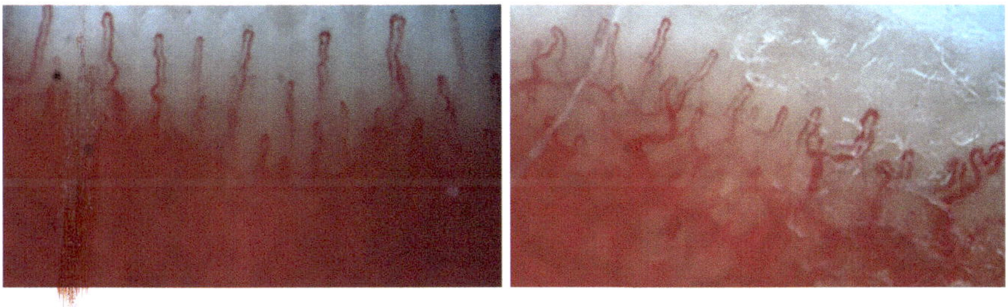

Fig. 15.76 Follow-up NFC demonstrated resolution of microhemorrhages

The corticosteroid dose was tapered. Over subsequent weeks, the skin lesions resolved and tingling subsided (Fig. 15.75). Follow-up NFC demonstrated resolution of microhemorrhages, with capillary morphology appearing improved (Fig. 15.76).

Discussion

Peripheral neuropathy in RA can result from vasculitic involvement of vasa nervorum. In RA, neuropathy may arise from axonal damage secondary to vascular injury [142, 143]. Rituximab has emerged as an effective therapy for refractory RA-associated systemic vasculitis, inducing remission in many patients and enabling steroid-sparing regimens [144].

Nailfold capillaroscopic findings in RA—including dilated and tortuous capillaries and microhemorrhages—are nonspecific but correlate with systemic microvascular involvement, especially in cases complicated by vasculitis [145].

Although NFC is better characterized in diseases like systemic sclerosis, this case illustrates its utility in monitoring microvascular alterations and treatment response in RA-related vasculitic processes. The NFC improvement parallel to clinical remission supports a dynamic microvascular response to immunomodulation—an area meriting further investigation.

This case exemplifies how nailfold capillaroscopy may reveal microvascular damage in RA-related vasculitis and how those changes can reverse following rituximab therapy. It underscores both the role of capillaroscopy in clinical assessment and rituximab's efficacy in treating complex RA phenotypes.

Learning Points

- Nailfold capillaroscopy can serve as a valuable, noninvasive biomarker for monitoring microvascular injury activity and therapeutic response in systemic vasculitic complications of RA.
- Rituximab is a highly effective, guideline-supported biologic agent for refractory, severe, systemic manifestations of RA, particularly RA-related vasculitis, and can induce both clinical and microvascular remission.

Case 28: Capillaroscopic Abnormalities in a Diabetic Patient with Retinopathy and Nephropathy: A Window to Systemic Microangiopathy

Rahma A. Elziaty
Internal Medicine Department, Rheumatology Division, Faculty of Medicine, Ain Shams University, Cairo, Egypt

Yasser El Miedany
Canterbury Christ Church University, Canterbury, UK

Rheumatology and Rehabilitation, Ain Shams University, Cairo, Egypt

King's College, London, UK

A 55-year-old male with a 12-year history of type 2 diabetes mellitus presented to the internal medicine clinic for routine follow-up. He complained of decreased visual acuity over the past year and mild lower limb edema. He denied Raynaud's phenomenon, digital ulcers, or skin changes. His glycemic control over the past few years had been suboptimal (HbA1c ranging between 8.5% and 9.5%).

Medical history included diabetic retinopathy (non-proliferative, confirmed by fundus examination), diabetic nephropathy (eGFR 58 ml/min/1.73 m^2, microalbuminuria 450 mg/day), and hypertension, controlled on ACE inhibitors.

On examination: Blood pressure: 138/84 mmHg, no joint swelling or deformities, no cutaneous signs of connective tissue disease, and no clinical features suggestive of systemic sclerosis, lupus, or vasculitis.

Laboratory data: HbA1c: 9.1%, serum creatinine: 1.4 mg/dL, urinary albumin-to-creatinine ratio: 350 mg/g, ANA and ENA panel: negative, and CRP and ESR: normal.

Nailfold capillaroscopy was performed as part of a vascular microcirculation assessment and showed: Dilated capillary loops, microaneurysms, increased tortuosity, and sparse areas suggestive of early capillary dropout. The findings suggested nonspecific but abnormal microangiopathic changes commonly observed in chronic systemic microvascular disease. No features consistent with scleroderma or

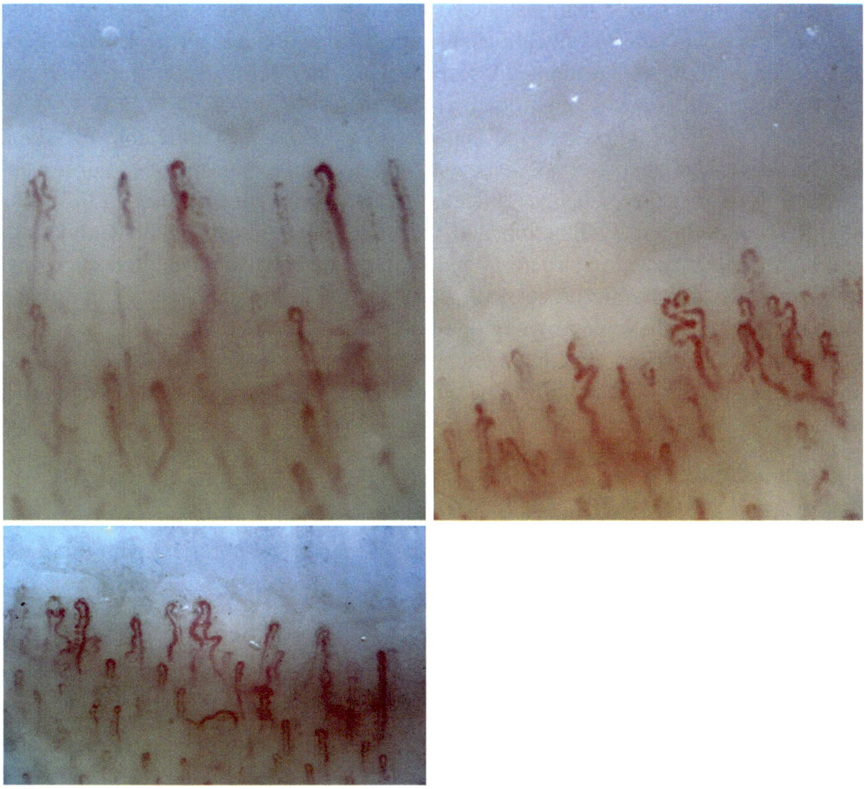

Fig. 15.77 Nailfold capillaroscopy was performed as part of a vascular microcirculation assessment and showed: Dilated capillary loops, microaneurysms, increased tortuosity, and sparse areas of capillary dropout

inflammatory capillaroscopic patterns were observed. The findings were consistent with a Diabetic Microangiopathy Pattern (nonspecific, non-inflammatory microvascular damage) and effectively ruled out a secondary autoimmune vasculopathy (Fig. 15.77).

Discussion

Diabetes mellitus is a chronic metabolic disease characterized by long-term damage to various organ systems, especially the microvasculature. Retinopathy and nephropathy are established complications, reflecting generalized microangiopathic damage. Nailfold capillaroscopy, though primarily used in rheumatology, is increasingly recognized as a tool for assessing microvascular health in non-rheumatic diseases [146].

In this case, capillaroscopy showed significant microvascular abnormalities—including tortuous and dilated capillaries and capillary dropout. These patterns correlate with chronic microvascular injury due to persistent hyperglycemia and oxidative stress.

Multiple studies have demonstrated a link between capillaroscopic changes and diabetic microvascular complications: Capillary dilatation and tortuosity have been associated with diabetic retinopathy severity. Capillary density reduction and drop-out correlate with diabetic nephropathy progression [147, 148].

Unlike scleroderma, where the capillaroscopy shows a predictable evolution (early, active, and late patterns), diabetes typically exhibits nonspecific microvascular alterations, yet these changes reflect systemic microvascular burden [147] This is due to endothelial dysfunction and the buildup of Advanced Glycation End-products (AGEs), causing structural and functional changes. Given that microvascular injury is a systemic process, the capillaroscopic findings may also correlate with the risk of diabetic neuropathy or cardiac microvascular disease.

Regular capillaroscopic assessments in diabetes may potentially serve as a non-invasive biomarker for monitoring microvascular involvement and guiding risk stratification.

Learning Points

- Capillaroscopic findings can reveal nonspecific but significant microvascular changes in patients with diabetic microangiopathy and correlate with the presence and severity of diabetic retinopathy and nephropathy.
- Differentiating capillaroscopic patterns of diabetes from those seen in systemic sclerosis or autoimmune diseases is crucial for accurate interpretation.
- The presence of microaneurysms, capillary dilation, and tortuosity on NFC strongly supports a diagnosis of Diabetic Microangiopathy, helping to rule out autoimmune connective tissue diseases in patients presenting with mild vascular symptoms like Raynaud's-like changes (which can occur in diabetes).

Case 29: Polyarteritis Nodosa Masquerading as Systemic Sclerosis: A Unique Case Challenging the Specificity of Scleroderma Patterns

Rahma A. Elziaty
Internal Medicine Department, Rheumatology Division, Faculty of Medicine, Ain Shams University, Cairo, Egypt

A 31-year-old male presented with a 7-month history of progressive Raynaud's phenomenon, painful digital ischemia, and nonhealing digital ulcers of the fingers. He reported intermittent burning dysesthesias in both feet, accompanied by difficulty walking due to sensory loss. Over the previous two months, she noticed a persistent violaceous, reticular-appearing rash on the left thigh, associated with mild tenderness (Fig. 15.78).

He denied joint swelling, morning stiffness, dysphagia, muscle weakness, breathlessness, or constitutional symptoms. There was no previous diagnosis of connective tissue disease.

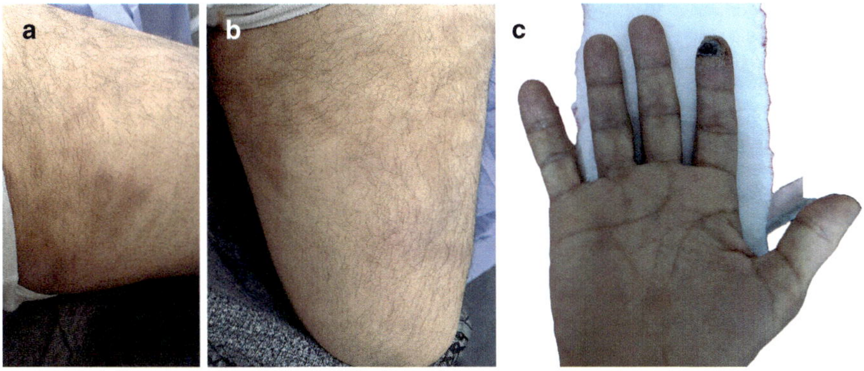

Fig. 15.78 Mottled violaceous rash on the lateral thigh suggestive of livedo-like vasculopathy (**a**, **b**). painful digital ulcer of the right index finger (**c**)

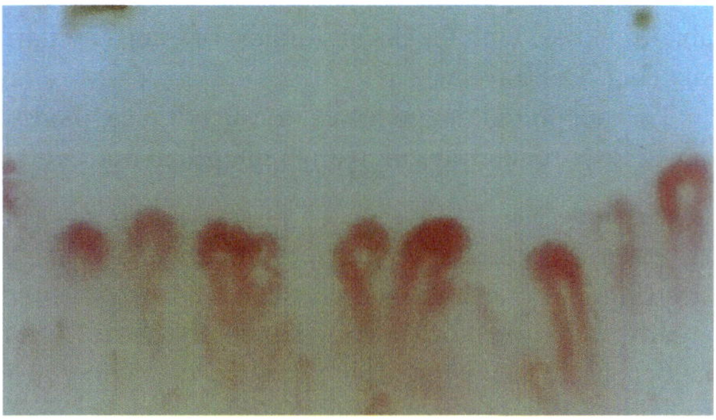

Fig. 15.79 NFC demonstrates early scleroderma pattern

Clinical examination: painful digital ulcer of the right index finger, periungual erythema, and cold fingers. Reduced pinprick and vibration sensation in a stocking distribution; distal weakness (MRC 4/5). Mottled violaceous rash on the lateral thigh suggestive of livedo-like vasculopathy. Vital signs were normal, with no organ-threatening manifestations (Fig. 15.78).

Baseline nailfold video capillaroscopy demonstrated: dilated capillaries, scattered giant capillaries and capillary dropout without ramified and bushy capillaries. This pattern was interpreted as an early scleroderma-type pattern (Fig. 15.79).

Investigations: CBC, renal, and liver function: normal. ESR 30 mm/hr and CRP 10 mg/L. ANA, ENA panel, anti-Scl-70, anti-centromere, and myositis panel: negative. Complement levels: normal. Hepatitis B/C: negative.

Nerve conduction studies showed asymmetrical axonal sensory-motor neuropathy. A sural nerve biopsy revealed transmural necrotizing inflammation of medium-sized arteries with fibrinoid necrosis, consistent with polyarteritis nodosa (PAN).

The patient was started on: High-dose oral corticosteroids, monthly IV cyclophosphamide for 6 months, then transitioned to rituximab (1 g × 2 doses two weeks apart, then every 6 months). Vasodilator therapy included nifedipine and iloprost infusions for Raynaud's and digital ischemia.

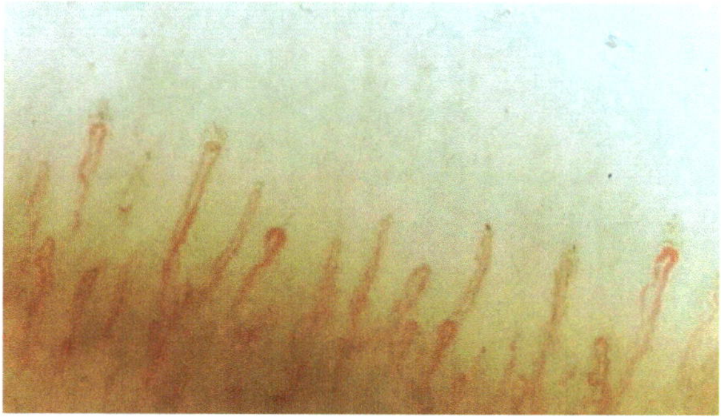

Fig. 15.80 NFC demonstrates a non-Scleroderma pattern of "nonspecific abnormalities"; the presence of dilated capillaries and dots of microhemorrages

Follow-Up: After 8 months: Digital ulcers healed, Raynaud's substantially improved, Neuropathic symptoms regressed, The thigh rash resolved, Inflammatory markers normalized

Capillaroscopy converted from an early scleroderma pattern to nonspecific abnormalities, with the disappearance of giant capillaries and improvement in density (Fig. 15.80).

This supported the interpretation that the capillaroscopic changes were secondary to PAN-related vasculopathy rather than true evolving systemic sclerosis.

Discussion

Polyarteritis nodosa (PAN) is a necrotizing vasculitis primarily affecting medium-sized muscular arteries and characterized by ischemic manifestations in multiple organs, including the skin and peripheral nerves. Digital ulcers and Raynaud's phenomenon are uncommon but recognized features in PAN, typically attributed to ischemia secondary to arterial inflammation and luminal narrowing rather than the microvascular dysfunction seen in systemic sclerosis (SSc) [149, 150]. The presence of Raynaud's and painful digital ischemia in this patient initially raised suspicion for an early connective tissue disease, particularly SSc. However, the absence of SSc-specific autoantibodies and the presence of systemic neuropathy helped widen the differential diagnosis toward a vasculitic process.

The patient's sural nerve biopsy, which demonstrated necrotizing arteritis of medium-sized vessels, was diagnostic for PAN. Mononeuritis multiplex, or asymmetric polyneuropathy, is one of the classical hallmarks of PAN due to ischemia of the vasa nervorum [151]. In parallel, the violaceous rash on the thigh likely represented livedo-like vasculopathy, a cutaneous manifestation frequently reported in PAN and related vasculitides. This constellation of neuropathy, skin involvement, and digital ischemia strongly supports systemic medium-vessel vasculitis rather than primary SSc.

One of the most intriguing findings in this case was the early scleroderma pattern capillaroscopic changes, including giant capillaries and capillary dropout. Nailfold capillaroscopy is classically used to differentiate primary Raynaud's from secondary causes such as systemic sclerosis, where a structured sequence of microvascular abnormalities is well described [152]. However, capillaroscopic abnormalities in vasculitides have been inconsistently reported. Some studies suggest that inflammatory vasculopathies such as PAN and ANCA-associated vasculitis can produce non-SSc-specific abnormalities, including tortuous, dilated, or hemorrhagic capillaries, reflecting endothelial injury and repair mechanisms [153]. The presence of giant capillaries and areas of dropout in this patient may represent severe microvascular damage secondary to PAN-related inflammation rather than hallmark scleroderma microangiopathy.

Importantly, the reversibility of the capillaroscopic abnormalities after effective immunosuppressive therapy and rituximab strongly argues against evolving systemic sclerosis. In SSc, capillary dropout and giant capillaries generally persist or progress over time, while in inflammatory vasculitis, microvascular damage may improve once inflammation is controlled. The return from an early scleroderma pattern to nonspecific changes suggests that PAN-related microangiopathy can transiently mimic scleroderma-like features, underlining the importance of integrating clinical findings, serology, and biopsy results when interpreting capillaroscopy.

Rituximab has emerged as a therapeutic option in refractory or atypical PAN, particularly in patients with significant neuropathic involvement. Although evidence is limited, case reports and small series show beneficial outcomes with rituximab in both HBV-negative PAN and ANCA-associated vasculitides with medium-vessel overlap features [154]. In this case, rituximab contributed to significant improvement of digital ischemia, neuropathy, and microvascular capillaroscopic abnormalities, emphasizing its role in disease modulation.

Overall, this case illustrates the complexity of diagnosing vasculitic syndromes presenting with Raynaud's phenomenon and capillaroscopic changes mimicking early systemic sclerosis. Clinicians should maintain a broad differential diagnosis when assessing Raynaud's with digital ulcers, especially when neuropathy or livedo-like rashes coexist.

Learning Outcome Points

- Raynaud's phenomenon and digital ulcers can rarely occur in polyarteritis nodosa, mimicking systemic sclerosis.
- Capillaroscopic abnormalities in vasculitis may transiently resemble a scleroderma pattern but can improve with treatment, unlike true SSc microangiopathy.
- A negative autoimmune panel and the presence of neuropathy should raise suspicion for vasculitis rather than primary connective tissue disease.
- Rituximab can be effective in PAN with refractory vasculopathy or neuropathy.
- Integration of clinical, serological, microvascular, and histopathological data is essential for accurate diagnosis.

Acknowledgments We extend our sincere gratitude to all contributing authors and clinicians who generously shared their cases, images, and clinical insights for this chapter. Their dedication to patient care, meticulous documentation, and commitment to advancing medical knowledge made this compilation possible. Their contributions will undoubtedly serve as a valuable resource for the medical community and foster further expertise in nailfold capillaroscopy.

References

1. Cutolo M, Sulli A, Smith V. How to perform and interpret capillaroscopy. Best Pract Res Clin Rheumatol. 2010;24(3):363–72. https://doi.org/10.1016/j.berh.2009.12.001.

Case 1

2. Avouac J, Fransen J, Walker UA, et al. Preliminary criteria for the very early diagnosis of systemic sclerosis: results of a Delphi Consensus Study from EULAR Scleroderma Trials and Research Group [J]. Ann Rheum Dis. 2011;70(3):476–81.
3. van den Hoogen F, Khanna D, Fransen J, et al. 2013 classification criteria for systemic sclerosis: an American college of rheumatology/European league against rheumatism collaborative initiative. Ann Rheum Dis. 2013;72(11):1747–55.
4. Bellando-Randone S, Del Galdo F, Lepri G, et al. Progression of patients with Raynaud's phenomenon to systemic sclerosis: a five-year analysis of the European Scleroderma Trial and Research group multicentre, longitudinal registry study for Very Early Diagnosis of Systemic Sclerosis (VEDOSS). Lancet Rheumatol. 2021;3(12):e834–43.
5. Lepri G, Guiducci S, Bellando-Randone S, et al. Evidence for oesophageal and anorectal involvement in very early systemic sclerosis (VEDOSS): report from a single VEDOSS/EUSTAR centre. Ann Rheum Dis. 2015;74:124–8.
6. Gotschy A, Jordan S, Stoeck CT, et al. Diffuse myocardial fibrosis precedes subclinical functional myocardial impairment and provides prognostic information in systemic sclerosis. Eur Heart J Cardiovasc Imaging. 2023;24(3):373–82.
7. Ross RL, Caballero-Ruiz B, Clarke EL, et al. Biological hallmarks of systemic sclerosis are present in the skin and serum of patients with Very Early Diagnosis of Systemic Sclerosis (VEDOSS). Rheumatology (Oxford). 2025;64(6):3606–17.
8. Bellando-Randone S, Del Galdo F, Matucci-Cerinic M. Insights into molecular and clinical characteristics of very early systemic sclerosis. Curr Opin Rheumatol. 2022;34(6):351–6.

Case 2

9. Smith V, et al.; EULAR Study Group on Microcirculation in Rheumatic Diseases and the Scleroderma Clinical Trials Consortium Group on Capillaroscopy. Standardisation of nailfold capillaroscopy for the assessment of patients with Raynaud's phenomenon and systemic sclerosis. Autoimmun Rev. 2020;19(3):102458. https://doi.org/10.1016/j.autrev.2020.102458. Epub 2020 Jan 10.
10. Santiago T, et al. Portuguese Recommendations for the management of Raynaud's phenomenon and digital ulcers in systemic sclerosis and other connective tissue diseases. ARP Rheumatol. 2024;3(2):84–94. English
11. Del Galdo F, Lescoat A, Conaghan PG, et al. EULAR recommendations for the treatment of systemic sclerosis: 2023 updateAnnals of the Rheumatic Diseases Published Online First: 11 October 2024. https://doi.org/10.1136/ard-2024-226430.
12. Smith V, et al.; EULAR Study Group on Microcirculation in Rheumatic Diseases. Fast track algorithm: How to differentiate a "scleroderma pattern" from a "non-scleroderma pattern". Autoimmun Rev. 2019;18(11):102394. https://doi.org/10.1016/j.autrev.2019.102394. Epub 2019 Sep 11.

Case 3

13. Cutolo M, Sulli A, Smith V. Assessing microvascular changes in systemic sclerosis diagnosis and management. Nat Rev Rheumatol. 2010;6:578–87.
14. Smith V, Vanhaecke A, Herrick AL, et al. EULAR Study Group on Microcirculation in Rheumatic Diseases. Fast track algorithm: How to differentiate a "scleroderma pattern" from a "non-sclerodern pattern". Autoimmun Rev. 2019;18(11):102394.
15. Patil A, Sood I. (2020). Nailfold capillaroscopy in rheumatic diseases. https://doi.org/10.5772/intechopen.92786.
16. Cutolo M. Capillaroscopy a safe and direct method for SSc diagnosis. The Rheumatologist; June 2011.
17. Cutolo M, Melsens K, Wijnant S, Ingegnoli F, Thevissen K, De Keyser F, Decuman S, Müller-Ladner U, Piette Y, Riccieri V, Ughi N, Vandecasteele E, Vanhaecke A, Smith V. Nailfold capillaroscopy in systemic lupus erythematosus: A systematic review and critical appraisal. Autoimmun Rev. 2018;17(4):344–52.
18. LeRoy EC, Medsger TA Jr. Criteria for the classification of early systemic sclerosis. J Rheumatol. 2001;28(7):1573–6.
19. Koenig M., Joyal F., Fritzler M. J., Roussin A., Abrahamowicz M., Boire G., Goulet J.-R., Rich É., Grodzicky T., Raymond Y., and Senécal J.-L., Autoantibodies and microvascular damage are independent predictive factors for the progression of Raynaud's phenomenon to systemic sclerosis: a twenty-year prospective study of 586 patients, with validation of proposed criteria for early systemic sclerosis, Arthritis and Rheumatism. (2008) 58, no. 12, 3902–3912, 2-s2.0-57349116070.
20. Makarem YS, Selim ZI, Ismail S, Imam Mekkawy A, Galal H, El Nouby FH. Nailfold capillaroscopy changes in systemic lupus erythematosus patients: Correlation with disease activity and anti-uridin1-ribonucleoprotein antibodies. Reumatol Clin (Engl Ed). 2025;21(3):501840.

Case 4

21. Mihai C, Landewé R, van der Heijde D, et al., incl. EUSTAR co-authors. Digital ulcers predict a worse disease course in patients with systemic sclerosis. Ann Rheum Dis. 2016;75:681-686.
22. Sulli A, Secchi ME, Pizzorni C, et al. Scoring the nailfold microvascular changes during capillaroscopic analysis in systemic sclerosis patients. Ann Rheum Dis. 2008;67:885–7.
23. Avouac J, Smith V, Wipff J, et al. Sequential nailfold videocapillaroscopy examinations have responsiveness to detect organ progression in systemic sclerosis. Semin Arthritis Rheum. 2017;47:86–94.
24. Ingegnoli F, Boracchi P, Gualtierotti R, et al. Nailfold capillaroscopy in systemic sclerosis: data from the EULAR Scleroderma Trials and Research (EUSTAR) database. Microvasc Res. 2013;89:122–8.
25. Gheorghiu AM, Oneata R, Ancuta I, et al. Capillary loss reflects disease activity and prognosis in patients with systemic sclerosis. Exp Ther Med. 2020;20:3438–43.
26. Del Galdo F, Allanore Y, Distler O, et al. EULAR recommendations for the treatment of systemic sclerosis: 2023 update. Ann Rheum Dis. 2025;84:29–40.
27. Lauterbach G, Dobrota R, Mihai C, Distler O, Calcagni M, Maurer B, et al. Evaluation of botulinum toxin A injections for the treatment of refractory chronic digital ulcers in patients with systemic sclerosis. Clin Exp Rheumatol. 2020;38(Suppl 125):S154–60.
28. Chiou G, Crowe C, Suarez P, Chung L, Curtin C, Chang J, et al. Digital sympathectomy in patients with scleroderma. Ann Plast Surg. 2015;75:637–43.

Case 5

29. van den Hoogen F, et al. 2013 Classification Criteria for Systemic Sclerosis. Arthritis Rheum. 2013;65(11):2737–47. https://doi.org/10.1002/art.38098.
30. Sebastiani M, Manfredi A, Vukatana G. Predictive role of capillaroscopic skin ulcer risk index in systemic sclerosis: a multicentre validation study. Ann Rheum Dis. 2012;71(1):67–70.
31. Hughes M, Allanore Y, Chung L, Pauling JD, Denton CP, Matucci-Cerinic M. Raynaud phenomenon and digital ulcers in systemic sclerosis. Nat Rev Rheumatol. 2020;16(4):208–21. https://doi.org/10.1038/s41584-020-0386-4.
32. Del Galdo F, et al. EULAR recommendations for the treatment of systemic sclerosis: 2023 update. Ann Rheum Dis. 2025 Jan;84(1):29–40. https://doi.org/10.1136/ard-2024-226430.

Case 6

33. Steen VD, Medsger TA Jr. Case–control study of corticosteroids and other drugs that either precipitate or protect from the development of scleroderma renal crisis. Arthritis Rheum. 1998;41(9):1613–9.
34. Maurizio Cutolo M, Pizzorni C, Sulli A, Smith V. Early diagnostic and predictive value of capillaroscopy in systemic sclerosis. Curr Rheumatol Rev. 2013;9(4):249–53. https://doi.org/10.2174/157339710904140417125010.
35. Ye W, Cao L, Zhou Y, et al. Active pattern on nailfold capillaroscopy in a patient with systemic sclerosis. Rheumatol Immunol Res. 2023;4(3):171–2. https://doi.org/10.2478/rir-2023-0025.
36. Vanhaecke A, Cutolo M, Distler O, et al. The EULAR Study Group on Microcirculation in Rheumatic Diseases. Nailfold capillaroscopy in SSc: innocent bystander or promising biomarker for novel severe organ involvement/progression? Rheumatology (Oxford). 2022;61(11):4384–96. https://doi.org/10.1093/rheumatology/keac079.
37. Raut S, Acharya S, Kumar S, et al. A case of diffuse scleroderma presenting as hypertensive encephalopathy due to scleroderma renal crisis. Cureus. 2024;16(6):e61732. https://doi.org/10.7759/cureus.61732.
38. Gigante A, Leodori G, Pellicano C. Assessment of kidney involvement in systemic sclerosis: From scleroderma renal crisis to subclinical renal vasculopathy. Am J Med. 2022;364(5):529–37.

Case 7

39. Smith V, Herrick AL, Ingegnoli F, Abignano G, Allanore Y, Damjanov N, et al. Standardization of nailfold capillaroscopy in systemic sclerosis: EULAR recommendations update. Ann Rheum Dis. 2020;79(6):745–53.
40. Sieiro Santos C, Ojeda Martínez J, Calzada Antolín S, Gómez Herrero J, de la Calle LJ, Sánchez Herránz L, Bollo de Miguel E, Rodríguez Guerrero M, Díez ÁE. Prognostic value of baseline nailfold videocapillaroscopy in predicting pulmonary decline and disease progression in systemic sclerosis. Rheumatology (Oxford). 2025;64:keaf361. https://doi.org/10.1093/rheumatology/keaf361.
41. Valera-Ribera C, Alegre-Sancho JJ, Lacasa-Molina J, Robustillo-Villarino M, Narváez J. Nailfold capillaroscopy as a predictor of major cardiovascular events and mortality in systemic sclerosis. Semin Arthritis Rheum. 2025;75:152845. https://doi.org/10.1016/j.semarthrit.2025.152845.

42. Pagkopoulou E, Soulaidopoulos S, Triantafyllidou E, Arvanitaki A, Katsiki N, Loutradis C, Karagiannis A, Doumas M, Garyfallos A, Kitas GD, Dimitroulas T. Peripheral microcirculatory abnormalities are associated with cardiovascular risk in systemic sclerosis: a nailfold video capillaroscopy study. Clin Rheumatol. 2021;40(12):4957–68. https://doi.org/10.1007/s10067-021-05795-4.

Case 8

43. Rodríguez Y, Novelli L, Rojas M, et al. Autoinflammatory and autoimmune conditions at the crossroad of COVID-19. J Autoimmun. 2020;114:102506. https://doi.org/10.1016/j.jaut.2020.102506. Epub 2020 Jun 16.
44. Fineschi S. Case report: systemic sclerosis after Covid-19 infection. Front Immunol. 2021;12:686699. https://doi.org/10.3389/fimmu.2021.686699. eCollection 2021.
45. Chandra A, Kahaleh B. Systemic Sclerosis (SSc) after COVID-19: a case report. Cureus. 2022;14(3):e23179. https://doi.org/10.7759/cureus.23179. eCollection 2022 Mar.
46. Oli P, Poudel P, Kc S, et al. Systemic sclerosis (positive anti-Ro 52 and anti-centromere antibodies) in a patient after COVID-19 infection: a rare case report. Ann Med Surg (Lond). 2024;86(6):3663–6. https://doi.org/10.1097/MS9.0000000000002032. eCollection 2024 Jun.
47. Spagnolo P, Balestro E, Aliberti S, et al. Pulmonary fibrosis secondary to COVID-19: a call to arms? Lancet Respir Med. 2020;8(8):750–2. https://doi.org/10.1016/S2213-2600(20)30222-8. Epub 2020 May 15.7.
48. Daoussis D, Liossis S-NC, Tsamandas AC, et al. Experience with rituximab in scleroderma: results from a 1-year, proof-of-principle study. Rheumatology (Oxford). 2010;49(2):271–80. https://doi.org/10.1093/rheumatology/kep093. Epub 2009 May 15
49. Tashkin DP, Roth MD, Clements PJ, et al. Mycophenolate mofetil versus oral cyclophosphamide in scleroderma-related interstitial lung disease (SLS II): a randomised controlled, double-blind, parallel group trial. Lancet Respir Med. 2016;4(9):708–19. https://doi.org/10.1016/S2213-2600(16)30152-7. Epub 2016 Jul 25

Case 9

50. Amaral MC, et al. Re-evaluation of nailfold capillaroscopy in discriminating primary from secondary Raynaud's phenomenon and in predicting systemic sclerosis: a randomised observational prospective cohort study. Expert Rev Clin Immunol. 2024;20(6):665–72. https://doi.org/10.1080/1744666X.2024.2313642.
51. Correia AM, et al. Differences in nailfold capillaroscopy findings between limited and diffuse cutaneous systemic sclerosis: a detailed analysis. RMD open. 2025;11(3):e005716. https://doi.org/10.1136/rmdopen-2025-005716.
52. Kubo S, Tanaka Y. Usefulness of nailfold videocapillaroscopy for systemic sclerosis. Inflamm Regener. 2016;36:5. https://doi.org/10.1186/s41232-016-0001-x.

Case 10

53. Parmar MS, Muppidi V, Bashir K. Gitelman Syndrome. [Updated 2024 Apr 7]. In: StatPearls [Internet]. Treasure Island (FL): StatPearls Publishing; 2025.
54. Nihtyanova SI, Ong VH, Denton CP, et al. Improved survival in systemic sclerosis is associated with better ascertainment of internal organ disease: a retrospective cohort study. QJM. 2010;103:109–15.

55. Launay D, Sobanski V, Hachulla E, et al. Pulmonary hypertension in systemic sclerosis: different phenotypes. Eur Respir Rev. 2017;26:170056.
56. Distler O, Hoffmann-Vold AM, Humbert M, et al. Performance of DETECT pulmonary arterial hypertension algorithm according to the hemodynamic definition of pulmonary arterial hypertension in the 2022 European Society of Cardiology and the European Respiratory Society Guidelines. Arthritis Rheumatol. 2024;76:777–82.
57. Masab M, Goyal A, Abrol S, Rangaswami J. Acquired Gitelman Syndrome associated with systemic sclerosis. Cureus. 2019;11(1):e3923.
58. Hinschberger O, Martzolff L, Ioannou G, et al. Syndrome de Gitelman acquis au cours d'un syndrome de Gougerot-Sjögren associé à une sclérodermie [Acquired Gitelman syndrome associated with Sjögren's syndrome and scleroderma]. Rev Med Interne. 2011;32:e96–8.
59. Lescoat A, Yelnik CM, Coiffier G, et al. Ulnar artery occlusion and severity markers of vasculopathy in systemic sclerosis: a multicenter cross-sectional study. Arthritis Rheumatol. 2019;71:983–90.

Case 11

60. LeRoy EC, Medsger TA Jr. Criteria for the classification of early systemic sclerosis. J Rheumatol. 2001;28(7):1573–6.
61. Torres Villarreal MC, Cajas Santana LJ. Prevalence and risk factors of interstitial lung disease in early systemic sclerosis and systemic sclerosis sine scleroderma: a cross-sectional study. ARP Rheumatol. 2025;4:5–12.
62. Smith V, Herrick AL, Ingegnoli F, et al. Standardisation of nailfold capillaroscopy for the assessment of patients with Raynaud's phenomenon and systemic sclerosis. Autoimmun Rev. 2020;19(3):102458.
63. Tashkin DP, Roth MD, Clements PJ, et al. Mycophenolate mofetil vs. oral cyclophosphamide in SSc-related ILD (SLS II). Lancet. Respir Med. 2016;4(9):708–19.

Case 12

64. Cutolo M, Smith V. State of the art on nailfold capillaroscopy: a reliable diagnostic tool and putative biomarker in rheumatology? Rheumatology (Oxford). 2013;52(11):1933–40. https://doi.org/10.1093/rheumatology/ket153. Epub 2013 Apr 25.
65. Santana-Gonçalves M, Zanin-Silva D, Henrique-Neto Á, Moraes DA, Kawashima-Vasconcelos MY, Lima-Júnior JR, Dias JBE, Bragagnollo V, de Azevedo JTC, Covas DT, Malmegrim KCR, Ramalho L, Oliveira MC. Autologous hematopoietic stem cell transplantation modifies specific aspects of systemic sclerosis-related microvasculopathy. Ther Adv Musculoskelet Dis. 2022;14:1759720X221084845. https://doi.org/10.1177/1759720X221084845. PMID: 35368373; PMCID: PMC8966069.
66. Miniati I, Guiducci S, Conforti ML, Rogai V, Fiori G, Cinelli M, Saccardi R, Guidi S, Bosi A, Tyndall A, Matucci-Cerinic M. Autologous stem cell transplantation improves microcirculation in systemic sclerosis. Ann Rheum Dis. 2009;68(1):94–8. https://doi.org/10.1136/ard.2007.082495. Epub 2008 Feb 28.
67. Burt RK, et al. Autologous non-myeloablative haemopoietic stem-cell transplantation compared with pulse cyclophosphamide once per month for systemic sclerosis (ASSIST). Lancet. 2011;378:498–506.
68. van Laar JM, et al. Autologous hematopoietic stem-cell transplantation in systemic sclerosis (ASTIS): a randomised controlled trial. JAMA. 2014;311(24):2490–8.
69. Sullivan KM, et al. Myeloablative autologous stem-cell transplantation for severe scleroderma. N Engl J Med. 2018;378(1):35–47.

Case 13

70. Shah AA, Rosen LC. Cancer and scleroderma: a paraneoplastic disease with implications for malignancy screening. Curr Opin Rheumatol. 2015;27(6):563–70. https://doi.org/10.1097/BOR.0000000000000222.
71. Gabriel POKHAI, Rino BUZZOLA, Adriana ABRUDESCU. Letrozole-induced very early systemic sclerosis in a patient with breast cancer: a case report. Arch Rheumatol. 2014;29(2):126–9.
72. Smith V, Herrick AL, Ingegnoli F, et al. Standardisation of nailfold capillaroscopy for the assessment of patients with Raynaud's phenomenon and systemic sclerosis. Autoimmun Rev. 2020;19(3):102458. https://doi.org/10.1016/j.autrev.2019.102458.
73. Pérez-Bucio C, Behere A, Landegren N. Mechanisms of autoimmune-mediated paraneoplastic syndromes: immune tolerance and disease pathogenesis. Front Immunol. 2025;9(16):1608934. https://doi.org/10.3389/fimmu.2025.1608934.
74. Tashkin DP, Roth MD, Clements PJ, et al. Mycophenolate mofetil vs. oral cyclophosphamide in SSc-related ILD (SLS II). Lancet Respir Med. 2016;4(9):708–19.

Case 14

75. Hamaguchi Y. Drug-induced scleroderma-like lesion. Allergol Int. 2022;71(2):163–8. https://doi.org/10.1016/j.alit.2021.08.005.
76. Guillot B, Bessis D, Dereure O. Mucocutaneous side effects of antineoplastic chemotherapy. Expert Opin Drug Saf. 2004;3(6):579–87. https://doi.org/10.1517/14740338.3.6.579.
77. Cozzani E, Iurlo A, Merlo G, Cattaneo D, Burlando M, Pierri I, et al. Essential thrombocythemia: the dermatologic point of view. Clin Lymphoma Myeloma Leuk. 2015;15(12):739–47. https://doi.org/10.1016/j.clml.2015.08.086.
78. Bouquet É, Urbanski G, Lavigne C, Lainé-Cessac P. Unexpected drug-induced Raynaud phenomenon: analysis from the French national pharmacovigilance database. Therapie. 2017;72(5):547–54. https://doi.org/10.1016/j.therap.2017.01.008.
79. García-Martínez FJ, García-Gavín J, Alvarez-Pérez A, Alonso-González J, Ginarte M, Toribio J. Scleroderma-like syndrome due to hydroxyurea. Clin Exp Dermatol. 2012;37(7):755–8. https://doi.org/10.1111/j.1365-2230.2011.04326.x.
80. Martín Guerra JM, Martín Asenjo M, Miramontes González JP, Prieto de Paula JM. Sclerodermiform Syndrome induced by hydroxycarbamide. J Clin Rheumatol. 2021;27(8S):S465. https://doi.org/10.1097/RHU.0000000000001230.
81. Stoica LE, Mitroi MR, Ică OM, Vîlcea AM, Fronie-Andrei LP, Vîlcea CI, et al. Dermatomyositis-like eruption induced by hydroxyurea-case report and literature review. J Clin Med. 2025;14(7):2192. https://doi.org/10.3390/jcm14072192.

Case 15

82. Tyndall A, Fistarol S. The differential diagnosis of systemic sclerosis. Curr Opin Rheumatol. 2013;25(6):692–9. https://doi.org/10.1097/01.bor.0000434599.51526.47.
83. Selva-O'Callaghan A, Trallero-Araguás E, Gil-Vila A, et al. Treatment and monitoring of eosinophilic fasciitis. Curr Treat Options in Rheum. 2025;11:3. https://doi.org/10.1007/s40674-024-00222-6.
84. Salam S, Dimachkie MM, Hanna MG, Machado PM. Diagnostic and prognostic value of anti-cN1A antibodies in inclusion body myositis. Clin Exp Rheumatol. 2022;40(2):384–93. https://doi.org/10.55563/clinexprheumatol/r625rm. Epub 2022 Jan 25

Case 16

85. Fett N, Werth VP. Update on morphea: part I. Epidemiology, clinical presentation, and pathogenesis. J Am Acad Dermatol. 2011;64(2):217–28; quiz 229-30. https://doi.org/10.1016/j.jaad.2010.05.045.
86. Denton CP, Khanna D. Systemic sclerosis. Lancet. 2017;390(10103):1685–99. https://doi.org/10.1016/S0140-6736(17)30933-9. Epub 2017 Apr 13.
87. Cutolo M, Pizzorni C, Sulli A. Nailfold videocapillaroscopy in systemic sclerosis. Z Rheumatol. 2004;63(6):457–62. https://doi.org/10.1007/s00393-004-0673-5.
88. Mostmans Y, Richert B, Badot V, et al. The importance of skin manifestations, serology and nailfold (video)capillaroscopy in morphea and systemic sclerosis: current understanding and new insights. J Eur Acad Dermatol Venereol. 2021;35(3):597–606. https://doi.org/10.1111/jdv.16813. Epub 2020 Aug 5
89. Duran J, Plaza JA. Morphea and systemic sclerosis. PathologyOutlines.com website. https://www.pathologyoutlines.com/topic/skinnontumorscleroderma.html. Accessed 18 Dec 2025.
90. Tharappel DCP, Ballal S, Kalegowda IY. Histopathologic study of morphea. Indian J Dermatol Venereol Leprol. 2025;91:257–60. https://doi.org/10.25259/IJDVL_316_2024.
91. Papara C, De Luca DA, Bieber K, et al. Morphea: the 2023 update. Front Med (Lausanne). 2023;10:1108623. https://doi.org/10.3389/fmed.2023.1108623. eCollection 2023.

Case 17

92. Cutolo M, Smith V. State of the art on nailfold capillaroscopy: a reliable diagnostic tool and putative biomarker in rheumatology? Rheumatology (Oxford). 2013;52(11):1933–40. https://doi.org/10.1093/rheumatology/ket153.
93. Smith V, Herrick AL, Ingegnoli F, et al. Standardisation of nailfold capillaroscopy for the assessment of patients with Raynaud's phenomenon and systemic sclerosis. Autoimmun Rev. 2020;19(3):102458. https://doi.org/10.1016/j.autrev.2020.102458.
94. Parker MJS, McGill NW. The established and evolving role of nailfold capillaroscopy in connective-tissue disease. In: Connective tissue disease – current state of the art. IntechOpen; 2020. https://doi.org/10.5772/intechopen.82386.
95. Wiąk-Walerowicz K, Wielosz E, Majdan M. The usefulness of nailfold capillaroscopy in scleroderma spectrum disorders: a single-centre observational study. Adv Dermatol Allergol. 2024;41(3):296–300. https://doi.org/10.5114/ada.2024.141158.
96. Hui X, Qian J. The role of nailfold video-capillaroscopy in the assessment of dermatomyositis. Rheumatology. 2025;64(5):2987–94. https://doi.org/10.1093/rheumatology/keae677.
97. Honda M, Shimizu F, Sato R, Nakamori M. Contribution of complement, microangiopathy and inflammation in idiopathic inflammatory myopathies. J Neuromuscul Dis. 2024;11(1):5–16. https://doi.org/10.3233/JND-230168.
98. Piette Y, Reynaert V, Vanhaecke A, et al. Standardised interpretation of capillaroscopy in autoimmune idiopathic inflammatory myopathies: a structured review on behalf of the EULAR study group on microcirculation in Rheumatic Diseases. Autoimmun Rev. 2022;21(6):103087. https://doi.org/10.1016/j.autrev.2022.103087.
99. Bogojevic M, Markovic Vlaisavljevic M, Medjedovic R, Strujic E, Pravilovic Lutovac D, Pavlov-Dolijanovic S. Nailfold Capillaroscopy changes in patients with idiopathic inflammatory myopathies. J Clin Med. 2024;13(18):5550. https://doi.org/10.3390/jcm13185550. Published 2024 Sep 19.
100. Chanprapaph K, Fakprapai W, Limtong P, Suchonwanit P. Nailfold capillaroscopy with USB digital microscopy in connective tissue diseases: a comparative study of 245 patients and healthy controls. Front Med (Lausanne). 2021;8:683900. Published 2021 Aug 6. https://doi.org/10.3389/fmed.2021.683900.

101. Fiorentino DF, Casciola-Rosen L. Autoantibodies and Cancer Association: the case of systemic sclerosis and dermatomyositis. Clin Rev Allergy Immunol. 2022;63(3):330–41. https://doi.org/10.1007/s12016-022-08944-y.
102. Betteridge ZE, Gunawardena H, Chinoy H, et al. Clinical and human leucocyte antigen class II haplotype associations of autoantibodies to small ubiquitin-like modifier enzyme, a dermatomyositis-specific autoantigen target, in UK Caucasian adult-onset myositis. Ann Rheum Dis. 2009;68(10):1621–5. https://doi.org/10.1136/ard.2008.097162.
103. Johnson D, van Eeden C, Moazab N, et al. Nailfold capillaroscopy abnormalities correlate with disease activity in adult dermatomyositis. Front Med (Lausanne). 2021;8:708432. Published 2021 Aug 10. https://doi.org/10.3389/fmed.2021.708432.
104. Doğantan Ş, Taşkın SN, Paç Kısaarslan A, Poyrazoğlu MH. Nail-fold capillaroscopic changes in children with juvenile dermatomyositis and specific autoantibodies. Med J Bakirkoy. 2025;21:39–47.
105. Mumtaz S, Phillipps J, Sullivan MM, et al. Microvascular abnormalities between anti-TIF1-γ-associated dermatomyositis with and without malignancy. BMC Rheumatol. 2025;9(1):50. Published 2025 May 6. https://doi.org/10.1186/s41927-025-00504-z.

Case 19

106. Sontheimer RD. Clinically amyopathic dermatomyositis: what can we now tell our patients? Arch Dermatol. 2010;146(1):76–80. https://doi.org/10.1001/archdermatol.2009.323.
107. Christen-Zaech S, Seshadri R, Sundberg J, Paller AS, Pachman LM. Persistent association of nailfold capillaroscopy changes and skin involvement over thirty-six months with duration of untreated disease in patients with juvenile dermatomyositis. Arthritis Rheum. 2008;58(2):571–6. https://doi.org/10.1002/art.23299.
108. Pachman LM, Morgan G, Klein Gitelman MS, et al. Nailfold capillary density in 140 untreated children with juvenile dermatomyositis: an indicator of disease activity. Pediatr Rheumatol. 2023;21(1):118. https://doi.org/10.1186/s12969-023-00903-x.

Case 20

109. Oldroyd AGS, Callen JP, Chinoy H, Chung L, Fiorentino D, Gordon P, et al. International Myositis Assessment and Clinical Studies Group Cancer Screening Expert Group. International guideline for idiopathic inflammatory myopathy–associated cancer screening: an International Myositis Assessment and Clinical Studies Group (IMACS) initiative. Nat Rev Rheumatol. 2023;19(12):805–17. https://doi.org/10.1038/s41584-023-01045-w.
110. Bica PF, Hysa E, Campitiello R, Sulli A, Pizzorni C, Gotelli E, et al. Nailfold videocapillaroscopy in juvenile dermatomyositis: detailed correlations between microvascular abnormalities with clinical and laboratory parameters from an observational retrospective single-center study. Clin Rheumatol. 2025;44(9):3615–27. https://doi.org/10.1007/s10067-025-07561-2.
111. Radzikowska E, Fijolek J. Update on cryptogenic organizing pneumonia. Front Med (Lausanne). 2023;10:1146782. https://doi.org/10.3389/fmcd.2023.1146782.

Case 21

112. Herrick AL. Pathogenesis of Raynaud's phenomenon. Rheumatology. 2005;44(5):587–96.
113. Barbacki A, Rached-d'Astous N, Pineau CA, Vinet E, Grenier LP, Kalache F, et al. Clinical significance of Raynaud phenomenon in systemic lupus erythematosus. JCR J Clin Rheumatol. 2022;28(2):e488.

114. Heimovski FE, Simioni JA, Skare TL. Systemic lupus erythematosus and Raynaud's phenomenon. An Bras Dermatol. 2015;90(6):837–40.
115. Cutolo M, Melsens K, Wijnant S, Ingegnoli F, Thevissen K, De Keyser F, et al. Nailfold capillaroscopy in systemic lupus erythematosus: a systematic review and critical appraisal. Autoimmun Rev. 2018;17(4):344–52.
116. Kuryliszyn-Moskal A, Ciolkiewicz M, Klimiuk PA, Sierakowski S. Clinical significance of nailfold capillaroscopy in systemic lupus erythematosus: correlation with endothelial cell activation markers and disease activity. Scand J Rheumatol. 2009;38(1):38–45.
117. Riccieri V, Spadaro A, Ceccarelli F, Scrivo R, Germano V, Valesini G. Nailfold capillaroscopy changes in systemic lupus erythematosus: correlations with disease activity and autoantibody profile. Lupus. 2005;14(7):521–5.
118. Ingegnoli F, Ughi N, Riccieri V, Stefanantoni K, Cracowski JL, Gutierrez M, et al. Distribution of nailfold videocapillaroscopy parameters in systemic lupus erythematosus and their association with disease activity: an international blinded case–control analysis on behalf of the EULAR study group on microcirculation in rheumatic diseases. RMD Open.

Case 22

119. Lambova SN. Scleroderma-like capillaroscopic pattern in SLE is not a sign of overlap syndrome in both adults and children. Lupus Sci Med. 2022;9:e000749. https://doi.org/10.1136/lupus-2022-000749.
120. Alexandru Caraba, Deiana Roman, Stela Iurciuc, Mihaela Nicolin and Mircea Iurciuc. Microvascular involvement in systemic lupus erythematosus assessed by nailfold capillaroscopy: correlations with clinical and biological parameters. IntechOpen. Lupus diagnostics and Developments. Published: 26 November 2024 https://doi.org/10.5772/intechopen.1005602
121. Ting Z, et al. Pattern of nailfold capillaroscopy in patients with systemic lupus erythematosus. Arch Rheumatol. 2020;35(4):568–74. https://doi.org/10.46497/ArchRheumatol.2020.7763.
122. Barreneche MFÁ, Franco CJV, Cuartas CEG, Navas MAM. Capillaroscopic abnormalities in systemic lupus erythematosus and its association with clinical manifestation. Revista Colombiana de Reumatología. 2024;31(3):304–10.

Case 23

123. Smith V, Ickinger C, Hysa E, Snow M, Frech T, Sulli A, et al. Nailfold capillaroscopy. Best Pract Res Clin Rheumatol. 2023;37(1):101849. https://doi.org/10.1016/j.berh.2023.101849.
124. Smith V, Herrick AL, Ingegnoli F, et al. Standardisation of nailfold capillaroscopy for the assessment of patients with Raynaud's phenomenon and systemic sclerosis. Autoimmun Rev. 2020;19(3):102458.
125. John KJ, Sadiq M, George T, et al. Clinical and immunological profile of mixed connective tissue disease and a comparison of four diagnostic criteria. Int J Rheumatol. 2020;2020:9692030.
126. Niklas K, Niklas A, Mularek-Kubzdela T, Puszczewicz M, Samborski W. Relationship between changes observed in nailfold capillaroscopy and serological profile, lung fibrosis, and elevated risk of pulmonary hypertension in patients with systemic sclerosis and mixed connective tissue disease. Postepy Dermatol Alergol. 2022;39(5):880–6.
127. Pizzorni C, Ferrari G, Schenone C, et al. Capillaroscopic analysis of the microvascular status in mixed versus undifferentiated connective tissue disease. Microvasc Res. 2022;142:104367.
128. Ferrari G, Gotelli E, Paolino S, et al. Antiphospholipid antibodies and anticoagulant therapy: capillaroscopic findings. Arthritis Res Ther. 2021;23(1):175.
129. Sulli A, Pizzorni C, Cutolo M. Nailfold videocapillaroscopy abnormalities in patients with antiphospholipid antibodies. J Rheumatol. 2000;27(6):1574–6.

Case 24

130. Cutolo M, Melsens K, Wijnant S. Nailfold capillaroscopy in systemic lupus erythematosus: A systematic review and critical appraisal. Autoimmunity Reviews. 2018;17(4):344–52.
131. Ting Z, et al. Pattern of nailfold capillaroscopy in patients with systemic lupus erythematosus. Arch Rheumatol. 2020;35(4):568–74. https://doi.org/10.46497/ArchRheumatol.2020.7763. eCollection 2020 Dec.
132. Smith V, et al. Nailfold capillaroscopy. Best Pract Res Clin Rheumatol. 2023;37(1):101849. https://doi.org/10.1016/j.berh.2023.101849. Epub 2023 July 6.
133. Desai SA, Nayak CS. Nailfold capillaroscopy as a prognostic marker for connective tissue diseases: an observational clinico-epidemiological study. Indian J Dermatol Venereol Leprol. 2024;90:283–90. https://doi.org/10.25259/IJDVL_205_2022.

Case 25

134. Miyakis S, Lockshin MD, Atsumi T, et al. International consensus statement on an update of the classification criteria for definite antiphospholipid syndrome (APS). J Thromb Haemost. 2006;4(2):295–306. https://doi.org/10.1111/j.1538-7836.2006.01753.x; José A. Gómez-Puerta, Ricard Cervera, Gerard Espinosa, et al. Antiphospholipid Antibodies Associated with Malignancies: Clinical and Pathological Characteristics of 120 Patients. Semin Arthritis Rheum. 2006;35(5):322–32. https://doi.org/10.1016/j.semarthrit.2005.07.003.
135. Kungwankiattichai S, Nakkinkun Y, Owattanapanich W, Ruchutrakool T. High incidence of antiphospholipid antibodies in newly diagnosed patients with lymphoma and a proposed aPL predictive score. Clin Appl Thromb Hemost. 2020;26:1076029620928392. https://doi.org/10.1177/1076029620928392.
136. Smith V, et al. Nailfold capillaroscopy. Best Pract Res Clin Rheumatol. 2023;37(1):101849.

Case 26

137. Movasat A, et al. Nailfold capillaroscopy in Behçet's disease, analysis of 128 patients. Clin Rheumatol. 2009;28(5):603–5. https://doi.org/10.1007/s10067-009-1106-2. Epub 2009 Feb 14.
138. Atienza-Mateo B, del Peral-Fanjul A, Pulito-Cueto V, Prieto-Peña D, González-Gay M, Blanco R. Microvascular involvement in Behçet's disease: study of nailfold capillaroscopy in patients from a national referral center [abstract]. Arthritis Rheumatol. 2022;74(suppl 9) https://acrabstracts.org/abstract/microvascular-involvement-in-behcets-disease-study-of-nailfold-capillaroscopy-in-patients-from-a-national-referral-center/. Accessed 18 Dec 2025.
139. Zontul S, Inanç E, Can A, et al. Can nailfold capillaroscopy findings be a marker for uveitis in Behçet's syndrome? Clin Exp Rheumatol. 2025;43(10):1742–7. https://doi.org/10.55563/clinexprheumatol/iunbq7. Epub 2025 Jul 25.
140. Tugal-Tutkun I, et al. Uveitis in Behçet disease: an analysis of 880 patients. Am J Ophthalmol. 2004;138(3):373–80.
141. Mirjam EJ Van Velthoven; Lisette Smid; Tom Missotten; Jan van Laar; Koenraad Arndt Vermeer. Retinal microvasculature in Behçet's disease measured with optical coherence tomography angiography. ARVO Annual Meeting Abstract | 2020;61(7)

Case 27

142. Upreti S, et al. Vasculitic neuropathy associated with Rheumatoid Arthritis, a case report. J Community Hosp Intern Med Perspect. 2019;9(5):430–2. https://doi.org/10.1080/20009666.2019.1676507.
143. Delia Tulba D, et al. Immune Axonal Neuropathies Associated With Systemic Autoimmune Rheumatic Diseases. Front. Pharmacol., 14 April 2021.Sec. Inflammation Pharmacology. Volume 12 - 2021 | https://doi.org/10.3389/fphar.2021.610585
144. Puéchal X, et al. Rituximab therapy for systemic vasculitis associated with rheumatoid arthritis: Results from the AutoImmunity and Rituximab Registry. Arthritis Care Res (Hoboken). 2012;64(3):331–9. https://doi.org/10.1002/acr.20689.
145. Anyfanti P, et al. Nailfold videocapillaroscopy for the evaluation of peripheral microangiopathy in rheumatoid arthritis. Life. Microangiopathy Rheum Dis. 2022;12(8):1167. https://doi.org/10.3390/life12081167.

Case 28

146. Maldonado G, Paredes C, Roberto G, Ríos C. Nailfold capillaroscopy a non-invasive tool for direct observation of microvascular damage in diabetes mellitus: review. JSM Atheroscler. 2017;2(4):1037.
147. Uyar S, Balkarlı A, Erol MK, et al. Assessment of the relationship between diabetic retinopathy and nailfold capillaries in Type 2 diabetics with a noninvasive method: nailfold videocapillaroscopy. J Diabetes Res. 2016;2016:7592402. https://doi.org/10.1155/2016/7592402.
148. Maldonado G, Chacko A, Lichtenberg R, et al. Nailfold capillaroscopy in diabetes mellitus: a case of neo-angiogenesis after achieving normoglycemia. Oxf Med Case Rep. 2022;2022(9):omac088. https://doi.org/10.1093/omcr/omac088.

Case 29

149. Pagnoux C, et al. Clinical features and outcomes in 348 patients with polyarteritis nodosa: a systematic retrospective study of patients diagnosed between 1963 and 2005 and entered into the French Vasculitis Study Group Database. Arthritis Rheum. 2010;62(2):616–26. https://doi.org/10.1002/art.27240.
150. Hernandez-Rodriguez J, et al. Diagnosis and classification of polyarteritis nodosa. J Autoimmun. 2014;48–49:84–9. https://doi.org/10.1016/j.jaut.2014.01.029. Epub 2014 Jan 28
151. Gwathmey KG, Burns TM, Collins MP, Dyck PJB. Vasculitic neuropathies. Lancet Neurol. 2014;13(1):67–82. https://doi.org/10.1016/S1474-4422(13)70236-9.
152. Cutolo M, et al. Nailfold video capillaroscopy in systemic sclerosis. Z Rheumatol. 2004;63(6):457–62. https://doi.org/10.1007/s00393-004-0673-5.
153. Bertolazzi C, et al. The current role of capillaroscopy in vasculitides. Clin Rheumatol. 2019;38(9):2299–307. https://doi.org/10.1007/s10067-018-4399-1. Epub 2019 Jan 5
154. Boukhris I, et al. Efficacy of rituximab in refractory polyarteritis nodosa: a case report. Pan Afr Med J. 2023;21(45):92. https://doi.org/10.11604/pamj.2023.45.92.36496.

Chapter 16
Test Yourself

Rahma A. Elziaty and Yasser El Miedany

The "Test Yourself" section provides an interactive learning part designed to enhance clinical reasoning and diagnostic interpretation skills in nailfold capillaroscopy (NFC). Through a series of short, case-based scenarios, readers are challenged to analyze NFC images, integrate clinical data, and apply theoretical knowledge in practical contexts. Each case is followed by targeted questions focusing on image interpretation, clinical decision-making, and multiple-choice questions to reinforce key concepts.

This self-assessment approach allows learners to actively engage with the material, identify areas for improvement, and consolidate their understanding of microvascular changes in various rheumatologic and systemic diseases. Ultimately, this chapter aims to bridge the gap between theory and practice, promoting confidence and competence in the use of NFC for diagnosis and follow-up in routine clinical practice.

By integrating visual interpretation with clinical problem-solving, this section serves as a practical tool for medical students, trainees, and clinicians who wish to strengthen their diagnostic skills. It also provides a valuable opportunity for self-assessment, ensuring readiness for both academic examinations and real-world clinical practice.

R. A. Elziaty (✉)
Internal Medicine Department, Rheumatology Division, Faculty of Medicine,
Ain Shams University, Cairo, Egypt
e-mail: drrahmaelziaty@med.asu.edu.eg

Y. El Miedany
Canterbury Christ Church University, Canterbury, UK

Rheumatology and Rehabilitation, Ain Shams University, Cairo, Egypt

King's College, London, UK

Y. El Miedany, R. A. Elziaty (eds.), *Capillaroscopy*, Contemporary Rheumatology,
https://doi.org/10.1007/978-3-032-22966-3_16

Case 1 A 22-year-old female presented with a history of episodic discoloration of the fingers triggered by exposure to cold temperatures. The attacks were symmetrical, involved both hands, and had been occurring for the past several months. There was no history of arthralgia, skin thickening, or systemic symptoms suggestive of connective tissue disease. NFC examination as illustrated in the figure, and there were no signs of cutaneous or musculoskeletal involvement. Laboratory investigations revealed a negative antinuclear antibody (ANA) test, with no other serological abnormalities detected.

Q1: Describe the NFC findings and interpret them.
Q2: How to manage this case?
Q3: Which NFC feature is typical in primary Raynaud's?

A. Giant capillaries
B. Hemorrhages
C. Avascular areas
D. Bushy capillaries
E. Normal morphology

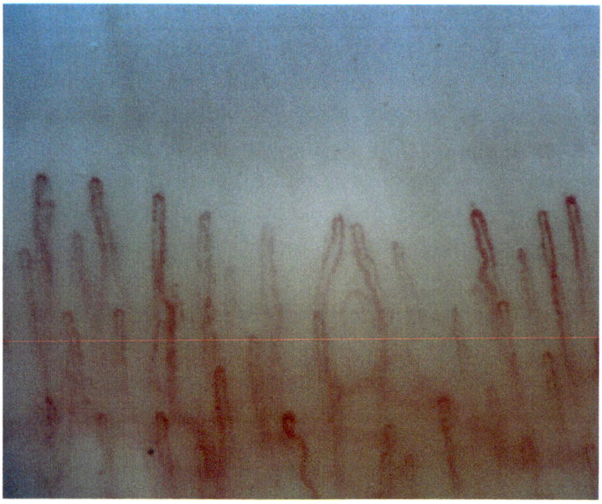

Case 2 A 29-year-old female presented with a history of Raynaud's phenomenon, characterized by recurrent cold-induced color changes of the fingers. She did not report any skin tightness, digital ulcers, or pitting scars on the fingertips. On examination, only puffy fingers and NFC as in the figure. Laboratory evaluation revealed a positive antinuclear antibody (ANA) test.

Q1: Describe the NFC findings and interpret them.
Q2: What is the most important next step?
Q3: Which feature differentiates secondary from primary Raynaud's?

A. Preserved density
B. Giant capillaries
C. Uniform hairpins
D. Absence of hemorrhage
E. Normal morphology

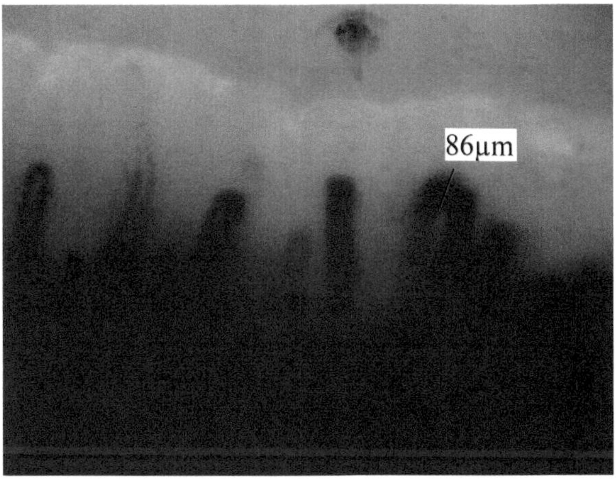

Case 3 A 35-year-old female presented with Raynaud's phenomenon, characterized by recurrent cold-induced finger discoloration, along with puffy fingers noted over the past 6 months. Clinical examination confirmed the swelling but showed no digital ulcers or skin tightening. Laboratory work-up revealed ANA positivity with a nucleolar pattern and positive anti-SCL 70 antibodies, both suggestive of an underlying systemic sclerosis spectrum disorder. Nailfold capillaroscopy (NFC) was performed, and the findings are shown in the figure.

Q1: Describe the NFC findings and interpret them.
Q2: What organs should be screened at this stage?
Q3: Early SSc NFC is characterized by:

A. Avascular areas
B. Bushy loops only
C. Giant capillaries with preserved density
D. Extensive neo-angiogenesis
E. Complete dropout

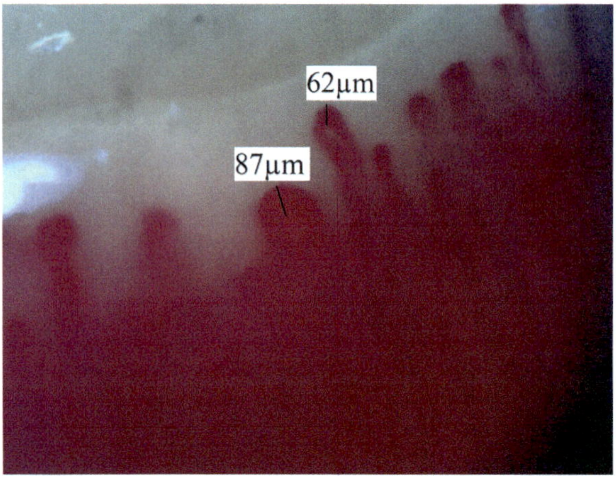

Case 4 A 40-year-old female presented with Raynaud's phenomenon, progressive diffuse skin thickening, and complaints of gastroesophageal reflux symptoms, heartburn, and regurgitation. Clinical examination confirmed widespread skin involvement, mainly affecting the hands and forearms. Given these features, she underwent nailfold capillaroscopy as shown in the figure.

Q1: Describe and interpret the NFC findings.
Q2: What would be your advice for the patient?
Q3: Active SSc pattern indicates:

A. Stable disease
B. Nonspecific changes
C. Progression of microangiopathy
D. Exclusion of interstitial lung disease (ILD)
E. Normal vessels

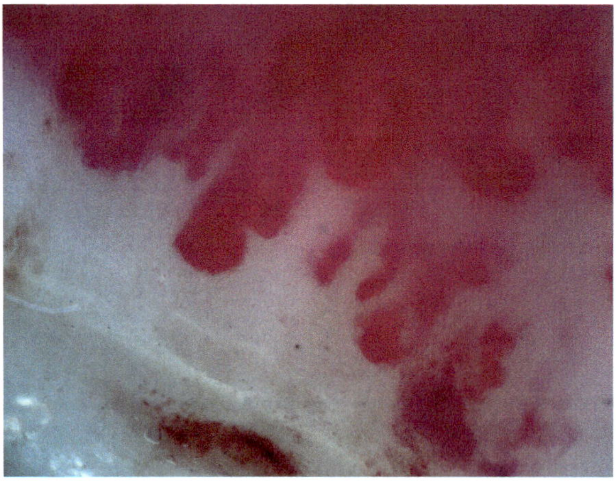

Case 5 A 45-year-old female with a history of long-standing systemic sclerosis attended the clinic for evaluation. She reported progressive hand stiffness and pain, and on examination, there were fixed finger contractures together with ischemic digital ulcers on the fingertips, indicating advanced vascular involvement. To assess microvascular changes, nailfold capillaroscopy (NFC) was performed, and the findings, illustrated in the figure, support the clinical impression of disease progression.

Q1: Describe and interpret the NFC findings.
Q2: What does this capillaroscopic pattern imply?
Q3: Which feature characterizes the late SSc pattern?

A. Presence of microhemorrhages
B. Normal capillary architecture
C. Presence of pericapillary edema
D. Neo-angiogenesis and Avascular areas
E. Preserved giant capillaries

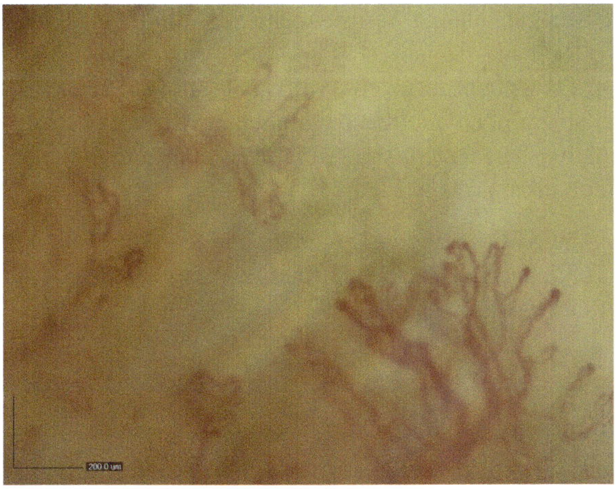

Case 6 A 32-year-old female, previously diagnosed with systemic lupus erythematosus, with a documented history of recurrent miscarriages, presented to the clinic with complaints of severe digital ischemia causing marked pain and discoloration of the fingertips. Clinical examination revealed evidence of critical vascular compromise, although no gangrene was noted. In view of her background and vascular symptoms, nailfold capillaroscopy (NFC) was requested to assess the extent of microvascular involvement and to aid in the evaluation.

Q1: Describe and interpret the NFC findings.
Q2: a. When would you expect to find this capillaroscopic pattern (diagnosis)? b. considering the clinical background of this case, what is the antibody profile expected?
Q3: Typical NFC feature in APS?

A. Giant loops
B. Avascular areas only
C. Comb-like pattern of hemorrhages
D. Bushy angiogenesis
E. Preserved morphology

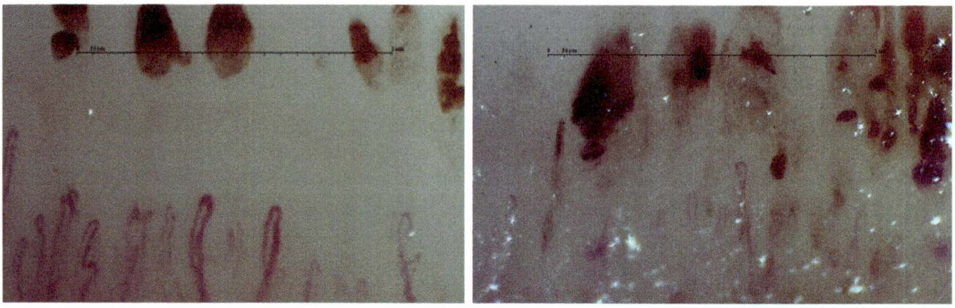

Case 7 A 28-year-old female was admitted to the inpatient department with an SLE flare (generalized polyarthralgia, anemia, serositis, and nephritis). On clinical assessment, there was severe Raynaud's manifestations. NFC was requested; it's results are shown in Figure a. The patient received a rituximab infusion according to the international protocols (1 gm, then another 1 gm after 2 weeks, then maintained on 500 mg every 6 months). The patient showed marked improvement clinically and follow-up NFC after 6 months, as in Figure b.

Q1: Describe and interpret the NFC findings in Figures a and b.
Q2: What is the clinical significance of microhemorrhages in this case?
Q3: NFC in active SLE often reveals:

A. A-V plexus
B. Giant loops only
C. Microhemorrhages and mild avascularity
D. Neo-angiogenesis only
E. Normal pattern

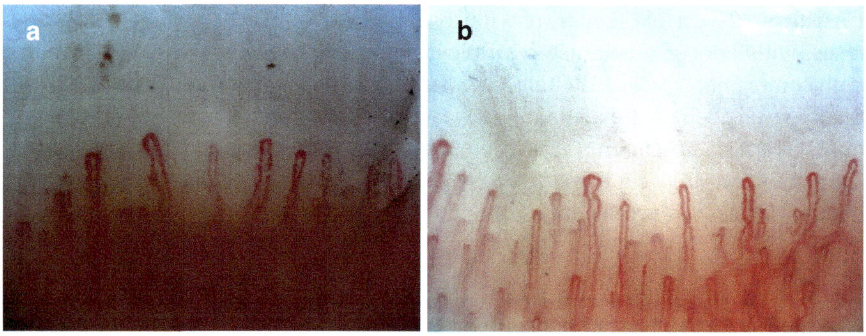

Case 8 A 40-years old female patient presented with muscle weakness. On examination, she had difficulty climbing upstairs, combing her hair, and standing up from a seated position. There was a heliotrope rash. Investigations revealed elevated ESR and muscle enzymes. NFC was done as shown in the following figure.

Q1: Describe and interpret the NFC findings.
Q2: Which systemic complication is important to screen for?
Q3: Most characteristic NFC finding in DM?

A. Normal loops
B. Extensive bushy capillaries + hemorrhages
C. Only tortuosity
D. Absence of changes
E. Preserved density

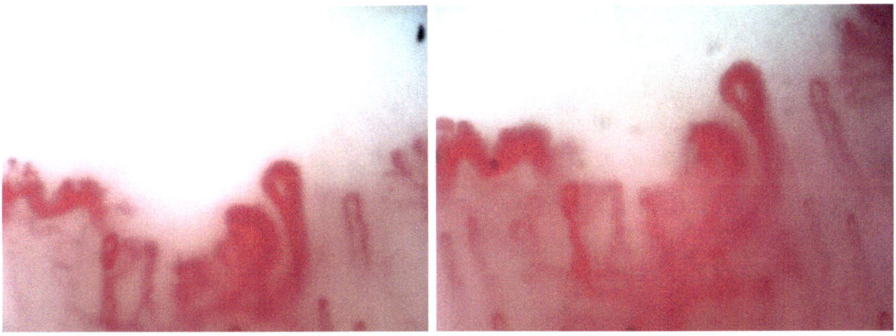

Case 9 A 36-year-old female with a history of inflammatory polyarthritis of hand and wrist joints for 2 years, who was maintained on oral steroids 30 mg daily, hydroxychloroquine 200 mg tab twice daily, and leflunomide 20 mg tab once daily. She started to develop Raynaud's 3 months ago. On examination, she had swollen hands with color changes. Investigations showed ESR 50 mm/hr., CRP 18 mg/L, ANA 1/80 speckled pattern, and anti-U1 RNP positive.

Q1: Describe and interpret the NFC findings.
Q2: What is the significance of capillaroscopy in such cases?
Q3: NFC in MCTD resembles mostly:

A. Scleroderma
B. Primary Raynaud's
C. Rheumatoid arthritis (RA)
D. Normal pattern capillaroscopy
E. Nonspecific abnormalities

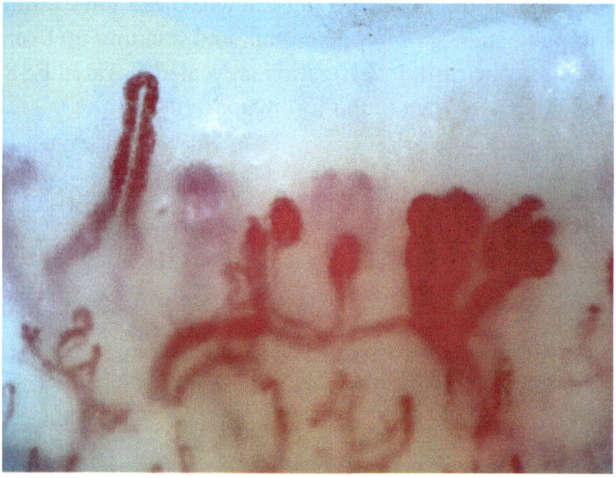

Case 10 A 45-year-old male with long-standing RA and joint deformities. Admitted with severe arthritis, vasculitic rash on both lower limbs, and Raynaud's. NFC was performed, and the result is as shown in the figure.

Q1: Describe and interpret the NFC findings.
Q2: What is the significance of NFC in such cases?
Q3: NFC in RA is usually

A. Normal
B. Giant loops
C. Nonspecific changes
D. Extensive neo-angiogenesis
E. Only avascular areas

Case 11 A 48-year-old female patient, known to have rheumatoid arthritis, presented with Raynaud's of 8 months' duration and progressive tightening of the skin of the hands, leading to sclerodactyly with difficulty in finger mobility and impaired hand function. On examination, the patient had swollen and deformed small joints of both hands, with a restricted range of motion. Skin thickening and sclerodactyly. Nailfold capillaroscopy was performed to evaluate the microvascular changes, as illustrated in the figure. Laboratory investigation: Rheumatoid factor: positive, Anti-CCP antibodies: positive, ANA: speckled 1/180, ESR: 55 mm/hr., and CRP: 14 mg/L

Q1: Describe and interpret the NFC findings.
Q2: What is the most probable diagnosis and the most important next step?
Q3: NFC in such cases usually resembles:

A. RA only
B. Scleroderma pattern
C. SLE pattern
D. Comb-like pattern
E. Nonspecific abnormalities

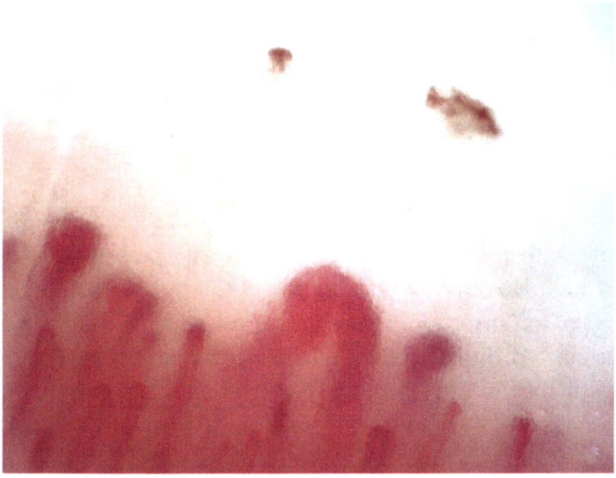

Case 12 A 13-year-old female with a history of oligoarticular juvenile idiopathic arthritis (JIA) with mild joint pain and stiffness, mainly affecting the knees and ankles. She presented with intermittent episodes of finger pallor and cyanosis on exposure to cold, suggestive of Raynaud's phenomenon. On examination, she had mild swelling of the right knee with limited flexion. Fingers showed no digital ulcers, but the skin was cool with periungual erythema, and nailfold capillaroscopy was performed. Investigations: ANA: positive, rheumatoid factor: negative, inflammatory markers: mildly elevated.

Q1: Describe and interpret the NFC findings.

Q2: What is the significance of capillaroscopy here, and which complication is important to be monitored?

Q3: NFC in JIA may reveal:

A. Giant capillaries with loss
B. Nonspecific dilations and hemorrhages
C. Always a normal pattern
D. Severe avascular areas
E. Exclusive tortuosity

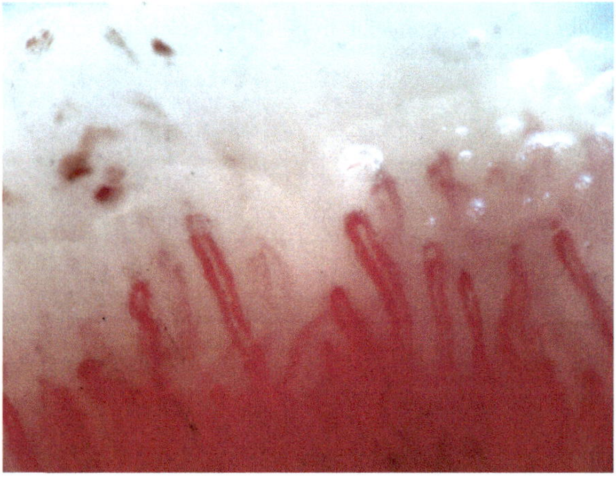

Case 13 A 35-year-old male with a 20-year history of psoriasis presented with joint pain, swelling, and stiffness. He developed dactylitis of the right index finger and enthesitis at the Achilles tendon insertion. Examination revealed psoriatic skin lesions over the extensor surfaces, diffuse swelling of the right index finger ("sausage digit"), and tenderness at the Achilles tendon. Nailfold capillaroscopy was performed to assess microvascular involvement. Investigations: Rheumatoid factor: negative, anti-CCP: negative, ESR: 45 mm/h, CRP: 14 mg/dl, and HLA-B27: positive.

Q1: Describe and interpret the NFC findings.

Q2: How can you differentiate between capillaroscopic findings in RA and psoriatic arthritis (PSA)?

Q3: Most common NFC finding in PSA?

A. Normal morphology
B. Bushy capillaries and mild loss
C. Giant loops
D. Severe avascularity
E. Exclusively hemorrhages

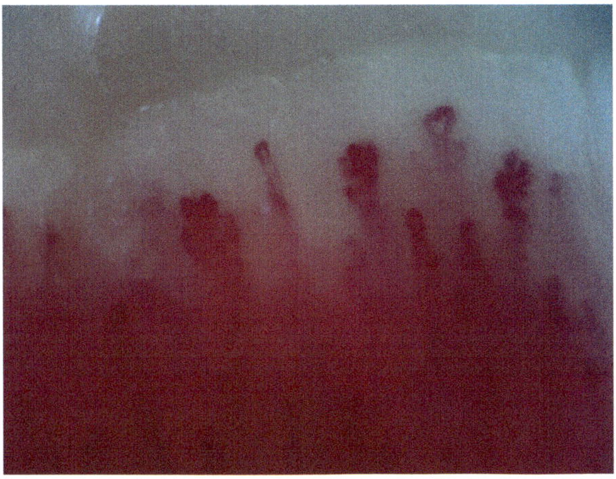

Case 14 A 47-year-old female with a known history of limited systemic sclerosis of five years' duration presented with painful fingertip ulcers. She reported progressive skin tightening of the hands and face, Raynaud's phenomenon, and digital pain interfering with daily activities. *Clinical Examination* revealed skin thickening and sclerodactyly were evident, with multiple ischemic fingertip ulcers. Facial skin appeared tight with reduced mouth opening. *Investigations:* ANA: positive 1/320; anti-centromere antibodies: positive. Nailfold capillaroscopy results are shown in the figure.

Q1: Describe and interpret the NFC findings.
Q2: How to manage digital and fingertip ulcers?
Q3: Digital ulcers correlate with:

A. Early scleroderma pattern
B. Reduced density and avascularity
C. Normal morphology
D. Abnormal morphology
E. Only hemorrhages

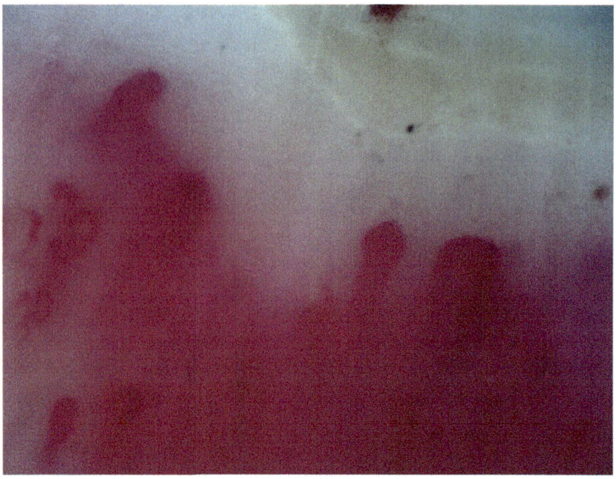

Case 15 A 60-year-old male with a 15-year history of type 2 diabetes mellitus presented with numbness and burning pain in both feet, consistent with peripheral neuropathy. He also reported occasional claudication and delayed wound healing. *Clinical Examination* revealed decreased sensation over the lower limbs with impaired vibration sense and reduced ankle reflexes. No active ulcers were noted, but the skin appeared dry with trophic changes. Nailfold capillaroscopy was performed to evaluate microvascular involvement in the context of long-standing diabetes. *Investigations:* HbA1c: 8.9%, inflammatory markers normal.

Q1: Describe and interpret the NFC findings.
Q2: What is the role of capillaroscopy in diabetes?
Q3: NFC changes in diabetes resemble:

A. Scleroderma
B. Normal pattern
C. Microangiopathy (tortuosity, microaneurysms)
D. Scleroderma-like pattern
E. APS pattern

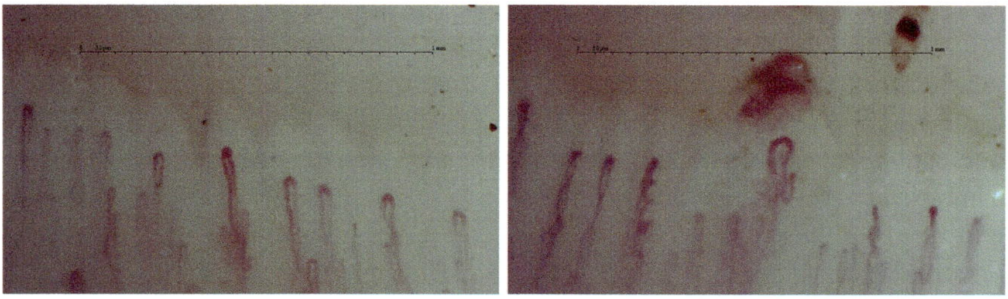

Case 16 A38-year-old female, previously healthy, developed a severe COVID-19 infection one year ago, requiring hospitalization. She now presents with persistent fatigue, diffuse joint pains, and reduced exercise tolerance. She also reports occasional cold-induced color changes of the fingers. *Examination* revealed no synovitis, but mild periungual erythema and cold peripheries were noted. Lungs were clear, and oxygen saturation was normal. Nailfold capillaroscopy was performed. *Investigations*: ANA: negative, complete blood count: normal, and ESR: 20 mm/h, and CRP: 9 mg/dl.

Q1: Describe and interpret the NFC findings.
Q2: What is the significance of capillaroscopy in this case?
Q3: NFC after severe COVID often shows:

A. Giant capillaries
B. Bushy angiogenesis only
C. Microhemorrhages and dilated capillaries
D. Normal vessels
E. Scleroderma pattern

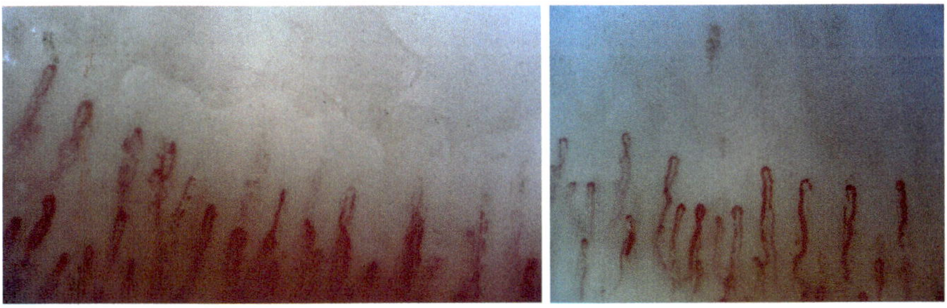

Case 17 A 44-year-old female with a known history of systemic sclerosis presented with progressive exertional dyspnea and dry cough. She reported Raynaud's phenomenon and progressive skin tightening over the hands and face. Clinical Examination Findings included sclerodactyly, digital pitting scars, and reduced chest expansion with fine basal inspiratory crackles on auscultation. NFC was performed, and the results are illustrated in the figure. Investigations: ANA: positive (nucleolar pattern), anti-Scl-70 antibodies: positive, ESR: 34 mm/h, CRP: 12 mg/dl, HRCT chest: interstitial lung disease with basal ground-glass changes and fibrosis.

Q1: Describe and interpret the NFC findings.
Q2: Which test is recommended for early detection of ILD?
Q3: Which NFC is mostly associated with ILD in SSc?

A. Reduced density and avascularity
B. Presence of microhemorrhages
C. Early scleroderma pattern
D. ILD is not related to any of the capillaroscopic abnormalities

E. More related to the presence of giant capillaries.

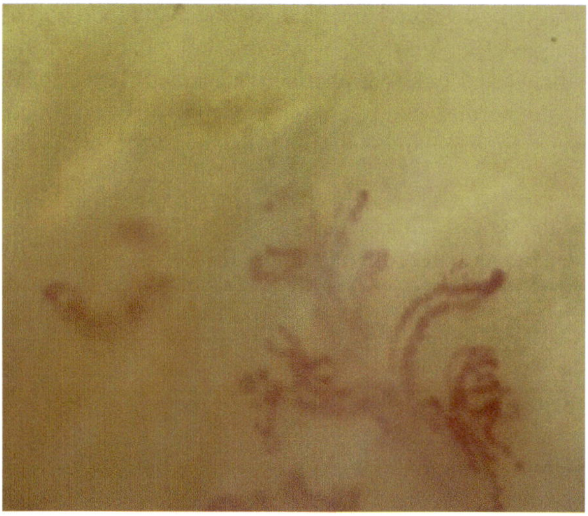

Case 18 A 39-year-old female presented with Raynaud's phenomenon, photosensitivity, and joint pain. Clinical examination revealed a malar rash and skin tightening of the fingers (sclerodactyly). Investigations: ESR: 50 mm/h, CRP: 12 mg/dl, ANA: positive 1/320 (homogeneous pattern), Anti-dsDNA: positive, Anti-Scl-70: positive. Nailfold capillaroscopy was performed.

Q1: Describe and interpret the NFC findings.
Q2: What is the significance of capillaroscopy in this case?
Q3: NFC in overlap usually resembles:

A. Scleroderma pattern
B. SLE with 2ry APS
C. Nonspecific abnormalities
D. Normal capillaroscopic pattern
E. Diabetes

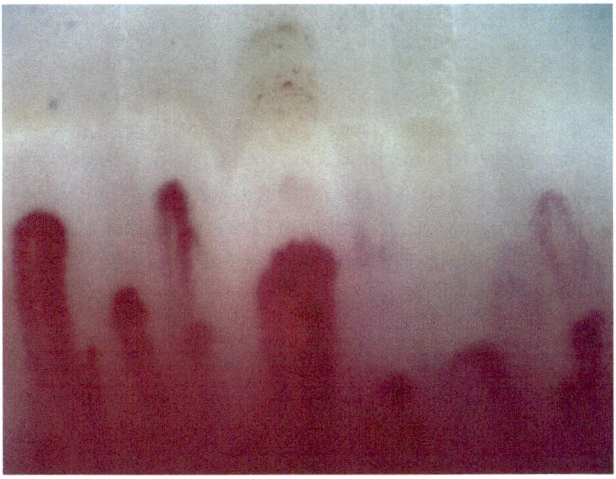

Case 19 A 42-year-old female presented with progressive dyspnea, myalgia, and arthralgia. She also reported Raynaud's phenomenon and mechanic's hands. Clinical Examination Findings included crackles at the lung bases and periungual erythema. Investigations: ANA: positive, anti-Jo-1 antibodies: positive, HRCT chest: interstitial lung disease with ground-glass opacities. Nailfold capillaroscopy: performed.

Q1: Describe and interpret the NFC findings.

Q2: What is the clinical significance and prognostic value of NFC in this case?

Q3: Which of the following nailfold capillaroscopy findings is commonly observed in anti-synthetase syndrome?

A. Normal capillary density and morphology
B. Tortuous capillaries without giant capillaries
C. Scleroderma-like pattern with giant capillaries, microhemorrhages, and capillary loss
D. Avascular areas without neo-angiogenesis
E. Nonspecific abnormalities

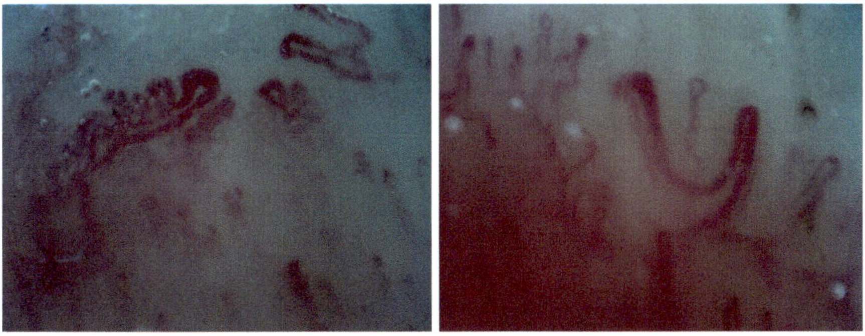

Answers to the "Test Yourself" Questions

Case 1 Answer:

Q1: Answer: **Description**; *Density:* normal >7 capillaries per linear mm. *Dimensions:* capillary with a diameter < 20 μm (normal apical width). *Morphology:* normal shapes of capillaries. *Microhemorrhages:* absent. **Interpretation**: normal capillaroscopic pattern in correlation with the history, clinical examination, and laboratory results suggestive of primary Raynaud's [1].

Q2: Answer: Only lifestyle measures (warming, smoking cessation); if still not responding, consider vasodilators (CCB, ….) *Discussed in detail in Chap. 3: Raynaud's phenomenon.*

Q3: Answer: e

Case 2 Answers:

Q1: Answer: **Description**; *Density:* normal; 7 capillaries per linear mm. *Dimensions:* capillary with a diameter > 50 μm (giant capillary). *Microhemorrhages:* present. **Interpretation**: abnormal capillaroscopic pattern (scleroderma pattern) suggestive of secondary Raynaud's [1].

Q2: Answer: By applying VEDOSS criteria, we can consider this case as very early systemic sclerosis (presence of Raynaud's phenomenon and puffy fingers as red flags, abnormal capillaroscopic pattern, and positive ANA). The presence of one or two VEDOSS criteria in patients with Raynaud's phenomenon confers a progressively higher risk for systemic sclerosis over time. Close monitoring of the patient for any progression and follow-up NFC after 6 months are recommended. Systemic sclerosis-specific antibodies are recommended in this case. Also, HRCT chest, pulmonary function tests (PFT), and ECHO for early detection of end-organ damage [2, 3].

Q3: Answer: b

Case 3 Answers:

Q1: Answer: **Description**; *Density:* preserved >7 capillaries per linear mm. *Dimensions:* capillary with a diameter > 50 μm (giant capillary). *Microhemorrhages:* present (recent hemorrhage). **Interpretation:** abnormal capillaroscopic pattern (early scleroderma pattern) [1].

Q2: Answer: [4–6]

- *Lung (ILD, Pulmonary arterial hypertension (PAH))*

- Interstitial lung disease (ILD): Pulmonary function tests (PFTs), including DLCO at baseline and follow-up. High-resolution CT (HRCT) is recommended in all early SSc patients or if PFTs are abnormal.
- Pulmonary arterial hypertension (PAH): echocardiography, proBNP, and RHC to confirm diagnosis.

• *Heart*
  - ECG in all patients.
  - Echocardiography to detect ventricular dysfunction, pericardial effusion, or pulmonary hypertension.
  - Cardiac MRI may be considered in suspected myocardial fibrosis or arrhythmias.

• *Kidneys*
  - The risk of scleroderma renal crisis (SRC) is highest early in diffuse cutaneous disease.
  - Monitoring includes frequent blood pressure measurements.
  - Serum creatinine, eGFR, and urinalysis for proteinuria.

• *Gastrointestinal Tract*
  - Early focus: symptom screening for reflux, dysphagia, and bloating. Endoscopy is used for severe GERD, dysphagia, or suspected Barrett's esophagus. Manometry may be used in specialized centers.

Q3: ☑ Answer: c

Case 4 Answer:

Q1: ☑ Answer: **Description**; *Density:* reduced; 5 capillaries per linear mm. *Dimensions:* capillary with a diameter > 50 μm (giant capillary). *Morphology:* abnormal shapes of capillaries. *Microhemorrhages:* present. **Interpretation**: abnormal capillaroscopic pattern (active scleroderma pattern) [1].

Q2: ☑ Answer: This patient with an active scleroderma pattern in capillaroscopy, further work-up should be performed, including a full history, clinical examination, laboratory investigations (ESR, CRP, scleroderma-specific autoantibodies, pro-BNP, urine analysis, and kidney function tests), and for organ involvement, baseline HRCT of the chest and pulmonary function tests, ECG, and ECHO [2–4].

Q3: ☑ Answer: c

Case 5 Answer:

Q1: ☑ Answer: **Description;** *Density:* markedly reduced (< 3 capillaries per linear mm). *Morphology:* abnormal shapes of capillaries with the presence of neo-angiogenesis. *Microhemorrhages:* absent. **Interpretation:** abnormal capillaroscopic pattern (late scleroderma pattern) [1].

Q2: Answer: The late scleroderma capillaroscopic pattern implies irreversible microvascular damage with long-standing disease, marked by capillary loss, neo-angiogenesis, and disorganized architecture. Clinically, it signals severe, established systemic sclerosis with a high risk of vascular complications such as digital ulcers, PAH, and organ involvement, "severe skin fibrosis and ILD." [7]

Q3: Answer: d

Case 6 Answer

Q1: Answer: **Description:** *Density*: normal, 7 capillaries per linear mm. *Dimensions:* Dilated capillaries with a diameter > 20 μm and < 50 μm. Morphology: presence of elongated, tortuous, and crossed capillaries. *Microhemorrhages:* present with a comb-like pattern. **Interpretation:** Abnormal capillaroscopic pattern suggestive of microvascular damage consistent with SLE 2ry APS.

Q2: Answer: **a.** antiphospholipid autoantibodies (aPL). **b.** It is suggested that the "comb-like" pattern may serve as a potential capillaroscopic biomarker in patients with APS. It is more frequently observed in these patients than its occurrence in healthy controls and aPL carriers (reported prevalence of, respectively, 50% vs 16% vs 20%) [7, 8].

Q3: Answer: c

Case 7 Answer:

Q1: Answer: Figure a; **Description;** *Density:* mild decreased capillaries per linear mm. *Dimensions:* Dilated capillaries with a diameter > 20 μm and < 50 μm. *Morphology:* presence of elongated, tortuous, and crossed capillaries. *Microhemorrhages:* present with point-shaped bleeding surrounding the capillary. **Interpretation:** Abnormal capillaroscopic pattern suggestive of microvascular damage consistent with Active SLE vasculopathy [1].

Figure b; **Description;** *Density:* normal >7 capillaries per linear mm. *Dimensions:* dilated capillaries with a diameter > 20 μm and < 50 μm. *Morphology:* presence of elongated, tortuous, and crossed capillaries. *Microhemorrhages:* Absent. **Interpretation:** Improvement of the follow-up NFC is suggestive of microvascular damage consistent with active SLE vasculopathy [1].

Q2: Answer: It is reported that the capillaroscopic changes in SLE—"dilated capillaries, microhemorrhages, reduced density, and abnormal shapes"—are related to disease activity and Raynaud's [7, 9, 10].

Q3: Answer: c

Case 8 Answer:

Q1: Answer: **Description;** *Density:* reduced with increased avascularity and dropout. *Dimensions:* Dilated capillaries with a diameter > 20 μm and < 50 μm, and giant capillaries with a diameter > 50 μm. *Morphology:* bushy capillaries and neo-angiogenesis. *Microhemorrhages:* present. **Interpretation:** the capillaroscopic changes reflect the microvascular changes in dermatomyositis, which may give a scleroderma-like pattern [1].

Q2: Answer: Interstitial lung disease. Also, you should consider searching for hidden malignancy.

Q3: Answer: b

Case 9 Answer:

Q1: Answer: **Description;** *Density:* reduced with increased avascularity and dropout. *Dimensions:* giant capillaries with a diameter > 50 μm. *Morphology:* abnormally shaped capillaries; neo-angiogenesis. *Microhemorrhages:* present. **Interpretation:** NFC shows mixed features—"giant loops, hemorrhages, drop-out"—which indicate a scleroderma-like pattern [1].

Q2: Answer: [11]

Nailfold capillaroscopy (NFC) is a valuable tool in MCTD, as it detects and characterizes microvascular involvement. Patients with MCTD often demonstrate a "scleroderma-like" pattern, although it is typically milder and more heterogeneous than in systemic sclerosis. Common findings include giant capillaries, capillary hemorrhages, moderate capillary loss, and disorganized architecture.

The main clinical significance is:

- *Diagnostic value*—NFC helps differentiate secondary Raynaud's phenomenon from primary, supporting the diagnosis of MCTD in patients with overlapping features.
- *Prognostic value*—The extent of capillary loss and vascular damage correlates with severe organ involvement, particularly pulmonary arterial hypertension, interstitial lung disease, and digital ulcers.
- *Disease monitoring*—Serial capillaroscopy allows assessment of vascular progression and therapeutic response.

Thus, capillaroscopy in MCTD is not only useful diagnostically but also serves as a noninvasive biomarker for prognosis and longitudinal follow-up, reflecting the systemic sclerosis spectrum vasculopathy that characterizes the disease.

Q3: Answer: a

Case 10 Answer:

Q1: Answer: **Description;** *Density*: normal; 7 capillaries/mm. *Dimensions:* dilated capillaries with a diameter > 20 μm and < 50 μm. *Microhemorrhages:* present "old and recent" microhemorrhages." **Interpretation:** NFC shows microvascular changes in this case, rheumatoid vasculitis and disease activity [1].

Q2: Answer: [12–14]

NFC plays several important roles in rheumatoid arthritis (RA), especially in disease activity or when complicated by vasculitic rash:

- *Detection of microvascular abnormalities*
  - RA patients can exhibit nonspecific NFC changes such as capillary dilatation, tortuosity, microhemorrhages, and capillary dropout.
- *Correlation with disease activity and severity*
  - Abnormal NFC patterns are more frequent in patients with long-standing and severe RA, and they correlate with extra-articular involvement, including vasculitis.
- *Prognostic implications*
  - Severe microvascular damage on NFC (avascular areas, extensive dropout) may predict risk of ischemic complications such as digital ulcers or systemic vasculitis.
- *Differential diagnosis*
  - NFC helps distinguish RA-associated vasculitis from systemic sclerosis or lupus, which have more disease-specific NFC patterns. This is particularly important in overlap cases.
  - Identifying peripheral microangiopathy (damage to small blood vessels), aiding in early diagnosis, and helping to differentiate RA from psoriatic arthritis (PSA).
- *Monitoring and follow-up*
  - Serial NFC can be used to monitor vascular changes and response to immunosuppressive therapy, providing a noninvasive biomarker of vascular health.

Q3: Answer: c

Case 11 Answer:

Q1: Answer: **Description**; *Density:* reduced; 6 capillaries per linear mm. Dimensions: capillary with a diameter > 50 μm (giant capillary). *Microhemorrhages:* present. **Interpretation**: abnormal capillaroscopic pattern (active scleroderma pattern).

Q2: Answer: [4, 5, 15, 16]

The most probable diagnosis is rheumatoid arthritis + systemic sclerosis overlap. Rheumatoid arthritis component: inflammatory arthritis affecting small hand joints, prolonged morning stiffness, RF + ve, and anti-CCP + ve.

Systemic sclerosis component: Skin tightness, sclerodactyly, and active scleroderma pattern in capillaroscopy.

In this case, you should ask for the systemic sclerosis-specific antibodies and screening for early detection of end-organ damage (ECG, ECHO, PFT, HRCT chest).

Q3: Answer: b

Case 12 Answer:

Q1: Answer: **Description**; *Density:* normal; 7 capillaries per linear mm. *Dimensions:* dilated capillaries with a diameter > 20 μm and < 50 μm. *Morphology:* presence of tortuosity, elongation, and A-V plexus. *Microhemorrhages:* present. **Interpretation**: Nonspecific abnormalities and the presence of microhemorrhages indicate early microvascular involvement in a case of JIA with secondary Raynaud's [1, 17].

Q2: Answer: Nailfold capillaroscopy provides valuable insight into microvascular involvement, helping to distinguish nonspecific changes in JIA from scleroderma-pattern abnormalities that may suggest overlap syndromes with juvenile systemic sclerosis. Also, it is reported that capillary changes in JIA highlight the possibility that capillary dilation is a specific finding in polyarticular and enthesitis-related forms [17].

The most important complication is uveitis, as the patient has JIA, is ANA positive, and has changes in capillaroscopy, which indicates microvascular involvement. Microvascular damage detected by capillaroscopy may precede clinical complications and end-organ damage, e.g., uveitis. Early recognition allows closer monitoring and preventive measures [17, 18].

Q3: Answer: b

Case 13 Answer:

Q1: Answer: **Description;** *Density:* reduced with increased avascularity. *Dimensions:* Dilated capillaries with a diameter > 20 μm and < 50 μm. *Morphology:* abnormal shapes of capillaries with the presence of bushy loops and capillary tortuosity. *Microhemorrhages:* recent microhemorrhages. **Interpretation:** Nailfold capillaroscopy was performed to assess microvascular involvement and to explore whether the patient shows changes typical of psoriatic arthritis (neo-angiogenesis, capillary dropout) [1, 18].

Q2: Answer: [13, 14]

Microvascular involvement reflects both inflammation and abnormal vascular remodeling and suggests that capillary structural abnormalities might reflect endothelial injury due to systemic inflammation during chronic arthritis. More angiogenesis-related changes (bushy, elongated, ramified loops) in PSA compared to RA.

NFC Pattern in Rheumatoid Arthritis (RA): Nonspecific changes, without a defined "RA pattern"; generally preserved capillary density, increased capillary tortuosity, mild dilatation of capillaries, occasional microhemorrhages, and sometimes a scleroderma pattern or scleroderma-like pattern on some occasions.

NFC Pattern in Psoriatic Arthritis (PSA): Reduced capillary density (capillary dropout), bushy/ramified/convoluted terminal capillaries, capillary tortuosity, and microhemorrhages.

Q3: Answer: b

Case 14 Answer:

Q1: **Answer: Description;** *Density:* reduced and increased avascularity; 4 capillaries/mm. *Dimensions:* presence of giant capillaries with a diameter > 50 μm. *Microhemorrhages:* present (recent and old). **Interpretation:** abnormal capillaroscopic pattern (active scleroderma pattern), which reflects the severity of microvascular damage, which correlates with the presence of digital ulcers and internal organ involvement [1].

Q2: Answer: [5]

Management for digital ulceration in SSc:

- Sildenafil (or tadalafil) is recommended as first-line agent in DU healing and secondary prevention and bosentan as second-line treatment.
- Intravenous prostanoids may be considered to promote DU healing
- Consider anti-platelet therapy in DU disease (particularly if local necrosis)
- Digital (palmar) sympathectomy (with or without botulinum toxin injection) may be considered in those intolerant to systemic vasodilator meds and recurrent DU at a single site.
- Debridement of DU may promote healing
- There should be access to SSc/CTD specialist wound care services to prevent and treat skin ulcers

Q3: Answer: b

Case 15 Answer:

Q1: **Answer: Description;** *Density:* normal; 8 capillaries/mm. *Dimensions:* presence of dilated capillaries. *Morphology:* tortuous capillaries and microaneurysms. *Microhemorrhages:* present. **Interpretation:** abnormal capillaroscopic pattern, which reflects the diabetic microangiopathy, which correlates with the risk of microvascular diabetic complications and end-organ damage [1, 19].

Q2: Answer: NFC detects early microvascular changes before the development of overt complications. Helps in assessing the severity of vascular involvement and stratifying patients at risk for chronic complications. May serve as a research and prognostic tool in evaluating diabetic microvascular disease [19, 20].

Q3: Answer: c

Case 16 Answer:

Q1: **Answer: Description;** *Density:* normal; 7 capillaries/mm. *Dimensions:* presence of a few dilated capillaries. *Morphology:* tortuous capillaries and microthrombosis. *Microhemorrhages:* present. **Interpretation:** abnormal capillaroscopic pattern (non-scleroderma pattern, nonspecific abnormalities) that reflects the post-COVID syndrome with evidence of microvascular involvement. [1, 21, 22]

Q2: Answer: To investigate possible post-COVID microvascular dysfunction and to explore whether her persistent symptoms are linked to endothelial dysfunction and damage or capillary abnormalities and micro-thrombosis. Also, to exclude evolving connective tissue disease in the presence of Raynaud's [21, 22].

Q3: Answer: c

Case 17 Answer:

Q1: **Answer: Description;** *Density:* markedly reduced; 2 capillaries/mm. *Dimensions:* absence of giant capillaries. *Morphology:* abnormally shaped capillaries "neoangeogenesis." *Microhemorrhages:* absent. **Interpretation:** NFC shows a late scleroderma pattern [1].

Q2: Answer: DLCO "Diffusing capacity for Carbon Monoxide," The amount of carbon monoxide that passes from the lungs into your blood determines DLCO. A low DLCO can indicate lung conditions that affect the alveoli or capillaries in the lungs.

Q3: Answer: a

Case 18 Answer:

Q1: **Answer: Description;** *Density:* reduced. *Dimensions:* presence of giant capillaries with a diameter > 50 μm. *Morphology:* hairpin, megacapillaries, and neo-angiogenesis. *Microhemorrhages*: present. **Interpretation:** active scleroderma pattern, which may indicate the presence of SLE+ SSc overlap [1].

Q2: Answer: [15]

Capillaroscopy was performed to evaluate microvascular involvement, confirm the presence of a scleroderma pattern, and help differentiate whether Raynaud's is secondary to SSc overlap rather than isolated SLE, especially in the presence of scleroderma-specific antibodies and sclerodactyly.

- Detects scleroderma-pattern microangiopathy in patients with features of multiple connective tissue diseases.
- Aids in early identification of overlap cases, especially in SLE patients with Raynaud's.
- Provides prognostic information, as severe microvascular damage is linked to digital ulcers, pulmonary hypertension, and organ involvement.

Q3: Answer: a

Case 19 Answer:

Q1: Answer: **Description**; *Density:* reduced. *Dimensions:* presence of giant capillaries with a diameter > 50 μm. *Morphology:* abnormal shape of capillaries and neo-angiogenesis. *Microhemorrhages:* present. **Interpretation:** NFC shows a scleroderma-like pattern, which indicates the presence of anti-synthetase syndrome with interstitial lung disease in correlation with the clinical and lab findings [1].

Q2: Answer: [23]

- Detects microvascular changes such as dilated loops, hemorrhages, and reduced density, which reflect endothelial dysfunction.
- Helps in differentiating from other CTDs, especially systemic sclerosis when Raynaud's is present.
- Provides prognostic information, as severe microangiopathy is associated with digital ischemia and increased risk of pulmonary hypertension.
- Useful for monitoring disease activity and vascular progression in follow-up.

Q3: Answer: c

References

1. Smith V, Herrick AL, Ingegnoli F, et al. Standardisation of nailfold capillaroscopy for the assessment of patients with Raynaud's phenomenon and systemic sclerosis. Autoimmun Rev. 2020;19(3):102458. https://doi.org/10.1016/j.autrev.2020.102458.
2. Bellando-Randone S, Del Galdo F, Lepri G, Minier T, Dörte Huscher, Furst DE, Allanore Y, Distler O, László Czirják, Bruni C, Guiducci S, Avouac J, Cutolo M, Smith V, Matucci-Cerinic M, Very Early Diagnosis of Systemic Sclerosis collaborators. Progression of patients with Raynaud's phenomenon to systemic sclerosis: a five-year analysis of the European Scleroderma Trial and Research group multicentre, longitudinal registry study for Very Early Diagnosis of Systemic Sclerosis (VEDOSS). Lancet Rheumatol. 2021;3:e834–43.

3. Lescoat A. Very Early Diagnosis of Systemic Sclerosis: deciphering the heterogeneity of systemic sclerosis in the very early stages of the disease. J Scleroderma Relat Disord. 2022;8(1):3–6. https://doi.org/10.1177/23971983221129211.
4. Varjú C, Pauling JD, Saketkoo LA. Multi-organ system screening, care, and patient support in systemic sclerosis. Rheum Dis Clin N Am. 2023;49:211–48. https://doi.org/10.1016/j.rdc.2023.01.002.
5. Denton CP, De Lorenzis E, Roblin E, Goldman N, Alcacer-Pitarch B, Blamont E, Buch MH, Carulli M, Cotton C, Del Galdo F, Derrett-Smith E, Douglas K, Farrington S, Fligelstone K, Gompels L, Griffiths B, Herrick A, Hughes M, Pain C, Pantano G, Pauling JD, Prabu A, O'Donoghue N, Renzoni EA, Royle J, Samaranayaka M, Spierings J, Tynan A, Warburton L, Ong VH. The 2024 British Society for Rheumatology guideline for management of systemic sclerosis. Rheumatology. 2024;63(11):2956–75. https://doi.org/10.1093/rheumatology/keae394.
6. Lazzaroni MG, Moschetti L, Breda M, Franceschini F, Airò P. Long-term organ damage accrual and late mortality in systemic sclerosis. Clin Exp Rheumatol. 2024;42:1541–8.
7. Smith V, Ickinger C, Hysa E, Snow M, Frech T, Sulli A, Cutolo M. Nailfold capillaroscopy. Best Pract Res Clin Rheumatol. 2023;37(1):101849.
8. Ferrari G, Gotelli E, Paolino S, et al. Antiphospholipid antibodies and anticoagulant therapy: capillaroscopic findings. Arthritis Res Ther. 2021;23(1):175.
9. Cutolo M, Melsens K, Wijnant S, Ingegnoli F, Thevissen K, De Keyser F, Decuman S, Müller-Ladner U, Piette Y, Riccieri V, Ughi N, Vandecasteele E, Vanhaecke A, Smith V. Nailfold capillaroscopy in systemic lupus erythematosus: a systematic review and critical appraisal. Autoimmun Rev. 2018;17(4):344–52. https://doi.org/10.1016/j.autrev.2017.11.025. Epub 2018 Feb 8.
10. Ting ZHAO, Fu-an LIN, Hong-pu CHEN. Pattern of Nailfold capillaroscopy in patients with systemic lupus erythematosus. Arch Rheumatol. 2020;35(4):568–74. https://doi.org/10.46497/ArchRheumatol.2020.7763.
11. Ornowska S, Wudarski M, Dziewięcka E, Olesińska M. Naifold capillaroscopy in mixed connective tissue disease patients. Clin Rheumatol. 2024;43(5):1703–9. https://doi.org/10.1007/s10067-024-06879-7. Epub 12 Mar 21.
12. Kuryliszyn-Moskal A, Kita J, Hryniewicz A. Raynaud's phenomenon: new aspects of pathogenesis and the role of nailfold videocapillaroscopy. Reumatologia. 2015;53(2):87–93. https://doi.org/10.5114/reum.2015.51508.
13. Graceffa D, Amorosi B, Maiani E, Bonifati C, Chimenti MS, Perricone R, Di Carlo A. Capillaroscopy in psoriatic and rheumatoid arthritis: a useful tool for differential diagnosis. Arthritis. 2013;2013(1):957480. https://doi.org/10.1155/2013/957480.
14. Lambova SN, Müller-Ladner U. Capillaroscopic pattern in inflammatory arthritis. Microvasc Res. 2012;83(3):318–22. https://doi.org/10.1016/j.mvr.2012.03.002.
15. Shenavandeh S, Azariyon Z, Nazarinia MA. Scleroderma-overlap syndromes: capillaroscopy, laboratory, and clinical manifestations and follow-up compared to scleroderma patients. Reumatologia. 2024;61(6):448–59. https://doi.org/10.5114/reum/175508.
16. Desinova O, Starovoytova M, Ananyeva LP, et al. AB0737 Capillaroscopic patterns in patients with Systemic Sclerosis- Rheumatoid arthritis (SSc-RA) overlap syndrome. Ann Rheum Dis. 2022;81:1495.
17. Uceda J, Velloso ML, Martinez R, Marenco JL. AB0688 Nailfold capillaroscopy (nfc) in children with juvenile idiopathic arthritis (jia): an observational study. Ann Rheum Dis. 2013;72:A998. https://doi.org/10.1136/annrheumdis-2013-eular.3010.
18. Abdelrahman MSI, Tohamy D, Osman NS, Saleh MGA. Nailfold capillaroscopic assessment in pediatric patients with autoimmune uveitis: a case–control study. Clin Rheumatol. 2024;43(12):3855–61. https://doi.org/10.1007/s10067-024-07183-0.
19. Maldonado G, Guerrero R, Paredes C, Ríos C. Nailfold capillaroscopy in diabetes mellitus. Microvasc Res. 2017;112:41–6. https://doi.org/10.1016/j.mvr.2017.03.001. Epub 2017 Mar 6.
20. Lisco G, Triggiani V. Computerized nailfold video-capillaroscopy in type 2 diabetes: a cross-sectional study on 102 outpatients. J Diabetes. 2023;15:890–9.

21. Wilkinson S, Wilkinson J, Grace A, Lyon D, Mellor M, Yunus T, Manning J, Dinsdale G, Berks M, Knight S, Bakerly N, Gebril A, Dark P, Herrick A, Taylor C, Dickinson M, Murray A. Imaging the microvasculature using nailfold capillaroscopy in patients with coronavirus disease-2019; A cross-sectional study. Microvasc Res. 2025;159:104796.
22. Gotelli E, Campitiello R, Pizzorni C, Sammorì S, Aitella E, Ginaldi L, De Martinis M, Carubbi F, Di Ruscio E, Cuomo G, Martinelli E, Marrone S, De Angelis R, Giuggioli D, Guiducci S, Ingegnoli F, Riccieri V, Sebastiani M, Sulli A, Smith V, Cutolo M, Study Group on Capillaroscopy and Microcirculation in Rheumatic Diseases of the Italian Society of Rheumatology (CAPSIR). Multicentre retrospective detection of nailfold videocapillaroscopy abnormalities in long covid patients. RMD Open. 2025;11(2):e005469.
23. Sebastiani M, Triantafyllias K, Manfredi A, et al. Nailfold Capillaroscopy characteristics of Antisynthetase syndrome and possible clinical associations: results of a multicenter international study. J Rheumatol. 2019;46(3):279–84. https://doi.org/10.3899/jrheum.180355. Epub 2018 Nov 15.

Chapter 17
Clinical Atlas in Capillaroscopy

Rahma A. Elziaty and Yasser El Miedany

Introduction

Over recent decades, nailfold capillaroscopy (NFC) has transitioned from a simple observational procedure into a fundamental diagnostic and prognostic tool for evaluating microvascular changes in rheumatic and systemic diseases. Once primarily associated with systemic sclerosis, NFC is now widely applied across various autoimmune, inflammatory, and vascular disorders, offering valuable insights into pathophysiological mechanisms, disease activity, and progression [1–3]. The ability to directly visualize and monitor microcirculation has made NFC an indispensable, noninvasive technique in modern rheumatology.

The concept of a clinical atlas in capillaroscopy arises from this growing recognition of NFC's importance. Unlike conventional manuals that often rely on schematic or idealized images, this atlas compiles authentic, high-resolution capillaroscopic images obtained from patients across different geographic regions and disease stages. This approach highlights the natural heterogeneity of microvascular findings and provides a practical visual guide that mirrors real clinical scenarios. Each section of the atlas focuses on specific disease entities or morphological categories, emphasizing the clinical context, temporal evolution of capillary changes, and their systemic correlations.

R. A. Elziaty (✉)
Internal Medicine Department, Rheumatology Division, Faculty of Medicine,
Ain Shams University, Cairo, Egypt
e-mail: drrahmaelziaty@med.asu.edu.eg

Y. El Miedany
Canterbury Christ Church University, Canterbury, UK

Rheumatology and Rehabilitation, Ain Shams University, Cairo, Egypt

King's College, London, UK

Y. El Miedany, R. A. Elziaty (eds.), *Capillaroscopy*, Contemporary Rheumatology,
https://doi.org/10.1007/978-3-032-22966-3_17

This project represents a collaborative international effort aimed at advancing education and consistency in capillaroscopic interpretation. By documenting and sharing diverse real-life examples, the atlas contributes to the establishment of a standardized visual and descriptive language for interpreting capillaroscopic findings. This harmonization supports improved diagnostic precision, facilitates research comparability, and promotes a deeper understanding of microangiopathy in systemic diseases.

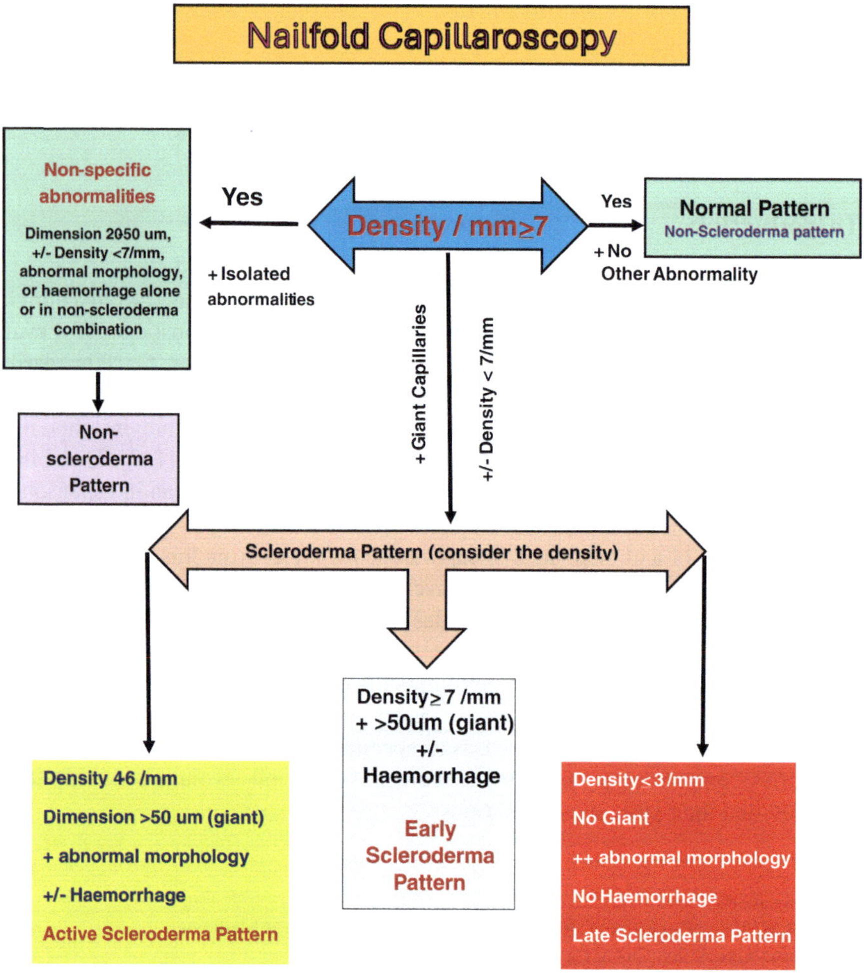

Fig. 17.1 Standardized quantitative capillaroscopy evaluation flow chart

Figure 17.1 presents the standardized parameters used to evaluate nailfold capillaroscopy findings. It defines the key morphological features, measurement criteria, and terminology to ensure consistency and reproducibility across clinical assessments and research studies. Each parameter—such as capillary density, morphology, dimensions, and presence of hemorrhages—is clearly described with corresponding normal and abnormal reference values. This standardization allows for uniform interpretation of microvascular changes, facilitates comparison between studies, and supports accurate diagnosis and disease monitoring in rheumatologic and microangiopathic conditions.

I- Normal Nailfold Capillaroscopy

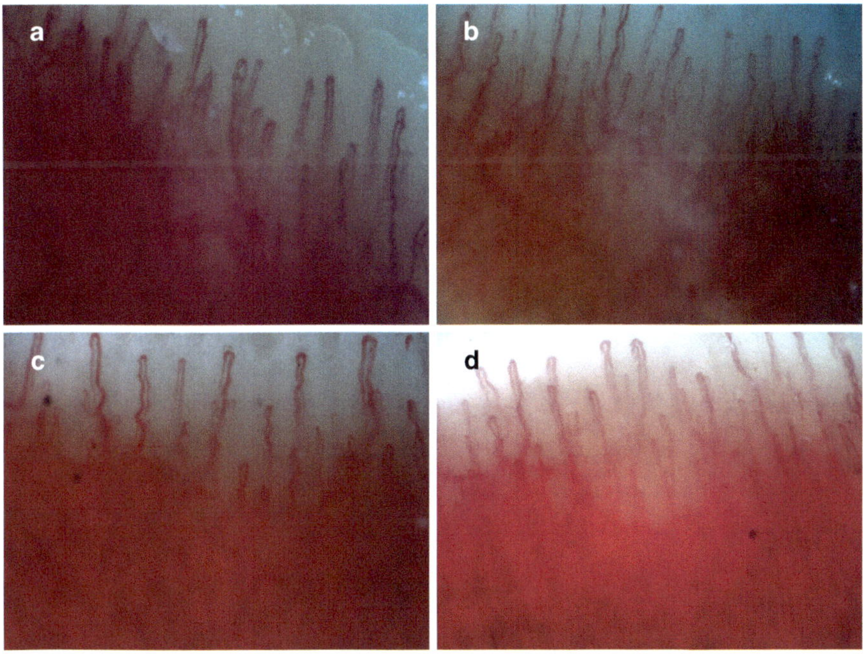

Fig. 17.2 Spectrum of normal-pattern capillaroscopy (**a**, **b**, **c**, **d**)

Rahma A. Elziaty
Internal Medicine Department, Rheumatology Division, Faculty of Medicine, Ain Shams University, Cairo, Egypt

Figure 17.2 illustrates a normal nailfold capillaroscopy pattern *(a, b, c, d)*, demonstrating a regular, organized arrangement of capillary loops. The capillaries are predominantly *hairpin- or U-shaped*, evenly aligned and distributed along the nailfold, with a *normal density of about 7–12 capillaries per millimeter*.

No *dilated loops, hemorrhages, avascular areas, or neoangiogenic formations* are observed. The *arteriovenous (A–V) plexus* is visible beneath the capillary loops, appearing as a normal subpapillary vascular network.

Occasionally, *tortuous or crossed capillaries* may be seen; these are considered *normal variants* and not indicative of pathology. Overall, the pattern reflects *preserved microvascular integrity and normal capillary morphology* (Figs. 17.3 and 17.4).

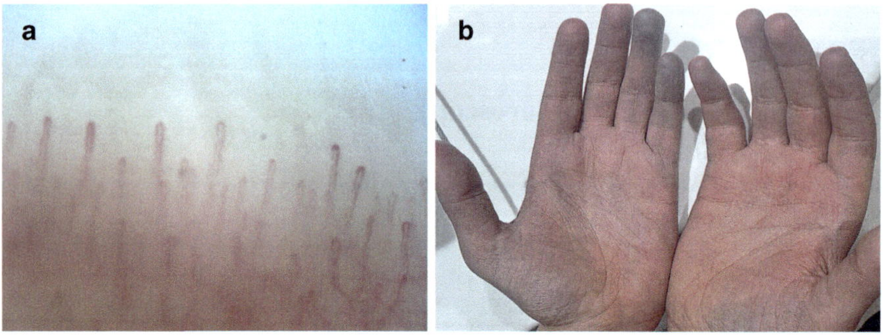

Fig. 17.3 Normal-pattern capillaroscopy (**a**) in a 35-year-old male patient presented with bluish discoloration of the fingers (**b**). No history suggestive of rheumatological illnesses with normal laboratory findings. Diagnosis: *primary Raynaud's phenomenon*
Rahma A. Elziaty
Internal Medicine Department, Rheumatology Division, Faculty of Medicine, Ain Shams University, Cairo, Egypt

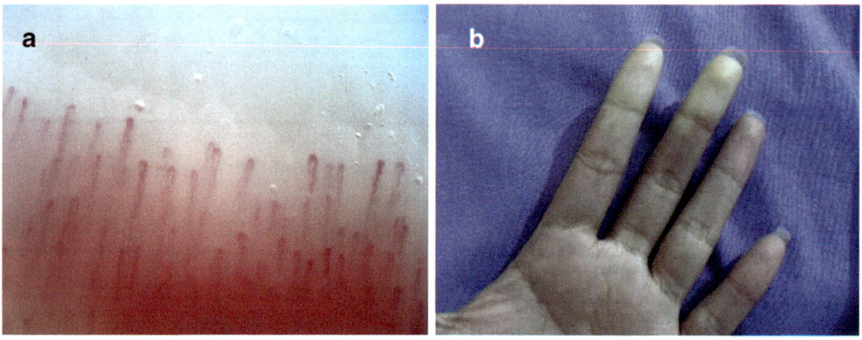

Fig. 17.4 Normal-pattern capillaroscopy (**a**) in a 27-year-old female patient presented with bluish discoloration of the fingers (**b**). No history suggestive of rheumatological illnesses, ANA: negative, ESR: 5 mm/h. Diagnosis: *primary Raynaud's phenomenon*
Rahma A. Elziaty
Internal Medicine Department, Rheumatology Division, Faculty of Medicine, Ain Shams University, Cairo, Egypt

A *normal capillaroscopic pattern* is not restricted to *primary Raynaud's phenomenon*. It may also be seen in various *rheumatologic and connective tissue diseases*, such as *systemic lupus erythematosus* (SLE), *Sjögren's syndrome*, *rheumatoid arthritis*, and other inflammatory arthritides. Therefore, careful *clinical assessment* and *laboratory correlation* are essential for accurate interpretation.

II- Scleroderma Pattern

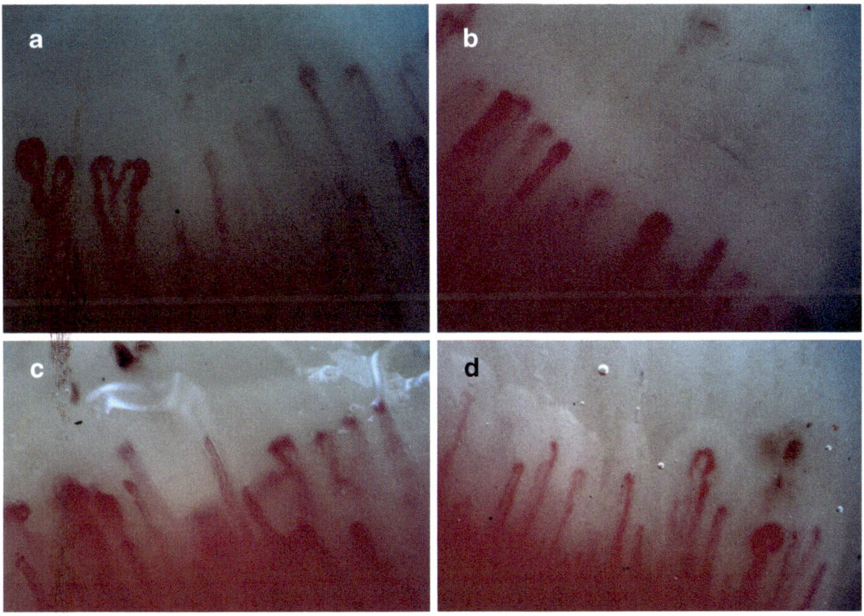

Fig. 17.5 Early scleroderma pattern (**a**, **b**, **c**, **d**)

Rahma A. Elziaty
Internal Medicine Department, Rheumatology Division, Faculty of Medicine, Ain Shams University, Cairo, Egypt

Figure 17.5 shows an *early scleroderma capillaroscopic pattern*, characterized by the presence of a few *giant capillaries* and *microhemorrhages*, with a generally *preserved capillary density and distribution*. The majority of capillary loops maintain their regular shape and alignment, but *focal areas of dilatation* can be observed, reflecting the initial stages of microangiopathy.

There are *no extensive avascular areas* or evident signs of neoangiogenesis at this stage. The coexistence of *normal, dilated, and giant capillaries* indicates an early vascular injury process, typical of the *initial phase of systemic sclerosis*, where endothelial damage has begun, but structural loss of capillaries is still limited.

Figure 17.6 demonstrates an *active scleroderma pattern*, marked by a *pronounced microangiopathy*. Numerous *giant capillaries* and *frequent microhemorrhages* are visible, indicating ongoing and significant endothelial damage. The *capillary density begins to decrease (4–6 capillaries/mm)*, with *avascular areas* appearing among the remaining loops.

There is a clear *loss of the normal orderly arrangement* of capillaries, with *heterogeneous loop sizes and shapes (C, D)* reflecting progressive vascular destruction. The coexistence of *giant, dilated, and missing capillaries*, together with recurrent hemorrhages, characterizes this *active phase* of the disease, during which microvascular injury and repair processes are simultaneously occurring.

Figure 17.7 depicts a *late scleroderma capillaroscopic pattern*, characterized by *severe microvascular damage* and *advanced structural disorganization*. There is a *marked reduction in capillary density (≤3 capillaries/mm)*, with extensive *avascular areas* replacing normal loops. *Giant capillaries and hemorrhages* are usually *absent or rare*, reflecting the exhaustion of active injury.

The remaining capillaries show *irregular shapes and ramified and bushy (neoangiogenic) loops*, indicating attempts at *vascular repair and remodeling*. The overall architecture is *highly distorted*, with a *loss of the normal parallel alignment*. This pattern represents the *chronic or late phase of systemic sclerosis*, in which capillary loss and neoangiogenesis dominate, signifying *irreversible microangiopathy*.

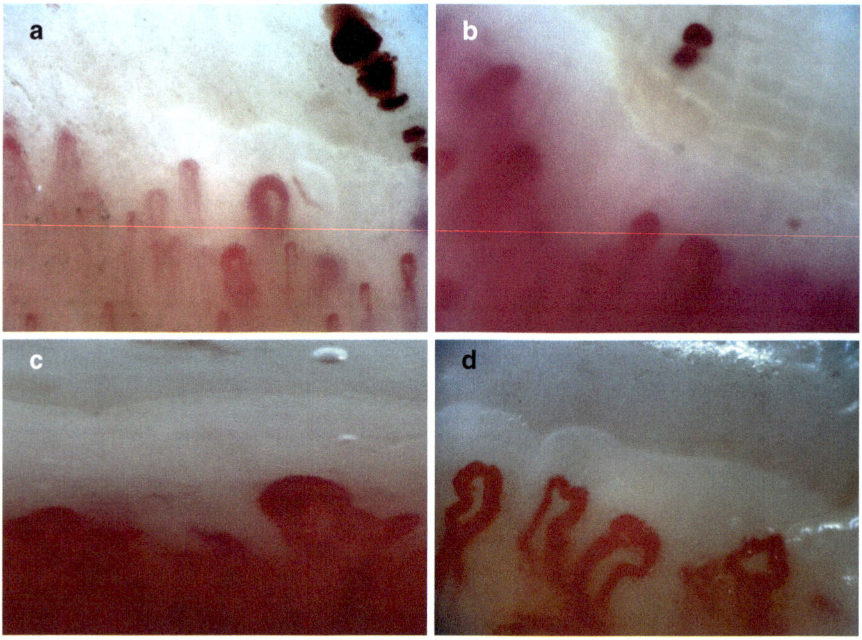

Fig. 17.6 Active scleroderma pattern (**a**, **b**, **c**, **d**)

Rahma A. Elziaty
Internal Medicine Department, Rheumatology Division, Faculty of Medicine, Ain Shams University, Cairo, Egypt

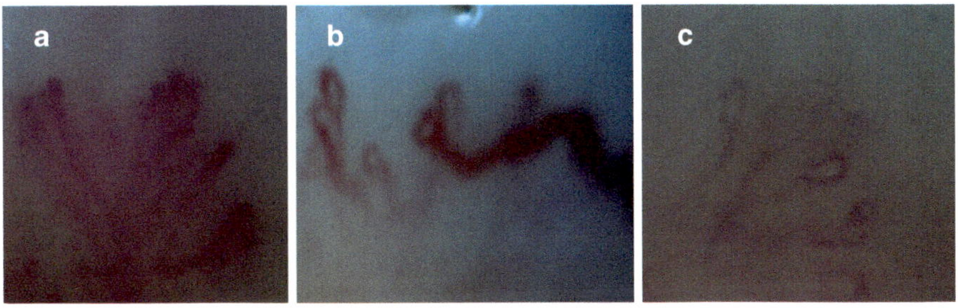

Fig. 17.7 Late scleroderma pattern (**a**, **b**, **c**)

Rahma A. Elziaty
Internal Medicine Department, Rheumatology Division, Faculty of Medicine, Ain Shams University, Cairo, Egypt

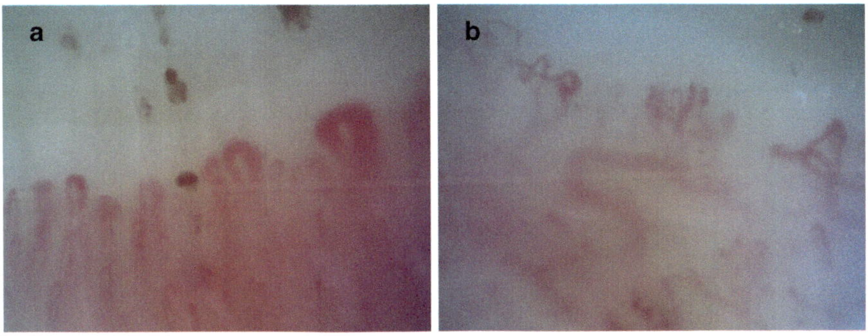

Fig. 17.8 Active and late scleroderma pattern. Two patients with SSc (**a**: 70-year-old female—active; **b**: 73-year-old female—late) exhibiting severe and widespread capillaroscopic abnormalities

Marco Di Battista[1, 2], Nicola Ortalli[1], Francesco Del Galdo[1, 3]
[1]Leeds Institute of Rheumatic and Musculoskeletal Medicine, University of Leeds, Leeds, UK
[2]Rheumatology Unit, University of Pisa, Pisa, Italy
[3]NIHR Leeds Biomedical Research Centre, Leeds Teaching Hospitals Trust, Leeds, UK

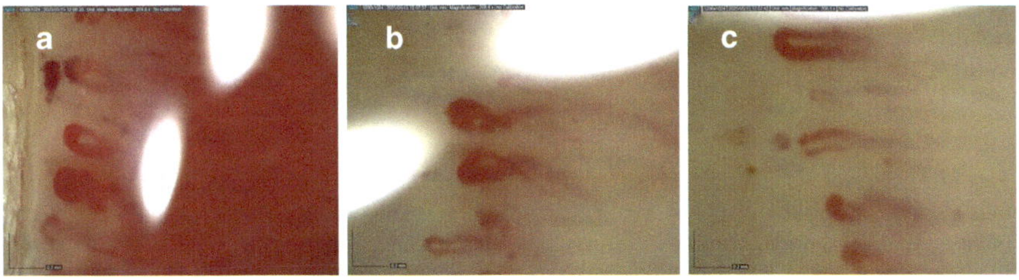

Fig. 17.9 Capillaroscopic picture with scleroderma pattern-like changes in the active phase (moderate-low capillary density, presence of megacapillaries and hemorrhages), lack of signs of neoangiogenesis. *Left hand (finger II)* (**a**)—density 4 capillaries/mm, size >50 μm (megacapillaries), normal morphology, present hemorrhage. *Left hand (finger III)* (**b**, **c**)—density 3 capillaries/mm, size >50 μm (megacapillaries), regular morphology, hemorrhages present

Maria Lungu[1, 2], Svetlana Agachi[1]
[1]Rheumatology and Nephrology Discipline, *Nicolae Testemițanu* University, Republic of Moldova
[2]*Timofei Moşneaga* Republican Clinical Hospital, Chişinău, Republic of Moldova

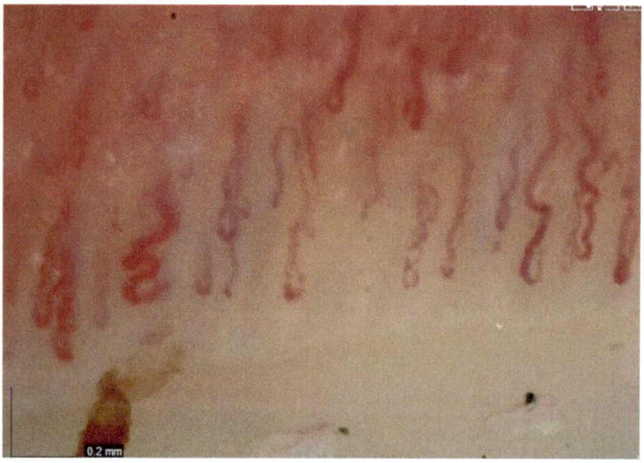

Fig. 17.10 Patient with anti-Scl70–positive limited systemic sclerosis showing an active scleroderma pattern. The capillaroscopy demonstrates elongated, tortuous, and ramified capillaries with mild capillary dropout and hemorrhages

Cristiana Sieiro Santos
University of Manchester, Center for Musculoskeletal Research, Manchester, UK

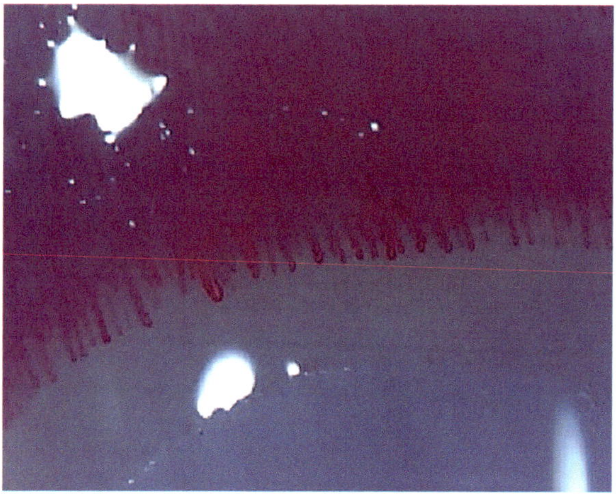

Fig. 17.11 Preserved capillary density and distribution with multiple tortuous and crossing loops. One elongated capillary displays asymmetric dilatation. In the absence of megacapillaries, microhemorrhages, or reduced capillary density, these findings are to be considered nonspecific abnormalities and do not fulfill the criteria for a scleroderma pattern. Diagnosis: Systemic sclerosis *sine* scleroderma

Carlos Valera-Ribera, MD. ORCID ID: 0009-0007-3059-4347
Department of Rheumatology, Hospital Universitario Dr. Peset, Valencia, Spain

III- Scleroderma-Like Pattern and Overlap Syndromes

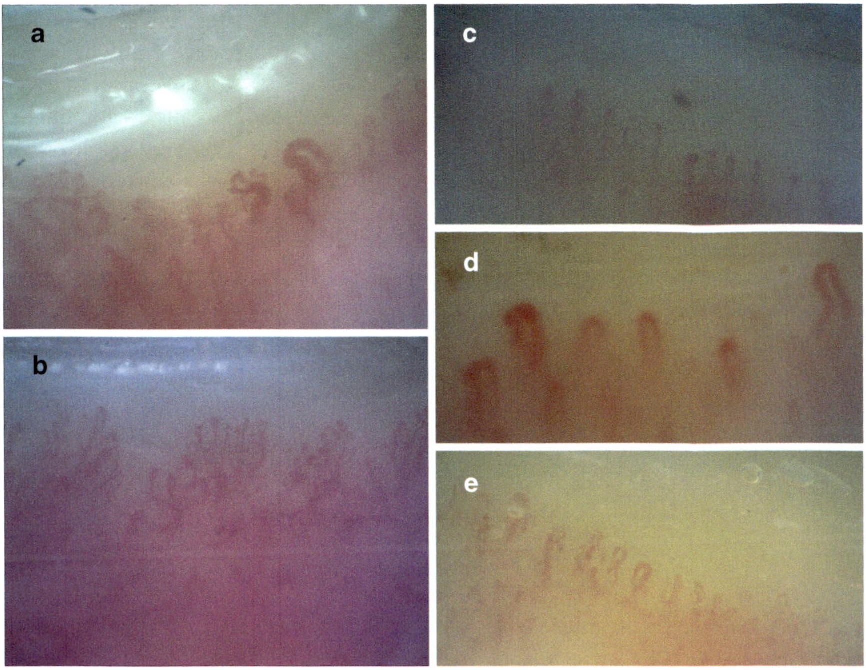

Fig. 17.12 In patients with dermatomyositis, NVC patterns resembling the scleroderma pattern can be observed (**a**: 63-year-old female), and in some cases, a characteristic bushy neoangiogenesis may be present (**b**: 79-year-old female). In contrast, patients with polymyositis and RP typically show absent or only mild nonspecific abnormalities on NVC (**c**: 67-year-old male). In mixed connective tissue disease, a wide spectrum of NVC findings can be observed, ranging from a scleroderma-like pattern (**d**: 59-year-old male) to normal findings (**e**: 60-year-old female)

Marco Di Battista[1, 2], Nicola Ortalli[1], Francesco Del Galdo[1, 3]
[1]Leeds Institute of Rheumatic and Musculoskeletal Medicine, University of Leeds, Leeds, UK
[2]Rheumatology Unit, University of Pisa, Pisa, Italy
[3]NIHR Leeds Biomedical Research Centre, Leeds Teaching Hospitals Trust, Leeds, UK

Figure 17.13 demonstrates a *scleroderma-like capillaroscopic pattern*, which shows microvascular *abnormalities resembling those seen in systemic sclerosis* but occurring in other diseases or conditions. The findings include *irregularly enlarged and few giant capillaries*, *microhemorrhages*, and *reduced capillary density*, often with *disorganization of the capillary architecture* and *bushy neoangiogenic formation.*

However, the *extent of avascular areas and neoangiogenesis* is typically *less severe* than in classic systemic sclerosis. This pattern may be observed in *dermatomyositis*, *mixed connective tissue disease*, and *undifferentiated connective tissue disease* and therefore requires clinical and laboratory correlation to confirm the underlying diagnosis (Figs. 17.14, 17.15, 17.16, 17.17, 17.18, and 17.19).

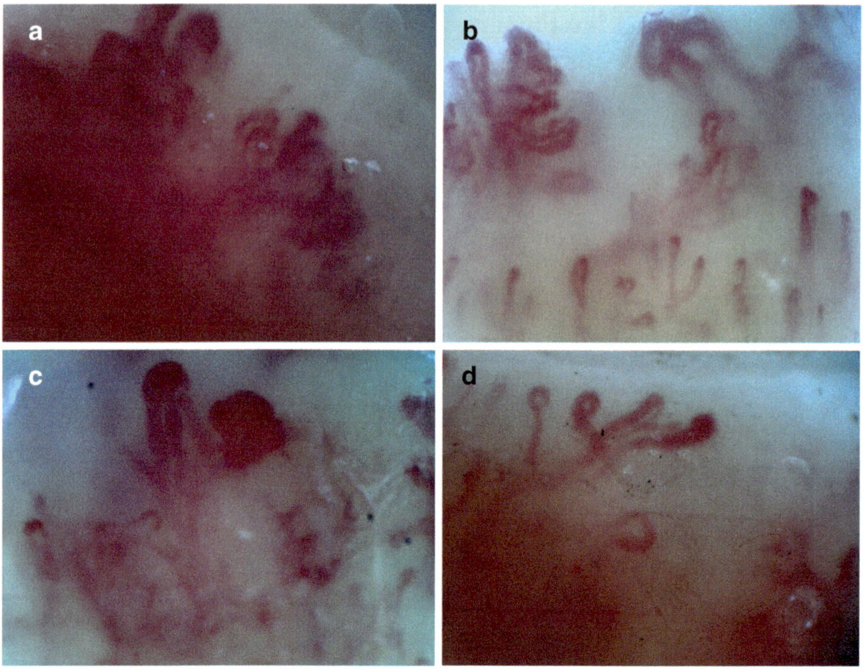

Fig. 17.13 Scleroderma-like pattern

Rahma A. Elziaty
Internal Medicine Department, Rheumatology Division, Faculty of Medicine, Ain Shams University, Cairo, Egypt

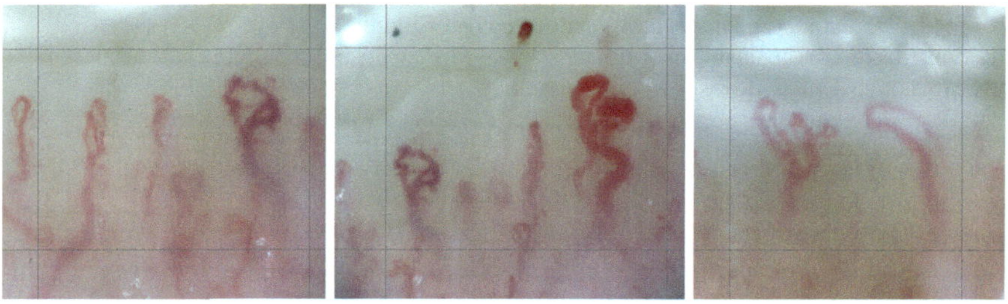

Fig. 17.14 Nailfold videocapillaroscopy (DS Medica, Italy, 200x) of a 16-year-old patient with amyopathic dermatomyositis (ANA 1:160, AC-4 fine speckled pattern, anti-TIF1γ (p155/140) antibodies positive) and no history of Raynaud's phenomenon. Videocapillaroscopic images demonstrate a scleroderma pattern with reduced capillary density, giant capillaries, and capillary aberrations and tortuosities. Hemorrhages were also found

Sara Alves Costa[1,2], Tânia Santiago[1,2]
[1]Rheumatology Department, Coimbra´s Local Unit Health
[2]Faculty of Medicine of the University of Coimbra

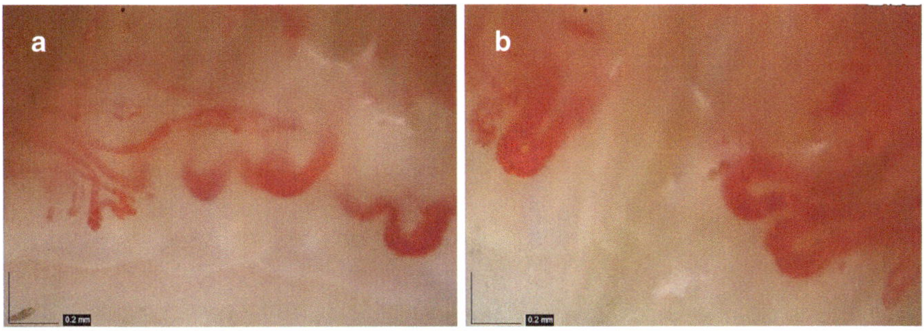

Fig. 17.15 Overlap systemic sclerosis–dermatomyositis patient with anti-MDA5 and anti-Ro52 antibodies, presenting with muscle involvement, diffuse cutaneous disease, and interstitial lung disease (ILD). The capillaroscopy demonstrates giant and markedly dilated capillary loops, areas of capillary loss, and bushy neoangiogenic formations, consistent with an active scleroderma-pattern microangiopathy typically seen in overlap syndromes (**a**, **b**)

Cristiana Sieiro Santos
University of Manchester, Center for Musculoskeletal Research, Manchester, UK

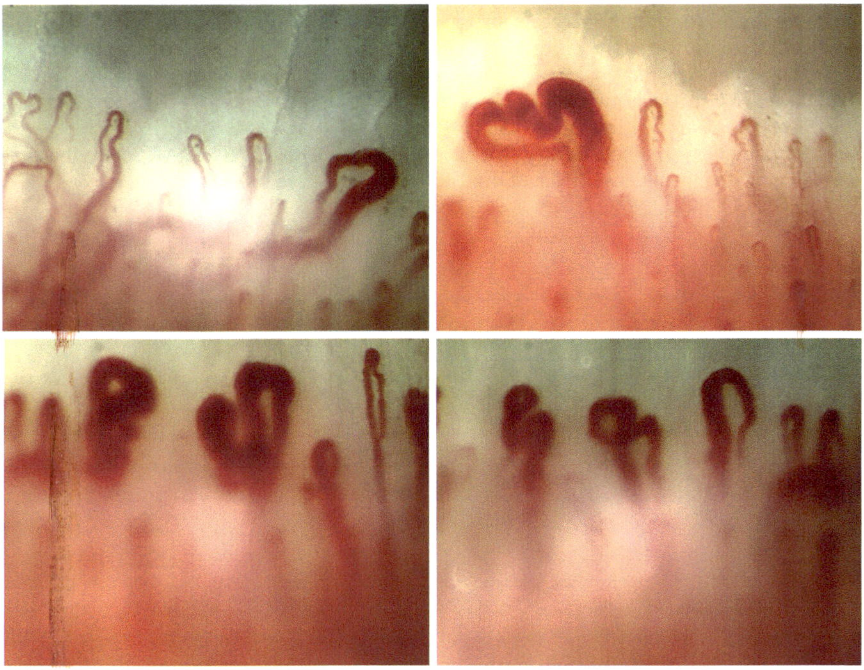

Fig. 17.16 A 65-year-old male was recently diagnosed with overlapping syndrome (SSc and myositis). Nailfold Capillaroscopy (NFC) showed reduced capillary density and enlarged/giant loops

Minrui Liang, M.D., Ph.D.
Department of Rheumatology, Institute of Rheumatology, Immunology and Allergy, Huashan Rare Disease Center, Huashan Hospital, Fudan University, Shanghai

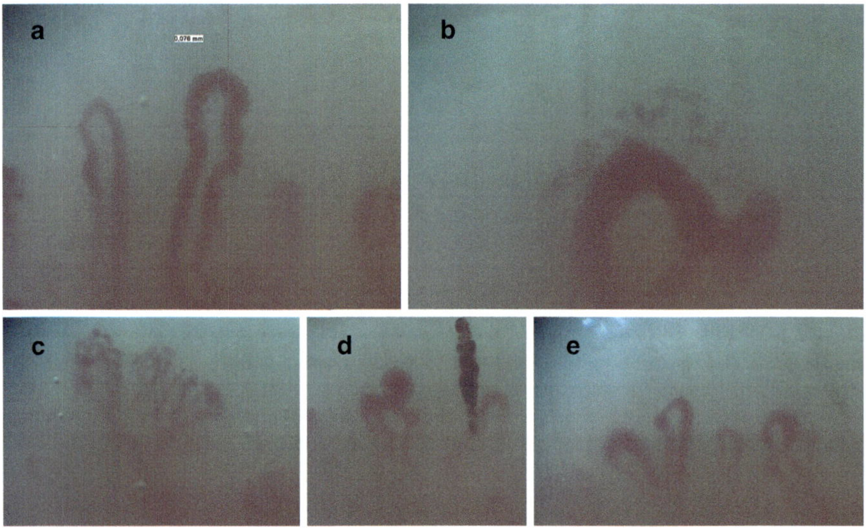

Fig. 17.17 A 65-year-old man with anti-Pm/Scl scleromyositis revealed by scleroderma-like capillaroscopy. (**a**): Megacapillary (diameter ≈ 76 μm) with only two capillaries visible in a 1-mm field. (**b**): Single megacapillary occupying the entire field. (**c**): Neoangiogenesis with branching capillary loops. (**d**): Megacapillary showing a microaneurysm and microhemorrhage. (**e**): Dilated, abnormally shaped capillaries with a characteristic "double-tip" morphology

Prof. Marco Matucci Cerinic and Veronica Batani
Vita-Salute San Raffaele University, Milan, Italy
Unit of Immunology, Rheumatology, Allergy and Rare Diseases (UnIRAR), Inflammation, Fibrosis, and Ageing Initiative (INFLAGE), IRCCS Ospedale San Raffaele, Milan, Italy

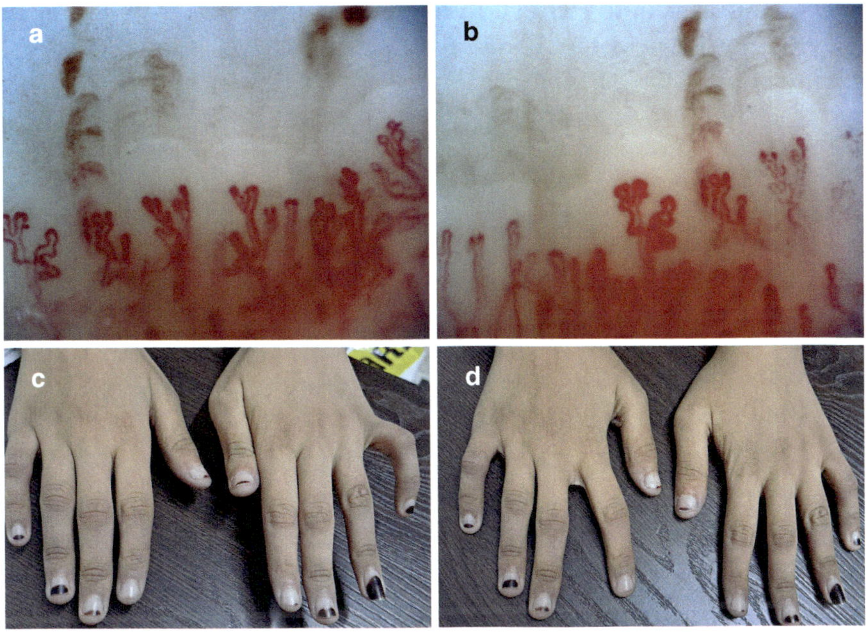

Fig. 17.18 Nailfold capillaroscopy (NFC) demonstrates characteristic bushy neoangiogenesis, capillary dropout, and microhemorrhages (**a**, **b**) in a 28-year-old female diagnosed with mixed connective tissue disease (MCTD). The patient presented with Jaccoud's arthropathy, as shown by the hand deformity in image (**c**), which was corrected in image (**d**), along with Raynaud's phenomenon and positive anti-U1RNP antibodies

Rahma A. Elziaty
Internal Medicine Department, Rheumatology Division, Faculty of Medicine, Ain Shams University, Cairo, Egypt

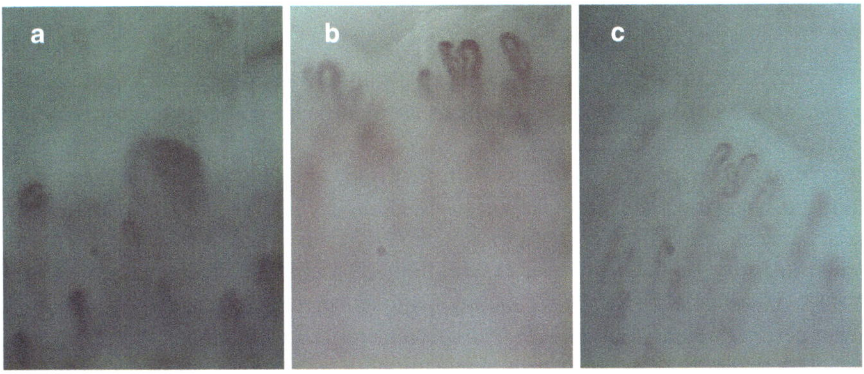

Fig. 17.19 46-year-old patient with ASyS, antinuclear and anti-PL-12 antibodies positive, with interstitial lung disease, myositis, arthritis, Raynaud's, and mechanic's hands. (**a**): Giant capillary, pronounced edema, reduced vascular density. (**b**): Avascular area, branched and ectatic capillaries, pronounced edema. (**c**): Avascular area, branched capillary, edema

Cansu Aglar and Konstantinos Triantafyllias
Rhineland-Palatinate Rheumatology Center, Bad Kreuznach, Germany

IV- Capillaroscopic Pattern in Systemic Lupus Erythematosus (SLE)

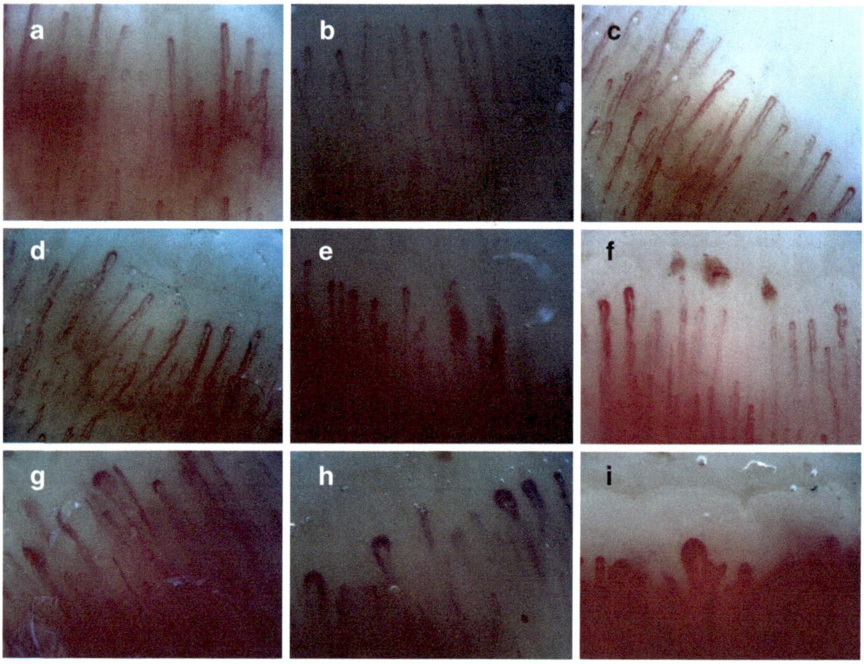

Fig. 17.20 Spectrum of NFC findings in SLE patients

Rahma A. Elziaty
Internal Medicine Department, Rheumatology Division, Faculty of Medicine, Ain Shams University, Cairo, Egypt

In *systemic lupus erythematosus (SLE)*, nailfold capillaroscopy findings are *variable*, ranging from normal appearances to significant microvascular alterations (Fig. 17.20).

Normal pattern: Many patients with SLE may show a *normal capillaroscopic pattern*, characterized by *regular, uniformly shaped capillary loops*, *normal density*, and *absence of hemorrhages or giant capillaries*. This reflects preserved microvascular integrity, particularly in cases with limited vascular involvement (**a**, **b**).

Nonspecific abnormalities: Some patients demonstrate *mild, nonspecific changes*, including *slight capillary dilatation*, *tortuosity*, *occasional microhemorrhages*, or *mildly reduced density*. These findings indicate *endothelial dysfunction or minimal vascular injury* but do not fit any specific diagnostic pattern (**c**, **d**, **e**, **f**).

Scleroderma-like pattern: A subset of SLE patients may exhibit a *scleroderma capillaroscopic pattern*, with *giant capillaries*, *microhemorrhages*, *capillary loss*, and *disorganization of the vascular architecture*. This pattern suggests *secondary microangiopathy*, often seen in *overlap syndromes* or patients with *Raynaud's phenomenon* and *vascular complications* (**g**, **h**, **i**).

Overall, SLE presents a *broad spectrum of capillaroscopic findings*, emphasizing the need for *clinical and laboratory correlation* to interpret their diagnostic and prognostic significance (Figs. 17.21, 17.22).

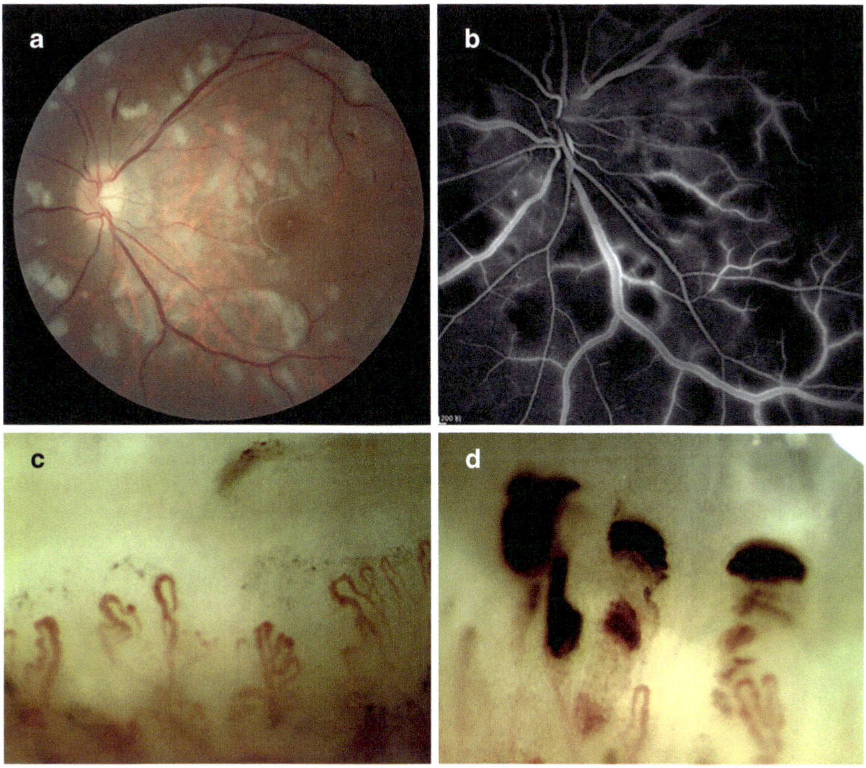

Fig. 17.21 A 26-year-old woman with recently diagnosed systemic lupus erythematosus (SLE) was referred to our hospital because of newly onset blurry vision and a dark shadow in her left eye despite ongoing glucocorticoid therapy (1 mg/kg/d). On admission, her SLE Disease Activity Index (SLEDAI) score was 12. Nasal visual field impairment was found in her left eye. Slit-lamp examination showed normal anterior segments. Funduscopic evaluation revealed widespread cotton-wool spots (**a**), while fluorescein angiogram (FFA) displayed typical frosted retinal periphlebitis and capillary drop-outs (**b**). Interestingly, her nailfold capillaroscopy (NFC) also showed ramification and capillary loss, as well as microhemorrhages (**c**, **d**). In this case, FFA and NFC results were parallel to each other, which suggested that focal capillary vasculitis may reflect systemic vascular damage. Diagnosis: Lupus Retinal Vasculitis
Minrui Liang, M.D., Ph.D., Chen Chen, M.D.
Department of Rheumatology, Institute of Rheumatology, Immunology and Allergy, Huashan Rare Disease Center, Huashan Hospital, Fudan University, Shanghai

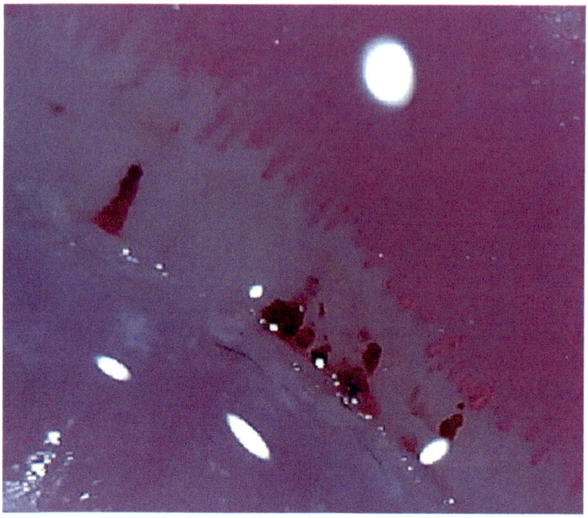

Fig. 17.22 Findings: Multiple microhemorrhages and several dilated capillary loops, with a small focal area of reduced capillary density in the upper-left quadrant. The overall architecture remains largely preserved outside the focal defect, consistent with an early scleroderma pattern. Diagnosis: Overlap syndrome between systemic sclerosis and systemic lupus erythematosus
Carlos Valera-Ribera, MD. ORCID ID: 0009-0007-3059-4347
Department of Rheumatology. Hospital Universitario Dr. Peset, Valencia, Spain.

V- NFC Pattern in Patients with Antiphospholipid Syndrome (APS)

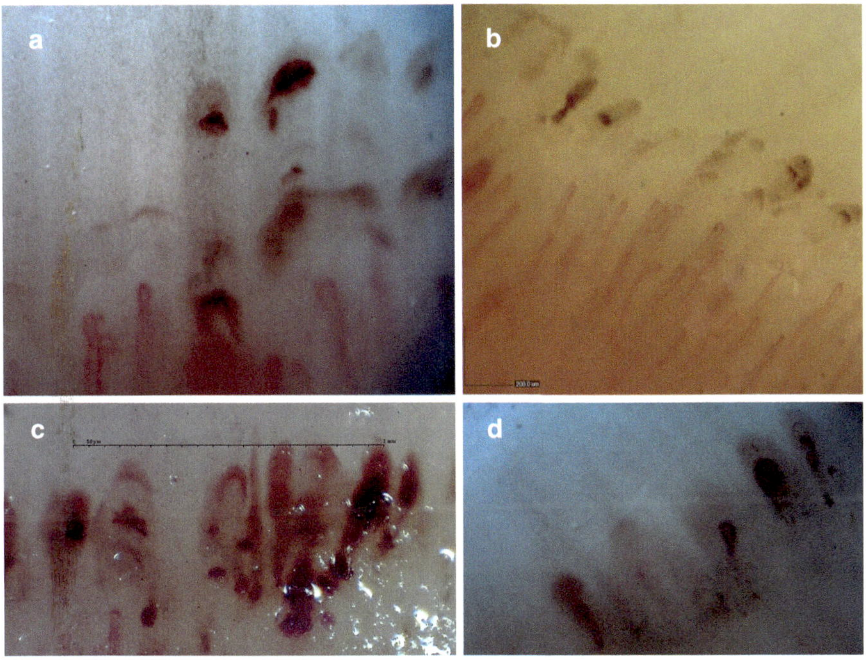

Fig. 17.23 Comb-like hemorrhage of APS

Rahma A. Elziaty
Internal Medicine Department, Rheumatology Division, Faculty of Medicine, Ain Shams University, Cairo, Egypt

The figure shows the characteristic *"comb-like pattern" of microhemorrhages* observed in *antiphospholipid syndrome (APS)*. This pattern is defined by the presence of *multiple, regularly arranged linear or punctate microhemorrhages* distributed along the nailfold, resembling the *teeth of a comb*. The hemorrhages are typically *aligned parallel to the capillary rows* and occur as a result of *repeated microthrombotic events* and *focal endothelial damage*.

Capillary morphology is usually *preserved*, with *normal or mildly reduced density* and *absence of giant or ramified capillaries*. The underlying *arteriovenous plexus* may be visible, but *no avascular areas or neoangiogenesis* are detected. This *comb-like arrangement of microhemorrhages* is considered a *distinctive microvascular feature* associated with APS-related microangiopathy (Figs. 17.24 and 17.25).

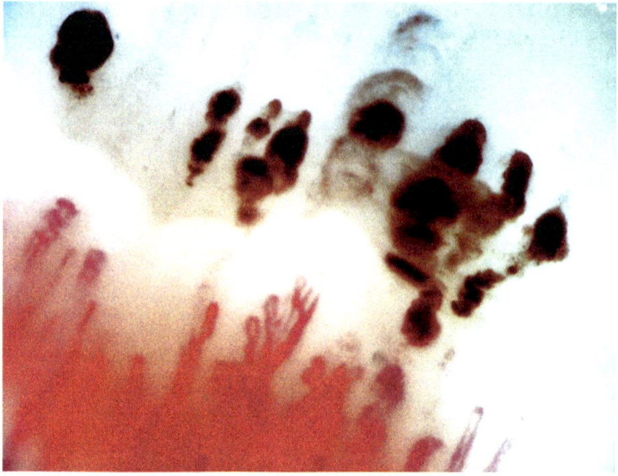

Fig. 17.24 Patient with mixed connective tissue disease (anti-U1RNP positive) and 2ry antiphospholipid (triple positivity autoantibodies). NFC shows decreased capillary density, presence of neoangiogenesis, branched capillaries, and *comb-like pattern* microhemorrhages
Rahma A. Elziaty
Internal Medicine Department, Rheumatology Division, Faculty of Medicine, Ain Shams University, Cairo, Egypt

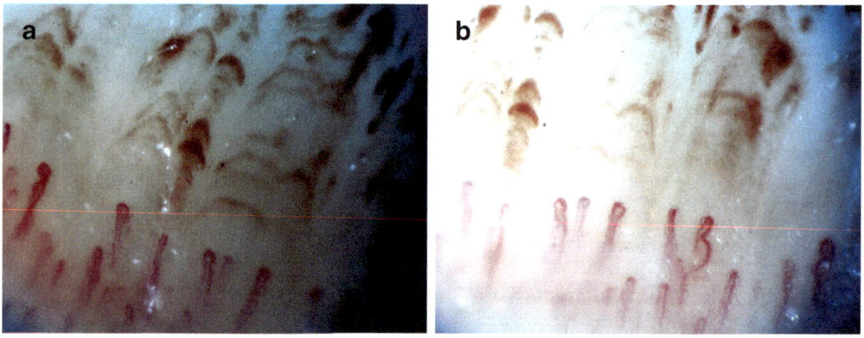

Fig. 17.25 A 35-year-old female patient with SLE and 2ry antiphospholipid (lupus anticoagulant and anti-cardiolipin IgM positive). NFC shows a mild decrease in capillary density, the presence of dilated, tortuous and crossed capillaries, and *comb-like pattern* microhemorrhages (**a**, **b**)
Rahma A. Elziaty
Internal Medicine Department, Rheumatology Division, Faculty of Medicine, Ain Shams University, Cairo, Egypt

VI- Nailfold Capillaroscopy Findings in Rheumatoid Arthritis (RA)

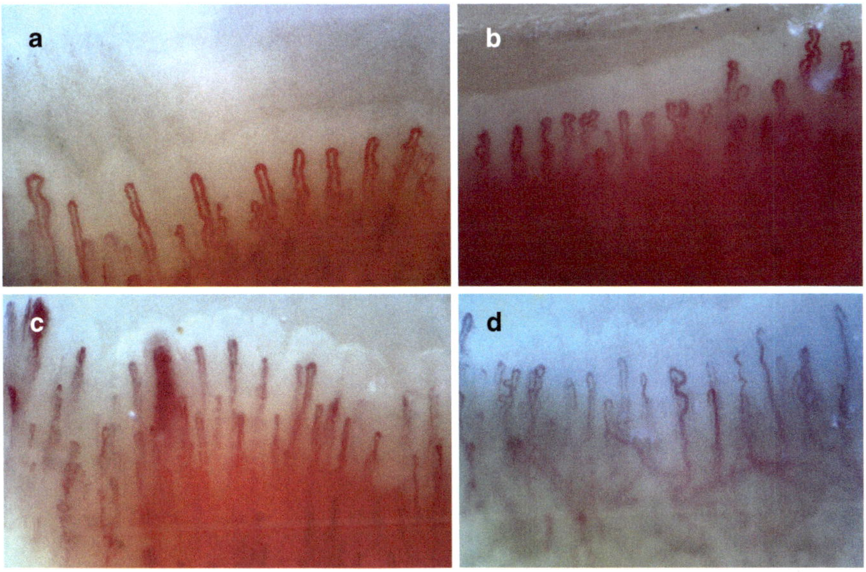

Fig. 17.26 Different nailfold capillaroscopy (NFC) presentations in rheumatoid arthritis. (**a**): Shows dilated, tortuous, and crossed capillaries. (**b**): Increased capillary tortuosity (**c**): Dilated, tortuous capillaries and microhemorrhages. (**d**): Tortuous capillaries and A-V plexus

Rahma A. Elziaty
Internal Medicine Department, Rheumatology Division, Faculty of Medicine, Ain Shams University, Cairo, Egypt

Capillaroscopic findings in *rheumatoid arthritis (RA)* are highly variable, ranging from a *normal capillary pattern* to *nonspecific microvascular abnormalities* and, less commonly, a *scleroderma-like pattern*. Many RA patients show *normal capillary morphology and density*, especially in early or well-controlled disease. However, *nonspecific abnormalities*—such as *capillary dilatation, tortuosity, elongation, microhemorrhages, or capillary crossing*—are frequently observed and reflect low-grade microangiopathy related to chronic inflammation or vasculitis. In a minority of cases, particularly in patients with *secondary Raynaud's phenomenon* or *overlap syndromes*, a *scleroderma-like capillaroscopic pattern* may appear, characterized by *giant capillaries, capillary dropout, and neoangiogenesis*, suggesting more severe or systemic microvascular involvement. Regular nailfold capillaroscopy assessment may help identify such transitions and guide further immunological and clinical evaluation.

VII- Role of Capillaroscopy in Follow-Up

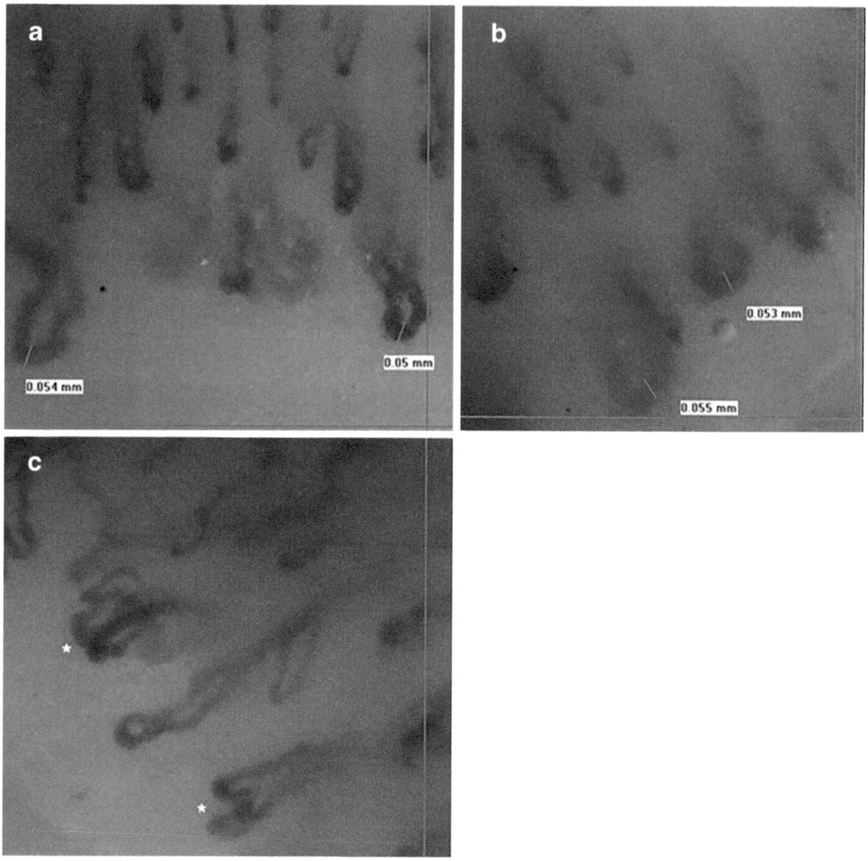

Fig. 17.27 (**a**, **b**, and **c**): Nailfold capillaroscopy (left hand, 200× magnification, VideoCap® 3.0 Rheuma) performed at the time of diagnosis of a patient with limited systemic sclerosis, anti-CENP-A and B positive, with severe Raynaud's phenomenon with a history of recurrent digital ulcers (DUs), particularly in the left hand, treated with bosentan and sildenafil (at maximum tolerated dose) with good response and prevention of new DUs. Nailfold capillaroscopy revealed reduced capillary density, with an average of 5–6 per 1 mm (1 mm grid placed on the image in light gray), multiple giant capillaries (apical size marked), and some dysmorphic capillaries (asterisks) consistent with an active scleroderma pattern

Nailfold capillaroscopy (NFC) is not only a diagnostic tool but is increasingly recognized as a *monitoring biomarker* in systemic sclerosis and related connective tissue diseases. It allows visualization of the microvascular changes over time—including capillary density, giant capillaries, hemorrhages, and neoangiogenesis—which may precede or parallel clinical progression. For instance, evolving from an *early* to *active* or *late* capillaroscopic pattern has been correlated with worsening disease activity and internal organ involvement in systemic sclerosis [1, 3].

In follow-up settings, serial capillaroscopy helps monitor both disease progression and therapeutic response. Some studies show that worsening capillaroscopic scores (e.g., increased avascular areas or drop in capillary density) are associated with declines in lung function (e.g., DLCO or FVC) or increased risk of interstitial lung disease or pulmonary hypertension. Conversely, stabilization or improvement of capillaroscopic features may reflect a positive response to therapy and slower progression of the organ [4, 5].

Progression of the Scleroderma Pattern Over 10 Years of Severe Vasculopathy in Systemic Sclerosis (Figs. 17.27, 17.28)

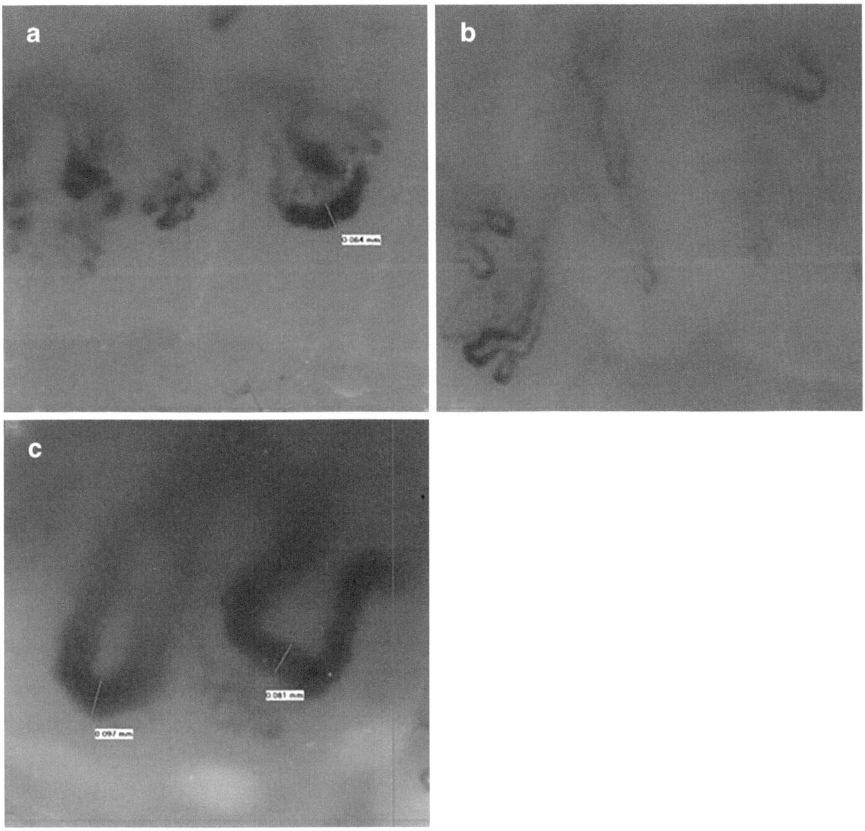

Fig. 17.28 3.0 Rheuma) from the same patient, performed 10 years after the one from Fig. 17.27. Images revealed severe capillary rarefaction (2–4 per 1 mm) with avascular areas, architectural disorganization, giant capillaries (apical size marked), and ramified capillaries, without microhemorrhages. These changes are suggestive of a transition from an active to a late scleroderma pattern. In comparison with Fig. 17.27, there is a reduction in the capillary density and an increase in dysmorphic capillaries as a result of dysregulated angiogenesis

Carolina Teles[1,2]
[1]Department of Internal Medicine, Hospitais da Universidade de Coimbra, Local Health Unit of Coimbra, Coimbra, Portugal
[2]Faculty of Medicine, University of Coimbra, Coimbra, Portugal

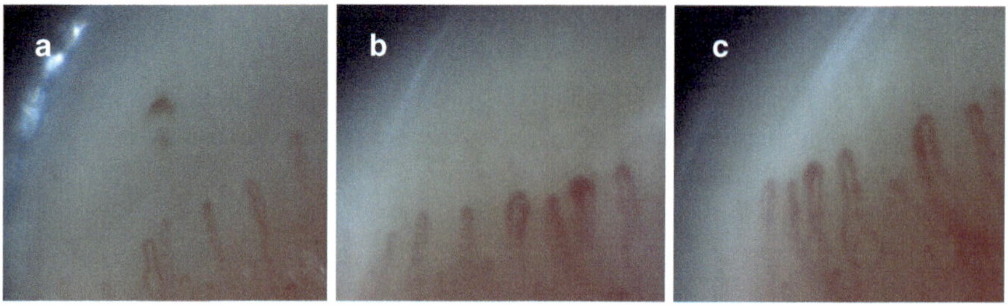

Fig. 17.29 (**a**) Baseline study (age 70): normal capillary density and morphology, one apical microhemorrhage. (**b**, **c**) Follow-up study (age 74): early scleroderma pattern with isolated giant capillaries

Prof. Marco Matucci Cerinic and Veronica Batani
Vita-Salute San Raffaele University, Milan, Italy
Unit of Immunology, Rheumatology, Allergy and Rare Diseases (UnIRAR), Inflammation, Ffibrosis, and Aagingeing Iinitiative (INFLAGE), IRCCS Ospedale San Raffaele, Milan, Italy

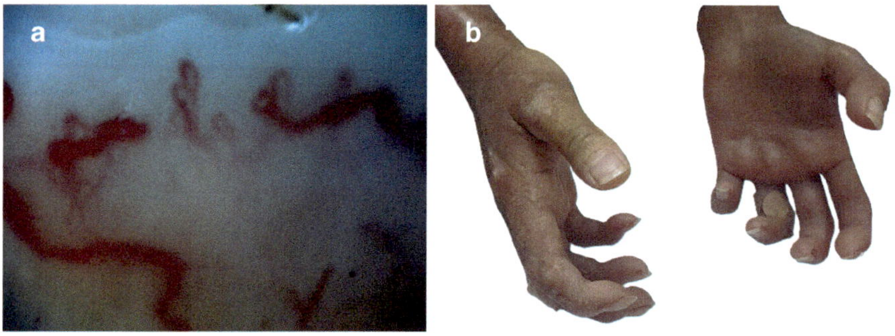

Fig. 17.30 Nailfold capillaroscopy of a 50-year-old female patient with a 13-year history of diffuse cutaneous systemic sclerosis (dcSSc) and anti-Scl-70 positive. The image demonstrates a late scleroderma pattern, characterized by severe capillary loss, extensive ramified capillaries, and evident neoangiogenesis (**a**). Clinically, the patient presents with marked sclerodactyly (**b**) (mRSS = 38), exemplifying the well-established correlation between progressive skin thickening, reduced capillary density, and the late capillaroscopic pattern in systemic sclerosis

Rahma A. Elziaty
Internal Medicine Department, Rheumatology Division, Faculty of Medicine, Ain Shams University, Cairo, Egypt

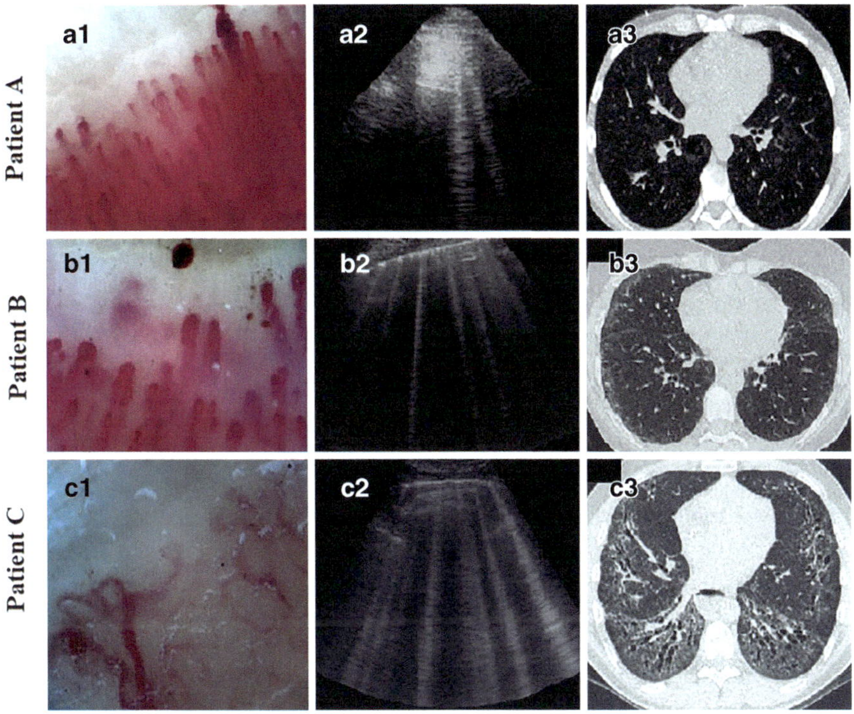

Fig. 17.31 This figure was captured from a study conducted by Elziaty et al., 2025 [4]

NVC, LUS, and HRCT corresponding changes in three participants with different grades of SSc-ILD. **Patient A**: **A1:** NVC shows an early scleroderma pattern with normal capillary density (8/mm), giant capillaries, and hemorrhage. **A2:** LUS shows minimal B-lines (2:3 per lung intercostal space (LIS)). **A3:** HRCT shows a few scattered ground-glass opacities. **Patient B**; **B1:** NVC shows an active scleroderma pattern with decreased capillary density (5/mm), an increased number of giant capillaries, and hemorrhage. **B2:** LUS shows moderate B-lines (5:8 per LIS). **B3:** HRCT shows dense ground-glass opacities and early bronchiectasis. **Patient C**; **C1:** NVC shows a late scleroderma pattern with a marked decrease in capillary density (2/mm) and neoangiogenesis; **C2:** LUS shows extensive B-lines (8:10 per LIS); **C3:** HRCT shows dense fibrosis, honeycombing, and traction bronchiectasis. NVC, nailfold video-capillaroscopy; HRCT, high-resolution computed tomography; LUS, lung ultrasound; LIS, lung intercostal space.

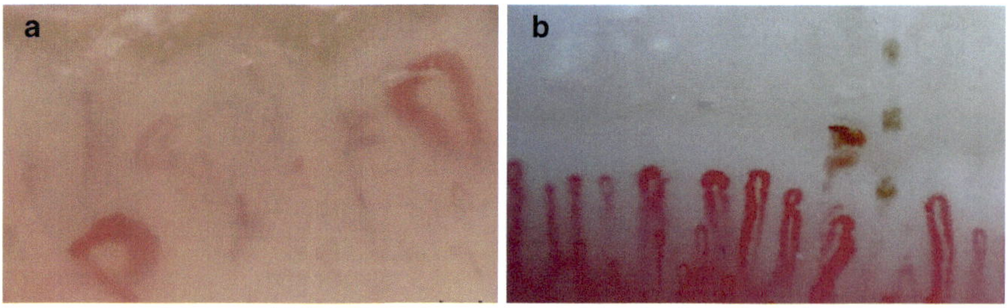

Fig. 17.32 (**a**) Nailfold capillaroscopy before autologous HSCT in systemic sclerosis. Late scleroderma pattern with marked capillary dropout, avascular areas, and a few giant/ramified capillaries, consistent with advanced microangiopathy. (**b**) Nailfold capillaroscopy after autologous HSCT in systemic sclerosis. Capillaroscopic image of the periungual area demonstrating an active pattern following HSCT. Compared with baseline, giant capillaries and microhemorrhages, together with a reduction in avascular areas, and partial restoration of capillary density compared with baseline

Cristiana Sieiro Santos
University of Manchester, Center for Musculoskeletal Research, Manchester, UK

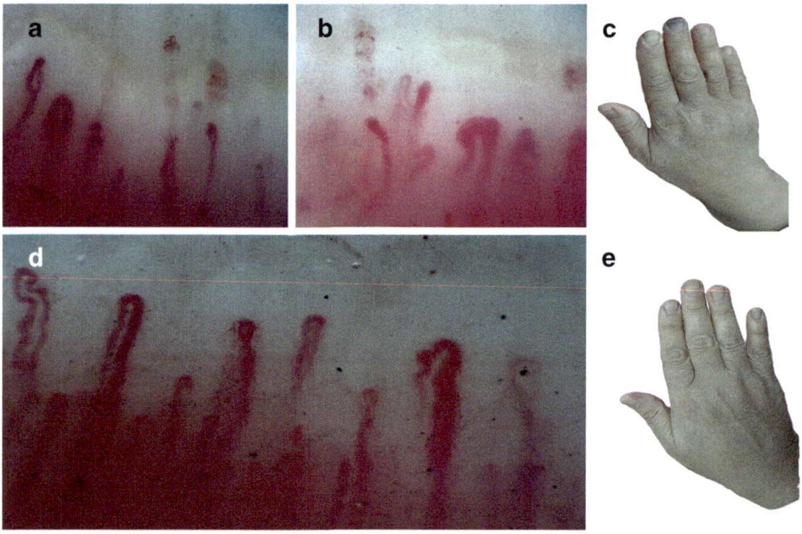

Fig. 17.33 Nailfold capillaroscopy (NFC) reveals an active scleroderma pattern, characterized by decreased capillary density, giant capillaries, and microhemorrhages (**a**, **b**) in a patient with systemic lupus erythematosus (SLE) who presented with a digital ulcer (**c**). Follow-up capillaroscopy after four months of treatment with pulse methylprednisolone followed by maintenance oral steroids and mycophenolate mofetil (2 g/day) demonstrates marked improvement, showing nonspecific abnormalities with elongated, dilated, tortuous capillaries and absence of microhemorrhages (**d**). Clinically, the digital ulcer had completely healed (**e**)

Rahma A. Elziaty
Internal Medicine Department, Rheumatology Division, Faculty of Medicine, Ain Shams University, Cairo, Egypt

Acknowledgments We express our sincere gratitude to all colleagues and collaborators who generously contributed their high-quality capillaroscopic images to this atlas. Your willingness to share your real-life experiences and findings has been invaluable in creating a comprehensive and representative visual collection.

Special thanks are extended to the participating rheumatology and capillaroscopy centers for their continuous collaboration, dedication to clinical excellence, and commitment to advancing education in microvascular assessment. This atlas stands as a reflection of our shared goal—to enhance understanding, promote standardization, and improve patient care through collective knowledge.

References

1. Cutolo M, Smith V. State of the art on nailfold capillaroscopy: a reliable diagnostic tool and putative biomarker in rheumatology. Rheumatology (Oxford). 2013;52(11):1933–40.
2. Smith V, Herrick AL, Ingegnoli F, et al. Standardisation of nailfold capillaroscopy for the assessment of patients with Raynaud's phenomenon and systemic sclerosis. Autoimmun Rev. 2020;19(3):102458.
3. Piette Y, Reynaert V, Vanhaecke A, et al. Standardised interpretation of capillaroscopy in autoimmune idiopathic inflammatory myopathies: a structured review on behalf of the EULAR study group on microcirculation in Rheumatic Diseases. Autoimmun Rev. 2022;21(6):103087.
4. Elziaty RA, Aboelyazeed AA, Hegazy SN, Khalifa AA, Khalil SA. Lung ultrasound for assessment of interstitial lung disease in systemic sclerosis: relationship with high-resolution computed tomography and nailfold capillaroscopy. Clin Med Insights: Arthritis Musculoskelet Disord. 2025:18. https://doi.org/10.1177/11795441251318050.
5. Corrado A, Carpagnano GE, Gaudio A, Foschino-Barbaro MP, Cantatore FP. Nailfold capillaroscopic findings in systemic sclerosis related lung fibrosis and in idiopathic lung fibrosis. Joint Bone Spine. 2010;77(6):570–4. https://doi.org/10.1016/j.jbspin.2010.02.019. Epub 2010 May 23.

Chapter 18
Conclusion: The Unfolding Horizon

Yasser El Miedany

The journey through the intricate microvascular world, as illuminated by nailfold capillaroscopy, reveals not just a diagnostic tool but a dynamic window into systemic health. This book has endeavored to consolidate the current knowledge, techniques, and diverse applications of capillaroscopy, demonstrating its invaluable role across a spectrum of rheumatic and microcirculation disorders. As we stand at the threshold of a new era in medicine, the insights gleaned from the nailfold offer a compelling vision for the future of patient care.

Recalibrating Our Lens: A Synthesis of Progress

Throughout this book, we have traversed the remarkable evolution of nailfold capillaroscopy. What began as a fascinating observation of microscopic blood vessels has matured into a sophisticated, noninvasive instrument critical for discerning the nuanced impact of microcirculation disorders. From the subtle shifts indicative of early disease to the profound architectural derangements seen in advanced conditions, capillaroscopy offers a tangible, visual representation of underlying pathophysiology. As explored in Chaps. 3, 4, 5, 6, 7, 8, 9, 10, 11, 12, and 13, its utility extends far beyond mere diagnosis, serving as a powerful aid in *early detection*, informing *prognosis*, and meticulously *monitoring disease progression* and response to therapy.

Y. El Miedany (✉)
Canterbury Christ Church University, Canterbury, UK

Rheumatology and Rehabilitation, Ain Shams University, Cairo, Egypt

King's College, London, UK

Y. El Miedany, R. A. Elziaty (eds.), *Capillaroscopy*, Contemporary Rheumatology,
https://doi.org/10.1007/978 3 032 22966-3_18

The true strength of capillaroscopy lies in *the power of patterns*. Each rheumatic and microcirculatory disorder, as meticulously detailed in Chaps. 3, 4, 5, 6, 7, 8, 9, and 10 and beyond, often presents with distinct capillaroscopic hallmarks. The "scleroderma pattern," for instance, with its characteristic giant capillaries, hemorrhages, and progressive avascularity, serves as a cornerstone in the diagnosis and classification of systemic sclerosis. Similarly, the specific patterns observed in dermatomyositis, mixed connective tissue diseases, and even inflammatory arthritis provide unique insights that complement clinical and laboratory findings. This visual language, once mastered, equips clinicians with a powerful diagnostic and prognostic vocabulary.

Furthermore, this book has aimed at *bridging the gaps* in the practical application of capillaroscopy. Chapter 12 delved into the critical nuances of *interpretation*, addressing the variability that can arise and providing a systematic approach to standardized reading. Chapter 13, focusing on *clinical applications*, illustrated how to effectively integrate capillaroscopy into daily practice, making this sophisticated technique more accessible and actionable for practitioners across various specialties. By demystifying the methodology and interpretation, we hope to foster wider adoption and better utilization of this indispensable tool.

Test Yourself: Knowledge Assessment and Application

To ensure effective knowledge translation and promote the successful implementation of these guidelines, a dedicated chapter (16), "Test Yourself," was included. This section provides readers, including physicians, residents, and allied health professionals, with "case-based scenarios and focused questions" designed to facilitate self-assessment. By actively measuring their grasp of the core diagnostic, treatment, and surveillance principles for nailfold capillaroscopy, users can confirm the successful attainment of the standardized clinical care protocols outlined in this document.

The Dawn of Digital Capillaroscopy: Innovation at the Forefront

The ongoing digital revolution is fundamentally reshaping the landscape of medicine, and nailfold capillaroscopy is at its vanguard. The integration of *Artificial Intelligence (AI) and Machine Learning (ML), which was discussed in* Chap. 14, is particularly poised to revolutionize the analysis and interpretation of capillaroscopic images.

Automated pattern recognition is rapidly advancing, moving beyond simple quantitative measurements like capillary density. Sophisticated AI algorithms are now capable of highly precise, automated classification of complex capillaroscopic patterns, mirroring and often surpassing human expert capabilities. This remarkable objectivity and speed significantly reduce inter-observer variability, a historical challenge in capillaroscopy, and profoundly streamline clinical workflow. Imagine a future where a comprehensive, AI-generated capillaroscopy report is available moments after image acquisition, providing immediate, unbiased insights. Studies like Lledó-Ibáñez et al. (2025) demonstrate the impressive accuracy of AI-driven models like CAPI-Detect in distinguishing scleroderma patterns and even identifying novel capillary variables previously overlooked by human analysis, highlighting the true potential of the "AI-powered capillaroscopist"—not as a replacement, but as a powerful augmentation to human expertise [1].

Beyond mere recognition, *predictive analytics* represents an exciting frontier. AI can leverage vast datasets of capillaroscopic images, combined with clinical, serological, and genetic information, to develop models that predict critical outcomes. This includes forecasting disease flares, anticipating specific organ involvement (e.g., interstitial lung disease in systemic sclerosis), or predicting individual patient responses to particular treatments. This shift toward proactive, rather than reactive, patient management promises truly personalized care. The ability of AI to analyze *big data and facilitate global collaboration* is also transformative. By processing immense datasets from numerous clinical centers worldwide, AI can identify subtle capillaroscopic biomarkers that might be imperceptible in smaller studies, leading to the refinement of existing patterns and the discovery of entirely new diagnostic and prognostic indicators.

The advent of *tele-capillaroscopy and remote monitoring* is democratizing access to this crucial diagnostic modality. Advancements in compact, handheld devices, USB dermatoscopes, and secure cloud-based platforms are enabling image acquisition in remote settings. This allows expert interpretation from afar, overcoming geographical barriers and improving access for patients in underserved regions or those with limited mobility. Furthermore, the concept of *continuous monitoring* through patient- or remotely-acquired images offers a tantalizing glimpse into the future. Envision patients with chronic conditions regularly submitting capillaroscopy images from home, allowing clinicians to track microvascular changes over time, detect early signs of disease activity, and make personalized, timely adjustments to therapy.

The scope of capillaroscopy is also expanding *beyond the fingernail*. While the nailfold remains the most accessible and well-studied site, ongoing research is exploring other microvascular beds, such as toenail folds, lip mucosa, and conjunctiva. These alternative sites may offer complementary or additional diagnostic information, particularly in cases where the fingernail folds are compromised due to trauma, infection, or anatomical variations [2]. This broader perspective enriches our understanding of systemic microvascular involvement.

Clinical Atlas: A Pioneering Visual Standard

This book proudly introduces the "Clinical Atlas" chapter—a groundbreaking, first-of-its-kind feature in the international literature. Recognizing the high value of visual pattern recognition in these complex diseases, this atlas sets a new benchmark for diagnostic education. By providing the field's first structured, dedicated collection of exemplary "Nail Fold Capillaroscopy (NFC) figures" and associated clinical imagery, we are not only supporting the text-based recommendations but are also establishing a "new visual standard" essential for advancing rapid and accurate diagnosis across all care settings.

By presenting high-quality visual examples of key microvascular changes and pathognomonic skin findings, this chapter aims to standardize the visual interpretation of complex diagnostic features and rapidly improve the clinical recognition skills of all guideline users.

Nailfold Capillaroscopy in the Landscape of Precision Medicine

Nailfold capillaroscopy is perfectly positioned to play a pivotal role in the burgeoning field of *precision medicine*. Its ability to provide individualized, real-time insights into microvascular health directly aligns with the goal of tailoring medical interventions to the unique characteristics of each patient.

In *personalized prognosis and treatment stratification*, detailed capillaroscopic patterns can become critical guides for individualized therapy. For instance, a patient exhibiting a rapidly progressive "active" scleroderma pattern, characterized by extensive giant capillaries and hemorrhages, might necessitate more aggressive immunomodulatory therapy compared to an individual with an "early" pattern. This allows for optimized resource allocation and minimizes unnecessary treatment burden. Moreover, capillaroscopy is increasingly recognized as a valuable, noninvasive *biomarker for drug development*. Its ability to visualize and quantify microvascular changes makes it an ideal tool for evaluating the efficacy of novel drugs specifically targeting microcirculation dysfunction in clinical trials, offering a direct measure of therapeutic impact.

The future of capillaroscopy also lies in its *integration with omics and systems biology*. The microcirculation, as observed through the nailfold, is a dynamic reflection of broader systemic processes. Future research will increasingly seek to integrate capillaroscopic findings with genetic, proteomic, and metabolomic data ("omics" data). This holistic approach will unravel the complex interplay between genetic predispositions, environmental factors, and the development of microvascular dysfunction, leading to a deeper understanding of disease pathogenesis. This integration forms the basis of the "digital twin" of microcirculation—a comprehensive, multidimensional model that allows for highly personalized risk assessment and intervention strategies. Furthermore, *multimodal imaging*, combining capillaroscopy with other advanced techniques such as high-resolution ultrasound or Optical Coherence Tomography (OCT) for detailed vascular assessment, promises to provide an even more comprehensive picture of microvascular health and pathology [3].

Indeed, capillaroscopy can be envisioned as a *"liquid biopsy"of the microcirculation*, providing real-time, noninvasive insights into active disease processes and therapeutic response, distinguishing it from traditional static biopsies. This moves us from a "snapshot" view to *dynamic monitoring*, allowing clinicians to track subtle changes over time and intervene proactively.

Challenges and Future Directions: Charting the Course Ahead

Despite its remarkable progress and immense potential, several challenges must be addressed to fully realize the promise of nailfold capillaroscopy.

Standardization and validation remain paramount. While significant strides have been made, particularly through efforts by groups like the EULAR Study Group on Microcirculation in Rheumatic Diseases, rigorous standardization of image acquisition techniques, analysis protocols, and interpretation criteria is crucial. This will ensure reproducibility across different centers and facilitate widespread clinical adoption, especially as newer AI-driven tools become more prevalent [4, 5]. Consistent terminology and reporting guidelines are also essential to enhance communication and data comparability [6].

Dedicated *training and education* programs are vital for clinicians, technicians, and even AI developers to effectively harness the potential of advanced capillaroscopy. This includes not only mastering the interpretation of complex patterns but also understanding the nuances of new technologies and integrating them into clinical decision-making.

The *cost-effectiveness and reimbursement* of advanced capillaroscopy also warrant attention. While the initial investment in high-quality equipment and training may seem significant, the long-term cost-benefits of early and accurate diagnosis, personalized management, and prevention of irreversible organ damage (e.g., in systemic sclerosis) are substantial. Advocating for appropriate reimbursement policies will be critical for widespread integration into healthcare systems [7].

Finally, as AI and big data play an increasingly central role, *ethical considerations* become more prominent. Ensuring patient data privacy and security, addressing potential biases in AI algorithms that could lead to disparities in care for marginalized populations, and maintaining transparency in how AI-driven insights are generated are crucial responsibilities [8]. Robust ethical frameworks must guide the development and deployment of these powerful tools.

The Unseen Worlds: A Call to Explore

In conclusion, this book has underscored the profound utility of nailfold capillaroscopy—that by peering into these seemingly small, intricate structures at the fingertips, we gain unparalleled insights into the largest and most complex systems of the human body. It is a testament to the fact that often, the most illuminating discoveries reside in the unseen worlds, just beneath the surface.

This book has presented capillaroscopy not only as a diagnostic modality but also as a clinical philosophy—one that emphasizes early detection, thoughtful pattern recognition, integrative reasoning, and continuous observation. Each case told a story: of microvascular pathology, of diagnostic uncertainty resolved, of disease silently evolving, or of therapeutic impact visualized. Taken together, these cases reflect the multidimensional power of capillaroscopy in modern medicine.

The journey of nailfold capillaroscopy is far from over; it is an evolving narrative of discovery and innovation. We stand at a pivotal moment where technological advancements, particularly in AI and digital imaging, are poised to transform their capabilities and applications. We invite all readers—clinicians, researchers, students, and patients—to embrace this evolving landscape, to continue pushing the boundaries of its application, and to recognize its critical and expanding role in unraveling the mysteries of rheumatic and microcirculatory diseases. Through continued curiosity, collaboration, and a commitment to precision, capillaroscopy will undoubtedly continue to illuminate pathways to earlier diagnosis, more effective interventions, and ultimately, vastly improved lives for countless individuals affected by these complex conditions.

We hope that this book has inspired confidence and curiosity in capillaroscopy. Whether you are a trainee, clinician, or researcher, the message is clear: learn the patterns, trust the images, and always consider the patient as a whole. The microcirculation may be small—but its message is vast.

References

1. Lledó-Ibáñez GM, Sáez Comet L, Freire Dapena M, Mesa Navas M, Martín Cascón M, Guillén Del Castillo A, Simeon CP, Martinez Robles E, Todolí Parra J, Varela DC, Maldonado G, Marín A, Pérez Abad L, Aramburu J, Vela L, Ramos Ibáñez E, Del Carmelo Gracia Tello B. CAPI-detect: machine learning in capillaroscopy reveals new variables influencing diagnosis. Rheumatology (Oxford). 2025;64(6):3667–75. https://doi.org/10.1093/rheumatology/keaf073.
2. Lambova SN, Müller-Ladner U. Nailfold capillaroscopy in systemic sclerosis - state of the art: the evolving knowledge about capillaroscopic abnormalities in systemic sclerosis. J Scleroderma Relat Disord. 2019;4(3):200–11. https://doi.org/10.1177/2397198319833486.
3. Wang H, Shi L, Qin J, Yousefi S, Li Y, Wang RK. Multimodal optical imaging can reveal changes in microcirculation and tissue oxygenation during skin wound healing. Lasers Surg Med. 2014;46(6):470–8. https://doi.org/10.1002/lsm.22254.
4. Amaral MC, Paula FS, Caetano J, Ames PR, Alves JD. Re-evaluation of nailfold capillaroscopy in discriminating primary from secondary Raynaud's phenomenon and in predicting systemic sclerosis: a randomised observational prospective cohort study. Expert Rev Clin Immunol. 2024;20(6):665–72. https://doi.org/10.1080/1744666X.2024.2313642.
5. Smith V, Vanhaecke A, Herrick AL, Distler O, Guerra MG, Denton CP, Deschepper E, Foeldvari I, Gutierrez M, Hachulla E, Ingegnoli F, Kubo S, Müller-Ladner U, Riccieri V, Sulli A, van Laar JM, Vonk MC, Walker UA, Cutolo M. EULAR Study Group on Microcirculation in Rheumatic Diseases. Fast track algorithm: how to differentiate a "scleroderma pattern" from

a "non-scleroderma pattern". Autoimmun Rev. 2019;18(11):102394. https://doi.org/10.1016/j.autrev.2019.102394.
6. El Miedany Y, Ismail S, Wadie M, Müller-Ladneru U, Giacomelli R, Liakouli V, Hermann W, Fathy N, El Gaafary M, Fouad NA, Saber S, Abu-Zaid MH. Development of a core domain set for nailfold capillaroscopy reporting. Reumatol Clin (Engl Ed). 2024;20(7):345–52. https://doi.org/10.1016/j.reumae.2024.07.003.
7. Smith V, Ickinger C, Hysa E, Snow M, Frech T, Sulli A, Cutolo M. Nailfold capillaroscopy. Best Pract Res Clin Rheumatol. 2023;37(1):101849. https://doi.org/10.1016/j.berh.2023.101849.
8. Herington J, McCradden MD, Creel K, Boellaard R, Jones EC, Jha AK, Rahmim A, Scott PJH, Sunderland JJ, Wahl RL, Zuehlsdorff S, Saboury B. Ethical considerations for artificial intelligence in medical imaging: data collection, development, and evaluation. J Nucl Med. 2023;64(12):1848–54. https://doi.org/10.2967/jnumed.123.266080.

Index

Y. El Miedany, R. A. Elziaty (eds.), *Capillaroscopy*, Contemporary Rheumatology,
https://doi.org/10.1007/978-3-032-22966-3

O

GPSR Compliance

The European Union's (EU) General Product Safety Regulation (GPSR) is a set of rules that requires consumer products to be safe and our obligations to ensure this.

If you have any concerns about our products, you can contact us on ProductSafety@springernature.com

In case Publisher is established outside the EU, the EU authorized representative is:

Springer Nature Customer Service Center GmbH
Europaplatz 3
69115 Heidelberg, Germany

Batch number: 10726133

Printed by Printforce, the Netherlands